T0221182

LIBER URICRISIARUM

A Reading Edition

Liber Uricrisiarum, bk. 1, ch. 1. © The British Library Board: London, British Library, Royal MS 17 D.i, f. 6r.

Liber Uricrisiarum

A Reading Edition

HENRY DANIEL

E. Ruth Harvey and M. Teresa Tavormina
General Editors

with

Sarah Star, Jessica Henderson,
and C.E.M. Henderson
Associate Editors

UNIVERSITY OF TORONTO PRESS
Toronto Buffalo London

ISBN 978-1-4875-0601-8 (cloth)   ISBN 978-1-4875-3312-0 (EPUB)
                                   ISBN 978-1-4875-3311-3 (PDF)

Library and Archives Canada Cataloguing in Publication

Title: Liber Uricrisiarum : a reading edition / Henry Daniel ; E. Ruth Harvey
    and M. Teresa Tavormina, general editors ; with Sarah Star, Jessica Henderson,
    and C.E.M. Henderson, associate editors.
Names: Daniel, Henry (Medical writer), author. | Harvey, E. Ruth, editor. |
    Tavormina, M. Teresa (Mary Teresa), 1951– editor.
Description: Includes bibliographical references and index. | Text in Middle
    English.
Identifiers: Canadiana (print) 2019020012X | Canadiana (ebook) 20190200197 |
    ISBN 9781487506018 (hardcover) | ISBN 9781487533113 (PDF) |
    ISBN 9781487533120 (EPUB)
Subjects: LCSH: Medicine, Medieval.
Classification: LCC R128 .D36 2020 | DDC 610.9/02 – dc23

University of Toronto Press gratefully acknowledges the financial assistance of
the Centre for Medieval Studies, University of Toronto in the publication of this
book.

University of Toronto Press acknowledges the financial assistance to its
publishing program of the Canada Council for the Arts and the Ontario
Arts Council, an agency of the Government of Ontario.

Canada Council   Conseil des Arts
for the Arts   du Canada

ONTARIO ARTS COUNCIL
CONSEIL DES ARTS DE L'ONTARIO
an Ontario government agency
un organisme du gouvernement de l'Ontario

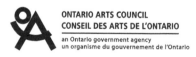

Funded by the   Financé par le
Government   gouvernement
of Canada   du Canada   Canada

In memory of Eric Stanley, who introduced us to each other's work

ERH and MTT

Contents

List of Illustrations and Tables

Illustrations

Tables

Acknowledgments

We are delighted to express our appreciation to the long list of people and institutions who have made this edition possible and encouraged us in pursuing it. Foremost are our colleagues and teachers, without whose early and ongoing advice and support we could neither have begun nor completed this project: the late Eric Stanley (with particular thanks for introductions to the Bodleian Library, Oxford hospitality, and bringing two of his students from different sides of the Atlantic together); Linda Voigts, George Keiser, Monica Green, and Peter Jones for their indispensable contributions to our understanding of the history of medicine, especially in England; the late A.G. Rigg for many years of help with Daniel's Latin and Greek sources; Ralph Hanna and Tony Edwards for their helpfully astringent advice at the beginning of the project and Laurence Moulinier-Brogi for her advice near its end; Jake Walsh Morrissey and especially Faith Wallis for their special contributions in relation to Daniel's beta text, herbal knowledge, astronomical and calendric interests, and more esoteric sources. We also gratefully acknowledge the help of colleagues on the MEDMED-L listserv, founded and maintained by Monica Green, in solving some of the knottier puzzles posed by Daniel's authority-citations, and an anonymous reader for University of Toronto Press for suggestions on linguistic aspects of the edition. Errors that remain are our own.

The general editors are also very grateful to the research team of graduate students at the University of Toronto: Lara Howerton, Shirley Kinney, Nora Thorburn, and Elise Williams, led by Sarah Star, Jessica Henderson, and C.E.M. Henderson. Working on a completely volunteer basis for over two years, the team made a full transcript of the base manuscript, tracked down many of Daniel's cited sources, and drafted thousands of potential glossary entries. Without their enthusiastic contributions, the project would never have stayed on track or reached completion. Of particular importance has been C.E.M. Henderson's work on the website for the ongoing Henry Daniel Project (https://henrydaniel.utoronto.ca)

and paleographic expertise; Jessica Henderson's codicological and digital photographic work on several of the manuscripts collated for the edition; and Sarah Star's logistical leadership, extensive work on variants and draft glossary entries, and final-stage proofreading and other editorial tasks.

No scholarly project whose sources are as diverse and far-flung as those associated with the *Liber Uricrisiarum* could succeed without the aid of librarians and their libraries. Our debts in this arena are many, beginning with our home institutions: the staff of University of Toronto Libraries; and Agnes Widder, Peter Berg, Patrick Olson, and the Interlibrary Loan staff at the Michigan State University Library, who have willingly and successfully tackled challenging problems in locating and providing rare or early texts.

We are also pleased to thank the ever-helpful staffs of the libraries that hold copies of the *Liber Uricrisiarum* and other uroscopic texts, both for access to the manuscripts and for providing images of manuscripts or permitting digital photography thereof: the British Library; the Bodleian Library; the Wellcome Library for the History and Understanding of Medicine (with special thanks to Elma Brenner for alerting us to the completed digitization of Wellcome MS 225); Cambridge University Library (and thanks to Suzanne Paul for assistance there); Gonville and Caius College Library (where Mark Statham has been a supporter of work on Middle English medical manuscripts for many years); Magdalene College Library (and particularly Catherine Sutherland in the Pepys Library); the libraries and librarians of St John's College and Trinity College, Cambridge, and of Merton College, Corpus Christi College, and Pembroke College, Oxford; the Royal College of Physicians Library in London; Glasgow University Library; the Massachusetts Historical Society Library; the Henry E. Huntington Library; and, for microfilm access to manuscripts of Isaac Israeli's *De urinis* and *De pulsibus*, as well as various commentaries on Giles of Corbeil, the Vatican Film Library at St Louis University (with special thanks to Susan L'Engle). We owe a particular debt to the late Chris Jeens, Librarian and Archivist of the Gloucester Cathedral Library, who personally supervised the digital imaging of the Gloucester manuscript by two generous Cathedral volunteers, and to his successor Rebecca Phillips.

For permission to publish text and reproduce images from British Library, Royal MS 17 D.i (ff. 6r, 18v, 49v, 51r, and 51*/52), we are grateful to the British Library Board. We are likewise pleased to acknowledge the Bodleian Library, University of Oxford, for permission to publish text from Bodleian Library, e Musaeo MS 187. Our use of Gloucester Cathedral's MS 19 in the textual apparatus is by permission of the Chapter of Gloucester Cathedral.

We are further indebted to the Centre for Medieval Studies at the University of Toronto and its Director, Suzanne Conklin Akbari, Associate Director (2016–18) Nicholas Everett, and Graduate Administrator Grace Desa for institutional and personal support of the Henry Daniel Project and for a publication subsidy for this edition; to the Pontifical Institute of Mediaeval Studies and the Editor-in-Chief of its Department of Publications, Fred R. Unwalla, for sponsoring the 52nd Annual Conference on Editorial Problems in 2017, which focused on issues in editing Henry Daniel and other English and Latin medical writers; and to the Social Sciences and Humanities Research Council of Canada for an Insight Development Grant in support of the ongoing Henry Daniel Project (2017–20). The Huntington Library provided Sarah Star and Jessica Henderson with Huntington Fellowships in 2015 and 2016 to consult HM 505; Henderson's work on several Daniel manuscripts in England was supported by a 2015 Mellon Foundation grant. Professor Alexandra Gillespie at the University of Toronto has given invaluable advice on matters paleographic, as well as providing space in the "lab" of her Old Books New Science Project, where members of the research team could work on manuscript transcriptions. The staff at University of Toronto Press, especially Suzanne Rancourt and Barb Porter, have made the production of this large and complicated book a smooth and pleasant process; it has also been a delight to work with Judy Williams, the book's copy editor.

Finally, we express deepest personal thanks to our families, friends, and mentors for their interest and unfailing support: Ruth Harvey to Dr Timothy C. Harvey and the late Mrs Mary Stanley, for many medical conversations over the years, and to Professor Stephanie Hollis for her generous invitation to talk about Giles of Corbeil in New Zealand; Tess Tavormina to the late Lister Matheson and to Professor Linda Voigts, both of whom put her on the trail of vernacular scientific and medical writing; Sarah Star to Jeff Espie, for listening to it all; Jess Henderson to her parents, Jon and Margaret Henderson, for their endless and unwavering support; and C.E.M. Henderson to Professors Linne R. Mooney and Alexandra Gillespie for their advice and encouragement.

Abbreviations

Editorial abbreviations are listed in the Editorial Practice section of the Introduction; grammatical abbreviations in the headnote to the Glossary.

a   column a
A-ND   W. Rothwell, D.A. Trotter, G. De Wilde, et al., eds. 2006– . *Anglo-Norman Dictionary.* 2nd ed. Online edition. http://www.anglo-norman.net
Aph.   Hippocrates, *Aphorisms*
appx.   approximately
attrib.   attributed
b   column b
BAV   Vatican City, Bibliotheca Apostolica Vaticana
BL   London, British Library
Bodl.   Oxford, Bodleian Library
c.   circa (with dates); chapter (in text)
cf.   compare
CUL   Cambridge, University Library
d.   died
des.   *desinit*, ends (with)
DMLBS   R.E. Latham, D.R. Howlett, and R.K. Ashdowne, eds. 1975–2013. *Dictionary of Medieval Latin from British Sources.* Oxford: British Academy. Online access at https://logeion.uchicago.edu
EETS   Early English Text Society
eVK2   Linda Ehrsam Voigts and Patricia Deery Kurtz. 2019. *Scientific and Medical Writings in Old and Middle English: An Electronic Reference.* Exp. and rev. ed. Online access at https://cctr1.umkc.edu/cgi-bin/medievalacademy
ex   in superscript: at the end (of a century)
f(f).   folio(s)
fl.   *floruit*, flourished, was active

G&C	Cambridge, Gonville and Caius College Library
in	in superscript: at the beginning (of a century)
inc.	*incipit*, begins (with)
LALME	Angus McIntosh, M.L. Samuels, and Michael Benskin. 1986. *A Linguistic Atlas of Late Mediaeval English.* 4 vols. Aberdeen: Aberdeen University Press. Electronic version, rev. and suppl. by Michael Benskin and Margaret Laing. 2013. http://www.lel.ed.ac.uk/ihd/elalme/elalme.html (*eLALME*).
LU	*Liber Uricrisiarum*
med	in superscript: in the middle (of a century)
MED	*Middle English Dictionary.* 1952–2001. Ann Arbor, MI. Online access at https://quod.lib.umich.edu/m/middle-english-dictionary/dictionary
MS(S)	manuscript(s)
Norri	Juhani Norri. 2016. *Dictionary of Medical Vocabulary in English, 1375–1550: Body Parts, Sicknesses, Instruments, and Medicinal Preparations.* 2 vols. London and New York: Routledge.
n.s.	new series
OED	*Oxford English Dictionary Online.* 2000–. Oxford: Oxford University Press. https://www.oed.com/
orig.	original(ly)
o.s.	original series
poss.	possible, possibly
prob.	probable, probably
Prog.	Hippocrates, *Prognostics*
r	recto
s.	*saeculum*, century
ser.	series
sig(s).	signature(s)
s.v(v).	*sub verbo (verbis)*, under the word(s)
TCC	Cambridge, Trinity College Library
v	verso
var(r).	variant(s)
vol(s).	volume(s)
Walther	Hans Walther. 1963–86. *Proverbia sententiaeque Latinitatis Medii Aevi.* 9 vols. Göttingen: Vandenhoeck and Ruprecht.
Wellcome	London, Wellcome Library
Whiting	B.J. Whiting. 1968. *Proverbs, Sentences, and Proverbial Phrases from English Writings Mainly before 1500.* Cambridge, MA: Harvard University Press.
1/4, 1/2, 2/2, 3/4, etc.	in superscript: first quarter, first half, second half, third quarter, etc. (of a century)

Sigils of Witnesses

The *Liber Uricrisiarum* and Its Adaptations

Sigils for Latin manuscripts cited in Appendix 2 (the *Regule Isaac*) will be found in the headnote to that Appendix.

A   Oxford, Bodleian Library, Ashmole MS 1404
B   Boston, Massachusetts Historical Society, MS P-361 (*olim* 10.10)
Br   Brussels, Bibliothèque Royale, MS IV.249 (now in private hands)
Cf   Cambridge, University Library, MS Ff.2.6
Cg   Cambridge, University Library, MS Gg.3.29
E   London, British Library, Egerton MS 1624
G   Gloucester, Cathedral Library MS 19
G3   Cambridge, Gonville and Caius College Library, MS 180/213
G5   Cambridge, Gonville and Caius College Library, MS 336/725
G6   Cambridge, Gonville and Caius College Library, MS 376/596
G7   Cambridge, Gonville and Caius College Library, MS 176/97
H   San Marino, Huntington Library, MS HM 505
Hu   Glasgow, University Library, Hunterian MS 328
J   Cambridge, St John's College Library, MS B.16
Jt   New York, Jewish Theological Seminary of America, MS 2611
Ju   *The Iudycyall of Vryns* (Southwark: P. Treveris, ?1527)
L   Glasgow, University Library, Hunterian MS 362
L6   Oxford, Bodleian Library, lat.misc. MS c.66
M6   Oxford, Bodleian Library, e Musaeo MS 116
M7   Oxford, Bodleian Library, e Musaeo MS 187
P   London, Royal College of Physicians, MS 356
Pe   Cambridge, Magdalene College Library, Pepys MS 1661
R   London, British Library, Royal MS 17 D.i
Ra   Oxford, Bodleian Library, Rawlinson MS D.1221

Sa   London, British Library, Sloane MS 1100
Sb   London, British Library, Sloane MS 1101
Sc   London, British Library, Sloane MS 1721
Sd   London, British Library, Sloane MS 1088
Se   London, British Library, Sloane MS 2527
Sf   London, British Library, Sloane MS 134
Sg   London, British Library, Sloane MS 2196
Sh   London, British Library, Sloane MS 5
Si   London, British Library, Sloane MS 340
T   Cambridge, Trinity College Library, MS O.10.21
T2   Cambridge, Trinity College Library, MS R.14.52
W   London, Wellcome Library, MS 225
W6   London, Wellcome Library, MS 226
W7   London, Wellcome Library, MS 7117
Y   New Haven, Yale Medical School, Cushing-Whitney Library MS 45

Daniel's Herbal

Add   London, British Library, Additional MS 27329
Ar   London, British Library, Arundel MS 42

Warning

The diagnostic methods and conclusions recorded in this book, along with the medical remedies described, are intended solely for historical, linguistic, and literary analysis. Any use of them for diagnosis or treatment could be dangerous.

LIBER URICRISIARUM

A Reading Edition

Introduction

I. The *Liber Uricrisiarum* in the Uroscopic Tradition

Henry Daniel's *Liber Uricrisiarum* (*LU*) is the most elaborate exposition in English of the ancient medical art of uroscopy, diagnosis by examination of urine. By the later fourteenth century there had been written comments on the significance of urine for medical diagnosis for well over a thousand years: the foundational texts were written in Greek, and built on them were works in Arabic and in Latin.[1] Daniel took the next logical step: he compiled and composed, out of the numerous Latin works available to him, a comprehensive explanation of the whole art in the English of his day.

Uroscopy was one of the few diagnostic tools available in early medicine: urine was one of the list of physical signs, like pulse, sputum, and cough, which required no instruments, only the evidence of the unaided senses. Urine came from deep within the body, and reported on its inner workings. Features of urine visible to the naked eye, for example its colour, turbidity, and the various stuffs found floating in it, appear as familiar diagnostic signs as early as Hippocrates' *Aphorisms*.[2] (Hippocrates himself is thought to have lived in the fifth century BCE; the Hippocratic writings are the product of a school, or schools, of thought deriving from his teaching.) The *Aphorisms* is a collection of brief diagnostic observations, and contains no overt physiological theory: the axioms are simply statements,

---

1 Moulinier-Brogi (2012) offers a detailed overview of medieval uroscopy, including its classical and Arabic roots, semiological implications, and an extensive bibliography; on vernacular uroscopic traditions, especially on the Continent, see Moulinier-Brogi 2008.
2 The Hippocratic writings are from various dates, most perhaps from 430–330 BCE. Section 4 of the *Aphorisms* contains the most influential remarks on urine.

such as "When the urine is thick, and with it is passed as it were bran, this means psoriasis of the bladder" (*Aph.* 4.77; Loeb ed. 4: 155–7). They suggest medical notes, conclusions drawn from the direct observation of patients. The Hippocratic writings carried enormous authority, and the *Aphorisms* in particular entered both the Latin-speaking and the Arabic-speaking worlds very early.[3] Hippocrates was "the father of medicine" to the Western world, and any statement bearing his name commanded automatic assent well into the period of the Renaissance and beyond.

Many of the Hippocratic writings were accessible to later physicians through translations into Latin and Arabic (some, like the *Aphorisms*, were translated several times), but they were usually seen through the commentaries and adaptations of Galen of Pergamum, who lived through most of the second century CE. Galen was a voluminous writer; he revered Hippocrates and made the Hippocratic ideas the foundation of his own lengthy series of books and treatises. Since he, like the Hippocratic writers, was a practising physician, his works are informed with his own observations of real patients. But Galen lived centuries after Hippocrates, and had the benefit of various anatomical discoveries, both from his own work with animals and from the research into human anatomy by Herophilos and Erasistratos at Alexandria. Hence his own physiological theories are far more complete and more elaborately developed. When he comes to deal with urine as a diagnostic sign, Galen incorporates Hippocratic remarks into his own discussion of signs, and relies upon his own interpretation of Hippocratic theory.

The main discussion is in his *De crisibus*, 1.12. There he first explains that the physician should familiarize himself with the appearance of the urine of healthy patients, so he can recognize unhealthy urine when he sees it. Healthy urine should be of a particular colour, something like a warm yellow shade, because that will indicate that the digestion is working properly. He is thinking of digestion as a kind of cooking process: if the digestive powers are weak, the urine will emerge "uncooked," or pale and watery; if the powers are overstrong or overheated, the urine will be dark, reddish or greenish or blackish. Urine should not be cloudy or turbulent, and flakes and sediment are signs of trouble. Galen recognizes the fact that when human urine is left standing for a while, it can show a kind of hovering "woolly cloud" of sediment (this is actually mucus); he notes exactly how this sediment should appear when the patient is in a healthy state. The fundamental principle is that of all Greek medicine: the body should be in balance – a balance of the four elements, earth, water, air, and fire,

---

3   Kibre 1985, 29–90.

which compose it – and any sign of imbalance, deviation from the mean composed of all the elements, is a token of ill-health. Because it is a result of the "cooking process" of digestion, urine is particularly significant in establishing the patient's position on the hot/cold axis. Like all early physicians, Galen had no knowledge of germs and only sketchy ideas about infection; he saw disease in the main as the result of poor digestion. Since the urine reports on the success of the whole process of digestion, a careful examination of the urine could reveal to the observer the correct diagnosis of the underlying physical condition.

Galen's writings include his remarks on uroscopy within the larger framework of diagnosis, signs, and treatment. But Galen was so verbose that after his death his numerous and often lengthy volumes began to appear in summaries and selections. *De crisibus* itself was translated into Arabic, and eventually into Latin, but it does not seem to have been especially well known in Latin. Galen's words on uroscopy were eventually distilled down into at least one short treatise devoted solely to urines. Here our evidence becomes rather scanty, and dates become difficult to determine. The next major figure in the tradition is Theophilos (Theophilus in Latin), but Theophilos says in his introduction that in the centuries between himself and Galen (and we do not know how many) a writer named Magnos wrote a separate treatise on urines. The text of the tract on urine by Magnos that survives in manuscript is very probably the same as a little treatise that appears in Renaissance prints of the works of Galen, but is now classified as one of the spurious books.[4] In general it summarizes what Galen had to say in *De crisibus*, in very much the same terminology.

Theophilos, a foundational authority on uroscopy, is very obscure indeed. His little treatise on urines is, like all of the works above, written in Greek. Theophilos was a Christian in the Byzantine empire; he considered himself to be at the end of a great and historic tradition of medical writers. He looked back to Hippocrates and Galen as the distant masters, and mentioned Magnos as their later follower. Modern scholars do not agree even on the century in which he lived; we know his work on urines was translated into Latin around 1100 CE, but that does not narrow the field very much. But once in Latin, his tract achieved enormous importance as an essential text for medical diagnosis.

---

4 *Galeno adscriptus Liber de urinis, Galeni de urinis compendium, De urinis ex Hippocrate Galeno et aliis quibusdam* (overlapping texts) are in Kühn, ed. 1821–33, 19: 574–628; some parts of this are reprinted in Ideler, ed. 1841–2, 2: 307–16.

What is strange and different about Theophilos's *Peri ouron* is that the author is far more interested in vocabulary than in medicine. It is easy to see the influence of Galen in the physiological description of digestion, the emphasis on under- and over-cooking, the description of ideal urine and of the various sediments; but what Theophilos mostly hands on to the Latin West is an enormous list of the names of seventeen separate urine colours, many in their own peculiar Greek. There is some overlap with Galen's terminology, but much of the detail about the paler colours is entirely new. *Peri ouron* is an oddly systematic little work, very far from the physician's practice. Many of the colours would be hard to determine, and some of them, once described, seem to be of little diagnostic value. Theophilos seems to have intended to make the art complete by systematizing Galen's discussion and incorporating, from an unknown source, a number of rare and technical terms. He divides his explanation into subheadings that eventually become standard categories. First he considers the "substance," by which he means the clarity, or the thickness or thinness of the fluid;[5] then he considers the urine under two main headings, its "colour" and "content," pairing each of these with "substance." He lists his seventeen different colours in a range from colourless, like water, to black. They are carefully arranged to show a progression: very clear and colourless urine signifies that no digestion has taken place, while the beginning of digestion is marked by pale hues such as "glaucos" and "karopos." These give way to the more healthy yellow and reddish colours, and then decline, through over-cooking, or "excessive digestion," to dark red, green, purple, and black. He describes the "thinness" or "thickness" of the fluid in each case, noting that the best digestion of all is indicated by a shade in the middle of the yellow-to-red range, appearing at the same time with a moderate "body" or "thickness." After completing the colours he moves on systematically through the "contents," the different floating bodies and bad signs, such as pus and blood, that may be seen floating around in the urinal. After Theophilos the "colours" and "contents" of urine, and the varying "substance" or "thickness" or turbidity of the fluid, become major mental categories.

Theophilos defined each colour by likening it to something natural: milk, onyx, flowers, wine, blood. The main ideas are recognizably Galenic, but there is nothing in the earlier texts corresponding to such

---

5 The Middle English *Dome of Uryne* helpfully explains that you can determine the kind of "substance" by holding the urine flask in front of your hand, and "ȝyf þe vryne be þynne, þan schal þou see thourgh þe vryne þe joyntis of þi fyngeris ... ȝyf hit be þikke ... þou may noȝt see þourgh" (BL, Add. MS 10440, f. 50r; ed. from BL, Sloane MS 374 in Tavormina 2019).

terms as *glaucos, karopos,* or *ochros.* Such shades serve no diagnostic purpose either: there seems, for instance, to be no useful difference between *glaucos* and *karopos,* or pallid and subpallid (*ochros* and *hypochros*) urines. It sounds as if Theophilos had found the words in the authorities available to him, and he included them for the sake of completeness.

In contrast, Theophilos's list of "contents" is much more recognizable. Galen mentions blood and flakes and fragments like bran, hairs, or vetch seeds appearing in urine, and draws various diagnoses from them. Theophilos dutifully includes these, but he is much more interested than Galen in the "woolly cloud" of mucus that can appear in urine that has rested for a while; he carefully classifies it into its various colours and positions within the urine flask, and once again his terminology, especially the word *hypostasis* as a general name for the cloud, becomes established as standard in the tradition. He records that the *hypostasis* may be differentiated into a *nephele* if it floats high in the flask, or an *eneorima* if it is in the middle.

A second route taken by uroscopy into the Latin West was through Arabian medicine. Most of the texts of Greek medicine were translated into Arabic in the eighth and ninth centuries, and scholars writing in Arabic studied, commented, and wrote extensively about them. Large and comprehensive volumes in Arabic followed, in which Greek medicine was systematized and organized. In the field of uroscopy nearly all of Galen's works, together with the text of Magnos, reappeared in Arabic; it seems, however, that Theophilos was never translated. (It is possible that he lived after the great wave of Arabic translation.) There were a number of texts on uroscopy written in Arabic, but the most famous and comprehensive of them all was that of Isaac Judaeus (also known as Isaac Israeli).

Isaac was a doctor and philosopher working in North Africa during the tenth century.[6] He wrote a number of works, among them *Kitāb fī'l baul,* "The Book of Urine," the most comprehensive of all medieval uroscopies (and perhaps of all uroscopies ever). It is a large and masterly work, in which Galen's rather casual observations provide the foundation for a systematic and inclusive scheme. Isaac is also credited with writing a treatise on the four elements, and a noteworthy aspect of his uroscopy is the careful way he matches up every colour and symptom with variations in the balance of the elements within the human body. He is deeply interested in medical theory, so instead of a simple list of colours and contents, Isaac explains exactly how and why each tint in the urine reflects an inner

---

6 For a recent collection of studies on Isaac and his works, see Collins, Kottek, and Paavilainen, eds. 2015.

physical condition. He is not concerned with a simple list of colours; his aim is rather to show how, within each major grouping of shades, what is manifest is the activity of the bodily humours. He mentions a very large number of colours, but they are arranged according to the hot/cold/moist/dry aspects of the four bodily humours, rather than in the simple light-to-dark list of Theophilos.[7] Isaac explains Galenic theory to the fullest degree, but he is not just theoretical: most important for the later tradition, he includes for the first time a careful description of the proper techniques for collecting and examining the specimen. This was the section of his work that was most profoundly influential.

The most momentous step in the development of the Western uroscopic tradition was perhaps the arrival from North Africa of Constantine the African (who died before 1098 or 1099) at Salerno in southern Italy. He brought with him a number of medical books in Arabic, including the works of Isaac. He became a Benedictine monk at the nearby monastery of Monte Cassino, the archabbey of Christendom, and there spent the rest of his life translating his Arabic medical authors into Latin. Salerno had had, for many years, a widespread reputation for medical arts,[8] and the new texts provided by Constantine's translations were received with enthusiasm. They were studied, developed, compared with other writings – some translated directly from Greek – and the ideas disseminated in new writings that spread throughout Europe. Constantine's work changed the whole nature of medical studies in Western culture.

One crucial volume associated with Salerno was the textbook known as the *Articella*. This is a collection of fairly short medical works considered essential to the beginner in the art. It included, among other works, Galen's *Art of Medicine* (known as the *Tegni*), a tract on pulses, and the *De urinis* of Theophilus, which must have been translated into Latin directly from Greek in Italy, at around the same time that Constantine was working with Arabic. There are hundreds of manuscripts of the *Articella*, and while some works appear in all copies, many of them also include extra texts, like Isaac's *De urinis*.[9] Any student of medicine after the early twelfth century would have read Theophilus in the *Articella*, and quite possibly Isaac's *De urinis* too.[10]

---

7   On Isaac's classification of colours, see Visi 2015.

8   For magisterial introductions to the School of Salerno and texts attributed to its masters, see Jacquart and Paravicini Bagliani, eds. 2007 and 2008.

9   Constantine's translation of Isaac's *De urinis* (also known as *Liber urinarum*) is edited in Peine 1919 and in Fontana 1966 (with Italian translation).

10   Veit (2015) surveys the reception of Isaac's *De urinis* in the Latin tradition and medical curricula, with an appendix listing known manuscripts of the *De urinis*.

A third book called *De urinis*[11] was often also included in the *Articella*, and was perhaps the most influential of all medieval works on uroscopy. A Frenchman, Giles of Corbeil (d. c. 1224?), went to Salerno in the later twelfth century to study medicine, and was enthralled by the learning of his teachers there. When he returned to France he found a position at the nascent University of Paris, and spent the rest of his life teaching Salernitan medicine. He owes his fame not to any originality or innovative discovery, but to his brilliant idea for instruction: he condensed his teaching into Latin verse, presumably in the expectation that his students would learn his poems by heart, and then the lectures would simply expatiate upon the subject. His first poem was devoted to urines: in 352 Latin hexameters he covered the most important features of the uroscopic art, just as he had learned it at the school of Salerno. The verse *De urinis* was extraordinarily popular: there are hundreds of manuscripts, and quotations and stray lines of verse from it often appear in the margins of other uroscopic texts, evidence of its mnemonic power. Because of its fundamental role as a textbook, Giles's poem had a powerful structural effect on the subject: the categories and subheadings he used become pigeonholes or moulds for most of the writers who came after him.

Giles's poem makes it apparent that considerable work on uroscopy had been done at Salerno in the century after the new texts had arrived from Arabic and Greek sources. Giles preserves the binary division between "colours" and "contents" laid down in Theophilus, but both categories have been enlarged and codified. The names of the colours are for the most part taken over directly from Theophilus: thus the highly specialized Greek terms *glaucos, karopos, ynopos* become standard terminology. But Giles asserts, in a famous line, "Bis deni urinam possunt variare colores," that there are twenty colours, not seventeen; and here it becomes apparent that the masters of Salerno, faced with two differing translations of Greek terminology, had accidentally doubled one of the pairs of "red" colours: Greek *pyrron* came into Latin from Theophilos as *rufus*, but through Isaac's Arabic as *citrinus*. Somewhere during the twelfth century the masters of Salerno, in trying to consolidate the subject from both texts, decided that

---

11 It is sometimes referred to as "*Carmen* (Poem) *de urinis*" to distinguish it from the other two works. For the text, see Choulant, ed. 1826 and Vieillard 1903 (the latter with French translation of the poem). Three other medical poems by Giles survive, on the pulse (ed. Choulant 1826), on compound medicines (ed. Ausécache 2017), and on symptoms of disease (ed. Rose 1907). On the pedagogical dimensions of Giles's texts, see Ausécache 1998. For the historiography of Giles's life, noting the limited evidence for past claims about his dates, status, and other details, see Ausécache 2017, 11–15 ("Une biographie incertaine").

they must be two different colours. The other extra colour arises from the hint in Theophilos that there is more than one kind of black urine: after Giles's popularization, uroscopists always distinguished between urine that was black-from-heat from urine that was black-from-cold. Thereafter the twenty colours of urine become canonical, even though there is very little to say about some of them (such as *subrubicundus*), and the characteristics of "good" or *pyrron* urine now have to be spread over *citrinus* and *rufus*. The twenty sometimes appear in rather beautiful circular illustrations, linked together in a colour wheel.

In the discussion on contents, Giles presents a simpler and more comprehensive list than Theophilus, even while including the usual bran flakes, scales, and vetch seed mentioned in Greek. He reduces Theophilus's remarks and Isaac's lengthy and complex discussion to a simple list of nineteen contents, one of which is the "woolly cloud" of mucus, often known by the Greek term *hypostasis*. The list now includes statements mined from Hippocrates' *Aphorisms* about foamy urine and things "like hairs," which must have been added at Salerno. More importantly, somewhere in this Salernitan interval a notable addition to the theory arrived: a new content, *attomi* or motes in urine, was determined to signify either gout or pregnancy. This addition introduced the whole topic of sex, conception, and pregnancy, and proved to be of great interest to later writers. A mere eleven lines in Giles (*Carmen de urinis* 287–97) established this doctrine as one of the major diagnostic features of uroscopy thereafter. Giles differs from Theophilus by ignoring the subject of digestion as such, but he does touch on new topics such as the etymology of the word *urina*; the regions of the body, to which the layers of the urine in the urinal correspond; and the doctrine of the bodily spirits. Most importantly, Giles reduces Isaac's lengthy account of the considerations the examining physician should bear in mind to three short and witty lines (10–12):

> Quale, quid, aut quid in hoc, quantum, quotiens, ubi, quando,
> Aetas, natura, sexus, labor, ira, diaeta,
> Cura, fames, motus, lavacrum, cibus, unctio, potus.

> (What kind, which, or what is in it, how much, how often, where, when,
> Age, kind, sex, work, anger, diet,
> Anxiety, hunger, activity, bathing, food, ointment, drink.)

These become known as the *conditiones* or questions that must be taken into account when making a diagnosis from urine; they form a preface to the lists of colours and contents that make up the rest of his poem.

Giles's *De urinis* seems to have been from the beginning accompanied by a commentary to expand upon the frequently cryptic verse and to gloss the technical vocabulary (referred to in this edition as the Standard Commentary, because of its ubiquity and influence). By itself the poem would be hard to follow: it is essentially a mnemonic, a collection of prompts for the proper understanding of the subject. The commentary includes all of Isaac's careful advice about how to collect and examine the specimen: the best light to examine it, the hand shading the flask behind, the careful shaking to observe the movement of the sediment, the spaced intervals for re-examination as it cools. This technique gave rise to the common iconographic convention in the Middle Ages by which a physician was usually identified by giving him a urine flask to hold or examine. Giles's work acquired other commentaries: a much more elaborate one by Gilbert the Englishman (Gilbertus Anglicus) was written by or in the 1230s, and was widely known.[12]

By the later fourteenth century all three of these very different texts called *De urinis* were well known in medical circles; they had been in circulation in Latin for some hundreds of years, and quite often were all included in copies of the *Articella*. Many other works had been written in Latin upon the foundation they provide. But there was an increasing demand for the learning available in Latin to be extended into the various European vernaculars, and this particularly applied to medicine. The art of uroscopy was the first stage in medical diagnosis and treatment, and the demand for medical knowledge far outran the small section of the population who could read Latin. In England, Henry Daniel responded to this need with his own book on urine, his *Liber Uricrisiarum*. He used many Latin sources – chief among them Giles, Isaac, and, to a lesser degree, Theophilus, but his great innovation was to render the whole subject most elaborately into the English language.

II. Henry Daniel and the *Liber Uricrisiarum*[13]

A close examination of the *LU* shows that the whole long book was, at bottom, constructed on the framework provided by Giles. The etymology

---

12 McVaugh 2010, 303–5.
13 Scholarly work on Daniel, like previous editions of his text, is sparse. Studies of his works, as well as passing references in scholarly articles of which we are aware, include Getz 1990; Means 1992; Jasin 1993a and 1993b; Friedman 1994; R.F. Green 1997; E.R. Harvey 1998; Walsh Morrissey 2014a; Star 2016, 2018a, and 2018b. Modern editions: Jasin, ed. 1983 (from the beta text manuscript Wellcome Library, MS 225); Hanna, ed. 1994 (bks. 1.1–1.3 only); Mäkinen, ed. 2002 (edition of Daniel's Rosemary treatise);

of *urina*, the *conditiones*, the twenty colours, the long list of contents, and many of the digressions come directly from Giles. All of Isaac's wise advice about how to handle the specimen is carefully recorded in the *conditiones*; Theophilus himself is quoted directly several times. Daniel made extensive use of the early Standard Commentary on Giles, and also of the much more advanced one written by Gilbert the Englishman. His book is not merely a compilation of his Latin sources, but an elaborate comparison and blending of different traditions. In addition, writing about an arcane medical skill in English required not only a mastery of the subject matter, but also the selection and creation of a specialized vocabulary of anatomical and technical terms. Daniel built his discussion on the scaffolding provided by Giles, but incorporated a wide survey of other related subjects by means of structured digressions: the longest of these by far is the excursus on astronomy included in *urina lactea*. Daniel manages to include a great deal of anatomy and physiology, notes on the pulse, other vital signs, fevers, sputum, the critical days, discussions on conception and pregnancy, as well as a large number of etymologies and arguments about names. Then he revised the entire book to make it even longer (we refer to this revision as the beta text). The *LU* is, in its knowledge and expertise, at the end of an ancient medical tradition; in its ambition and language, it stands at the beginning of academic medicine in English.

There are no records of Daniel outside his own books.[14] Besides the *LU*, he wrote a large text on herbs and simple medicines,[15] and that text contains a little tract on rosemary, which also circulated independently.[16] Daniel was a compulsive reviser, and both of his long books exist in multiple versions. We can follow to some degree the development of his career

---

Johannessen, ed. 2005 (the seventeen-chapter abridgment of the *Liber Uricrisiarum*, from Gonville and Caius College MS 336/725). Studies of the Herbal and Rosemary treatise include J.H. Harvey 1972; 1974, 17, 135; and 1987; Keiser 1996, 2008; Walsh Morrissey 2014b. Recent reference texts that mention Daniel or his works include Kaeppeli 1970–5, 2: 192; Talbot and Hammond 1965, 79; Keiser 1998, 3661, 3851–2 (with citations of earlier notices); eVK2; J.H. Harvey 2004; Tavormina 2014, 87–92. Norri's recent dictionary of Middle English medical terminology (2016) draws extensively from the BL, Royal 17 D.i copy of the *Liber Uricrisiarum*, the principal base text for this edition.

14   The "tentative obit" of 1379 suggested by Hanna (ed. 1994, 187) cannot stand: in the record he cites there is a misreading of *ferour* "farrier" as "friar." Also, 1379 does not account for the dates provided by the later revision of the *LU*.

15   The work is entitled "Aaron Danielis" (after the first herb) in BL, Additional MS 27329; it is untitled in the version found in BL, MS Arundel 42. We use the sigils Add and Ar to refer to these manuscripts respectively.

16   Keiser 1996; Mäkinen, ed. 2002.

and the course of his life from what he tells us in his books, but we are completely without any corroborative documents.

The most informative piece he gives us is the prologue to the *LU*. Written formally in Latin, with a number of rhetorical flourishes, it was revised and elaborated at least twice. Two manuscripts (R, M7) contain a version in which the prologue is translated into English, but the English translation does not have any of Daniel's characteristic stylistic turns (series of synonyms, onomatopoeic word-formation, alliteration, etc.), and is probably not by him. Some features of the prologue are constant, but differing versions show Daniel's typical elaborations. In all versions he names himself and states that he is a Dominican friar. He explains that he has recently written something about the study of urine in Latin, but, at the urging of a friend and colleague named Walter Turnour of Keten (modern Ketton, Rutland), he has decided to take the unprecedented step of putting the same material into the English language. English, he says, is his mother tongue; but he is more comfortable in Latin. He worries – perhaps conventionally – about the propriety of putting a learned subject into the vernacular; and, in the earliest version of the prologue (M6G3 GTSaSc), he explains that he will have to use some strange words and Latinate coinages to convey the appropriate anatomical and technical vocabulary. He justifies his project as an act of charity and pity for the unlearned who have no access to proper instruction in medicine. He asserts his own qualifications: he has never been formally instructed in medicine, but he has worked on his book at least two years, and consulted books by Galen, Isaac, Giles, Theophilus and others, together with commentaries upon them.

In the next version of the prologue (HBCfCg; in English translation in RM7), he rearranges the same material, alters the time he has worked on the book to three years, and elaborates on his concern for instructing the ignorant practitioner and the profit to be gained from his work. His list of authorities is replaced by a more general statement, and a complaint that he has been much hampered by serious illness. In the next revision, witnessed by only two manuscripts (AG6), there are fewer changes; one alters the number of years for which Daniel has been working on his book to five (witnessed by G6 only; A omits the number), and another notes that his ill-health has prevented him from searching out more books than the eleven authors and commentators he has at hand.

The dates between which Daniel lived are unknown, but he does tell us when he was writing. Within the body of the text of the *LU*, in the course of a long astronomical digression, he provides an explanation of how leap years are calculated, and initially notes that he is writing in the year 1377 (M6G3). Then, in a number of manuscripts, the date in the leap year passage is changed to 1378. Four of these manuscripts (GTSaSc) contain a text that has been revised and slightly expanded, but still preserves the prologue in a form which is essentially the same as the first version; these four manuscripts are also linked textually in other minor variants. Most of the "revised text" manuscripts, however, have a revised prologue, where the material is rearranged, and Daniel declares that he has been working on his book for three years (HBCfCgRM7). Finally, in the major revision and expansion of his book (our "beta" version), he changes the prologue as well as the text once again. In the prologue (included in only two "beta" manuscripts) the time spent writing is now five years (G6, omitted in A); the passage on leap years within the text is reworded so that no date is given (AG6EWP). Some manuscripts conclude the text with a set of Latin verses, dating the book to the second year of the reign of Richard II, i.e., June 1378–June 1379. Extra lines are added in later revisions, noting major contemporary events; the latest reference is to the great earthquake of 1382. And Daniel tells us that he is getting old: he suffers, he says, from *eelde* and poverty, not to mention kidney disease and depression.[17]

Daniel's other big book is a herbal-cum-medical dictionary, which exists in two different versions. He must have written it after the *Liber Uricrisiarum*, because several times he gives cross-references to the previous work. Sometimes these references (which appear in both versions of the herbal) are quite specific: they cite individual chapters of the longer, or beta, revision of the *LU*. So it is a safe inference that Daniel wrote the *LU* first, and then revised it; the herbal came afterwards. The herbal appears to have been partly rearranged, but the later version is incomplete; either the rest of the manuscript has not survived, or Daniel did not live to finish it.

Within this collection of texts, Daniel does give us a fair amount of information about his life. Since he claims in the preface to the *LU* to be more comfortable writing in Latin than in English, and proceeds to deck out his argument with a rhetorical flourish from Aristotle's *Metaphysics*, it seems apparent that he must have had a university education, though no records of his presence at either Cambridge or Oxford survive. The *Metaphysics* is not exactly common reading: it was one of the more advanced university textbooks. Daniel was certainly very bookish, and had access as he worked to a large number of books: he quotes from at least half a dozen

---

17 "Diversisque infirmitatibus etiam quandoque fere ad mortem frequenter interceptus" (often interrupted also by various sicknesses, sometimes almost to death; Bodl., Ashmole MS 1404, Prol., f. 3v); "nefresy gret and huge dissese and þys fele I well also in my self alle tymys of þe ȝere continuelly" (Bodl., e Mus. MS 116, bk. 3.5, f. 129v); "the seed þerof abated in me þe colre and melancolie, and made me glad and ligth" (Add, Ar: ERBUS); see also note 21, below.

different authorities in the herbal,[18] as well as the impressive range of medical texts in the *LU*. He isn't working from memory; he translates some of his authors into English "nerhand word for word," names his sources with great care, notes when he is using an abridged text instead of a full one, and distinguishes between material he has found in the text from that found in glosses. It all suggests that he is working in a library of some consequence, probably, since he is a friar at the time, in his own Dominican convent.[19]

It seems apparent, however, that Daniel was not always a friar. In the herbal there are a number of references to the time "when I might maintain me," when he kept a herb-garden in Stepney,[20] east of London. This was in his past: it is paired with a remark about his current old age and poverty[21] (a remark that is repeated from the *LU*). And, while Daniel was careful to say that he had no formal training in medicine, he does claim to be an authority on herbs. He says he studied the subject for seven years, and acknowledges various teachers. He makes the astonishing claim that he had cultivated 252 different herbs in his garden at Stepney, including *garofilus* (pinks?) and a cutting of rosemary, which came from Queen Philippa's garden.[22] He describes taking cuttings, transplanting, and problems in growing particular plants (Ar: CIPRESSUS, CUCURBITA; Add: CROCUS), and records the particular places in England where he found them (he mentions Shaftesbury in Wiltshire, Chatham in Kent, and Bruton, near Bristol);[23] he firmly corrects those who misidentify their plants. It is noteworthy that in his herbal he sometimes mentions knowing or helping various personages, such as Lady Zouche or "a worthy gentilman,"[24] in the preparation of ointments and remedies, whereas in the case histories in the *LU* he claims to have been a bystander rather than an authority. Friars were not supposed to practise medicine,[25] but we do not know how seriously this prohibition was taken; in any case, Daniel writes as if his

---

18 This number refers to books he certainly had; there are many references to other authors, but in most cases they are almost certainly nested in quotations included in the books in front of him.

19 Friedman 1994 and R.F. Green 1997 have suggested the Dominican convent at Stamford, but there is no documentary evidence.

20 Ar: ANEMICON, ERBUS, ESULA, GAROFILUS.

21 "Þese 2 hadde Y in my gardyn, but eelde and pecunie onweelde now arn ryche with me" (Ar: ESULA).

22 Ar: ANTHUS, GAROFILUS.

23 Particular places where he found herbs are mentioned in Add: AMIFRUCTUS, ANACROCUS; Ar: ALTEA, AMYAMIA, CACULUS, CIPRESSUS.

24 Daniel says he helped "a worthy leche" (Ar: ADACTIS) and "a lady" (Add: CELIFOLIA, AMARISCUS; Ar: CERFOLIUS, ERISIPILA); he cites Lady Zouche in Ar: AMBROSIA; see also Add: ARNOGLOSSA.

25 On medical practice and writings by friars, see Montford 2003, 2004; Jones 2008, 2011, 2016.

herbalist days are behind him. It seems quite likely that he became a friar after he considered his days of practice were over. If the phrase "Y sawe at ey" is a reference to the secular medical establishment at Eye, in Suffolk, it might mean that he spent some time working there before he became a friar, but we have no other evidence. It might simply mean, "I saw with my own eyes."

As to where he was working: we do not know when he became a friar, nor do we know which convent he belonged to. Among the number of places in his works, his garden at Stepney, very close to London, is the most significant, but that was in his past; the *LU* itself is addressed to Walter Turnour, a *socius* or colleague, of Keten. We have no knowledge of Walter, but Ketton is a village in the old county of Rutlandshire, not very far from Stamford in Lincolnshire, where Daniel saw the very sick man in the "Great Hostel" (2.7.49). Daniel was familiar with that part of the world. He found a rare herb on the left hand side of the road "when you are within a mile of Stamford" (Ar: CACULUS). The area is not far from the forest of Rockingham, where he noted that you could find a rare kind of wild mallow (Ar: ALTEA). If we are to look for Daniel's convent, somewhere in that region is perhaps the most likely.

III. Daniel's Circle and Audience

What we do get from Daniel's works is an animated picture of medical practice in fourteenth-century England. We know that learned university doctors were few and far between; Daniel shows us how medicine was actually practised by a wide variety of amateurs. There are great ladies preparing their own ointments and skin-care products; a high-ranking man who grew his own herbs especially to treat his gout; and herb-gatherers and apothecaries of various levels of attainment.[26] Some he praises, others are "bonglers and smaterers" who cannot tell argentilla from water betony. He mentions the people he learnt things from: a converted Jew gave him information about gentians and lunaria; "a Cristene man þat longe haued woned amonge Saracenus and Juys" told him an interesting thing about comfrey.[27] He heard of a dubious method of trapping spiders with centonica juice from an earl's servant (Add: CENTONICA); and witnessed

---

26   See above, note 24; also Add: ABROTANUS; Ar: ARGENTILLA, BISARA.
27   Add: GENCIANA, LUNARIA; Ar: ANAGALLA. Perhaps the same man mentioned in Ar: ATHANASIA; he could also be the same man ("Maister Gyles") who was both illiterate and almost blind, but had learned medicine from the Saracens and practised uroscopy on the locals in the *LU*, beta text, 1.11 (Ashmole 1404, f. 21r).

the diagnostic skills of a wealthy young man who had no need to practise medicine, but gave free advice anyway (*LU*, beta text, 2.16; Ashmole 1404, f. 64r). He noted that a man with some local fame as a lecher was reputed to avoid getting his women pregnant by giving them catmint (Daniel is careful not to vouch for this) and records that the common people believe the rowan tree is effective in protecting babies from elves and witchcraft.[28] He is wary of endorsing such views, but he finds them interesting enough to record. He tells a very odd little story of how once in his youth he met an old man who carried a mandrake root around, which was said to make him rich; he saw the root with his own eyes, and a penny lying beside it, but he does not really know what to make of the tale.[29]

Herb lore would not have been taught at university, but Daniel does claim to have had a serious education in the subject: "In my ȝonge ȝeres Y travalyed 7 ȝer to lernyn and knowyn and han swuche þynges." While he appears to have acquired some knowledge by working as an assistant, he also cites "a wise master" who taught him the properties of borage, possibly the same man as the "mayster, wysest of al þe est quarter of Bryȝtlond in þis science and in alle 7 sciencis," who clarified for him the names of various kinds of mullein.[30] "Wise in all seven sciences" suggests, for once, training at a university, where the curriculum was theoretically based on the classical seven liberal arts; though it is not clear which of the arts, if any, would have made the master so knowledgeable about varieties of mullein. Daniel is proud to mention a pupil of his own, who became his master (Ar: ADARASTA). If Daniel did not learn his medicine formally at university, it sounds as if he spent years travelling around the country, discovering plants, talking to people, observing, assisting, inquiring, as well as planting and growing things for himself. It seems particularly endearing that, in his discussion of comfrey's power to knit bones, he cites his own attempts at mending the bones of sparrows and cranes; and that he brings his own experience in raising baby otters into his discussion of beaver's testicles.[31] His range of sources, from Queen Philippa down to the peasant mother putting her "plusk" of rowan berries into the cradle, sets him quite apart from the academic doctors at the universities. And all these sources are used to supplement the row of Latin texts arrayed before him, from which he translates the bulk of his herbal, "nerhand word for word."

---

28 Ar: ACALIFA, BEEN.
29 Ar: APOLLINARIS.
30 Ar: APIARIA; Ar: BARBASTUS; Add: BORAGO; Add: CUSTOS ORTORUM.
31 Ar: ANAGALLA, CASTORIUM; Add: CASTORIUM.

The page or so in the *LU* concerning the meanings of the terms "diuretic" and "styptic" (1.4.757–87 below) throws some light both on Daniel's method and on his potential audience. He is considering the effects of various kinds of drinks on the urine: some fluids are traditionally known as "diuretic" in effect, and others as "styptic." From the start he was unsure of how to define these terms exactly, and he worked over the passage in different revisions. Daniel describes how he went about looking for their meanings. First, he says he consulted fourteen different authors, and found no definitive answer, so he consulted the practical, professional knowledge of "þise droggeris and þise apothecaries þat beste schulde wyten" including "one of þe wisest droggers of al Engelonde" (1.4.761–3). They proved to be at odds with each other: some said diuretic meant "dry" and styptic meant "thick"; but others said that diuretic meant "binding or constricting," and styptic meant "sour or loosening," like sour pears, while others said just the reverse. Yet another group held that diuretic meant old and "stale" (= settled, clarified), like stale beer, or old and matured like wine, but styptic meant raw or cloudy, like new wine or ale. Daniel then turned to a traditional literary man's source of meaning, and considered etymologies: he explained in detail how an examination of the Latin words suggests support of this last pair of meanings: "diuretic" contains the Latin word *diu*, "a long time," whereas "styptic" derives from *stipes*, "a trunk," "a stem," and suggests fresh fruit. But that does not settle the question entirely, because the etymological method can also be used to suggest that diuretic means hot and dry, and styptic cold and moist. In this light, the contrast is between the hot sharpness of old wine or ale and the cooler sweetness of spiced wine and other such confections. Daniel cites the author John of St Paul in support of this view.

In the beta revision of the *LU* he was still not satisfied with this passage. He replaces his authority John of St Paul with yet another group of authorities; these he called "ryght cunnyng men in many diuers science, and eke in this faculte had ryght mykel of the speculatyf & ryght mykel of the practyf" – that is, knowledgeable professionals who know both theory and practice of medicine – and he added that he thought these men had more knowledge "than sum that wer lettyn & know gret maistres & covth lechys" (beta text, 1.19; Ashmole 1404, f. 27r). They agreed with John of St Paul: both diuretic and styptic drinks are hot and moist, but styptic ones are sweet, and provoke more urine. Despite this professional opinion, Daniel points out that all medical authors agree that the effect of diuretic drinks is loosening, and of styptic ones, binding.

From Latin textbooks to a variety of people – those in the apothecary business, knowledgeable and practising physicians, and famous and celebrated society doctors – this passage shows some of his resources, and his methods of research. Daniel considered all of them his acquaintances and suitable for questioning. Even after all this inquiring, he confessed himself still not clear on the exact reasoning behind the usage of the technical terms: he simply puts the all the evidence before his readers, "But þe ground of the vnderstondyng of the termes rede I not, ne noon fynd þat men kan sey" (beta text, 1.19; Ashmole 1404, f. 27r).

What we know of Daniel's life highlights the obvious inference that the *LU* was not written for learned academic medical doctors: they had their Latin books. He set out to translate his own Latin researches into English at the request of Walter Turnour, a "colleague" (*socius, felowe*), who presumably felt the need for more academic medical knowledge, but did not have the Latin to pursue it. As the novelty and the scale of the enterprise grew on Daniel, he turns his thoughts to all those who are, presumably, in the same state as Walter: practising uroscopy without any understanding of the fundamentals. They needed to know human anatomy and physiology, what questions they ought to ask the patient, and what observations they ought to make before pronouncing judgment, so Daniel acknowledges that he will have to explain a great deal of material for which there is as yet nothing in English. He wants to use the best authorities, and to make them available to an audience which must have included many of the kinds of people Daniel had met in his life: the gentry who could read, the apothecaries and herbalists, physicians, travellers, and probably even those intelligent but illiterate folk who could afford to have someone read to them, people, like his various informants, who practised "medicine" of a sort at all levels of society.

The *LU* was the first, rather tentative step. Daniel thought that there should be a "Book of Remedies" to accompany it, and promised to write one if he had time and leisure.[32] And, as he revised his uroscopy, he saw several more areas that he would like to bring into English: a treatise on astronomy and astrology, a book on pulses and other bodily signs, possibly a book on diseases. The herbal was probably his "Book of Remedies," and in that text he refers to a translation – his own? – of the "Commentary on Nicholas" in such precise terms that it suggests this was actually completed;[33] but we do not have any manuscripts of it. The increasing

---

32 Ashmole 1404, f. 4r: "Nec miretur quis si morbis et egritudinibus in hoc libro tactis medicinas non subsequor pertinentes quod vtique non facio ... Quapropter iuuante deo et vita comite et ordinis mei obedientia promittente vnum opus ad hoc me facturum promitto" (Do not be surprised that I do not append medicines for the diseases and sicknesses mentioned in this book, which I do not do ... wherefore, with the help of God, and if I live long enough, and my duty to my order permits, I promise I will make a work by itself on the subject). Cf. Prol.83–6 below.

33 Ar: ABIES, BISARA, BISTORTA, BRASICA, CASTORIUM, ELIDRIUS, EPITHIMUS. Wellcome Library, MS 559 includes a brief preface to a Latin text entitled *Dosis medicinarum*

number and ambition of these remarks show Daniel's growing enthusiasm for his plan to establish medicine in the English language.

IV. The Manuscripts[34]

General Overview

The *Liber Uricrisiarum* survives in various forms in more than thirty-five manuscript witnesses, as well as a print edition (?1527), reset with minor changes perhaps in the same year. Twenty manuscripts either contain or probably once contained the whole work; the present location of one of these (*olim* Brussels, Bibliothèque Royale IV 249) is unknown. A twenty-first manuscript, London, Royal College of Physicians MS 356, 1r–64r, ends just after the astronomical digressions in book 2, chapter 35, with the phrase "Explicit liber" centred below the end of the text, so its scribe or commissioner may have deliberately chosen to end the treatise at that point (creating an unabridged excerpt, rather than an amputated but originally complete copy).

In her extensive studies of all witnesses to the *Liber Uricrisiarum*, Harvey has identified two main forms of the text, distinguished in part by the division of their content into relatively few longer chapters or many shorter chapters, as well as by significant expansions to the text in the later, shorter-chapter version. Aside from the organizational differences and the expanded content in the latter version, language and style in the two versions is generally consistent, and the second version appears to be Daniel's own revision to his original text. We have labelled the long-chapter textual type the "alpha version" and the short-chapter type the "beta version." Complete or near-complete copies of the alpha text appear in RM7 GTSaSc; complete or near-complete copies of the beta text in AG6 EW. At least three complete copies (M6G3 H) begin with an alpha text (or a variant thereof in M6G3, which appears to be slightly earlier than the standard alpha form,[35] and which we refer to as the "proto-alpha" text). However,

---

quem tractavit Henricus Dauid, which could possibly be related to a similar lost work of Henry Daniel, though the work that follows the preface is the Walter Agilon-based uroscopy "Cum secundum auctores."

34   The information provided in this section supersedes the list and groupings of witnesses given in Tavormina 2014, 87–92 (item 15). For the manuscript sigils used in the Introduction, apparatus, and Explanatory Notes, see the Sigils of Witnesses list (pp. xvii–xviii above).

35   As noted in section II above, M6G3 refer to the current year as 1377 in the discussion of leap year, whereas other alpha witnesses give 1378 as the date. The Latin prologue to M6G3 says that Daniel has been working on the *Liber Uricrisiarum* for two years, though that prologue is also used to introduce the standard alpha text in GTSaSc, which otherwise largely agrees with the alpha text in RM7 and the alpha section of

they switch over to a beta text and beta chapter structure partway through the work, albeit at different points. Three more witnesses (CfCgB) switch from an alpha to a beta text at the same point as H, but retain the alpha chapter structure. The form of the beta text in the latter parts of M6G3 H CfCgB is distinctive, and appears to be a further, relatively minor revision of the standard beta version as found in AG6EW; we have labelled this further revision beta*. More subtle influences or hybridizations between the two versions may also exist, but are not within the scope of this introduction to elaborate fully. Daniel also produced a condensed Latin version of his treatise, which survives in only one manuscript (Glasgow, University Library, Hunterian MS 362). For more details on the manuscripts and textual tradition of the full *Liber Uricrisiarum*, see Harvey's chapter in the volume of companion essays that will follow this edition.

Some seventeen manuscripts contain excerpts or adaptations of Daniel's work, discussed more fully in Tavormina's chapter in the companion volume. Many of these spin-offs can be identified as being adapted specifically from an alpha or a beta text, based on particular phrases or content unique to one or the other version. It is possible that other excerpts or adaptations of the *LU* remain to be discovered, though they are more likely to be short than long.

Many of the full-text copies of the *Liber Uricrisiarum* were written by single scribes, in a substantial investment of time and labour. Copies on paper are slightly more common than those on parchment. The manuscripts of the complete (or likely originally complete) work fall into two principal size categories: ten fit into Ralph Hanna's "half-skin octavo" category, all of them very similar in size, mostly measuring from about 210–20 x 143–53 mm (in one case, 200 x 140 mm). Six manuscripts appear to fall into Hanna's "half-skin quarto" category, though sometimes at the small end: four measure from 285–300 x 190–225 mm and two from 250–65 x 175–90 mm.[36] A sixteenth-century paper manuscript falls somewhere between these two groups, at 238 x 167 mm. Only one witness is noticeably larger than the rest (H: 345 x 242 mm), and only one is noticeably

---

HCfCgB. The prologues to the latter six witnesses give three years as Daniel's period of work on the book. For further changes to the period of work and current date, see section II.

36 Hanna 2015, 183–7. Hanna characterizes the larger of these two half-skin sizes as "the standard literary format" and the smaller as typical of "small-format books of devotional materials" (which does not exclude the size from appearing in other genres). Hanna limits his analysis to parchment manuscripts and a relatively narrow time frame, but his findings apply quite well to the *Liber Uricrisiarum* manuscripts, copied from c. 1400 to c. 1525, on both parchment and paper.

smaller (B: 155 x 108 mm); the latter belongs to Hanna's "quarter-skin quarto" or "mini-volume" category.

A significant number of the manuscripts are professional productions, with clear and handsome scripts, navigational aids in the text and the margins, and occasional tables of contents or indexes. Others appear to have been written by individuals for their own use, some of them surviving in what Hanna has called a "tatty" state, "grime-encrusted, on cheap paper" (ed. 1994, 185), with more and less successful attempts at structural markup. Elaborate decoration is rare, though the scribes often use dropped or decorated capitals and rubrication as organizational signals. Most of the copies include a program of diagrams in books 1 and 2 that appear to be related to figures in John of Sacrobosco's computistical treatise, *De computo ecclesiastico*. These diagrams, when completed, usually include some or all of the following items:

1. A circular diagram of the correspondences of cosmic and humoral quaternities (elements, directions, complexions, winds, etc.);
2. A circular diagram for calculating the dominical letter and leap year, sometimes with an associated piece of English instructional doggerel;
3. A circular diagram of the concentric celestial and elemental spheres, often referred to in the text as *rota celi*;
4. A table of lunar positions within the zodiac during the course of a lunar month, sometimes labelled *tabula lune*;
5. A table of planetary hours during the week, sometimes labelled *tabula planetarum*.

We have reproduced these diagrams from British Library, Royal MS 17 D.i, on plates 1–5 (see List of Illustrations); the first also serves as our cover illustration.

Another noteworthy feature of some complete or originally complete copies of the *Liber Uricrisiarum* is a pair of framing Latin texts, a prose prologue and a verse epilogue. Daniel must have kept tinkering with this frame, as each of the texts has a history of its own, with revisions and expansions (see section II above). For the Latin prologue and for a translation of the Latin verse epilogue, see Appendices 1 and 3; on possible dialectal differences between the English translation of the prologue and the main scribal dialect in our base text R, see the final paragraph of Appendix 5.

Table 1 lists all known complete or likely originally complete witnesses to the *Liber Uricrisiarum*. Atelous copies are labelled "inc." (incomplete), while copies with missing or mutilated leaves within the text are labelled "impf." (imperfect); copies that are both imperfect and atelous are simply labelled "impf."

Table 1. *Liber Uricrisiarum*: Complete or Likely Originally Complete Copies

Sigil	Shelfmark	Date†	Dialect (if known)	Version	Material; Size (mm)	Remarks
Alpha Texts						
R	BL, Royal MS 17 D.i	c. 1400	Northern Norfolk or border of S. Lincs. and Ely, Rutland, Leics., SE Notts.	α (impf.)	Parchment; 260 x 190	A few lost and mutilated leaves, but one of the most carefully copied and organized witnesses to the alpha text
M7	Bodl., e Musaeo MS 187	c. 1450	Similar to R, possibly slightly further north (see Appendix 5)	α	Parchment; 215 x 145	Textually very close to R, including cross-referenced internal citations; probably a daughter MS; useful for supplementing R
T	TCC, MS O.10.21, part I	s. xv	Oxon.	α	Paper; 295 x 225	
G	Gloucester Cath. Lib., MS 19	c. 1450		α (impf.)	Paper; 209 x 143	A few mutilated leaves and ff. 82–8 lost; large spaces left for illustrations at beginnings of bks. 2 and 3, finally filled in by Henry Fowler (MS owner) in 1614
Sa	BL, Sloane MS 1100	c. 1450		α	Paper; 220 x 152	Textually close to Sc
Sc	BL, Sloane MS 1721	c. 1475		α (inc.)	Paper; 218 x 150	Textually close to Sa; missing a few leaves at end
W6	Wellcome Library, MS 226	s. xv²ᐟ⁴	N Cent Mdld	α (inc.)	Parchment; 300 x 195	Ends incomplete in 2.8

(continued)

Table 1 (*continued*)

Sigil	Shelfmark	Date†	Dialect (if known)	Version	Material; Size (mm)	Remarks
Beta Texts						
A	Bodl., Ashmole MS 1404	s. xv$^{1/4}$		β	Parchment; 200 x 140	The best of the beta witnesses
G6	G&C, MS 376/596	s. xv	Cambs.	β	Mixed; 216 x 152	Textually close to A; badly damaged by water and rodents
E	BL, Egerton MS 1624	s. xv^{med}	Ely, NME	β (impf.)	Paper; 215 x 150	Plus vellum insert (ff. 109–21), not in orig. foliation
W	Wellcome Library, MS 225	c. 1425	Northumberland	β (impf.)	Paper; 216 x 146	Textually close to E
Br	*olim* Brussels, Bib. Roy., MS IV.249 (now in private hands)	c. 1480 (Kaepeli)		inc.?	??	Not seen; ends in 3.26 (Hanna, ed. 1994, 190), so it may be an incomplete β or β* text (with more than 20 chapters in bk. 3)
Hybrid Texts††						
M6	Bodl., e Musaeo MS 116	s. xv^{med}		proto-α + β*	Parchment; 265 x 180	1377 = current year in leap year discussion; transition to β* text in 2.37
G3	G&C, MS 180/213	s. xv	some northerly features	proto-α + β*	Parchment; 213 x 145	1377 = current year in leap year discussion; transition to β* text in 2.37
H	Huntington Library, MS HM 505	s. xv$^{3/4}$		α + β*	Paper; 345 x 242	Transition to β* text in 2.70
B	Boston, Massachusetts Hist. Soc., MS P-361 (*olim* 10.10)	s. xv$^{1/4}$		α + β*	Parchment; 155 x 108	Retains alpha chapters after transition to β* text in 2.12/2.70

Cf	CUL, MS Ff.2.6	s. xv		α + β*	Paper; 295 x 210	Retains alpha chapters after transition to β* text in 2.12/2.70
Cg	CUL, MS Gg.3.29	s. xv		α + β*	Paper; 286 x 208	Retains alpha chapters after transition to β* text in 2.12/2.70
Sb	BL, Sloane MS 1101	c. 1450	Some northerly, some E Anglian features	β + β*? (impf.)	Paper; 218 x 148	many gaps; possibly with alternating β and β* exemplars
J	St John's College Cambridge, MS B.16	s. xvi$^{1/4}$		α + β? α + β*?	Paper; 238 x 167	1517 "current year" in leap year discussion; scribe or his exemplar(s) regularly condenses the text

† Dating in Table 1 is drawn from several sources, including Keiser 1998, 3851; Kaeppeli 1970–5, 2: 192; Ker 1969–2002; eVK2; *LALME/ eLALME*; library catalogues; and consultation with Professor Alexandra Gillespie of the University of Toronto. Dialect identification is based on *LALME/eLALME*, our own analyses, and other studies of the manuscripts.

†† We assume that the "proto-alpha" text in M6G3 (to near the end of Lacteus chapter) is earlier than the remaining alpha witnesses because of its 1377 date for the current year in the leap year discussion, accompanied by the earliest version of the Latin prologue and the assertion in the prologue that Daniel had been working on the book for two years, in contrast to the 1378 date given in all other alpha texts and the three-year period of work noted in the revised Latin prologue in HBCfCg and its English translation in RM7.

The beta* (β*) text is a distinct form of the beta version, with a large number of relatively small divergences from the main beta version found in AG6EW. It only survives as the second part of the hybrid texts M6G3 (from 2.37 on), HBCfCg (from 2.70 on, though the beta chapter numbers appear only in H; BCfCg shift textual allegiance at the same point as H, but preserve the alpha chapter structure already established), and in parts of the idiosyncratic witnesses Sb and J, whose precise points of transition between source-versions have yet to be fully determined.

Manuscripts Used in This Edition

In the following section, we provide a full description of R, the base text of the edition, and abbreviated descriptions of the five manuscripts collated for the apparatus, M7 GSc CgH. The last two manuscripts are used only up to their transition to the beta version at the start of bk. 2.12, the chapter on Rubicundus colour.

1. R   London, British Library, MS Royal 17 D.i

s. xiv[ex]/xv[in].[37] Parchment, except for paper flyleaves. Ff. iv + 120 + iv.

Ff. 8, 9 mutilated (text almost entirely lost); bottom third of f. 67 cut away. Five leaves lost between ff. 42 and 43; one leaf lost between ff. 94 and 95; at least one leaf lost at the end of the text (after f. 118). A volvelle appx. 130 mm in diameter (referred to as a "pacche" in the text, at f. 48rb, 2.6.278 below), with a diagram for calculating dominical letters and leap year, is attached to a modern half-leaf of parchment mounted between ff. 50 and 51. The volvelle is numbered 51* on its recto and 52 on its blank verso, both in modern pencil.[38] Ff. 1–3, 119–20 are old parchment flyleaves.

DIMENSIONS. c. 250–60 x c. 185–90 mm. WRITING AREA: c. 175–80 mm x 120–2 mm (total); column width: 55–8 mm; space between cols. appx. 10 mm. LINES/PAGE: 40–1.

HANDS. One scribe, writing an anglicana formata script. Uses yoghs, thorns, $y \neq þ$.

CONTENTS.

ff. 4ra–5ra *Liber Uricrisiarum*, prologue. *Inc.* "Frere Henry Danyel of the ordre of ffrerez prechoures."

---

37   Keiser 1998, 3851 ("ca 1400"); we are grateful to Professor Alexandra Gillespie for confirmation of this date (personal communication). For a later dating (c. 1450), provided by Malcolm Parkes, see Norri 1992, 67 and 71.

38   The verso number "52" is older than the number "51*" on the recto of the volvelle; Warner and Gilson (1921) report that the "calendar-wheel is inserted as f. 52" (2: 250), and the old black and white microfilm of R shows only the number "52" on the volvelle. The *pacche* has a hole at its centre, through which a knotted string could have been threaded, and smaller prick-holes in two concentric circles below the inner circle of letters. It is creased along several diameters, suggesting that it has been folded over at some periods of its history. Another hole occurs at the centre of the *rota celi* diagram on f. 49v, but it seems unlikely that the volvelle would have been attached on top of the diagram, even if it could be folded over to reveal the image underneath, as it would have covered all or most of the *rota*. See Plates 2 and 3.

ff. 5ra–5va *Liber Uricrisiarum*, table of contents, keyed to the original foliation system. *Inc.* "1. Of significacion i. of knowyng of this worde vrina . lef .j."

ff. 6ra–118vb *Liber Uricrisiarum. Inc.* "Uryn is as mykel for to say in englis as on in þe reynes." Ends incomplete in bk. 3.20, the "Rules of Isaac"; probably missing only one more page of text. *Des.* "a party drubli but litle wiþ sperme of the man."

COLLATION. 1^6 (wanting 6), $2–5^8$, 6^8 (wanting 6–8), 7^8 (wanting 1–2), 8^8 (not including the parchment insert with attached volvelle between the second and third leaves of the quire), $9–12^8$, 13^8 (wanting 6), $14–15^8$, 16^8 (wanting 7–8). Catchwords on ff. 13v, 21v, 29v, 37v, 48v, 57v, 65v, 73v, 81v, 89v, 96v, 104v, 112v. A system of signatures survives in part, though sometimes cropped or skipping letters, and written in different colours of ink (brown, red, blue). Modern rebinding has slightly obscured the original quire structure.

TEXTUAL PRESENTATION. Double columns; running heads in red giving book numbers; original foliation in red; three- to five-line blue initials, pen-flourished in red; alternating paraphs in red and blue; red underlining, often for cross-references to other parts of the text; leaf numbers of those cross-references also in red. Diagrams on ff. 18v (quaternities), 49v (*rota celi*), 51*/52 (sun-cycle diagram and verses on volvelle numbered 51* and 52 on front and back), 51r (*tabula lune; tabula planetarum*). In later hand(s): a few early modern marginal notes *passim*, often the single word "mark"; 120v: faint cropped diagram of five roundels arranged around a central roundel, with room for two more roundels in cropped region (possibly an attempt at drawing a urine wheel organized by digestion groups); page also contains other arcs and circles, some of them possibly water-rings from cylindrical vessels.

LANGUAGE. The scribe's spellings can be localized to a region that includes the northern part of Norfolk and a narrower band reaching west from Norfolk, running along the border between Lincolnshire and northern Cambridgeshire (Isle of Ely), Northamptonshire, Rutland, and Leicestershire, and possibly a small part of southeast Nottinghamshire. He tends to eschew narrowly regional spellings available in this area (e.g., East Anglian *xal-/xul-* for SHALL/SHOULD; *-lk-* spellings in forms of SUCH and WHICH; and *qu-/qw-/qwh-* for WH-), perhaps from a desire to reach a wider audience. For more detailed discussion of this localization, see Appendix 5.

PROVENANCE, OWNERSHIP, OTHER NAMES AND DATES. F. 120r: s. xvi note on medical treatment (so Warner and Gilson 1921) of Dorothy Ferys: *Inc.* "M^d that <I> was with dorothe fferys at adam ?sky< ... > howsse," much crossed out but with some day and time details still visible ("on Sunday"; "at ij off clocke"; etc.). F. 120v: *sideways near gutter:* "pretium – 15ˢ || 1579." F. 2: "Mr. John Sherly at þe Golden Pellican in Litle Brittaine" (in John Theyer's hand, according to Warner and Gilson 1921, 2: 250). John Sherly was a London bookseller who sold books at the "Golden Pelican in Little Britain, 1644–1666" (Plomer 1907, 163), which may suggest that Theyer (1597–1673) bought the MS from Sherly at some point in the mid-seventeenth century. Theyer's books, including this manuscript, were purchased by Charles II c. 1678 and thereby passed into the Old Royal Library, becoming one of the four foundation collections of the British Library in 1757.

DESCRIPTIONS. Warner and Gilson 1921, 2: 250; Hanna, ed. 1994, 187, 190–1; Norri 1992, 71; Norri 1998, 101. Noted in Kaeppeli 1970–5, 2: 192; Keiser 1998, 3851; J.H. Harvey 2004; Tavormina 2014, 90.

2. M7   Oxford, Bodleian Library, MS e Musaeo 187
s. xv$^{1/4}$. Parchment. Ff. v + 83 + i; c. 213–15 x c. 143–5 mm.

CONTENTS.

f. i *blank*.

ff. ii recto–iv verso. Legal document, concerning a claim against the estate of William Penyfader, ostler of Wells.

ff. v recto–v verso. *Liber Uricrisiarum*, prologue. *Inc.* "Frere henry danyel of þe ordre of frerez prechoures."

f. 1r *Liber Uricrisiarum*, table of contents. *Inc.* "1. of significacion i. of knowyng of þis word vrina . lef j."

ff. 1v–78v *Liber Uricrisiarum. Inc.* "Uryn as mykel for to say in englis as on in þe reynes." With Latin verse epilogue.

f. 78v "Explicit liber vricrisiarum a fratre . henrico . daniel . ordinis fratrum predicatorum ex latino in wlgare translatus Deo gratias."

ff. 79r–83r Miscellaneous recipes, notes, verse, and copies of legal documents, in several later hands.

3. G   Gloucester, Cathedral Library MS 19
s. xv^{med}. Paper. Ff. iii + 200 + iii; 209 x 143 mm. F. 1 was misbound for many years with MS 23 but has now been rejoined to MS 19.

CONTENTS.

ff. 1r–2r *Liber Uricrisiarum*, prologue. *Inc.* "Dilecto socio in christo Waltero Turnuro de ketene ffrater henricus Daniele ordinis predicatorum."

ff. 2r–189v *Liber Uricrisiarum. Inc.* "Urine is als myche to say in Englyssh as on the reynys." With Latin verse epilogue.

f. 189v "Explicit liber vricrisiarum ex latino in vulgare translatus a fratre henrico Daniell ord[i]nis fratrum predicatorum omnium doctrinarum ac scripturarum . &c."

ff. 190r–195r Table of contents and index for *Liber Uricrisiarum. Inc.* "Presens tractatus in 3^{es} paraticulas [*sic*] diui[di]tur."

ff. 195v–199v Notes on urines by Alexander Ramsey, friend of Henry Fowler (s. xvii owner and extensive annotator of the MS), dated 24 Feb. 1616. *Inc.* "It were goode that all men had some knowledge in there owen vrynes/that therby they may be \þe/ better able to instruct the phisition."

f. 200 *blank.*

4. Sc   London, British Library, MS Sloane 1721

c. 1475. Paper. Ff. iv + 216 + v; 218 x 150 mm (ff. 1–213), 152 x 105 mm (ff. 214–16).

CONTENTS.

f. 1r s. xvi^{ex}/xvii^{in} note identifying the work and author.

f. 1v *blank.*

ff. 2r–3r *Liber Uricrisiarum*, prologue. *Inc.* "Dilecto socio Waltero Tornar de Keten ffrater henricus Danyell ordinee [*sic*] predicatorum."

ff. 3r–213v *Liber Uricrisiarum. Inc.* "Uryne is as \mech/ to sey in English as on the reynys." Ends incomplete in bk. 3.20, the "Rules of Isaac." *Des.* "and ake & peyn in þe hedd and stopping in þei [= 'the'] [*catchword*: nose & þe]."

ff. 214r–216v "De Vrinis in genere." *Inc.* "There be 20^{tie} coloures in vrine that is to say Niger, Lividus, Albus, … " (in s. xvi hand).

5. Cg   Cambridge, University Library, MS Gg.3.29

s. xv. Paper (one parchment flyleaf). Ff. iv + 171 + ii; c. 286 x 208 mm.

CONTENTS.

f. i verso s. xvii biographical note relating to David Harris, Jr, and David Harris, Sr, apothecaries of Bristol, and collectors of medical books.

f. ii *originally blank.*

f. 1r–2r *Liber Uricrisiarum*, prologue. *Inc.* "Dilecto socio in christo Magistro Waltero de Ketene frater Henricus Daniel Ordinis fratrum predicatorum."

ff. 2v–169r *Liber Uricrisiarum. Inc.* "Uryn is as mykyl to seyne in englissh / As on in the Reyns." With Latin verse epilogue.

f. 169r "Explicit liber vricrisiarum ex latino in vulgar' editus a fratre henrico Danyell . Ordinis ffratrum predicatorum omnium sciencarum et doctrinarum lingue latine yperapiste et translatorie [*sic*]/Amen."

f. 169v   s. xvi Latin luxury recipe "pro vxore mea." With s. xvi signature in
different hand next to recipe heading: "Dauid: Harris . apothecarie."

6. H   San Marino, Huntington Library, MS HM 505

s. xv³/⁴. Paper (with one parchment leaf, f. 60). Ff. iv + 134 + iv; c. 345 x
242 mm.

CONTENTS.

ff. 1r–2r *Liber Uricrisiarum*, prologue. *Inc.* "Dilecto socio in christo
Magistro . Waltero de Ketene Ffrater henricus Daniell Ordinis ffratrum predicatorum."

ff. 2r–134v *Liber Uricrisiarum. Inc.* "Uryne is as mekyll for to sayne in
Anglish as on in þe reynes." With Latin verse epilogue.

f. 134v "Explicit liber vricrisiarum ex ex [*sic*] latino in ?vulgato editus a
ffratre" [*breaks off incomplete, possibly after the first stroke of an* H].

V. A Reading Edition

The following work is not a critical edition in the usual sense of the phrase.
It is our considered view that putting a good representative version of
Daniel's work into the hands of scholars and students in a relatively expe-
ditious manner is of higher priority than the far more unwieldy task of
creating a traditional critical edition for a long text with a complicated
textual history. Even if limited to one or the other of the two main versions of the text, such an edition would require many years to prepare, and
entail a critical apparatus of daunting complexity, arguably with rapidly
diminishing returns.

Instead, we have chosen to provide a "reading edition" of the *Liber Uricrisiarum* in its earlier, alpha version, as represented by British Library MS
Royal 17 D.i, one of the earliest and most carefully produced witnesses
to either version of the text.[39] Emendations are limited almost entirely
to corrections of obvious medical and verbal errors (e.g., dittographies,
eyeskips) in the text, supported by collation with a select group of only
five other witnesses to the text. These witnesses are M7, a possible direct
descendant of R, which is also used to supplement R where the latter is
wanting text (about ten leaves); GSc; and CgH up to the point where they

---

39 For the general rationale behind the production of reading editions for long texts
with complicated textual histories, see Hanna 2013; for examples of such editions, see
Hanna, ed. 2008 and Hanna and Wood, eds. 2013.

and their textual subgroup switch over to a beta exemplar in book 2.12. These copies represent the three principal subfamilies of the alpha version, with a strong case for R as the best text among them all, despite the minor losses that can be supplemented from M7. In relatively rare cases, we have corrected somewhat more complex errors in content, even when the grammar and syntax of R's text are unremarkable, based on variants in the select group of collated witnesses, but with additional support from the broader textual tradition. We address such additional variation in the Explanatory Notes as necessary.

Approaching the text in this way allows modern readers to approximate – admittedly rather roughly – their medieval predecessors' experience of encountering the *Liber Uricrisiarum* in a well-made copy, especially if those earlier readers had sufficient professional expertise to recognize and compensate for occasional scribal errors. We leave to future scholars the projects of editing and analysing Daniel's beta revision and of further elucidating relationships between the two main versions, their hybrids, and possible draft or cross-contaminated witnesses.

VI. Editorial Practice

The edition below uses British Library, Royal MS 17 D.i (R) as its base manuscript, supplemented by the very closely related witness, Bodleian Library, MS e Musaeo 187 (M7), for approximately ten leaves that have been lost or mutilated.[40] M7 may well be a direct descendant of R, based on common errors, linguistic forms, and often identical marginal cross-references to other leaves, usually correct for R but nearly always, unavoidably, incorrect for M7.

Abbreviations and contractions in the text are usually expanded silently, aside from retention of scribal *i.*, *s.*, and *c./ca(p).* for *id est*, *scilicet*, and *capitulum/chapitre/chapitle*.[41] Italicization, capitalization, word-division, and punctuation follow modern practice where possible, though some attention has been paid to the scribe's use of paraphs to indicate shifts in topic.[42] Daniel's prose style runs to long, loosely concatenated clauses and

---

40   The mutilations occur at ff. 8–9 (almost entirely cut away) and f. 67 (lower third cut away); the losses between modern ff. 42/43 (five leaves lost), 94/95 (one leaf), and after f. 118 (one leaf).

41   Examples of common abbreviations: vr' = vryn (*urina* in Latin contexts); fe. = febre (*febris* in Latin contexts); angl/an^ce = *anglice*; h(u), c(a), s(ic), f(ri) = *humidus, calidus, siccus, frigidus* (and their forms); etc.

42   In books 2 and 3, for purposes of emphasis, we have capitalized the English terms for the urinary colours and contents derived from Giles of Corbeil, at points where they

sentences. In response to this complexity, we have been deliberately generous with punctuation, both within and between sentences, perhaps to a degree unnecessary in modern prose but helpful in negotiating Daniel's meaning.

The letters *u/v* and *i/j* follow the scribe's usage, except that the identical capital letter used for *I/J* is transcribed according to its vocalic or consonantal intention (thus, *I* for the first-person singular pronoun, but *Jupitre* for the planet).[43] The graph *ff* in word-initial position is transcribed as *f* or *F*, depending on modern capitalization conventions. The "yogh/tailed z" graph is used by R's scribe for both the traditional phonemes represented by ȝ (e.g., /j/, /ɣ/, /x/, etc.) and for the sounds more commonly represented by *z* (notably in *zodiac* and the Arabic loan *zirbus*, and as a sibilant plural marker on certain nouns). For the sake of clarity and ease of reading, we interpret it as ȝ or *z* depending on its context, but students of Middle English spelling systems should be aware that all *z*'s in the text below are written with the same letter-form as that used for yogh (ȝ). The scribe of M7 uses the graph *y* for phonemes represented in R by *þ* and *y*; for text taken from M7 because of its loss in R, we have interpreted M7's *y* as *þ* or *y* based on context, again for clarity's sake.

Bold font signals the scribe's rubricated chapter headings. We have treated most small tags and flourishes at the end of words as otiose; we likewise ignore the relatively rare occurrence of the nasal suspension over a final -*n* in words like *vppon* "upon," *on* "one" or "on," *ben* "be/been," and so on. However, for final -*r* with an upward curl, we have used both the scribe's spelled-out forms and our judgment to decide whether the curl is large enough (or too small) to warrant expansion to -*re*. The *per/par* contraction (a barred *p*) is expanded to match the scribe's spelled-out forms where those provide guidance;[44] then following etymology for Latin loan words (e.g., *superfluites*, *partie*); otherwise with *per*.

Emendations are normally restricted to manifest verbal and medical errors, spelled in the orthography of R, and indicated by square brackets in the text for additions or substitutions. Omissions are recorded solely in the apparatus. Individual words and short phrases supplied by the editors

---

are applied to urine proper (thus, *vryn Whit* but not *whit fleume*; *Blode in vryn* but not *herte blode*).

43 The scribe almost always uses *j* for the single-digit number 1; in arabic numerals with the digit 1 in any position (e.g., 14, 61, 117, etc.), he writes that digit with a single minim (an undotted *i*). We retain the *j*, but represent the minim as an arabic *1*.

44 In words where the scribe spells out the syllable with both *per* and *par*, the predominant form is used to expand the abbreviated form, but spelled-out minority spellings are retained, preserving the scribe's occasionally inconsistent practice.

to fill in lost or illegible material are indicated by angle brackets, both in the text and in the apparatus: < >. Cancellation of text by the scribe of R or a corrector is recorded in the apparatus; cancellations and self-corrections in the collated witnesses are silently incorporated. Interlinear insertions of words (which are rare) are signalled by backward and forward virgules: \ /. The most common uncorrected errors in the text are minor dittographies, corrected in the edition and recorded in the apparatus.

Variants are extremely selective, not only in the restriction to manifest errors but also in the limitation to only six manuscripts, representative of the three principal families of the alpha version: the base text R and its likely descendant M7; Gloucester Cathedral Library MS 19 (G) and British Library, MS Sloane 1721 (Sc); and the alpha sections of Cambridge University Library MS Gg.3.29 (Cg; to bk. 2.12) and Huntington Library, MS HM 505 (H; to bk. 2.12). M7 is used for its filial proximity to R; the others for their careful production and high legibility (within their familial groups). Variants are cited in order of closeness to the lemma; for each variant, supporting witnesses are cited in the order RM7CgHGSc. Other witnesses, including copies of the beta version, have been consulted for particularly problematic passages, but are mainly cited in the commentary rather than the apparatus, if their readings shed light on R's version of the text. (See the list of manuscripts in Table 1 above for identification of these secondary witnesses.) The following abbreviations are used in the apparatus: *abbrev.* "abbreviated"; *canc.* "cancelled"; *char(s).* "character(s)"; *illeg.* "illegible"; *corr.* "corrected"; *eras.* "erased, erasure"; *foll.* "followed"; *marg.* "(in the) margin, marginal"; *om.* "omitted"; *poss.* "possible, possibly"; *prec.* "preceded"; *susp.* "suspension."

Marginal notes by the original scribe (but not the few notes in later hands) are included in the apparatus, except for the numerical cross-references to folios on which specific topics are discussed, typically cited within the text by book, chapter, and the word *lef*, sometimes followed by a space, and with the leaf-number usually written in the margin in red. Those numbers are keyed, generally accurately, to the original foliation of the manuscript; we have indicated them within the text using curly brackets: { }. In some of these cross-references, the scribe or rubricator (possibly the same person) who added these numbers failed to give a specific number in the margin; for some but not all of those cases, the word *lef* is cancelled, presumably because the book and chapter number or topic were deemed sufficient to locate the reference. Where the word *lef* has not been cancelled, we mark the omission of the marginal number thus: {*om.*}. Many of these internal cross-references, as well as some other passages, have been underlined by the rubricator; we have retained that underlining.

Two unusual spelling practices are common enough in the text that the scribe may have considered them acceptable orthographic variants, and we have left them unemended: 1) the omission of final *-t* after *-gh-* or *-ʒ-* in the words *brigh, brygh, mygh, taugh, (vn)wrogh, nogh, strengh, lengh, riʒ,* and *noʒ,* alongside more standard forms ending in *-ght* and *-ʒt*; and 2) the omission of the nasal suspension in some instances of the word *comunly,* to yield *comuly.* These forms seldom cause problems in comprehension; selected instances are listed in the Glossary.

The text of this edition is based on two independent transcriptions, one made by Harvey in the 1990s and one by the University of Toronto team of research assistants (Lara Howerton, Shirley Kinney, Nora Thorburn, and Elise Williams, led by C.E.M. Henderson, Jessica Henderson, and Sarah Star) in the academic year 2015–16. Those transcripts were then proofed against the manuscript and each other and copy-edited by Tavormina. In 2016–17, the research team identified sources and drafted glossary entries; the final glossary was compiled by Tavormina from those draft entries. Star and Tavormina compiled the apparatus; Star proofread the final edited text against the manuscript and helped to edit the notes, appendices, and glossary. The general editors prepared the introduction (parts I–III: Harvey; IV–VI: Tavormina) and reviewed and completed the apparatus, notes, and glossary.

Liber Uricrisiarum

HENRY DANIEL, O.P.

[Prologue]

[f. 4ra] Þis prolog was first made in Latyne, bot afterward it was translate into Ynglisch.

Frere Henry Danyel of the ordre of Frerez Prechoures, þe seruant of Jhesu Crist & of þe Virgine his moder, vnto his belouede felowe in Crist, Walter Turnour of Ketoun.   5

Moste belouede felowe, þou haste praiede me oftymez & besily þat Y shulde gadre to þe one handeful of flourez of þe domes of vrines, and þat I shulde write þe it shortly and þat in wlgare, i. comune langage. Þe which forsoþe to be done, þou haste put me to an harde wark and opne to the barking & to the scornyng of detractours; bothe for that þat is gyffen into   10 teching by wrytyng, but if it be softening þe eres of men and passing þe witte of meny men, it is al arectede into scorn. And also for Y haue noȝt mynde that I haue redde ne harde neyþer þis science giffen in English; and also for Y am nouþer witty ne wise of this tonge; and also for after Aueroys (and it is had of Gilbert in his Coment vpon Giles), that this   15 faculte mai noȝt be schewede by tonge. For whie, as it is opne schewede to konnyng men, no science may sufficiently be schewede in þis tonge, s. English, and þis as Y trowe is þe resoun: ouþer for the langage is vnsufficiant in itselfe, or for þat we kane it noȝt parfitly. And also for noþer haue I take it ne lerede it of man but as in oþer sciences of interpretacions by þe   20 gifte of the Holy Gost, which departeþ to euery man vnto helþe as he will.

But certeynly, riȝt wel belouede broþer, loue & charite ouercommeþ simple men, but couetouse of temporal lucre or of praysing or of fauour ouercometh **[f. 4rb]** hem þat bene childer of þis worlde. And what so eny man coueyteþ moste, þat praiseþ he moste. We rede in Scriptures   25 meny holy men for þair saiingez & þair writyng ful greuousely haue bene

punysshede & suffrede meny eueles, but noȝt but of euel men. Also Holy
Writte makeþ mynde þat þe selfe aposteles of Crist were arectede reprouabli wiþouten letres and ydiotes. Þerfor if so grete men & so holy men,
ȝa, þat were inspired wiþ þe Holy Goste, myȝt no waies eschewen the   30
cont[um]elez,¹ i. myssayingz or vpbraidinges, of proude men, scornyngz
of presumptuouse men, and þe setting at noȝt of enuyouse men & corrupt
in soule and þe hissingz & detraccions of serpentes tonges, how shal I,
þat am so litle as þe leste of the seruantz of Criste, and þe first article (as
I trowe) þat techeþ þis faculte in English tonge, how shal I inow eschewe   35
euel spekingz & vpbraidyngz? Certeynly in no waiez, for I do it noȝt for
cause of lucre of fauour as oþer men doþ, þat þai be sene wise onely in
myche speche of speking men þat bene nowe. But certeynly, while þat
þe euyles þat ar done to gode men of euel men ar gadrade into þe merite
to þe same gode men, gode warkes ar demede of discrete men noȝt to be   40
wiþdrawen for þe maneres of schrewede men.

   Therfor dere frende, I considerand meny men & diuerse þat couaiteþ to
be experte of demyng of vrines, forþi þat þe science is faire & wonderful,
and also sich a science is as it were propurly mych [**f. 4va**] profitable vnto
men, and also I seand ful meny men – ȝe, as it were alle men – languishand   45
doutously aboute þe sothfastnesse or trewþe of it. And forþi þat euery
þing in how mich it is more openly taghte, in so myche it schal be take
more liȝtly & of moo men; þerfor þat I be noȝt made a liȝtede lantern hide
vnder a busshel, but þat I condescende vnto þi praiers, & noȝt only to þine
& þam þat be like þe, but þat I eke & encresce in Gode þe knowlich of al   50
þam þat coueteþ for to profite in þis faculte, I haue gadrede as I myȝt wiþ
grete labour by 3 ȝere þis presente werk of þe bokes of meny auctoures
& þe sayingz of þe comentours of þam, oftetymes lettede or take þerfro
noȝt only for þe labour of þe obediens of myn ordre, but also for diuerse
infirmites and somtyme almoste to þe deth. For which causes more þan   55
for scarsenes of þe langage I lefte meny þingz or addede to myne owen þat
som auctoures affermeth noȝt.

   In whiche werke forsoþe ar schewede certeynly rewles of demyng of
vrynes after giffyng & teching of auctours and of comentoures of þis sciens wiþ diffiniciouns and exposiciouns of termes of sekenes or infirmites   60
& of membres wiþoutforth & withinforþe & wiþ meny oþer þingez notable in þis crafte, which I demede to be callede *Liber Vricrisiarum*, "Þe
Boke of Demyng of Vryn."

---

1   contumelez] M7, contumelias CgHGSc, conti(*line end*)nuelez R (*misinterpretation of
    minims*)

Forsoþe he þat biholdeþ wel and parfitely þis boke made in wlgare, i. in comune tonge, he [**f. 4vb**] shal mowe be a parfite domesman in this   65 crafte and wiþoute doute he schal gete gode & richez and helthe of his soule; neuerþeles if he mysvse noȝt a pompouse lif or bostful, ful of wordes, ful of fables & ful of lesingez, as leches þat bene now ar wonte to done.

Wise Aristotel forsoþe, as it is openly schewede _ex fine primi & prin-_   70 _cipio secundi Methaphisice,_ he þankeþ þaym þat bifore him gaf or taght in writyngz noȝt only wisely but also þam þat dede noȝt wisely, for he fonde meny more subtil þingz of þo þinges þat oþer wrote bifore. For after þe same Aristotel _in fine 2ᶦ libri Elenchorum,_ þo þinges þat ar fonden labored afore of oþer men ar particulerly ekede or encresede of þam þat toke þam   75 afterwarde. _& sequitur,_ þo þingz forsoþ þat ar first fonden ar wont for to take but litil encresyng in þe first tymes, but þe encresyng þat is done afterward of þam is more profitable, _hec ille._ For whie I saie noȝt þis of myself þat I am to write newe þinges, but þat I do it newely. I haue gadrede now late for þam þat kan take it in Latyn a schorte tretice conteynyng   80 fully þe marowe of þis faculte, and I wrote it in þe tong þat forsothe is riȝt dere to me.

Ne wonder noȝt eny man if I sewe noȝt medicynes perteynyng to þe sekenes & þe infirmites tochede in this boke. For God helping and þe obedience of myn ordre noȝt agaynstanding, I bihete me for to make   85 a werk by itselfe þerto. Therfor in þis werk I aske euermore a trewe [**f. 5ra**] reder, I desir a meke herer, I biseke euermore a lele & a benigne correctour, for charite broght me more herto þan hardines. Ouer þat I praie euery writer or compiler of þis, þat he kepe my writing, but if he be of þe langage of annoþer contre. For whie as for þe langage of Englissh   90 tong, as anentz a discrete man & him þat hath þe gift of tunge, trewe & parfite craft of ortographie is taugh in þis bok; he that vnderstondes it noȝt, praie he þat he maye interpretate it, seiþ þe trompe of Criste, i. Seynt Poule.

Therfor þis present tretis of Englisshe is diuidede into 3 bokes or elle   95 3 particules. In þe j bok is taught of vryn wherof it is saide & what it is, wherof and how it is gendrede, what þinges and how meny ar to be considerede of a leche, & howe þat he owe to haue himself in demyng, & it hath 4 _capitula._ In þe 2 bok of domes & significacions of coloures & of bodies of vryn, & it hath 14 _capitula._ In þe 3 boke forsoþ of domes &   100 significacions of contentez of vrynes, & it hath 20 _capitula._ In þe laste of which 20 _capitula,_ it is tretede of þe reules of Ysaac, which himself giffeþ in þe 10 partie of his _Boke of Vryns._

Explicit prologus

---

2 *Running heads for chapters in the following edition are drawn from the chapter titles
   given in this contents list, which vary slightly from the titles given within the text at the
   beginning of each chapter.*
3 wherof] M7, wheof R, *no Table of Contents* CgHGSc
4 he] M7, he he R, *no Table of Contents* CgHGSc
5 pallido] M7, plallido R, *no Table of Contents* CgHGSc
6 11] M7 (*written to the left of other chapter numbers*), om. R, *no Table of Contents*
   CgHGSc

[*rest of the folio blank*]

Book 1

[1.1]

[f. 6ra] Here bygynneþ the firste chapitre of significacioun, i. of knowyng, of þis worde *vrina*

"Uryn" is as mykel for to say in Englis as "on in þe reynes," *reyns* Freynche, *renes* Latyn, "lendes" in Englisch. If þou wilt wete wytterly what arne þe reyns, <u>se in þe 2 boke, þe 4 chapitre, *de albo colore*</u>. And   5
vryn is callede "on in þe reyns" for þer it is kyndely and formely causede and formed. And vnderstonde þat vryn is gendrede & made[1] in 2 places of mannes body: first in þe lyuer and syþen in þe reynes, but principaly in þe reynes. For in þe lyuer he takeþ first his body and his substance. His coloure he takeþ when he entriþ þe reyns and kynde hete bygynneþ for to   10
wyrken into þe humours, but in þe reyns it is decocte and digestede, þat is for to say soden and defiede, and þere he takeþ his fynal forme and his laste colour. And þerefor it is callede "on in þe reyns."

Also it is callede "vryne" of þis worde of Grewe <u>*vrith*</u>, þat is as mykel to say as a demonstracion, a schewyng, for more certeynly & more verreyly vryne   15
scheweþ & telleþ þe disposicion of þe reynes þan of eny oþer partyes of þe body. For when we wil wete and knowe þe state & þe disposicioun of mannes body wiþin and namely in þe reyns, we take rede and conseile at þe vryn.

Also vryne is saide of þis Latyn worde <u>*vrere*</u>, þat is to say **[f. 6rb]** "bryn-nyng os fyre," which þat is be way of kynde hote and drye.[2] Be resoun of   20
his dryhede he is desiccatif, þat is for to say dryand, and be cause þat he is hote and drye he is saide boþe desiccatif & vrytif, i. dryand and brennande. And it haþ also in him kyndly a saltischhede, be cause of whiche it is desic-catif, vrytif, and mordificatif, i. dryand, brennand, and bitand, for þo þre bene þe propurtes of salt.[3]   25

And þerfor vryn is medycynable souereynly to hem þat haue sekenes of þe splene [i.][4] þe mylte, agayne þe ydropisi and ȝyche & scabbe and pusshes and kyns, and aȝeyn al maladies þat neden desiccacioun, if a clene wollen cloþ be wel dippede and dappede þerein and þe place wel wesschen þerwith.

Also as saiþ þe Comentoure vpon Gyles, if an oyntment be made   30
þerof and of haukes galle, it fordoþ sores and maladyes þat oncomen in

---

1 gendrede & made] *marg.*: <u>Wher vryne is gendrede & made</u>
2 hote and drye] *marg.*: þe qualit\<e\> of vryn
3 propurtes of salt] *marg.*: <u>The propurtes of salt</u> & of vryn
4 i.] CgG, and R, & M7, *damaged leaf* H, *om.* Sc

mannes ȝerde and womennes membres. Also men seyn þat it fordoþ þe webbe & þe pyn in þe eye. And as Gilbert seyþ, it fordoþ also þe webbe in þe eye þat women cachen of here chyldyng. Also if *spleneticus*, i. he þat haþ sekenes of þe splene, drynke his owen fastande water, he beyng   35
fastande, it helpeþ him myȝttely. What þat splen is, se in þe 2 boke, þe 7 c. *de karopos.*

Also ageyne þe colde goute, tak whit clay or elles blake clay and his owen fastande vryn 7 or 9 daies [**f. 6va**] olde, and þat þe clay be clene piked, and menge hem togeder in a wollen cloþe clene and new wasshen   40
and lay emplastre alse ferre as þe peyne lastiþ, and þe peyne schal abate but noȝt þe maladie. & do þus as often as þe peyne comeþ. Also a wollen clout, clen awasshyn⁵ & dippede in his owen fastand vryn 7 or 9 daies, wonden & wappede alse fer as þe peyn lastiþ doþ þe same effecte. Also a potel of his owen vryn 7 or 9 daies stonden wiþ halfe a quarte of Peyto salt, boiled   45
half or 3 part, doþe þe same.

[1.2]

What vryne is, whereof, and how it is made: the secunde chapitre

Os saiþ Giles in his texte and alle auctores and comentoures, þis is descripcioun of vryn (descripcioun of a þing is þe telling what a þing is): vryne is a late and a subtil meltyng & clensyng of blode & of humores. And take hede þat Y say "late" for this skyl: for somtyme þe water passeþ oute of   5
þe body sone after þat i[t] is¹ dronken, and þat owen noȝt to be callede "vryn" propurly, but it owe to be callede "pisse." For when it is pissede sone, noþer it is decocte ne digestede in þe veyns and in þe reyns, ne þe coloure of him is noȝt profundet, i. noȝt depede ne dyede as it schulde be, and al is be cause þat he haþ noȝt his tyme in þe body kyndely as he   10
schulde haue.

Also Y say "subtile" for þe more² þat he is decocte and dygestede in þe body, þe more subtile he is in hymself and þe [**f. 6vb**] bettre profundet in colour as þou myȝt se in þe 2 boke. "Subtil" is as mykel to say as þen, clere, and bright.   15

---

5   wollen clout clen awasshyn] wollen clout clena wasshyn RM7, wollen clowt clene wasshin CgH, clene clowte wollyn wasshen G, clene wollen clothe weshed Sc

---

1   it is] M7CgHGSc, is is R
2   for þe more] *foll. by* for þe more *canc.* R

Item, i. also, Y say a "meltynge," a "clensyng of þe blode and of þe humores" for þis skyl: for ry3t as whei is wrongen & clensede and press-ede oute fro þe mylke þrogh wirkyng and trauaylyng and þristyng out of þike matere, i. fro þe cloddres & þe clompres and þe cruddes, ri3t so þe vryn is pressede and wrongen and clensede out fro *massa*[3] *sanguinis*, i. fro   20
þe clode and clompre of blode. Vnderstonde þat *massa* is no3t elles but a colleccioun, i. a gaderyng togedre, of þe 4 humores and þat is *epar*, i. þe lyuer, which is noþing but *sanguis coagulatus* (*anglice*: a colleccioun of blode clumprede and cruddede togedre), and þ[r]ou3[4] my3t and vertu of þe 4 humores causede and wroght, helpeand kynde hete as þou may se in   25
þe nexte chapitre folweand.

And[5] þis forsaide descripcioun of vryn þat Gilbert 3eueþ accordeþ wel to þe diffinycioun þat Ysaac and Theophile 3euen (diffinicioun and descripcioun ar al one to say): vryn is a clensyng of blode and of alle oþer humores wro3t be way of kynde in mannes body. <u>Which and how meny</u>   30
<u>and what be þe humores of man, se in þe 4 c. nexte sewyng.</u>

For I spake of mylke in þe firste diffi- **[f. 7ra]** nicioun of vryn, vnder-stonde þat in mylke ar foure þinges: *serum*,[6] i. whei, and þat is *frigidum* and *humidum*, colde and moyste; *butirum*,[7] butter, and þat is *calidum* & *humidum*, hote and moyste; *caseus*,[8] chese, & þat is *frigidum* & *siccum*,   35
colde and drye; þe 4 is þat ilke wete and white substance *lac*,[9] mylk, and þat is *frigidum* & *humidum*, colde and moyste.

Item, anoþer similitude, i. exawmple, of causyng and of genderyng of vryn in man putten auctoures also, for þai calle vryn a "cribracioun," i. a siftyng, a clensyng þrogh a syf. And for þis skyl: for ri3t as þou seste þat   40
þorou þe cribre (þe syue) is separate and diuisede, i. atwynnede and depart-ede, þe smal mater fro þe grete, þe clene fro þe foule, and þe couenant fro þe vncouenant, ry3t on þe same wise in þe 2 digestioun, i. in þe lyuer, is sequestracioun and diuisioun of þe fode and of þe 4 humores. Which sequestracioun and diuisioun is in maner of a siftyng in þe 2 digestioun þat   45
we callen in Latyn *epar*, þe lyuer in Englisshe. <u>Of þis maner of wirkyng &</u> <u>syftyng, se in þis folwende chapytre.</u>

---

3 massa] *marg.*: Massa sanguinis, i. epar, þe lyuer
4 þrou3] CgHGSc, þou3 RM7
5 And] *foll. by* to *canc.* R
6 serum] *marg.*: whey
7 butirum] *marg.*: Butter
8 caseus] *marg.*: Chese
9 lac] *marg.*: mylke

[1.3]

Of generacioun of vryne: c. 3

For to wete and knowe howe & in what wise þe vryn is gendred and made in man, and also how þe fode, s. mete and drynk, þat man ys sustened by is digestede [**f. 7rb**] and defiede in man, vnderstonde þat digestion[1] is in 3 places in þe body: in þe stomac, in þe lyuer, and in alle þat oþer membres   5 and lymes of man. And þerfor þe stomac is callede þe first digestioun;[2] þe lyuer i[s][3] callede þe 2 digestioun; and alle þat oþer parties of þe body is callede þe 3 digestioun.

The firste digestion[4] Y saie is in þe stomac, for euery maner fode – be it mete or be it drynke – þat kyndely entriþ þe body for to norisch it, ferste it   10 draweþ kyndely to þe stomac, & þere it is decocte and digestede. And þan þe iowse of þe fode is sewede and soken & dryllede riȝt as it were a maner of drynke þat we callen "pthisan." And þis doþ *epar*, þe lyuer, fro whom þe stomac haþe his kynde hete. Se in þe 2 boke, de colore karopos. And al þis is þrouȝ wirkyng & helping of kynde hete.   15

When þe stomac haþ þus done, he draweþ & takeþ to hym, i. to his kyndely fode and norischyng,[5] þat þat is moste like and answeryng to his kynde and to his complexioun, and lateþ þe remenant passe oute awaie be an hole in his botume, i. in þe neþer ende of þe stomac. Whiche issue or hole is callede in phisik *porta stomachi*[6] (*anglice*: mawe ȝate). And for þis   20 skil: for it is [s]hote[7] til þat nede of kynde delyuereþ þe fode oute of þe stomac. And as sone as it is oute, it schetteþ hymselfe a- [**f. 7va**] gayne as he was biforne. Galienus in *Libro anathomiarum suarum*, in þe *Boke of His Anathomy*, calleþ it *portonarium* (*anglice*: þe portonarie).

To þis portonarie is knyte and tyede a therme þat is callede *duodenum*,   25 þe duodene,[8] and for þis skil: for he bereþ in lengh 12 fyngerbrede, i. vppon þe proporcioun of euery man, woman, or childe; and it is of quantite euen with portonarie. Þan, when þis *duodenum* haþ vnderfongen & receyued þe fode fro maw ȝate, he takeþ þerof þat him nedeþ to his kyndeli fode. &

---

1 digestion] *marg.*: þe 3 diges\<tiouns\>
2 first digestioun] *marg.*: þe first digesti\<oun\>
3 is] M7CgHG, in R, *om.* Sc
4 firste digestion] *marg.*: þe first digestioun
5 norischyng] CgHGSc, *foll. by* and RM7
6 porta stomachi] *marg.*: porta stomachi, i. mawe ȝate
7 shote] shet CgH, schette G, schite Sc, hote RM7
8 duodene] *marg.*: þe duodene

þat þat beleueþ, þe duoden wringeþ it riȝt os it wer a pressour & deliuereþ   30
it forþ into anoþer gut knyt and tyed to him, þat is clepede *ieiunum*,[9] ieiune or fastand gut, \þat/ vnderfongeþ þe fode oute fro *duodenum*. And
he draweþ oute al þe iowse and þe moystour of þe fode, riȝt as a magnete
stone draweþ yren to hym, [& kepeþ to hym][10] þat þat falleþ to his kynde;
and sendeþ forþ þat iowse, þat humydite, to *epar* be certeyn veyns þat   35
gone fro him to *epar*. Which veynes ar callede *meseraice*,[11] meserays. & þis
is þe skil whi it is callede *ieiunum*: for when he haþe soken vp al þe iouse,
þe humidite, to *epar* be certeyn veyns and sent it to *epar* os Y saide, right
as it were in maner of a swete (for it haþe none issue where þe iows and
þe moysture may gone oute), it is as it were fastande and voide and empty.   40
For it is noȝt sene where it passeþ awaie.

[f. 7vb] This ieiune is globbede and rounde and bostuse, as seiþ Isaac
and þe auctour of *Anathomys*, for þis skil: þat þe iowse and þe moystour
may swete oute be diuerse smale waies and pores of hym. But *duodenum*,
to whom ieiune is tyede, is pleyn and smoþe, & þat for 4 skyles: þat þe   45
fode may þe more liȝtlier descende, i. go doun, into ieiune; also þat þe
places schulde noȝt be lettede, which place is necessarie to certeyn veyns
and diuisen hem þerfro by a veyne comende fro þe lyuer; also be enchesoun of smale skynnes and buddy fleissche þat arne þer nere; and also þat
þe fode mai haue his kyndely dwellyng þer til *epar*, when his tyme comeþ,   50
may take & draw fram hym þat ilke ious and þat substancial humidite.

Item, þe forseide ieiune, os som seyn, is callede *porta lactis* or *lactea
porta* (*anglice*: mylke ȝate).[12] And þis is þe philosophie, i. þis is[13] þe skyl:
for as Y saide, al þe iows, al þe humydite, sweteþ and sweltiþ oute of it
[into þe lyuer, ryght][14] as þe mylke swetiþ and sweltiþ oute of þe kowes   55
body vnto þe vdder. Item, *lactea porta* or *porta lactis* is anoþer þing. Se in
þe 2 bok, *de liuido colore*.

Þe forseide meseraices arne 8 in nombre. On of hem is knyte to þe ouer
mouþe of þe stomac, s. to þe ouer ende of þe stomac, [M7, f. 2v][15] anoþer
faste by þat ouer ende of þe stomac, & þe þrid of hem is festenede to þe   60

---

9 ieiunum] *marg.*: Ieiune
10 & kepeþ to hym] CgHGSc, *om.* RM7
11 meseraice] *marg.*: Meseraice
12 mylke ȝate] *marg.*: Milk ȝate
13 is] CgHGSc, in is RM7
14 into þe lyuer ryght] M7HGSc, *words barely visible under erasure in* R, *om. due to
    eyeskip* Cg
15 *Ff. 8–9 in* R *are almost completely cut away; from here to f. 10ra in* R, *the text is taken
    from* M7, *with the* þ/y *character transcribed according to phonetic intent; otherwise,*
    M7's *spelling (which is very close to* R's*) is retained. The very few lines of text in* R *that
    have survived the mutilation of these leaves correspond closely to* M7's *readings.*

botume of þe stomac, i. to þe neþer ende of þe stomac. And al þat oþer 5
arne knyt & [ti]ede[16] to ieiun, þat semeþ so alwai fastande, os I saide. &
be þo 5 meserayces passeþ þe iowse & þe humidite to *epar*, os I saide. &
al þe remenant, s. drestes & þe grounde-soppes & þe þik mater, i. dryt,
descendeþ doun to a gutt þat is callede in Latyn *saccus ventris* (*anglice*: þe 65
wombe sak), for þerin is alle þe relef of þe mete.

Also it is callede *orbus*, i. rounde,[17] for it is rounde. Also it is callede
monoculus, i. on-eyede, for it haþ but one hole. & þerfor, þer þe mater
comeþ in, þer it most go oute. & þat may it noȝt but þorgh mordicacioun,
i. þorgh bytyng & fretying, of *sista fellis*, i. of þe galle. For hys myȝt comeþ 70
[**M7, f. 3r**] to hym be certeyn pores, & he bit it & constreyneþ it & casteþ it
oute, & so it passeþ into *yliones*, into þe ylions, þe smale ropes þat lewede
folk callen "þe guttes." & so forþ into *colon*, fro *colon* into *longaoun*, & al
forþ. Of *colon* & of *colica passio*, se in þe 2 bok, c. *de albo colore*. Of ylioun
& of *ylica passio*, se in 2 bok, c. 7 *de colore karapos*. 75

Þan vnderstonde þat *longaon*[18] is þe laste gutt in þe body & it is tyede
vnto þe tayle ende. Som folke calle it þe "erse-þerme" & "tail end," or "þe
erse-bubble." Vnderstonde þat *cista fellis* is propurly noȝt elles but þe skyn
of þe galle. & it is taken here also often tyme boþe for þe skyn & for þe
matere þat is þerin. 80

And tak hede þat þogh Isaac say þat *duodenum* is on & *ieiunum*
[anoþer],[19] os said now beforn, noȝtforþan þe *Bok of Anathomis* saiþ
þat þai arne boþe on. And þis þe werkyng of þe fyrst digestioun, i. of þe
stomac.

Þan[20] when *epar* haþ vnderfongen þat iouse & humidite fro þe stomac 85
in his wyse, he sendeþ forþ þe remenant aboute to his veynes, for to be
soden & boylede in hem. For fro hym comeþ veynes al about to euery
menbre & lyme in þe body & to al þe extremitees of þe body, as to þe
armis, þe ligges, hondes & fete, fyngres & toose. And in þis sendyng
aboute, *epar* wyrkeþ & makeþ & gendreþ þe blode of þe humydite. & 90
þan he twynneþ & dyuiseþ þe clere fro þe þyk & þe clene fro þe vnclene,
& kepeþ hym hys fode of þe blode, for his kind norissyng & fodyng is
blode. For he [is]²¹ noȝt but blode himself, as I saide in þe 2 chapitre. And
in þis sendyng forþ, alle þo oþer parties of þe body taken here kynde &
here norissching. 95

---

16 tiede] nede M7, *om.* CgHGSc, *wanting* R
17 rounde] *marg.*: orbus i. rounde
18 longaon] *marg.*: longaon
19 anoþer] CgGSc, *om.* M7H, *wanting* R
20 Þan] *marg.*: þe 2 digesti<oun>
21 is] CgHGSc, *om.* M7, *wanting* R

Cor, þe hert, be resoun þat he is most noble menbre of beste – for he is
grounde & wel & spryng of kynde hete in al þe body of man – & þerfor
he draweþ to hym þe moste worthy party of þe fode, for to confort &
noryssch him & encresen his kynde hete & diuisen & yifen & senden it to
al þe menbres & partyes aboute be al þe body. & namely to þe most worþi   100
places ferst, as to þe breste & to þe heuede. & þerfor þe lyuer & þe stomac
& alle oþer menbres in þe body haue here kynde hete fro þe herte. And
þerfor riȝt as þe son wirkeþ in alle creatures here beneþen, riȝt so þe hert
in man.

But vnderstonde þat *stomachus* haþ his kynd hete fro þe hert noȝt *inme-*   105
diate, i. noght first & principaly & by non noþer, fro þe hert; but he haþ it
mediate fro þe hert, i. *secundarie* & by anoþer or elles be mene of anoþer.
F[or]²² þe hete þat þe stomac haþe of þe herte, þe stomac takeþ of þe lyuer,
f[or]²³ *epar* takeþ hete fro þe herte & ȝiffeþ to þe stomac.

Epar,²⁴ þe lyuer, lith vnder þe botime of þe stomac, noȝt euen vnder but   110
more on þe ryȝt halfe, as Galien saiþ in his *Anatomis*. *Et* so *epar* is as fire
to þe stomac, & þe stomac is to hym as pot or calderon standond al hote
ouer þe fire. Þus speken auctoures & bokes of phisic. <u>*Cor*: in þe 2 bok, *de*</u>
<u>*karapos*.</u>

Þan *pulmo*,²⁵ þe longe, & alle þe toþer spirituale membres drawen to   115
hem here fode & noryschyng, to þo menbres & places þat bene vpwarde as
here parties, wiþ þo parties of þe fode þat beleueþ hem. <u>*Pulmo* & spirituale</u>
<u>menbres: se in þe 2 bok, *de liuido colore*.</u>

When²⁶ *pulmo* takeþ his parte, he takeþ also & draweþ to hym kyndely
þat mater of þe fode þat is moste answering to *fleuma*. & þer, s. in þe longe,   120
& of þat mater is fleume causede & genderede. Þan *felle*,²⁷ þe galle, draweþ
his parte to hym and þerweþ mater þat onswereþ most **[M7, f. 3v]** to colre
and turneyt into colre. And *splen*,²⁸ þe mylt, takeþ to him his fode & gendreþ melancolie. But *epar* takeþ to him þe mater & blode, & mundefieþ
& clenseþ him, as I saide. And þus & on þis wise & þis places & menbres   125
ar þe 4 humores causede & gendrede. What are þe 4 humores: se in þe 4
chapitre.

And when *epar* mundefiede, i. purgede or clensede, þe mater of þe blode,
þan descendeþ þe moste substance, i. vryn, þe which is but a clensyng fro

---

22 For] CgHGSc, fro M7, *wanting* R
23 for] CgHGSc, fro M7, *wanting* R
24 Epar] *marg.*: epar i. þe lyuer
25 pulmo] *marg.*: pulmo i. þe lunge
26 When] *marg.*: þe generacion <of> þe .4. humo<res>
27 felle] *marg.*: fel þe ga<ll>e
28 splen] *marg.*: spleen þe mylte

þe blode into norisschyng & fode of blode in þe reynes, beryng be veyns   130
which ar callede *vene capillares* (*anglice*: smale veyns as heres). For þai ar
smale as heuede heres, for þai mow vneþes be seyne wiþ eye for smalehode, for þai ar knyt to þe bak and to þe rigebone aboute þe myddes of þe
rigebone wiþin þe body. Þat it bereþ wiþ him of þe blode & of þe rudyhede, it is for to norisshe þe reyns.   135

And þan when *epar* haþ on þis wyse purgede & clensed þe þik fro þe
þin & þe clene fro þe vnclene, & also after þat he haþ sent aboute to euery
party þat þat longeþ to him, þan þat beleueþ is *purus sanguis* or *humor
sanguinis* (*anglice*: fyn blode or elles þe humore of blode) – þai ar al on to
seyn. Item, when *pulmo*, þe lunge, haþ taken to hym, as I saide, þat þat is   140
moste answerande to hym, þe remenant þat beleueþ is pure *fleuma*. Item,
when *fel* haþ taken so, þe remenant is pure colre. Item, when splen haþ
taken so, as I saide, þe remenant is pure melancolie & blak colre (blak colre
& melancolie ar al one).

Þan when alle þise poyntes arne þus done, þe superfluytes of þe fode, i.   145
þe refus, þe oute-castes & þe bleuynges of al, ar sente oute by þe pores of
þe skyn & by oþer issues of þe body, as be þe eyȝen by gownd & bleredе-
hede, by þe eres wiþ droppyng and sap, by þe noseþirle thorog filþe, by
þe mouþ þorgh sputyng, and by þe pores of þe hide þorgh fumosites &
swetyng. & on þis wise euery menbre takeþ of þe fode þat that is hym like: 150
clene clennes, foule foulness.

Þan when þe vryn comeþ to þe reyns be *venas capillares*, as I saide, þer
he duelleþ til he is kyndely bulede & decocte and defi\e/de, and þer he
takeþ his kynd and hys fynal coloure, al be it so þogh he take his body, i.
his substancialhede, befornhond in *epate*, i. in þe lyuer. And þerfor sai alle   155
auctoures þat vryne takeþ [his substaunce]²⁹ in þe lyuer, but his forme, i.
colour, he takeþ in þe reynes. & þan when he is decocte & digested as he
schal bene, þe reyns sent it forþ be tuo smale waies to þe vesye, i. to þe
bledder, & at hys tyme passeþ forþe by þe ȝerde. Þise tuo smale pissing
places be which þe vryn passeþ fro þe reynes into þe vesie bene called   160
vrythides or elles *vrythides pory*.

Þe þridde digestioun,³⁰ as I said, is in alle þis oþer menbres of þe body,
for þer kynde digesteþ into fleisch and into sinow & into bone. And
þe residu, i. þe remanant, of þe fode & also þe residu of þe 4 humores
bleuand stille in þe menbres is called *tercia* [*super*]*fluitas*³¹ or *superfluitas*   165
3ᵉ digestionis (*anglice*: þe þrid superfluyte or elles þe superfluite of þe 3

29 his substaunce] CgHGSc, *om.* M7, *wanting* R
30 þridde digestioun] *marg.*: þe 3 digestioun
31 superfluitas] CgHGSc, fluitas M7, *wanting* R

digestioun[32]). Þe which superfluyte, if it be so þat kynde be stronge &
myȝty & þe menbres of þe body also, þai schewe & delyuereþ it oute
by þe poris & þe issues of þe hyde. If it be kyndely moyste, be swete.
If it be kyndely drie, be diuerse fumositees, as I saide while ere. Fumo-   170
site in Englisshe: "smokishede" & "smoþerhede." And vnderstonde þat of
fumosites[33] in þe body is cau- [M7, f. 4r] sede here & ruggedhede, as we se
in trees, þat thorogh kynde hete þai putten & casten oute here superfluites
and þerof comeþ here rynde & here bark & here mosse.

  And if kynde hete be noȝt sufficient ne myȝty to cachen oute þe super-   175
fluytes by þe pores, þan kynde ledit it aȝeyn to *epar* be þo same waies,
i. weynes, be þe which it cam to þe menbres, as I saide. And þan *epar*,
þe lyuer, sendeþ þ\i/se superfluities forþ to þe reynes wiþ clensyng of
blode, & so kynde delyuereþ hem forþ wiþ þe vryn, & þat is propurly
ypostasis[34] in þe vryn. For *ypostasis* in þe vryn is noþing but superfluite of   180
þe þridde digestioun. *Et* þerfor saiþ Galien þat vryn of hole folke, when
it haþ stonden & restede, it haþ but a lytil *ypostasis* or none. & philoso-
phi is: for þe kynde[35] is myȝty in hemselfe & putteþ oute þe superfluites
by þe pores of þe body, & þerfor when *ypostasis* scheweþ in þe vryn, it
telleþ how mykel kynde & þe humores wirke in þe 3 digestioun. Item,   185
þe lycoure of þe vryn, i. þe selfe vryn, telleþ & scheweþ þe wirkyng of
kynde in þe 2 digestioun, and also how þe humores ar decocte & digeste
in þe veynes. Item, þe superfluite of þe first digestioun, s. þat þat goþ
oute at þe tayle ende, scheweþ þe wyrkyng of kynde in þe firste digestioun & also how þe fode is decocte & digestede in þe fyrst digestioun.   190
Ypostasis: in þe 2 boke, þe 2 c. *de nigro colore* & in c. *de pallido colore* &
in þe pride boke, þe laste c.

  Vnderstond þat euery of þe 3 digestions which I haue said haþ his owen
propur purgacioun for to purgen & clense himself fro his superfluites. The
first digestioun[36] haþe purgacioun to hys superfluytes þe ouer hole & þe   195
neþer hole, s. þe mouþ & þe tail ende: [þe mouþ be golpyng & rospyng
& brakyng; þe tail ende][37] be egestion, i. schytyng, crakkyng, & fysting
beneþe is[38] purgeyng propurly of þe guttes & of þe ropis.

---

32 digestioun] CgHGSc, digestiouns M7, *wanting* R
33 fumosites] *marg.*: þat here comeþ <?of> fumositez
34 ypostasis] *marg.*: de ypostasi
35 þe kynde] CgHGSc, þe kynde þe kynde M7, *wanting* R
36 first digestioun] *marg.*: purgacion of þe first digestion
37 þe mouþ be golpyng … tail ende] CgH, the mouth by galpyng & rospyng & brakyng
    (gapynge Sc) The ers hole GSc (*phrases about oral and anal purging transposed in* Sc),
    om. M7, *wanting* R
38 is] CgHG, his M7, *om.* Sc, *wanting* R

The 2 digestioun[39] haþe vryn makyng.

And þe þridde digestioun[40] haþe ypostasy & swetyng by þe pores & 200
þe essues of þe hide. Than if it be so þat þe kynde of þe menbres & lymes
be vnmiȝty for to leden & bryngen agayne þe forsaide superfluytes of
þe fode to *epar*, þan for alse mychyl as þai may noȝt h[a]ue[41] here kynde
course agayn to *epar*, þai beleuen stille closede & sparede [**R, f. 10ra**] in
the membres or elles in the blode of þe veynes or elles in boþen. And 205
þan is þis superfluyte callede *cruditas humorum*[42] (*anglice*: þe rawhede
of humores or elles rawe humores), and for þis skyl: for þe membre[s][43]
sethen noȝt parfitely, ne digesten þe fode, ne turnen it noȝt into here
substance and into here kynde os þai schulde done. Or elles for alse
mykil as þe fodes or þe fode is noȝt necessarie ne noteful ne couenant 210
to þe membres. Or elles because þat þe stomac and þe lyuer noȝt defyen
hem parfitely, for but if þe fode be parfitely decocte and digestede in þe
stomac and in þe lyuer, it is impossible to be kyndely dygestede into
þe oþer membres of þe body or for to be turnede into here substance
and norysshyng. For ellez þe membres vnderfongeþ hem noȝt kyndely, 215
but refusen hem and so þai tornen noȝ into gode substance but leuen
stille rawe and vnwrogh, in hendryng of þe kyndely substance of þo
membres.

Verbi gratia, i. se by example: when *stomachus*, þe stomac, haþe receyuede þe fode and wroȝt into þat fode as his kynde and myȝt and power 220
is, so he digestiþ for þe tyme, and þan when it passeþ oute of þe stomac
noȝt parfitely digestede and wolde come into þe lyuer, þer may he noȝt
haue his kynde duelleng ne receyuen his kynde decoccioun [**f. 10rb**] ne
digestyoun in the stomac, ne haue his kynde chaungeyng and turnyng into
parfite blode, be resoun þat he hade noȝt first his kynde decoccioun and 225
digestioun in þe stomac as he schulde haue hadde. And so it beleueþ stille
in þc membres, i. in þe veynes and in þo partyes.[44]

And þan if it be so þat þe veynes and þe placez bene myȝty and stronge
and vertuouse in kynde, þan þai cacchen and dryuen it oute by þe pores
and oþer issues of þe body. And elles it beleueþ stille þer, as Y said, schet 230
and closede in þo membres or in þo veynes or elles in boþe. And þan it

---

39 2 digestioun] *marg.*: purgacioun of þe 2 digestioun
40 þridde digestioun] *marg.*: purgacioun of þe 3 digestioun
41 haue] HSc, have G, han Cg, hue M7, *wanting* R
42 cruditas humorum] *marg.*: þe crudite of humors
43 membres] CgHGSc, membre RM7
44 partyes] *foll. by* I saide afore clere and rody as rose and crudus and indigestus, i. rawe
    and vndefiede *canc.* R, *om.* M7; CgHGSc *retain the clause with minor modifications*

turneþ into mater and corrupcioun, whiche is cause[45] of dyuerse sekenes
& maladies and passions in man, and vppon þe kynde & þe complexioun
of þe fode.

For *cibus calidus*, fode þat is kyndely hote & moyste, causeþ sekenes   235
of blode; *frigidus* & *humidus*, colde & moiste, fleumatic; *frigidus* & *siccus*,
colde and drye, melancolic; *calidus* & *siccus*, hote and dry, colrik. Than
if swyche materes maken duellyng in þe body and wickede aire or colde
takyng, and greuance or myskepyng, or swyche oþer poynts comyng, þo
helpen, conforten, and strenghen þose wickede humores, and þan ar þai   240
more feruent and more [f. 10va] perilouse. And þan þai flowen aboute in
þe body and in þe veynes and so þai ar cause and mater of dyuerse febres
and sekenes. If be so þat þai turnen noȝt into mater of diuerse febres,
þan þai heten and enchaufen þe skyn and þe pores. And þan is þe blode
enchaufede þorȝ ham, and þat enchaufyng of þe blode causede a febre etik.   245
Se febre etik in þe 2 boke, *de liuido colore.*

If it be so þat sum of þat mater passe to oþer membres and placis in þe
body, þan vppon his kynde and his qualites it gendreþ in þo membres and
places in þe body dyuerse maladies and sekenes of sores and of apostemes.
If it so be þat þat mater be confortede and stre[n]ghede[46] and it be of myȝt   250
for to schouen and putten oute himselfe be þe pores, and þanne myȝt of þe
skyn fayle hem, þan þat mater beleueþ stille sperde and closede vnder þe
hide. And þerof comen corrupciouns and sores, as iche and pusshes and
scabbes and þe morphe and siche oþer. If it be so þat þe mater hyde himself
in þe fleisshe, þan he causiþ and gendereþ *carbunculos, vlcera, antraces,*   255
scrophulas, & *cancros* and swych oþer. *Carbunculus*[47] is a sore þat is in þe
bigynnyng, i. in þe growynge, rede as a carbuncle stone; afterward, i. when
it is rype, it [f. 10vb] is blak as a quenchede cole. And be cause of rodehede, it bereþ þe name of a carbuncle. *Vlcus*[48] is a bole or a boche. *Antraxa,*
feloun.[49] *Scrophula*[50] is a sore þat is like a swynes wortyng. *Cancer,*[51] þe   260
ca[n]cre.[52]

Nerehonde al þat I haue sayde in þis chaptire, Isaac techeþ nyȝ worde
for worde.

---

45   is cause] *foll. after line break by* is cause *canc.* R
46   strenghede] strengthid CgSc, strenthed G, streynthed H, strereghede RM7
47   Carbunculus] *marg.*: Carbuncle
48   Vlcus] *marg.*: boche
49   feloun] *marg.*: feloun
50   Scrophula] *marg.*: Scroful
51   Cancer] *marg.*: Cancre
52   cancre] M7CgHGSc, carcre R

[1.4]

Whyche and how many bene of a leche to be considerede and how he schulde behaue him in demyng: c.^m 4[1]

Affter þat þou haste vnderstonden alle þise forsaide þinges, if þou wilte be
wise and war in þis faculte, s. in demyng of vryn,[2] ȝitte þe moste knowe 20
condicyons,[3] as techeþ Giles & Gilbert and auctours and nyȝ alle comen-   5
toures, i. expositoures, and arn þise: Whilke it is; What it is; Which þinges
bene þerin; How mykil it is; How fele siþes; Where; When; Age; Complexioun; Kynde, s. wheþer it be man or woman; Trauayl; Ire, i. wraþe;
Diete; Besynes; Honger or þerste; Mouyng; Wasshyng; Etyng; Drynkyng;
and Enoyntyng. If þou wilt wise-man be in demyng of vryn, this poyntz   10
moste þou knowe boþe wel and fyne.

Than for to knowe parfitely alle þise poyntes and condicions, vnderstonde þat when Y say <u>whilk</u>,[4] be þat is vnderstonden þe qualyte of vryn.
Qualitas vrine, þe qualite of [f. 11ra] vryn, for to speken in þis purpos
is þe coloure of þe vryn. The coloures of vryn ar 20 in nombre, <u>as þou</u>   15
<u>schalt se in þe 2 bok</u>. The coloure of vryne is causede principaly of þise 2
qualites: *calidite* and *frigidite*, hete and colde, for þe more hete þat regneþ
in þe body þe more depe is þe vryn, and þe lesse hete þe lesse depe, as þou
mayste see be alle þe 2 boke.

But take hede þat þogh I sai þat þe qualite of vryn is causede and   20
genderede of 2 qualites, s. *calidite* and *frigidite*, as I saide right nowe,
noȝtforþan it is none of þe 4 qualites. For euery þing þat is bodely and
erþely is made and componed of 4 elementz and of 4 humores and of 4
qualites, and þai ar made of ryȝt noȝt but of [hym] þat [all] saue [hym]-
selfe[5] made of noȝt. And þerfore þai ar callede *qualitates prime*, þe first   25
qualites. <u>Whiche bene þise 4 elements & þe 4 humores and þe 4 qualites,</u>
<u>se in þe 9 condicioun.</u>

Item, by þis worde <u>what</u>,[6] vnderstonde þe substance of þe vryn. Take
hede þat þise 4 ar al on: *substancia vrine, corpus vryne, liquor vrine, et*
ipsa vrina (*anglice*: þe substance of vryn, þe body of vryn, þe liquour of   30

---

1 c.^m 4] *marg.*: 4
2 vryn] *foll. by* of vryn *canc.* R
3 20 condicyons] *marg.*: 20 condicions
4 whilk] *marg.*: þe first condicion
5 but of hym þat all saue hymselfe] CgH, but of hemself save of himself GSc, but of þat
   saue of hemselfe RM7
6 what] *marg.*: þe 2 condicioun

vryn, and þe selfe vryn). *Et* riȝt as qualite is causede by þis 2 qualites,
calidite & frigidite [**f. 11rb**] as Y saide riȝt nowe in þe ferst condicioun,
ryght so þe substaunce, þe body of þe vryn, is causede of þise 2 qualites:
siccyte and *humydite*, dryhed and moisthede. *Caliditas*[7] and *frigiditas*
arne callede *qualitates actyue*, þe qualites actif, i. qualites of wirching   35
& doyng, for þinges þat ar made and componede of 4 elements wirken
and done by þo qualites. And *siccitas*[8] and *humiditas* ar callede *quali-*
tates passiue, þe qualites passyue, i. of tholyng and suffryng, for þingz
þat ar componede of 4 elementz thole and suffre by hem. Actyf, i. þat
wirkeþ and doþ; passif, þat suffreþ and þoles. <u>*Verbi gratia:*</u> *siccitas* kynd-   40
ely constreyneþ and halt togeder and late noȝt passe awaie fro hym in
as mykel as in him is, and þerfor he spereþ and wiþhalt humydite; but
þat þat is more nesche and more meltande and more watry, þe humores
melten and swelten it into a þyn and subtile substance. And þan when
humydite diffundeþ þe mater, i. sokeþ him and dilatiþ hym, þan he   45
makeþ it obedient and able to wirchyng. And so qualite actif ouercomeþ
it and wirkeþ into hym hete or colde, wheþer it be more and somtyme
of boþe alike.

   Item, vnderstonde þat *substancia vrine* is in 2 wise, for somty- [**f. 11va**]
me it is þik, and sometyme it is þenne. Thik it may be in 2 wise, for some-   50
tyme it is þikk and somtyme menely þik and so of þenhede.

   Be þe þrid worde, <u>which þinges bene þerin,</u>[9] s. in þe vryn, vnderstond
þo þinges þat þou seste in þe vryn of <u>which spekeþ al þe þrid bok</u>.

   Item, be þis worde <u>how mykel,</u>[10] vnderstond boþe coloure and also þe
body, for ferste þou moste take hede at þe quantite of þe colour, for þe   55
depper þat þe coloure be the more it meneþ and seiþ in þe body causand
swich colour. For when eny of þe 4 humores *regnat & dominatur in cor-*
pore (*anglice*: regneþ & haþe the mayst[r]y[11] in mannes body), i. when þe
body stant moste by þat humour, i. moste be þe kynde and þe[12] complexioun of þat humour which of alle 4 humores it stant more by þan by eny   60
oþer of alle þe 4 humores – for euery body þat is made of the 4 elementz
stant moste by two of ham, of þe which humores þe body stant moste
by þat on of hem 2, and þat same humour is maistre in þe body – þan þat
humour fyndeþ none þat may him wiþstonde. & þan þat is þe skil whie þat
humour multiplieþ his spice, i. causeþ and makeþ swych colour in þe vryn   65

---

7   Caliditas] *marg.*: þe qualites actif
8   siccitas] *marg.*: þe qualitez passif
9   which ... þerin] *marg.*: þe 3 condicioun
10   how mykel] *marg.*: þe 4 condicioun
11   maystry] CgHGSc, maysty RM7
12   þe] *foll. by* þe *canc.* R

as þe kynde and þe com- [f. 11vb] plexioun of þat humour askeþ. <u>Qualites</u>
<u>and complexions of þe 4 humores, se afterward in þe 9 condicioun.</u>

Item, quantite of þe vryn is in 3 wise. Somtyme it is mykel, sumetyme
litil, and somtyme mene. *Et* þerfore þou moste take hede to the quantite,
for one maner of vryn boþe in colour and substance sumtyme seiþ, i. sig-   70
nifieþ, boþe dethe and lif. <u>*Verbi gratia:*</u> vryn blak and mykel in quantite in
woman þat trauaileþ in her floures, i. seke in þe malady þat women callen
her "floures," it saiþ warschyng of þat sekenes, for it saiþ þat sche is ful of
wickede mater and corrupcioun, but kynde is of myȝt for to maistrie it and
ouercome it and purge it and kacche it oute and delyuer hymself þerof.   75
Bot þe same vyrn in a woman þat noȝt trauaileþ on þe floures, it seyth deþ
but þe more grace be. Womanes floures ar called in Latyn *menstrua* (in
Englissch: womannes euyl). <u>Se in þe 2 bok, *de liuido colore.*</u>

Item, be þis worde <u>how fele siþes,</u>[13] vnderstonde þise 3 poyntz: how
ofte tymes þe vryn ow to be made, how often gadred, and how ofte tymes   80
lokede. The vryn owe to be made al at onys alse fer forþ as one may. And
for þis skil: þat it may be seyne and dempte & knowen how mykel of myȝt
[f. 12ra] þat kynde is and how mykel wirkyng þe kynde haþ. But somtyme it byfalleþ þat on may noȝt at onys, as in passions of þe vesie, as in
stranguiria, in *flegmon*, in *elcosis*, in *pitiriasis*, *trichiasis*, *dissuria*, *emorogia*,   85
& in *paralisis.*

Stranguiria[14] *est guttatim vrine effusio* (*anglice*: when þe vryn gutteþ
and droppeþ awaie now & now, litil and litil).

Flegmoun[15] is a bolnyng in þe necke of þe vesie wiþ a peyn in longaoun,
and þerwiþ comunely comeþ a rysyng vp of þe stomac and in þe wombe   90
and aboute þe score. And þan þai braken and mowe noȝt slepe. Item, flegmon is a maladye when a colde comeþ aboute þe hert. *Sincopis*[16] is propurly the coth, but *flegmoun* is þe colde þat comeþ biforne. *Flegmon* in
Greke tunge, *frigus* in Latyn, "colde" in Englisshe. In flegmone somtyme
þe vryn is constreynede, i. lettede and wiþholden, and sumtyme noȝt.   95

Helcosis[17] *est vulneracio vesice* (*anglice*: hurtying or blemysshyng and
wastyng of þe vesie). Þai þat han þis sekenes, þai felen oþerwhile when þai
pyssen huge peyne. And when þai felen no peyn, þan þai li[s]ten[18] gretely
for to pysse and purgen hemselfe benoþen and þan mow þai [noȝt].[19] And

---

13 how fele siþes] *marg.*: þe 5 condicioun
14 Stranguiria] *marg.*: þe strangury
15 Flegmoun] *marg.*: Flegmoun
16 Sincopis] *marg.*: Sincopis
17 Helcosis] *marg.*: helcosis
18 listen] CgH, lyke GSc, liȝten RM7
19 noȝt] CgH, not purge thayme GSc, *om.* RM7

when þai haue made water and þe vesie is empty & ydel þerwhiles, þai fele   100
no peyn. **[f. 12rb]** Somtyme þai pyssen as it were wel corupte and roten
atter and quytter, somtyme as it were blody mater, & somtyme as it were
þe scuddes and þe rasynges of a bile or of a sore, and all is be cause of
scabihede and blemesshing of þe vessy.

Trichiasis,[20] *i. capillositas* (*anglice*: herihede), for here vryn apperiþ as   105
þer were in heuede heres, and þai þat hauen þis two passions, *trichiasis* and
pitiriasis, þai felen grete ych aboute þe vesye, wiþ ȝykyng abouten þe tayl
end. Wherfor him likeþ tochyng þeraboute, and cold þinges, be cause of
bytyng and ychyng & tykelyng.

Pitiriasis[21] is as mykel for to saie as "brenne," for þai þat haue þis malady,   110
here vryn scheweþ him wiþ bodies moste like brenne or scuddis or rouus
of a soore, and þat is be cause of scabbyhede & scuruyhede of þe vesye.

Lityasis[22] and *calculus* ben al one. Calculus in þe 2 boke, *de lacteo colore.*

Dissuria[23] *est vrine retencio ita vt omnino vrina negatur* (*anglice*: a con-
streynyng, a crepyng, a gederyng & schrynkyng togeder of þe ȝerde so   115
mykel þat he may noȝt make water wiþoute grete peyn).

Emorogia[24] *est per secretum membrum, s. virgam vel vuluam, in myn-
gendo sanguinis emana-* **[f. 12va]** *cio* (*anglice*: when one pisseþ blode).
And it is saide of þis worde, *emac,* i. blode, & of þis worde *roys,* a flode or
a rynnyng.   120

Paralisis[25] is þe pallesie and it is taken here as when þe vryn rynneþ fro
on þat he feleþ it noȝt or elles þat he wote noȝt; *haec Breuiarius medicine*
(*anglice*: þise þenges seith the auctoure þat is callede *Breuiarie of Medycyn*). Men are somtyme so smyten wiþ þe palasye in here priue membres
þat here vryn passeþ from þat þai witen it noȝt. Item, some folk, as namely   125
elde folk, ar so feble in kynde þat þai mow noȝt witholde hem.

Þan in swiche cas, if it may noȝt be taken at ones, it oweþ, os techeþ
Isaac,[26] be taken in diuerse tymes & in dyuerse vessailes (& noȝt 2 ma-
kyngez in on vesseil), þat euerych colleccioun may be seyn & dempt which
is most miȝti. And þerfor as it owe for to be made at onis & in on vesseil,   130
if it may riȝt so, it owe to be collecte, i. gadrad, at ons in a vesseil, for al
scheweþ bettre and more verayly þe myȝt and þe wirkyng of kynde in þe
body þan doþ but one part of the vryn.

---

20 Trichiasis] *marg.*: trichiasis
21 Pitiriasis] *marg.*: pitriasis
22 Lityasis] *marg.*: litiasis
23 Dissuria] *marg.*: dissuria
24 Emorogia] *marg.*: Emorogia
25 Paralisis] *marg.*: paralisis virge
26 os techeþ Isaac] M7CgH, as Isaac techith GSc, os techeþ os techeþ Isaac R

Item, the vryn owe to be lokede 3 atte þe leste. First,[27] anone as it is made, stoppe þe vrynal þat þe kynde hete and þe spirit passe noȝt oute 135 þerof, and þan alse blyue loke it þat þou maiste se and know what and how mykel kynde wirkeþ in þe bo- [f. 12vb] dy. For oþerwhile þe vryn is then when it is newe made and dwelleþ stil þen, and[28] þat seiþ fordoyng of digestioun of humores in þe body, and so vnhelþe. Somtyme also þe vryn is made then and turneþ þik, afterward turneþ þenne aȝeyn, & þat 140 seiþ mene digestioun. And somtym it is made þik & turneþ þen, & þat seiþ complet, i. pleyn & ful, digestioun. *Et* þerfor vnderstond þat euery vryn þat changeþ fro þen to þik is bettre þan þat þat doþ *e contrario*, i. agaynward. *Et* þerfor þat vryn þat is made thenne & turneþ þik is best of al vryns, & namely if it be clere or clere himself abouen after þe changyng. 145 Þe beste after þat is þat is made þik & changeþ into þenne. After þat, þat is made þik & chaungeþ noȝt but kepeþ himself stille. Þe werst of alle þat is made then & lastiþ stille þenne.

Þan when þou haste first wel biholden it & sette it in þi soule wheþer it [is][29] mykel or litil in quantite, what colour, body þik or þenne or elles 150 mene atwene boþe, swart or bryȝt, clerc or droubly, equal or inequal, i. wheþer oueral alike þik or more in one place þan in anoþer, and also what maner bodyes schew hem in þe vryn (as þou schalt se be al þe 3 boke), set it vp softely and clene hilede þat it may kepe his kynde coloure as it came fro þe body, and also þat it may haue his kind resydens, i. his kyndely restyng. 155 And þat [it][30] be noȝt pourede oute of vesseil into vesseile, for þan þe ayre wil make it corupte and chaunge it. Ne þat it be noȝt schaggede ne borne from place to place, for þorgh schaggyng and bos- [f. 13ra] touse tretyng may cause droblyhede and þikhede, and so may þe dome be deceyuede.

Þan[31] þre houres after, or 2 hours, or on hour, or 3 quarteres of an houre 160 at þe leste, biholde it eftesones, if be as þou leftest it or if it be chaungede fro þik to þen or *e contrario*. And eftesones late it resten, & þan þe þrid tyme,[32] an hour or more after, take gode hede if it be as when þou seye it laste or elles it be turnede. And þan ȝif dome as þou schalt be enformede in boþe þe laste bokes.   165

When an vryn is broȝt bifore a leche for to deme,[33] if he se þat þe vryn be chaungede, he takeþ and chaufeþ it atte þe fire, or in hote water, and þat

---

27 First] *marg.:* þe first inspeccioun
28 and²] *foll. by* and *canc.* R
29 is] CgHSc, y G, *om.* RM7
30 it] CgHGSc, *om.* RM7
31 Þan] *marg.:* þe 2 inspeccion
32 þrid tyme] *marg.:* þe 3 inspeccion
33 for to deme] *marg.:* þat vryn shuld noȝt be chaufed

is bettre. But Ysaac in his texte techeþ þat þe maner of doyng is noȝt, and
for þis skil: for sometyme when vryn comeþ fro man, it is þik and droubly,
& þat saiþ grete ventosite and destemperour of humores in the body, and   170
þat is be cause of þat grete ventosite and also be resoun of þe dilacioun, i.
spredyng, of humores in þe body. Þe vryn is grosse, i. thikke, by resoun
of indigestioun. And al is be resoun þat kynde hete is slowe and nouȝt ȝit
redy ne nouȝt ȝit of myȝt for to fulfille his kyndely wirkyng. And when
þe vryn is chaffede, þan þrouȝ myȝt and vertue and helpe of þe hete is þe   175
decoccioun of crudite of hu- [f. 13rb] mores in the vryn [made]³⁴ complete, i. fulfillide. Which fulfillyng of decoccioun of crudite of humores,
kynde hete was noȝt of myȝt ne of power for to wirken ne maken whil þe
vryn was in þe body. *Et* þerfore chaufyng of vryn makeþ a false significacioun. Þus seiþ Isaac word for word.   180

   Item,³⁵ by þis word "[w]her,"³⁶ vnderstond þo þingz þat ar conteynede
in þe vryn, i. þo bodies þat aper in þe vryn, wheþer þai appere abouen in þe
vryn, or in þe myddes, or beneþe, or elles oueral in þe vryn as þou schalt
se in þe 3 boke.

   And also vnderstond be þis 6 condicioun, the place³⁷ where þe vryn   185
owe to be collecte, i. gaderede and taken. And also þe place where it owe to
be lokede: the place þere þe vryn owe to be collecte and taken in oweþ for
to be a vesseil of glas, clene, white, and þen, clere and rounde, and schapen
alse like þe vesie of man as it may bene, þat ryȝt as þe parties of þe vryn
haue ham in þe vesie wiþin þe body of man, ryȝt so be cause of the forme   190
and þe figur of þe vesseil, the vryn may schewe hem holy in his kynde.

   For in þise wise, alle þe vryn and al his parties schewe hem plenerly in
þe site and to þe dome of man in ordre of kynde and elles noȝt. Kynde
so ordeyneþ and schapeþ and disposeth in swyche wyse in þe body and
in alle þise³⁸ membres of [þe]³⁹ [f. 13va] body þat among þo þinges that   195
ar callede *contenta vrine* (*anglice*: þe bodyes þat ar in þe vryn), as al þe 3
boke spekeþ, whiche bodies ar desisede and departede fro the membres in
þe body, he diuiseþ and departeþ and putteþ hem into þe vryn ryȝt as þai
ben causede and genderede in the body: þe neþer byneþe, þe myd in þe
myddes, and þe ouereste abouene.   200

   The parties of the ouereste membres in þe body of man ar kyndely moste
liȝt by þis skil: be cause þat þe ouereste parties of þe body ar fodede and

---

34   made] GSc, is RM7, *om.* CgH
35   Item] M7CgHGSc, Item (*line break*) Item R; *marg.*: 6 condicion
36   wher] CgHGSc, her RM7
37   place] *marg.*: þe place of collecioun of vryn
38   þise] *foll. by* oþer *canc.* R
39   þe] CgHGSc, *om. at page break* R, *om.* M7

kepte and norisshede of þe blode þat is in the herte, which blode is more
liȝt and more clene & more bryght be way of kynde þan eny oþer blode
in the body of man or of beste. Þe myd parties of þe body also but lesse,   205
and þe neþer parties ȝit lesse. & þerfore þat is þe skyl why þo resolucions,
þo decisions, i. þo parties þat ar chippede of (þat comen of) þo membres
and falle awaie fro hem and of þo placis which in þe body of man schewen
hem *proporcionaliter* in þe vryn wiþouten man where þaie be caused and
gendrede in þe body wiþin man.   210

   The place[40] þere vryn schal be lokede oweþ for to be in place clere &
bright, noȝtforþan noȝt ouerdone bryght, for ouerdone briȝtnes makeþ
þe vryn to seme of the same coloure & brighnes **[f. 13vb]** and þere þow
mayste be deceyued.

   And þerfor in þis w<ise>[41] schal þou done: holde þe vrynal in þi ryȝt   215
hand, & if þe liȝt be bryȝt & radiouse aboute þe, as be cause of glas or of
bryghtnes of wyndowez or of oþer þinges þat gefen agayneward liȝt and
refleccioun of lyȝt, putt þyn hande betwene þi face & the liȝt, þat þe spiritz
of þi siȝt be noȝt diuisede ne disperplede thorgh radyouse lyght or refleccioun or ayre, or elles what it be, and also þat þe droblyhode or elles þe   220
clerehode may þe bettre be seyn or aparceyuede and dempte. And if þe
aire be mykyl bright aȝeynes þe, haue þyn honde byhynde þe vrynal and
the bryght eyre, diuisand and schedant þe stroke of þe ayre.

   Þan when þou haste wytterly auysede þe þeron, vppon alle þe poyntz
and condicions þat I haue sayde beforn, þan moue it and schagge it a litil   225
softely and liȝtly and helde it stil a litil. And in þe meuyng take hede if
þer apere þerin *ypostasis*, and wheþer *ypostasis* moueþ hym heuyly or
liȝtly, and also in þe restyng wheþer it drawe aȝeyn to þe place þere it was
byforne and into þat same figure and forme as it was biforne, or elles þat
he diuise hym and desperple hymselfe in diuerse parties of þe vryn. Of alle   230
þise poyntz, se parfitely in þe 3 boke in þe laste chapitre. Also of *ypostasis*,
se in[42] **[f. 14ra]** the places þer I saide aforne. After al þis poyntz smel þerto
wiþ þi nose: if it stynk or if it haue eny wickede sauour oþer þan vryn
schulde haue.

   Item, Isaac techeþ þat it oweþ to be lokede at candel-liȝt whan it nedeþ,   235
and on þe same wise as be day.

   Item, be þis word "when,"[43] vnderstond boþe tyme when vryn oweþ
to be made and also þe tyme when it oweþ for to be lokede. As anenþes

---

40   place] *marg.*: place of inspeccioun
41   wise] M7CgHGSc, w(*blot*) R; *marg.*: þe maner of inspecc<ion>
42   se in] *catchword*: the places
43   when] *marg.*: þe 7 condicioun

þe first poynt,[44] vnderstonde þat it oweþ to be made in þe mornyng or
ellez aӡeynes þe day, when it is wel and parfitely [digestede] as kynde wil   240
and may[45] and wel gaderede in þe vesie, and after þat he haue hade his
kynde slepe and reste and kynde be redy for to delyuer it oute, for þan ar
wirkyngz of kynde complete.

Et þerfor vryn þat is wrogh and digestede kyndely be nyght, as I saie,
is for to ӡeuen certeyn dome of – and none oþer vryn but swiche vryn.   245
And þis is the philosophie: for when man wake[þ],[46] his kynde is mouede
and wanderand and vnquiete and haþ noӡt his kynde reste, but man is
doand and besy and ocupiede by þe 5 wittes in þoght and dede vtwardes
þat man haþe for to done. And þerfore as longe as man is ocupiede more
owteward þan in- [f. 14rb] ward, þe kynde hete is lesse myӡty and of lesse   250
wirkyng wiþin; but when man hath his reste and slepe, þan kynd haþ his
rest & is noӡt letted thoroӡ oþer ocupacions fro wiþoutewarde, and þat
tyme he wirkeþ moste myӡtely abouten decoccion and digestioun of þe
fode and of þe humours. And þerfor is þe mornyng vryn bettre in alle
maner poyntez þan oþer. When it owe to be lokede and how fele syþes   255
it is said.

Item, be þe 8 word, when Y say "age,"[47] vnderstonde þat o maner of
vryn oweþ for to be in a childe and anoþer maner of vryn in ӡonge folk.
Also o maner of vryn in agede folk and anoþer maner in folk failend for
elde, and þat vpon intensioun and remissioun of kynde hete in hem, i.   260
vppon þat þat kynde hete is mykel or litil in hem.

Childer[48] hauen vryn palesch and þennysch, for þoӡ it so be þat þai
be *naturaliter*, i. kyndely, *calidi* and *humidi* (*anglice*: hote and moyste),
and be resoun of here hete here vryn schuld be clere & intense, i. high in
coloure, and be cause of moystnes he is þikk. Noӡtforþan, for alse mychil   265
as þai bene reulesse and kepe no certeyn diete, þerfor here hete is stranglide and chekede. And þat is þe cause whi þat here vryn comunely apereþ
whitissch and palissch and þennyssch as[49] [f. 14va] it were a feynt white.
That childe[r]ne[50] ar so alday etyng is be cause of possibilite of here mater

---

44   first poynt] *marg.*: þe tyme of þe makyng of vryn
45   parfitely digestede as kynde wil and may] parfitly as kynde wille & may digeste it (be
        digestid Sc) GSc, parfitely as kynde wil and may RM7CgH (*see note*)
46   man wakeþ] Cg, men walkith or wakith G, men walkith Sc, man waken R, man uaken
        (*corr. from* maken) M7, maketh H
47   age] *marg.*: þe 8 condicioun
48   Childer] *marg.*: vryn & complexioun of childerne
49   as] M7CgHGSc, as (*page break*) as R
50   childerne] childryn CgH, childre GSc, childene RM7

and nede of here encresing and waxing, and be cause principaly of st[r]eyt-   270
tehede[51] of þe waies of here vryn is her vryn þinnysshe.

Ȝong folke[52] arn kyndely *calidi* and *sicci* (*anglice*: hote and dry). Be
cause of here[53] hete, here vryn [oweþ][54] to be depe in coloure, s. *citrine* or
subrubicundus.[55] & be cause of siccite, þenne and clere and bright. *Citrin*
and *subrubicundus*, se in here propre chapitres.   275

Olde folke[56] be comune course ar *frigidi* and *sicci* (*anglice*: colde and
dry), and vppon þat complexioun here vryn is feynt of colour: subcitrinysshe or ȝelowisshe, whitisshe or palisshe. Feynt in colour be cause þat
here kynde hete bigynneþ to failen, and colde begynneþ to regnen in hem
and þan be cause of dryhede for melancolie, i. þat ilke humour þat is call-   280
ede so, swych humour is colde of kynde and begynneþ to regne in hem.

Folke failand & bedred[57] for elde ar *frigidi* and *humidi* (colde & moyste).
And þerfor here kynde vryn is *alba* and *spissa* (*anglice*: white and þik):
white be cause of colde and þik be cause of humidite and also be cause of
plente of superfluytes of fleume, which superfluytes rennen and flowen   285
in hem wiþ **[f. 14vb]** þe vryn and causeþ þikhede in þe vryn, and so is it
noȝt ȝit in olde folk. Of humores and of complexions and of ages of man,
se anone.

Item, be þis worde "kynde,"[58] vnderstonde complexioun of man. For
ryȝt as age causith vryn of man, riȝt so doþ complexioun of man. And   290
for to knowe what is complexioun, vnderstonde þat þer ar 4 elementz:
ignis, aier, aqua, & *terra* (*anglice*: fier & eyre, water and erþe). Also þer
ar 4 humores: *sanguis, colera, fleuma,* and *melancolia* (blode and colre,
fleume & melancolie). Now[59] ar þer 4 qualites answerand kyndely to þe 4
elementz and to þe 4 humours: *caliditas, siccitas, frigiditas,* and *humiditas*   295
(hete and dryhede, coldehede and moystehede). Þis worde "answerande in
kynde" is in þis mater as mykel to mene as "acordand in kynde."

Now þe 4 qualites answere boþe to þe 4 elementz and to þe 4 humores:
for blode answeriþ to eyre, colre to fire, fleume to water, & melancolie to
þe erþe. For *aier* and *sanguis* ar *calidus* & *humidus; ignis* and *colera, calidi*   300

---

51 streyttehede] CgHGSc, steyttehede RM7
52 Ȝong folke] *marg.*: vryn & complexioun of ȝonge folk
53 here] here *canc.* (*line end*) here R
54 oweþ] CgHGSc, *om.* RM7
55 subrubicundus] CgHG, subrubicunde Sc, subrurubicundus R, subrubic M7
56 Olde folke] *marg.*: vryn & complexioun of olde folk
57 bedred] *marg.*: vryn & complexioun of bedrede folk
58 kynde] *marg.*: 9 condicioun
59 Now] *marg.*: 4 elementz, humours and qualites

& *sicci; aqua* & *fleuma, frigide* and *humide; terra* and *melancholia, frigide* and *sicce*. And þus mayste þou se how þe **[f. 15ra]** secunde 4 answere to þe first 4, and þe þrid 4 answereþ to boþe 4. And of þise 3 4, euery þing þat is bodely and erþely is componede & made, and vppon þe temperure and disposicioun or indisposicioun of þis 3 4 stant euery maner helþe or 305 vnhelþe of man.

And se how *sanguineus*[60] is he þat is sanguyne complexioun, for he haþ moste of eire and of blod and so his complexioun is *calida* & *humida* (hote and moyste), and swych ar white and rede in þe face and bright wiþ auburne here.   310

Colericus[61] stant moste be fier and colre and so he is *calidus* and *siccus* (hote and dry), blake here, and skilfuly faire & brygh and some wiþ a rudihede in þe chekes and þat is þe most token of þe complexioun of colre, and þat is moste clene.

Fleumaticus[62] be watre and fleume, and so he is *frigidus* and *humidus*, 315 heer auburne or blake, riȝt white face.

Melancolicus[63] be erþe and melancolie, and þerfor þat complexioun is *frigida* and *sicca* (colde and dry), blake here and saloȝwy face.

Nowe vnderstonde þat þe coldeste man of þe worlde is more hote þan þe hotest[64] woman of alle þe world. Also þer is noþing þat is bodely and 320 erþely þat it ne **[f. 15rb]** is boþe hote and colde and moist and drye, al foure, for it is – as I sayde – made of alle þ[r]e 4.[65] But vppon þat þat it haþe moste of, what elementz or of what humores it be of, þo stant þe kynde by and of hem schal he bere þe name of complexioun.

Now[66] for to speke of a man, þere is no man ne no woman in þis world 325 þat he ne is *calidus* and *humidus*, but noȝtforþan one more and anoþer lesse. *Verbi gratia*: perauenture þis man is *calidus* & *humidus* and in euen temperure atwene þe 4 qualites, but for alse mykel os in cas þe kynde of his compleccioun appeireþ and lesseþ and feyntiþ and feblisscheþ, and befalleþ perauenture þat his hete encreseþ and his moystehede vanissheþ and so he 330 falliþ to be *colericus* þere he was afornhand *sanguineus*. For *colericus*, as I saide, is *naturaliter calidus* and *siccus*, and *sanguineus* is *naturaliter calidus* and *humidus*. If *humiditas* be more and *caliditas* lesse, þan is he *fleumaticus* & þan is he *frigidus* and *humidus*. If *siccitas* be more and *caliditas* lesse,

---

60   sanguineus] *marg.*: Sanguine complexioun
61   Colericus] *marg.*: Colrik complexioun
62   Fleumaticus] *marg.*: Fleumatik complexioun
63   Melancolicus] *marg.*: Melancolik complexioun
64   hotest] CgHGSc, hotestest RM7
65   þre 4] 3 4 G, thre fowres CgHSc, þe 3 4 M7, þe 4 R
66   Now] *marg.*: chaungeyng of complexions

þan is he *melancolicus, frigidus* and *siccus.* But if *calor* and *siccitas,* hete &   335
drie, be *equaliter,* i. boþe alike euen in proporcioun, þan is he *sanguineus.*
If *calor* and *humiditas* be in euen proporcioun, sanguine [f. 15va] also.
If *caliditas* and *frigiditas,* sanguine also. But be cause of inequalite of þe
humores, i. be resoun of vneuenhede of humours in proporcioun of hem,
we be in euyl disposicioun and vnheyle, and þerfor in euery complexion   340
may man waxen noȝtforþan more in on þan in anoþer.

   Thise ar þe states of complexion.[67] *Sanguinei* comunely ar longe and
fatte. Longe be cause of hete, for hete is liȝt be waie of kynde and þerfor
kyndely it draweþ vpward; fat be reson of humidite, for humidite kyndely
delateþ and goþ on brode.   345

   Colerici longe and sk[len]dre.[68] Longe be cause of colre, for colre kyndly draweþ vpward be cause þat it is hote in kynde; and sclendre be cause
of siccite, for as it wel semeþ by þat þat Y saide in þe 2 condicioun, siccite
noght dilateþ ne sp\r/edeþ noȝt himself abrode, but raþer *e conuerso,* i.
agaynward.   350

   Fleumatici litil and fatte. Litil, i. schorte, be cause of colde, for colde is
constr[i]ctif,[69] i. schrynkand and drawand togederward; fat be cause of
humydite, os Y saide.

   Melancolici ar litil and sclendre. Litil be resoun of frigidite, as I saide;
and sclendre be resoun of siccite, also as I saide.   355

   But oftetyme, state of complexioun varieþ and chaungeþ *per accidens,* i.
be diuerse enchesons & chaunces & cases þat befallen alday. For [f. 15vb]
somtyme þo þat ar *colerici* and þai þat ar *melancolici* ar fatte and þat is be
cause of plente of gode mete and drynk or of mykel reste and ese and swich
oþer þinges. Item, somtym *sanguinei* and *fleumatici* ar *graciles* (*anglice:*   360
smal and sclendre) be cause of abstinence & trauailyng and swich oþer
poyntz. Item, som are more litil þan þai schulde be be kynde of complexioun and þat may be be cause of litilhede of þe matrice or be cause of litilhode of þe sperme of þe fader or of þe moder or of boþe, or elles be cause
of wickede kepyng in ȝouthe. *Sperma: se in þe 2 bok, de liuido colore ca°.*   365
   This are þe condicions of complexions of man *et cetera:*

Sanguineus

   large or curteis, louyng, glade, louȝhyng, rede colour,[70]
   Largus amans hillaris ridens rubeique coloris

---

67 complexion] *marg.*: the states of complexioun
68 sklendre] CgH, sclender GSc, skeldre RM7
69 constrictif] CgHGSc, constructif RM7
70 *English glosses inserted above Latin lines in smaller letters.*

syngand, poble, hardy, bonere   370
Cantans carnosus satis audax atque benignus

Colericus

rowgh, false, wroþþi, wastour, hardy,
Hirsutus fallax irascens prodigus audax
slygh, sklendir, drye at breste, ȝelow coloure   375
Astutus gracilis siccus croceique coloris

Fleumaticus

slepy, slowe, spittand often or mykel,
Hic sompnolentus piger in sputamine multus
dulle wytte, fatte þe face, colour whyte   380
Ebes hinc sensus pinguis facies color albus

Melancolicus

enuyious, ferde or carful, couetouse in gode, hard or togh
Inuidus atque tristis cupidus dextroque tenaci
gyle, dredeful, modie coloure   385
Non expers fraudis timidus luteique coloris

Nowe as þer are 4 elementz and 4 humores and 4 qualitees, [f. 16ra] so be
þere 4 ages of man:[71] *puericia* & *iuuentus*, *senectus* and *decrepita* (*anglice*:
childehode and ȝouthe, mannes age and elþe). *Puericia* is to þe 14 ȝere.
Iuuentus bigynneþ in þe 15 ȝere and endeþ wiþ þe 49 ȝere. *Senectus* begyn- 390
neþ wiþ þe 50 and endiþ in þe 79 ȝere. *Decrepita* bigynneþ in the 80 ȝere
and endiþ at deþes dai. Þus diuiseþ phisik þe ages of man.

No3tforþan Holy Writ and diuinite,[72] i. doctoures of Holy Cherche
and þe comunate of Cristen men, putten 7 ages of man: *infancia*, *puericia*,
adolocencia, *iuuentus*, *virilitas*, *senectus*, & *decrepita* (*anglice*: infantehede, 395
i. while he can no3t speken, chilþe, ȝouthe, bachiler ȝonge man, sadde man,
olde man, and crekede and bedred for olde). *Infancia* is til the 7 ȝere, *pueri-*
cia bygynneþ wiþ þe 8 ȝere and endith wiþ þe 14 ȝere, *adolossencia* in þe 15
ȝere and endeþ in þe 25 ȝere, *iuuentus* in þe 26 and endeþ in þe 49, *virilitas*
fro 50 to þe 79, *senectus* fro þe 80 to þe 100, *decrepita* fro þat he waxeþ 400
lame for elde to his dede day. And som sayn þat þer ar 7 ages as þou seste
wel, and som wil haue but 6 ages. Þai þat sayn but 6, þai acompten *senectus*

---

71 ages of man] *marg.*: þe 4 ages of man
72 diuinite] *marg.*: 7 ages after diuines

and *decrepita* al on, and her skil is þis: for in oure daies vn- **[f. 16rb]** eþes a man may come to 100 þat he ne is firste bederide or elles dede or boþe.

Item, riȝt as þer ar 4 ages of man, so ar þere 4 ages of þe ȝere[73] (al be it   405 so þat it is[74] more in vs to calle hem 4 tymes of þe ȝere þan þe 4 ages of þe ȝere) and arn þise: *ver, estas, autumpnus, yemps.* *Ver* is þe first quartere of þe ȝer, s. þe tyme atwene wynter and somer, and it bygynneþ when þe son entreþ in *Arietem*, s. 15 *Kal.* April, þe 18 day of Marche, and þat is þe firste day þat euer was, and in þat day was þe worlde made and it lastiþ til   410 þe son entreþ *Cancrum*, 15 *Kal.* July, s. þe 17 day of June. *Estas* bygynneþ when þe sone entreþ *Cancro* and lasteþ til þe sone entreþ *Libram*, s. þe 15 *Kal.* of October, þe 17 dai of September. *Autumpnus* bigynneþ on þat same day, s. 15 *Kal.* of October and lasteþ til þe so[nn]e[75] entreþ in Capricorn, s. 15 *Kal.* of Januare, þe 18 day of December. *Hyemps* bygynneþ þe same   415 day, s. þe 15 *Kal.* Januarij and lastiþ til þe sone entreþ *Arietem*, s. þe 15 *Kal.* of [Aprilis].[76] Þus phisik and philosophie and astronomie bygynne the 4 tymes of þe ȝere, *vnde versus:*

Marcius a medio ver incipit, Junius estas,
autumpn[us][77] Septembri medio, brumaque Decembri.   420

Holy Chirche diuiseþ þe ȝere into 4 quadres. Þe firste begynneþ in *Cathedra Sancti Petri* and **[f. 16va]** endiþ on Seynt Vrbanes euen. *Estas* on Seynt Vrbanes day and endiþ on Seynt Bartholomeus euen. *Autumpnus* on Seint Bartholomeus dai and endiþ in Seynt Clementz euyn. *Hyemps* begynneþ on Seynt Clementz day and endiþ in þe euyn of þe *Cathedra Sancti Petri.*   425 *Vnde versus:*

Ver Cathedre detur Vrbanum estasque sequetur
autumpnus Bartho Clementis yemps quoque festo.

Than se howe þai answere togeder in qualite. Thise 4 acorden togyder in qualite: *aer, sanguis, puericia,* and *ver:* hot and moyste. Þise 4 in calidite   430 & siccite: *ignis, colera, iuuentus,* and *estas.* Þise 4 in frigidite and humidite: *aqua, fleuma, decrepita,* & *hiemps.* And þise 4 in frigidite & siccite, s. *terra, melancolia, senectus,* & *autumpnus.* And vnderstonde when Y speke of hote and colde, moyste and drye, I speke noȝt of swich maner hete, colde,

---

73 ȝere] *marg.:* þe 4 ages of þe ȝere
74 þat it is] *foll. by* þat it is *canc.* R
75 sonne] CgHG, son M7, some R, *om.* Sc
76 Aprilis] CgHG, Aprile Sc, Januarij RM7
77 autumpnus] G, autumpn RM7, autumpni CgH, Autumni Sc

moysthede, & dryhede as we se att bodyly ey3 and fele wiþ honde. For so   435
for to speke, be a þing neuer so hote it is neuerþelesse colde and neuer so
colde it is nerþeles hote, and wete is dry and dry is wete. But I speke of
hote and colde, moyste and dry, vppon þe kyndes & qualites of complexioun, i. vpon þe qualites of 4 elementz & of the 4 humours þat þe þing is
made of. And in þise wise be a þinge neuer so brennand or chilland or dry   440
or moyste þerfor, it is neuerthemore hote ne colde ne wete [f. 16vb] ne
drie. And þerfor þe 4 qualites aforsaide ar callede *qualitates prime* (*anglice*:
þe first & the principale qualitees of alle þe qualitees þat bene), *quia primo*
& *principaliter insunt omni element*[*at*]*o*[78] (*anglice*: for þai ar firste and
principaly in euery maner þing þat is made of þe 4 elementz). Item, I   445
vnderstonde þat þe 4 tymes of þe 3ere ar neyþer hote ne colde but onely
þorgh course of þe son, for þe ferþer þat þe sone is fro vs þe more colde,
and þe more nere to vs þe more werme.

Than if þou se an vryn whiche þou wiste no3t who made it, wite trewly
wheþer it is man or woman or childe, of what age and of what complex-   450
ioun, if þou my3t & alse slely as þou mayste. As anenþes man or woman
or oþer beste, se anone in þe nexte condicioun folowing. As anenþes what
age, þou hast aforn in þe [8][79] condicioun.

As anenþes what complexioun, wite wel þat if *caliditas* & *humiditas*
dominatur in þe body,[80] i. if þe body stonde by þe 2 qualites, os it is in   455
on þat is sanguine complexioun and hole, þe vryn is rede or redisshe and
menly þike. Rede be cause of calidite and þik be cause of humidite, for sanguine complexion makeþ swyche vryn, s. rede and þik. *Et* vnderstonde þis
redehede and þis þikhede as for a bright [f. 17ra] rudihede wiþ a menely
þikhede. *Et* when an vyrn scheweþ him so and he or sche þat made it be of   460
sanguine complexioun, it seiþ helth.

If þe vryn[81] aperyn golden or citrine and þenne and clere and he be
coleric complexioun, it sayþ helthe. Þat it is goldyn or citrine i[s][82] be
cause of hete, thenne and clere be cause of siccite. For *colericus* is *calidus*
and *siccus* and þerfor he makeþ swich vryn.   465

If þe vryn[83] be *alba* and *grossa*, i. white and grete, i. þik, and he be fleumatik, it seiþ þat he is heyle and hole. White be cau[se][84] of frigidite and
þicke be cause of humydite, for *fleuma*, i. *fleumatica complexio*, is *frigida*

---

78   elementato] CgH, elemento RM7GSc
79   8] *only in beta witnesses; alpha witnesses read 7, in error ("age" is condition 8)*
80   body] *marg.*: vryn of sanguineus
81   vryn] *marg.*: vryn of colrik
82   is] CgHGSc, it RM7
83   vryn] *marg.*: vryn of fleumatik
84   cause] M7CgHGSc, cau R

and *humida*. And þerfor suche is þe vryn of þat complexioun, or elles pale
& þik by that same skyl.   470

If ȝelow[85] or white and þen and subtile, i. clere and bright in on þat is
melancolic complexioun, it seiþ þat he is hole. It is ȝelow or elles white
be cause of frigidite, then and subtile be cause of siccite. For *melancolica
complexio* is colde & drye, siccite alwaie causeth clerehede and brighthede
in the vryn, as humidite causeth þickehede. <u>Of þise forsaide coloures in</u> 475
<u>vryn, se in here owen propre capitles in þe 2 boke.</u>

Item, by þis 10 word "<u>he or</u> [f. 17rb] <u>sche</u>,"[86] vnderstonde wheþer þe
vryn is of a man or of a woman. *Et* vnderstonde þat þe vryn of a man and
þe vryn of a woman ar ful like if þai be boþe of on complexioun and ful
harde to knowe asundre, and also vryn of an hole man colrik & vryn of an 480
hole woma[n][87] sanguine. But euermore and in euery complexioun and in
euery sekenesse, but if it be so þat man be seke and þe woman hole, be þe
vryn of a man[88] neuer so þik or neuer so þenne and womannes vryn neuer
so þik or neuer so þenne, noȝtforþan þe mannes vryn is euermore kyndely more liȝt & more bright þan womannes vryn. And womannes vryn is 485
more swartisshe & derkissh and more dymmysshe þan manes vryn. And
þe cause is of what complexioun þat sche be, sche is *frigida & humida*.
And man of what complexioun so he be, he is kyndely *calidus* and *siccus*
more þan woman. And also be cause of filþes & corupcions þat brede in
hem more þan in man – for mykel of here corupcioun of filþes of super- 490
fluytes of humores in hem gadereþ and draweþ kyndely donwarde to here
matrice for to purge and delyuer hym oute by þat membre, s. be þe
[f. 17va] matrice and so oute by þe value, i. by þe ȝate of here body, i.
by her priue membre and of such filþes and corupcions comeþ here malady þat is callede "womannes malady," for no bodi haþe it but woman. 495
Women calle it here "floures." This sikenes is callede in Latyn *menstruum*.
The matrice of a woman is þe centyne of a womannes body. *Sentina* is propurly þe guter[89] of a ship or of a kichyn or þe issue of a gong þere þe filþe
goþ oute. Ryȝt so al þe filthe and corupcioun þat is in womannes body
draweþ þider as to here goter. <u>Of þe matrice and propurtes þerof and of</u> 500
<u>womannes malady, in þe 2 bok. c. *de liuido colore*.</u>

And wite wel þat nouþer phisic ne auctoure of phisic ȝeueþ oþer lore or
oþer reule for to haue discresioun or knowyng bitwene man & woman in
vryn, but os Y saide riȝt nowe, for þere is no phisik ne auctour þat ȝeueþ

---

85 ȝelow] *marg.*: vryn of melancolik
86 he or sche] *marg.*: þe 10 condicioun
87 woman] M7CgHGSc, womam R
88 vryn of a man] *marg.*: vryns of man or of woman
89 guter] gutter M7HSc, goter CgG, gurter R

eny skyl, if þis⁹⁰ woman be wiþ childe, wheþer þis childe be colrik or 505
melancolik, and so of alle þe toþer, ne if þis kowe be wiþ calf, wheþer a
blake or a don or a white bole or a braynede. Oþer lore þere is þat is vsede
þerfore and for oþer poyntz eke, of which maner lore wil Y noȝt write.

If þou wilt haue lore for to deme bestes water fro mannes water &
[f. 17vb] womannes, þus techeþ Auicen in his *Bok of Vrynes*:⁹¹ þe more 510
nyhe þat mannes vryn is to þi sight, the more þik it semeþ to þi sight, but
oþer bestes vryn *e contrario*, i. þe more ner, þe more þen to þe sight. Also
vryn of man hathe euermore a lymyng of briȝtnesse in him, bi which it is
alwaie eþe for to knowe. For bestes vryn, if it be in an vrynal, it is euermore whitisshe or ȝelowisshe and no brightnes þerin, and be it neuer so 515
clere oute of þe vrynal, it semeþ þik in the vrynal and neuermore briȝt. If
it so be þat þe water of a man be mengede wiþ water of a beste, mannes
vryn haþ him abouen and bestes beneþe or elles þai drawe al in plottez by
hemself, for kyndely þat on wil noȝt wiþ þat oþer.

Item, by þis worde "trauayl,"⁹² vnderstonde besynes, os stodie, 520
thought, trauayl, weryhede, and swich poyntz. For be cause of trauail &
besines comeþ mouyng and steryng, and be cause þerof þe body cacheþ
chaufyng. And be cause of chaufyng of þe body, þe humores heten, kachen
chauf[yng]⁹³ and boylicioun, i. bolying and plawyng & rullyng and hurlyng. And þat chaufyng and bulicioun subtileþ and makeþ thenne þe blode 525
and so causith redehede and þynhede in the vryn. For [blode of his owen]⁹⁴
kynde is hote [f. 18ra] and when grete hete fro wiþoutward achaufeþ him,
he is more hote and so is he hote *per accidens*, i. vnpropurly & vnkyndly
hote. For þan is he hote be oþer waie þan be his owen kynde and þan þat
accidentale hete, i. þat vnkynd hete, parbrakeþ and discraseþ þe body, i. 530
distempereþ & vndisposeþ þe body and mynuseþ, i. lesseþ þe humidite of
þe blode, and þan þe vryn is rede be cause⁹⁵ of swich vnkynde hete and þen
because of minusshing of þe kynde humidite.

Item, be trauail vnderstond his contrarie, s. reste and ese,⁹⁶ for reste
þere it is ouerdon, it congeleþ & constreyneþ & byndeþ and wiþhalt the 535
kynde hete & refreiþ, i. coliþ, þe complexioun. And þat causiþ in þe vryn
a þikhede and wan colour & rawe and indigeste.

---

90 if þis] *foll. by* if þis *canc.* R
91 Bok of Vrynes] *marg.*: vryn of bestes
92 trauayl] *marg.*: 11 condicioun
93 chaufyng] CgHGSc, chaufen RM7
94 blode of his owen] CgHGSc, the doyng of our RM7
95 be cause] *foll. by* be cause *canc.* R
96 reste and ese] *marg.*: reste & ese

Item, ouerdone reste & ese maken þat superfluytes & corupcions of wikede humores gendren in þe body and ar cause þat þe body may noȝt delyuer him of hem by fumosites[97] by þe poris and by swete. For ryȝt os 540 exces of trauayl harmeþ & noyeþ þe kynde, ryȝt so exces of reste and ese noyeþ and greueþ þe kynde. For in al þing kynde loueþ mene and hateþ exces.

If it so be þat one take colde fro wiþoutward, þan is þe vryn whitisshe and crude, i. [f. 18rb] raw. If grete colde, it entriþ þe inder partyes of þe 545 body and perissheþ þe places of digestioun and congeleþ þe kynde hete, os Y saide ryȝt nowe. *Congelare* is for to congelen propurly, in Englisshe for to fresen, and also it restreyneþ, i. letteþ and wiþholdeþ, þe colour fro his kynde decoccioun and digestioun. Litil colde entreþ the poris and stoppeþ hem and letteþ þat þe moystoures may noȝt haue here kynde issue be þe 550 pores of þe body. And þerfor þai beleuyn stille closede vnder þe hide and þer[98] þai encresen and waxen & in som folk it causith febre and feyntnesse and wickede disposicions. And such folk nede boystyng and gode kepyng. In som is kynde myȝty and draweþ and turneþ hem to þe lyuer, and þe lyuer – if he be myȝty and [kene][99] – sendiþ it forþe to þe reynes and so it 555 passeþ oute wiþ þe vryn & causeþ in þe vryn a whitehede.

Item, by þis word "ire,"[100] vnderstonde eny maner passioun in soule, as wraþ, sorwe, noy & ten, drede, kare, thouȝt and studie, and such poyntz. For in euery swyche passioun, þe kynde hete and the *spiritus* and þe blode ar calefacte, i. achaufede, or fro wiþinward or fro wiþoute or elles boþe. 560 & also þe hert is calefacte and þan is al þe blode of þe body mouede and chaungede and distempred, [f. 18va] and be cause þerof, alle þe humores. And so þe vryn kacheþ depehede in coloure.

Item, by þis worde "diete,"[101] vnderstonde reulyng and kepyng in leuyng. For in wel rewelyng stant moste þe helthe or vnhelthe in man, 565 os etyng and drynkeyng noȝt but in tyme when kynde axeþ it, i. when þe appetite wille, and þat him leue alwaie some apetite. Also in metes and drynkes answering to his complexioun. Also cloþing and trauaile noȝt in exces, & reste also, and in slepyng and waking vpon skil and so of al oþer poyntes. For if alle suche poyntz be kepte, þe body is heil and sowne. And 570 þan þe vryn sheweþ him after þe kynde complexioun of þe body and elles

---

97 fumosites] CgHGSc, fumemosites RM7
98 þer] þerfor *with* for *canc.* R
99 and þe lyuer if he be myȝty and kene] CgH, and þe lyuer if he be myȝty and clene
    RM7, iff it be myghty & kynde G, if it be myghty kind Sc
100 ire] *marg.*: 12 condicioun
101 diete] *marg.*: 13 condicioun

þe body is vnhele and þerafter scheweþ him þe vryn. But [s]omwhile[102]
þe kynde is myȝty and ouercomeþ swich poyntz, but nerþeles, þow kinde
ouercomeþ & maistri som swich poyntz, noȝtforþan not al & þow som-
tym, not alweie.   575

Item, gode eire helpeþ myche. Wode contre is beste of aire, after þat
medwy and hilly cuntre; nexte þat, heþi contre; nexte þat, medwy and
playn. Alþerwerste fennyche and morisshe contre & contre þat is ful of
woses and lakes. Contre þat is stony[103] is kyndely *frigida & sicca*. Gorry
and mody, *frigida & humida*. Fat and tough and clayisshe, *calida &*   580
humida. Sondisshe, *calida &* [f. 18vb] *sicca*. Item, high contre is comunly
frigida & sicca, lowe contre *e contrario*.

Item, þer ar 4 principal wyndes:[104] *Eurus, Auster, Zepherus*, and *Borea*.
Eurus, the este wynd; *Auster*, þe soþerne wynd; *Zephirus*, þe westerne
wynde; and *Borea*, þe norþerne wynde. *Eurus* is *calidus & siccus. Auster*,   585
calidus & humidus. Zephirus, frigidus & humidus. Borea, frigidus & siccus.
And euerych of þise 4 forsaid wyndes hauen on vpon þe riȝt halfe and
anoþer vpon þe lefte halfe. *Eurus* hath on his riȝt side *Wlturnus*, on his lefte
side *Subsolanus. Auster, Affricus & Nothus. Zephirus, Chorus* and *Fauo-*
nius. Borea, Circius & Aquilo. Wlturnus is þe este-northest wynde. *Sub-*   590
solanus, þe est-soutest wynde. *Aufricus*, soutwest-south wynde. *Nothus*,
southest-south wynde. *Chorus*, weste-soutwest wynde. *Fauonius*, west-
northwest wynde. *Aquilo*, northest-north wynd, þat we calle in Englisshe
"pirnale wynde."

Þan how þe 4 elementes & þe 4 ages of þe ȝere & þe 4 wyndes & his 8   595
wyndes & þe 4 parties of þe wolde answere togeder in qualite, se in þis
figure [Plate 1]:

[f. 19ra] Item, for to diete hymselfe wel vpon þe 4 tymes of þe ȝere is
ful helplich to man. Ver, of whiche Y spake aforn, is a tyme of ȝere þat
comunely is vnstabil, for nowe it is reyny be cause of neȝhede of wyn-   600
ter þat goþ bifore, and now dry be cause of nyȝhede of somer comand
anone after. And be resoun þerof,[105] folk ofte seken in þat tyme of þe
ȝere, and also for þis skil: for in wynter tyme ar gadrede & gendrede in
mannes body wicked humores and moystures be cause of colde, be cause
of wicked eyre and wicked kepyng, & swich oþer poyntz. *Et* þo wicked   605
moystoures þat ar so causede in þe body, þei dilaten & spreden hem and
flowyn and walmyn aboute in þe body, and be cause of hem and of þe frigidite of hem arn þe kind humores constreynede and stopped and lettede

---

102 somwhile] otherwhyle CgHGSc, omwhile RM7
103 stony] *marg.*: qualites of erthez
104 wyndes] *marg.*: qualites of wyndes
105 resoun þerof] *marg.*: of þe effecte of ver

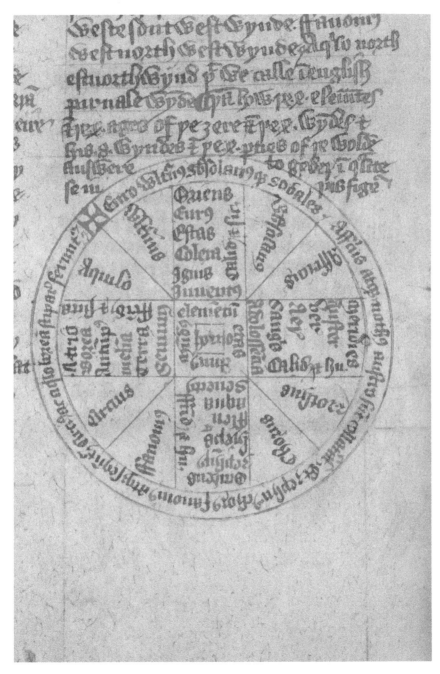

Plate 1. Quaternities Diagram. © The British Library Board: London, British Library, Royal MS 17 D.i, f. 18vb (detail).

fro here kynde course þat þai mowe noȝt sprede hem about in þe body for
to wirch vppon here kynde.[106]   610

And when ver comeþ, hete of þe sonne þat bygynneþ þan for to wirk
vppon here kynde dissolueþ, i. vnbynt, & openeþ & vnduþ hem both. Þan
for alse mykil os þe kynd humores han, os **[f. 19rb]** Y saide, be speride
and stopped and wickede humores and moystoures han had here wil and
here fredam, þai ar the more stronge & more wicked. & when þai be þus   615
dissoluede, þai rennen and plawen al abouten in diuerse places of þe body
& þan vpon þat þai ar meny and wickede and litil restyng, than takeþ man
sekenesse. In þis tyme of þe ȝere, s. in vere, *melancolici* arn in gode poynt,
i. in gode helthe, *sanguinei* wers. Also *senes* wel, childern werse.

Item, in þis tyme, folke schuld vse metes and drynkes *frigidis & siccis*.   620
And in þis tyme is sekenes þat comeþ of blode werste, leste wicked of
melancoli. <u>When *ver, estas, autumpnus,* and *hyemps* begynne, þou hast
beforne in þe 9 condicioun.</u>

In estate,[107] *fleumatici* arn best, *colerici* worst; *decrepiti* wel, *iuuenes*
werse. Moste perilouse is sekenesse of colre, lesse wicked of fleume.   625

In þis tyme, folk shulde vse *frigida* and *humida*. Item, in þis tyme, folk
schulde drenke wel and ete litil. For in þis tyme þe pores of þe body ar
open be cause of hete, and þerfor by ham vaporeþ kynde hete oute, and
so mete þe les defieþ. And also for drynke passeþ and turneþ into blode in
[somer] soner[108] þan in oþer tymes of þe ȝere.   630

In autu[m]pno[109] arn *sanguinei* heil, *melancolici* sekeisch; **[f. 19va]** *pueri*
heyle and *senes* sekisshe. Moste perilouse sekenesse is of melancoly, lesse
perlouse of blode. In þis tyme, vse *calida* & *humida*. Þis tyme is vnstedefast
os ver is, by cause þat *estas* goþ so nygh byforne and *hyemps* comeþ hastilik after. In þis tyme mykil folk taken gret sekenesse be cause of vnsta-   635
blenes of þe tyme by þe same skil os in ver, for þan is wynter nyghonde
and somer is passand, and also be cause of fruyt etyng. For nyh al fruytes
and namely apples ar *frigida* and *sicca*.

Item, *in hyeme,*[110] pores of þe erþe ar sperede and closede þorȝ colde. Þat
hete is besperde in þe grounde and be cause of absence of þe sone may noȝt   640
vapurne oute. But so he duelleþ þere and norischeþ and fodeþ þe rotes of
herbes and trees, os þe moder childe in here body byforne þe birthe. Ne

---

106 kynde] *foll. by* course þat þai mowe noȝt sprede hem about in þe body for to wirke
vpon here kynde *canc.* R
107 estate] *marg.:* þe effecte of somer
108 blode in somer soner] blode soner CgHGSc, blode in somer M7, blode in soner R
109 autumpno] M7, autumpus CgHG, autumno Sc, autupno R; *marg.:* þe effecte of
auctumpn
110 hyeme] *marg.:* The effecte of wynter

þer comeþ noþing [vp]¹¹¹ in þat tyme, for neþer hete ne humour – wherof
al maner grond of lyf is – may none comen fro beneþe, be cause of absence
and prolongacioun of þe sone. In þis tyme arn *colerici* in gode poynt, *fleu-*   645
matici seke; *iuuenes* heil and *decrepiti* feble & febre seke.

   In þis tyme vse *calidis* & *siccis*. Item, in þis tyme ete wel and drynke
lytil, for þe pores of mannes body ar constreynede, i. narouȝ & streyte,
wherfore the hete wiþin wastith and **[f. 19vb]** defieþ more þan in oþer
tymes. Wherfore it is noteful for to myȝten þe body wiþin agayn coldes   650
and wickede eyre and moystoures fro wiþoutward. The werste and þe
moste perilouse sekenes in þis tyme is sekenesse of fleume, os comunely a
febre cotidien. Malady of colre is noȝt so wickede as comunely a febre tercien. And vnderstonde þat in what tyme of þe ȝere malady moste perlouse
befalle, it cometh of hete answeryng to þat tyme of þe ȝere. For vppon þe   655
qualites of þe tymes of þe ȝere regneth þe mater of þe ma[la]dy.¹¹²

   Item, by þis word <u>cure</u>,¹¹³ vnderstond trauail & besines in soule, as I
saide in þe 12 condicioun vppon þis worde ire. For besynesse and þoght
and kare mouyn and styreyn¹¹⁴ and desturbleyn the humores in the body
and be cause þerof takeþ vnkynde hete. And þat vnkynd hete desturbleþ   660
and destempereþ þe body. And vppon þat is þe vryn more tynct, i. more
depe in coloure. And principaly vnderstonde by þis worde cure, stodie
and þouȝt and kare. For stodie, if it be in exces and namely wiþ mykel syt-
tyng, is destruccioun and fordoyng to þe body.

   Item, vnderstond by þis worde <u>hunger</u>,¹¹⁵ fastyng and abstynence and   665
nedyng of mete and drynke. For fasting **[f. 20ra]** and grete abstynence
makeþ swonge wome and Aristotil saiþ þat swonge wombe achaufeþ þe
vryn and replete wombe remytteþ þe vryn. Wherfor it semeþ wel þat þai
þat eten litil and drynkyn litil maken vryn wel colourede, s. citrin or elles
rede, & þenne. For when [hete]¹¹⁶ is ouermaystryde and ouercomen wiþ   670
siccite, os it is in hem þat ete litil & drynken litil, þat ilk siccite (þat ilk
dryhede) multeplieþ colour in her vryn. But þai þat ar replete and ful
and fatte, þai make vryn crude and whitisshe; but þai þat suffre mykel
hunger or þirste or bene mykel abstynent and folke lene and swonge don
e contrario. For hunger and abstynance and þirste and penance dryeþ þe   675
body and schorten the lif. *Et* man schal lengh his lif for to leue and serue
his God.

---

111 vp] CgHGSc, *om.* RM7
112 malady] M7CgHGSc, mady R
113 cure] *marg.*: 14 condicioun
114 styreyn] *corr. from* storeyn R, steryn CgH, sterith GSc, storeyn M7
115 hunger] *marg.*: 15 condicioun
116 hete] CgHGSc, it RM7

Item, by þis worde <u>meuyng</u>,[117] vnderstonde riȝ as Y <u>saide be</u>forne in þe 11 condicion.

Item, by þis worde <u>wasschyng</u>,[118] vnderstonde baþeing. For bath of freis- 680
she water refreteth, i. coleþ, þe body and moysteþ kyndely and feyntiþ þe colour in þe vryn. Bath of hote water chaufeþ and warmeþ þe body and multeplieþ coloure in the vryn; colde water refreteþ þe body. Item, bath of salt water and bittre watre [**f. 20rb**] dryeþ þe body and multeplieþ colour in vryn, as watre of þe se and water of sulphur and swhich maner water. 685
After bath, kepe þe hote; after mete[119] go or stonde; after veyn blode, kepe þe cole, as techeþ þis verse: *Lote cale sta paste vel i frigesce minute.*

Item, be þis word <u>etyng</u>,[120] vnderstonde qualite and quantite of fode. For grete plente & namely exces in mete and drynk causeþ vryn white and schire, and þat for 2 skiles, as Isaac techeþ. One is þis: for þourȝ exces 690
of mete and drynke, þe kynde is ouerchargede and agreuede and so be cause þerof is digestioun stuffede and stoppede and letted; and til þe fode be parfitely defiede, þe blode is noȝt parfitely complete ne eke þe vryn may noȝt haue parfite dyeng as he schuld haue. And þerfor it comeþ *alba* and *cruda*, white and rawe, whitisse and raw schirisshe. And swich maner 695
vryn[121] maken þise glotons and þise dronken folk.

Anoþer skyl is þis: for exces in mete & drynk moisteþ þe body & when it is excessif in þe body, i. when it is ouerdon mykel, þe kynde of þe blode is minussede þerþrough. And so is þe blod congelede and kynde hete faileþ in myȝt in his wirkyng and þerfor þe vryn passeþ oute crude and indigeste, 700
i. whitisshe, wannyssh, waterisse, & sherish.

[**f. 20va**] Item, litil fode[122] makeþ þe vryn rody and bryȝt & clere, for litilhede of fode fordoþ þe humidite in þe body. And þe more þat humidite is wastede, þe more dry moste þe body be, and dryhed euermore causeþ rudihede and clerehede in the vryn, as it is in hem þat eten litil and drynken 705
litil. But fode when it is taken in mene quantite,[123] i. in skilful mesure, it hetith kynde in al þe body and moysteþ and fodiþ and susteyneþ and tem-preþ alle þe lymes & parties of mannes body and holdeþ and norissheþ þe lif. & in alse mykel as in him is, is caused such vryn as þe complexioun of þe body askeþ. And ryȝt as the fode diuerseþ the vryn vppon diuersite of 710
quantites of fode, s. vppon þat it is mykel or litle or ellez mene, riȝt so it

---

117   meuyng] *marg.*: 16 condicioun
118   wasschyng] *marg.*: 17 condicioun
119   after mete] *prec. by* after mete *canc.* R
120   etyng] *marg.*: 18 condicioun
121   vryn] *marg.*: vryn of glotons
122   litil fode] *marg.*: þe effecte of litle mete
123   mene quantite] *marg.*: þe effecte of mesurable fode

varieþ & diuerse þe vryn vppon diuersites of his qualites, s. vppon þat he
is hote or colde, moyste or drie in complexioun.

Verbi gratia: fode þat is kindeli hote[124] causeth rudyhede & clerehede
in þe vryn, as þai þat eten hote metes and drynkes & delyte. And swyche   715
maner hete of suche fodes first achaufe þe lyuer, and so it achaufeþ þe
blode þat þoruȝ þe chaufyng, þe blode of þe lyuer[125] cacheþ gode coloure
and hete and makeþ him able for to wirke. And þan þe spiritz of þe hert
tak of þat hete and ȝilden and ȝeuen a[g]eyn,[126] and so þe vryn is calefacte
and **[f. 20vb]** wel coloured.   720

Colde mete[127] or fode in comp[l]exioun[128] makeþ þe vryn crude and
i[n]digest,[129] for frigidite lesseþ þe hete in þe lyuer and also þe hete of þe
spiritus of þe hert and so mykel fordoþ and letteþ digestioun.

Item, fode þat is moyste[130] makeþ þe vryn þik, for þe kynde humidite
of þe fode kyndely encreceþ þe moystehede of þe lyuer. And the more   725
þat þe moystehede of þe lyuer be, the lesse moste the hete of þe blode and
þe spiritz of þe hert bene. But if þe fode be *calida & humida*, so þat it be
more *calida* þan *humida*, þan it hetiþ þe blode and causith rudihede and
þikehede in þe vryn.

Item, fode þat is dry[131] causeþ vryn þinne and clere, and often rede and   730
somtyme citrine, for siccite of fode kyndely dryeþ þe humidite of blode
and so it causiþ dryhede in þe body and dryhede causeþ rudihede in þe
vryn or elles citrinehcde. But noȝtforþan if þe stomac be so colde þat be
cause of his coldenes he swageþ & lesseþ þe hete and þe feruoure of þe
blode, and so be cause þerof letteþ the depenes of þe colour in þe vryn,   735
þan if þe mannes or wommanes complexioun be hote, þat dry fode turnyth the vryn into citrine colour or elles into white colour. If his complexioun be colde, into white colour.

[f. 21ra] Johannicius in his boke *De ysagogis* seiþ þat sum metes causen
gode humores in man & som wikede. Brede of clene whete newe and wel bake,   740
flesche of one-ȝeres lombes flesch, & kyde-lambes flesch maken gode blod and
equal, i. euen in commixtioun, i. in mengeyng of blode wiþ oþer humores.
Wickede blode maken mowlede brede and elde baken and euyl baken; þe
same doþ netis fleisch and rammys fleisch and gotes fleisch and olde flesch.

---

124 hote] *marg.* þe effecte of hote mete
125 þe blode of þe lyuer] CgHGSc, of þe blode of þe lyuer RM7
126 ageyn] CgH, aȝayn G, again Sc, aneyn RM7
127 Colde mete] *marg.*: þe effecte of colde mete
128 complexioun] M7CgHGSc, compexioun R
129 indigest] M7CgHGSc, idigest R
130 moyste] *marg.*: þe effecte of moyste fode
131 dry] *marg.*: þe effecte of drie fode

Item, pork and bef ar heuy metes; pulle[tt]es[132] and wilde foule & fis-   745
sches \þat ar/ note wel grete and not ouer fate and ar squamouse, i. skalide, ar liȝt metes. Heuy metes comuly causiþ fleume and blak colre; liȝt
mete causith rede colre. And som metes causen onely fleume, as lombes
flesche and pigges flesch & porke & skirwhittes and arages. *Et* som melancolie as lentlyes and fechis and wortes and olde roþer flesch and flesch   750
of bugle. *Et* som rede colre, os crescis, seneuey, likes, oynons, and garlik.
Þus seiþ he.

Item, <u>drynk</u>[133] diuerseþ þe vryn in 4 wise: be cause of quantite and also
be cause of qualite, be cause of þe substance of þe drynke and be cause of
colour of drynk. Be resoun of qualite and quantite of drynk, as I seide ryȝt   755
nowe of mete; be resoun **[f. 21rb]** of substance of drynke, os if þe drynke
be mykel diurytik or mykel stiptik. For drynke suptil and diuritik multiplieþ þe vryn, i. makeþ for to pisse mykel in quantite; spis and stiptik, litil
vryn. Subtile is þenne and clere, spis is þik.

"Diuretik" and "stiptik": of 14 autoures fynde Y none þat me wil tell-   760
en what it arn. But þise droggeris and þise apothecaries þat beste schulde
wyten, sum seyn me þat diuretik is drye and stiptik þik. Þus taȝght me one
of þe wisest droggers of al Engelonde. Sum seyn þat diuretik is byndand,
as wyn byndyth at þe breste, and stiptik sooure and harsche, os peres or
þai be rype. Som seyne me þat diuretik is constrictif, i. byndyng, and stip-   765
tik solutif, i. lesnend & vnbyndand. *Et* sum seyn þat *e contrario* diuretik
solutif and stiptik constrictif.[134] *Et* some seyn þat diuretik is longe kepte
and stale, as syþer of 2 ȝere olde or 3 and as stale ale and swich oþer, and
stiptik newe and vnstalede, newe wyn, newe siþer, newe ale, and swyche
maner þinges. And þat is seid gramerly, for so for to speken, "diuretik"   770
is sayde of þis word in Latyn *diu*, i. longe, and of þis word *retinere*, i.
wiþholdyng & byndyng, as þing þat is longe tyme kepte. It may be saide
[f. 21va] of þis worde *stipes*, and in this wise for to speken, "stiptik" is no
more for to sayen but new as it comeþ of þe stoke, for *stipes* is þe stok þat
bereþ þe fruyt.   775

Item, som seyn þat diuretik is hote and drye and stiptik cole and moste,
and so is "diuretik" saide of þis worde *de*, i. of, and of þis worde *vrere*, i.
brennyng; and "stiptike" comeþ of þe stok, i. of *stipes*. Item, some seyn
þat *diureticum* is hote and moyste wiþ a maner of scharphede, as wyne &
syþer and scharpe ale and ale þat is ouer-olde & swich maner, for swych   780
maner drynkes causen mykel vryn. *Et stipticum* hote and moyste wiþ

132 pullettes] CgHGSc, pullecces RM7
133 drynk] *marg.*: 19 condicioun
134 constrictif] M7CgHGSc, constructif *with one minim of* u *underpuncted* R

swetehede or liciouste, os pyment and drinkes þat ar made wiþ spices &
noble fyne alle. For fyn ale[135] is *calida* & *humida* and chaufeth if it be noȝt
ouerdone taken. And wiþ þis laste opinioun acordeþ mykel in sentence
John de Sancto Paulo in his *Boke of Phisik Medycynal.*   785

    Diureticum schal be wryten wiþ "di" but noȝt souned wiþ "di," but it
schal be saide *dureticum* "duretik."

    Item, drynk diuerseþ þe vryn be cause of colour, as white wyne[136]
makeþ þe vryn scher and waterish, for be resoun of þe subtilte of his substance and also be cause þat it is glidand as water, it passeþ swiftely and   790
myȝtely to þe vesie. Item, wyne rede and [f. 21vb] clere causith vryn white
& clere but noȝt fully as white wyne, for it is more hote þan is white wyn
and noght so glidond as white wyne. And þerfor it drencheþ more or it
come doun into the vesie þan doþ white wyne þogh it litil be. If þe wyne
be spisse, droubly, þik, and swart rede, it makeþ þe vryn þik & swart, s.   795
mykel toward. Swete wyne, þogh it be þik, it makeþ vryn þen & clere.
For if it be swete wyne, þe brest anon (be cause of þe swetehed) dr[a]w-
eþ[137] him to him for þe likyng þat þe brest hath þerto. For þe spirituales
of man kyndly desireþ metis & drynkes þat arn delicat. And þan onely
þe aquosite, i. the watrihede, and þe moysthed þerof duelleþ a while in   800
epate and alse blyue passeth forth vnto þe vesy, as Y saide in þrid chapitre.
Gilbertus in his Coment vpon Giles saiþ þat al maner wynes[138] causen
vryn white & thenne, and namely if it be take in exces and so doþ al maner
drynk þat is ordeynede for mannes body. And vnderstond þat al maner
wynes ar hote & moyste in complexion and be cause of calidite þai ar   805
desiccatif. White wyne is moste tempre for it hath moste of humidite &
leste of calidite and þerfor it is most humectif and leste desiccatif, i. moste
moystand and leste dryand. Item, tak hede þat euermore the depper wyn
in colour,[139] [f. 22ra]] i. þe more swart rede þat it be and þe more þik þat
it be and þe more swert it be, þe more hote it is and þe lesse moyste in   810
effecte, i. in myȝt and in vertu of kynde. And þerfor alle wynes & namely
swete wyn noyȝen þe brest.

    Item, by þe 20 condicioun,[140] i. be þis worde <u>enoyntyng</u>, vnderstonde
þat enoyntyngz of oynementz þat arne hote of kynde, os *oleum laurinum*
& *vnguentum dampnaleoun* and swich oþer, achaufe þe body and cau-   815
sen coloure in the vryn intens or elles remis, i. hygh or lowh, vppon here

---

135 ale] *marg.*: qualites of ale
136 wyne] *marg.*: þe effecte of wyns
137 draweþ] drawith CgHGSc, drweþ R, drewþ M7
138 wynes] *marg.*: qualites of wynes
139 colour] *catchword* i. the more swarte
140 condicioun] *marg.*: 20 condicion

qualites, and also vpon þat þe iows or þe mayn of hem þrilleþ & entreth the veynes and the synowes of þe body.

If þou wilte be wise & ware and discrete and noȝt deceyuede in dome of vrynes, þe behoueþ to knowe þise 20 forsaide condicions wiþ þe poyntz 820 þat arne bifore put, but principaly þe 4 firste, for þo 4 ar moste nedeful and necessarie. For þai be moste principal and moste substancial and moste fro wiþinward and þat oþer 16 ar but accidental and secundarie toward þo 4. For þai more certefien the leche in demyng and more verayly schewen the state & þe disposicioun of þe body þan þe remanant. Thise arne þo 4: the 825 qualite of vryn, þe substance of vryn, þe þingez þat ar conteynede in the vryn, [f. 22rb] and quantite of vryn. And in alle þe poyntz þat I haue saide or schal saie in þis faculte, vnderstonde generally þat vryn euermore signi-fieþ 3 þingz,[141] s. disposicioun of complexioun of þe body, disposicioun of humores of þe body, & disposicion of myȝt and kynde in þe body. 830

The colour of þe vryn[142] seiþ euermore disposicioun of þe complexioun, for color in vryn is causede principaly of complexioun of man and prin-cipali of calidite, for calidite is principal wirker and maker of digestioun in man.

The body of þe vryn[143] seiþ alwaie disposicion of þe humores of man, 835 for when the humores arne discaterede & disperplede aboute in the body and destourblede and distemprede, þai causen a þikhede in þe vryn, and *e contrario* whan þai arne oþerwise.

But both togeder,[144] s. þe coloure of þe vryn and þe body of þe vryn, seyn þe state of þe body of man. And take gode hede whie Y sai both þe 840 colour of þe vryn and the body of þe vryn boþe togeder: for þough þe coloure of an vryn schewe hym neuer so gode, but if þe body of þe vryn be gode also, it is no gode token, ne þogh þe body of þe vryn be neuere so gode, but þe colour be eke gode. But neuertheles bettre is one [f. 22va] gode þan neyþer. But if boþe be gode, bothe body and colour, it seyt helth 845 and myȝt & vertu in kynde. And by þe grace of God I schal teche by þe 2 bokes folowende os bokes & auctoures of þis faculte speken and techen.

Here endeþ þe first boke &c.

---

141 þingz] *marg.*: Vryn signifieþ vpon 3 þinges
142 colour of þe vryn] *marg.*: Colour of vryn
143 body of þe vryn] *marg.*: body of vryn
144 both togeder] *marg.*: bothe body & colour

Book 2

[2.1]

Here bygynneþ þe 2 boke, þe first chapitre: of colours in ordre

Affter þise þinges þat bene saide in the first trete, for to go to our purpos, vnderstonde þat þere be 20 couloures of vryn. *Et* þogh it so be þat som saie 40, som 48, som 50, & som 52, noȝtforþan þe more partie of auctoures and most autentik and moste couþe maken destinccion but of 20 couloures and   5 seyne þat þis nombre sufficeþ. For all oþer couloures of vryn, if þere mo be os þai saie, arne comprehendede in þise 20. Ne þou schalt no colour fynde in vryn þat it ne is like to some of þise 20 couloures.

And arne þise al bedene, as auctour[s][1] put and as þou schalt se be ordre be al þis 2 boke: þe ferste is *niger*; þe 2 *liuidus*; þe 3 *albus*; þe 4 *lacteus*; þe   10 5 *glaucus*; þe 6 *karapos*; þe 7 *pallidus*; þe 8 *subpallidus*; þe 9 *citrinus*; þe 10 *subcitrinus*; þe 11 *subrufus*; þe 12 *rufus*; þe 13 [f. 22vb] *subrubeus*; þe 14 *rubeus*; þe 15 *subrubecundus*; þe 16 *rubecundus*; þe 17 *ynopos*; þe 18 *kyanos*; þe 19 *viridis*; þe 20 *niger*. What alle þise couloures be in Englisshe, and how þai schulde be knowen, and what þai betoken and in what wise, þou   15 schalt haue in here propre chapitres by and by.

And haue no wonder þat nyghand alle auctourse bygynne at Blak colour and ende at Blak colour. For þere is on maner of Blak colour in vryn þat is causide of mortificacion, and þat maner of blachede is moste like a blake horne schynand or like a rauenes feþer or like a man of þe londe of Ethiop.   20 *Et* anoþer maner of blakhede þer is þat is causede of adustion complet. Of whiche maner blakhede, se in þe laste capitre of þis 2 boke. And so auctoures make proces, as who so go aboute a cercle and com agayn þere he began.

And vnderstonde þat þis terme "mortificacioun"[2] is þus mykil for to   25 saye in þis faculte: wastyng, quenchyng, and fordoyng of kynd hete in man throuȝ exces of colde. For when þe body is ouercomen wiþ exces of colde, þan ar þe humores of þe body al desolat and destitut and refte fro her kynde hete, þat kynde may noȝt wirk ne rewelen in the body. And [f. 23ra] ryȝt as þis terme "mortificacioun" is for to be vnderstondyn alwaie   30 in regard of colde, riȝt so, *e contrario*, þis terme "adustioun"[3] is euermore to be vnderstonde in regarde of hete. Schortely to speke, mortificacioun is

---

1 auctours] CgHG, doctours Sc, auctoure RM7
2 mortificacioun] *marg.*: mortificaciou\<n>
3 adustioun] *marg.*: adustioun

fordoyng of kynde hete be cause of exces of colde & adustioun complete
is fordoyng of hete be cause of exces of vnkynd hete.

And vnderstonde þat difference is betwene þise 2 termes, "adustioun"   35
and "adustioun complete":[4] "adustioun" is on Englisshe "brennyng," os
when þe humores, or elles some of þe humores, is trauaylede and distemperede throgh exces of vnkynde hete. But "adustioun complete" is when
exces of vnkynde hete is so mykel þat þer is none helpe or vneþes eny.

Than þise forsaide 20 coloures, som auctours diuisen[5] hem vpon þe dis-   40
posicioun of digestioun þus. Of coloures, som betokne mortificacioun of
digestion, os *niger color* & *liuidus color*. What is mortificacioun, I saide
riȝt nowe. <u>*Niger & liuidus*: se in here propre chapetres</u>. *Et* som coloures
betoken priuacioun of digestioun, os *albus* and *lacteus, glaucus* & *karopos*.
Priuacioun, i. reneyng & benymmyng, and is saide of þis worde *priuare*,   45
reneyng and fornymyng. And priuacioun is taken here for lessyng and
vanisshing and feblesshing & litil- **[f. 23rb]** hede of digestioun.

Item, som coloures betoken bygynnyng of digestioun, as *pallidus* and
subpallidus & *subcitrinus*. And som, digestioun complete, as *citrinus, sub-*
rufus, rufus. And som, exces of digestioun, os *rubeus* & *subrubeus, subru-*   50
becundus, rubecundus. And som colours seyne adustioun of digestioun, os
ynopos and *kyanos*. *Et* som, adustioun complete and mortificacioun also,
as Blak colour moste like[6] þe lefe of a blak cole þat we calle þe rede cole,
and Grene colour moste like þe leef of a grene cole þat we calle þe white
cole. And so þer is two maner of blakhed in vryn, os I saide & as þou schalt   55
sene. <u>Which is *mortificacio* and *adustio* and *adustio completa* is seyde</u>.
Mortificacioun, i. fordoyng of kynd hete. Adustioun, i. brennyng. Adustioun complete, when it is alle fullike brennede.

Som diuise[7] þise 20 coloures of vryn vpon disposicioun of humores of
man. For some humore arn mater and cause of þe colour in vryn. And þis   60
is þe more verray diuisioun, as meny seyn. *Et* þai sayn þat alle coloures fro
Citrine dounward signifien þat mykel melancoly wiþ litil fleume regneþ
in the body. Vnderstonde þat þis terme of "melancolie" is taken in 3 wise:
sumtyme it is **[f. 23va]** taken[8] for on of þe 4 humores (*sanguis, colera,*
fleuma, & *melancolia*), of which it is saide sufficiently in þe j boke, 4 c.   65
And somtym it [is][9] taken for exces of þe same humour, as Y spak in þe j
bok, 4 c., 4 condicioun, lef {*om.*}, þer þou hast of þise 2 termes *regnat &*

---

4 adustioun complete] *marg.*: adustioun complete
5 diuisen] *marg.*: þe diuisioun of colours
6 like] M7CgHGSc, li (*line end*) like R
7 diuise] *marg.*: anoþer diuisioun of colours
8 taken] *marg.*: melancolie is on 3 wise
9 is] CgHGSc, *om.* RM7

dominatur, and in þis wise it is taken here, þer I saie mykel melancoli wiþ litle fleume. & somtym it is taken for a passion in þe soule, i. ire, wraþ.

Citrin colour, colre & fleume, but more of colre. *Rufus color* wiþ a mene 70
body, somdel more þen þan þik, saiþ þat þe arteries & þe blode of þe
artaries ar gode & myȝti, & namly þe blode of þe arteries, which blode is
cause and mater of kynde hete of þe spiritz of lif.

Arteries[10] propurly be þo veynes be whiche þe spiritual membres drawen
to hem her eyre and spiritz be þe pipes of þe lunges. And þerfor arteries 75
ar alse myche for to seyn os *aertrarie*, or elles *aertraharie*, i. drawend eyre.
Herewiþ acordeþ Galienus in his *Boke of Anathomyes*, þere he seiþ þus:
Arteries ar certeyn veynes by which þe hert is tyede and knyt to þe lunges
and draweþ to him eyre by þe pipes of þe lunges. And þo arteries passe
forþ by oþer parties of þe body þer þe pouces bene. "Pouces" in Englissh, 80
pulsus[11] in Latyn, ar þe veynes in þe wristes. *Et pulsus* is often taken for þat
place þer þe poucis lyue, s. for þe wirst of þe honde. Which be the [f. 23vb]
spiritual membres, se in c. *de liuido colore*, lef {28}, and in c. *de karopos*,
lef {om.}; þe pypes of þe lunges, in c. *de karopos.*

Item, *rufus color* wiþ a body sumdel more þik þan þinne, but noȝt fullik 85
þik, seyþ þat *sanguis epatis*, i. blode of þe lyuer, *dominatur* in þe body.[12]
And when *sanguis dominatur*, þan is *epar* heile & sounde and in gode temperour, and þat is cause and token of gode helthe and nurisshing of lif. For
in helþe of þe lyuer stant helþe of þe blode, and in helþe of þe blode stant
helth of þe body principaly. 90

Subrubeus and *rubeus*, wiþ a body clere and þenne, seyth \os/ *rufus*,
but noȝt so parfitely, for *rufus* seiþ more euen temperur þan *rubeus* or
subrubeus. For *rubeus* & *subrubeus* seyn more exces & destemperure of
hete þan doth *rufus*. Item, *rubeus* and *subrubeus* colour, wiþ a body þik
and drubly, seiþ grete rouryng and rollyng and desturblyng of humours 95
in þe body.

Rubecundus & *subrubecundus* seiþ þat colre is maistre in þe body out
of mesur, and ouergoþ þe blode and enflammeþ þe blode and brenneþ and
distempreþ him. *Et* if þe colour in þe vryn be so mykel rubecunde þat it be
moste like purpur, it seiþ þat þe blode is þik & dry, þat þe moystour of þe 100
blode is soken oute and drawen awaie fro [f. 24ra] him þurgh distemperur
of exces of hete.

Ynopos: þat þe blode is þik and clammyde and clodded togedre and
corrupt, and al forscolkerede and forbrynt and menkt wiþ foule corrupt

---

10 Arteries] *marg.*: Arteries: what þai ben
11 pulsus] *marg.*: pulsus
12 body] *marg.*: Wherein stant helþe of body

fleume. *Kyanos* þe same, saue þat *kyanos* is riȝt werse þan *ynopos*, for it   105
seiþ riȝt more skolkeryng and adustioun þan doþ *ynopos*.

Viridis color in vryn seiþ euermore þat melancoly is maistre in the body,
and þat kynde humidite of þe body is wastede and fordon & destroiede.
And also þat þe blode haþ lorn his owen kynde colour. For þe kynde
colour of blode is rudihede.   110

Liuidus colour seiþ þat fleume and melancolie ben maystres & regne in
þe body.

[2.2]

Here begynneþ þe secunde chapiter, *de nigro colore*, i. of Blak colour

Vnderstonde þat þou schalt knowe Blak vryn euermore by a swerthode,
a dirkehode, and a dymhede in vryn, acordyng moste to a blakhede, sumtyme moste like an horn blakishe, schinond and glirond; somtyme moste
like a rauennes feþer; and somty[m]¹ moste like þe face of a man of Ethiop.   5
And swich maner blakhede in vryn, þat is for to saye, swiche maner
blakhede as þis chapitle spekeþ of, is euermore causede and gendrede in
þis wise: first þe vryn is in þe body, hete wirkyng into **[f. 24rb]** moyste,
and so it causiþ a dymhede and a swarthede [in]² þat moyst body, s. in þe
vryn, for hete lesseþ and vanessheþ awaie þat [þat]³ is subtil & eyrissh.   10
And þat þat is gros and terrestre, i. þik and erþisshe, bleuiþ stil, and hete
scaldiþ it and scolkeriþ it and brenneþ it, and so causeþ swarthede and
blakhede in þe vryn. And in þis wise is blakhede⁴ in vryn causede.

Som saie þat Blak colour in vryn is caused in 6 wise:⁵ be cause of
adustion,⁶ as Y seide riȝt nowe, and also as it is in folke of Ethiop þat ar   15
son brennede. Item,⁷ be cause of mortificacioun of kynde hete. <u>What is
mortificacioun Y saide in þe nexte chapitle biforne.</u> For þan þe kynde hete
is noȝt of myȝt ne of vertu for to coloure þe blode as he schulde done.
Wherfore þe blode leseþ and forgoþ his owen kynde colour and turneþ

---

1   somtym] M7CgGSc, sumtyme & sumtyme H, somty (*end of line*) R
2   in] CgH, and RM7GSc
3   þat þat] CgHGSc, þat M7, þat it R
4   is blakhede] *foll. by* is blakhede *canc.* R
5   6 wise] *marg.*: blak colour is caused in 6 wyse
6   adustion] *marg.*: j maner
7   Item] *marg.*: 2 maner

into blakhede. Item,[8] be cause of congelacioun of þe blode, os when on   20
takeþ colde be his extremytes of his body, as we sene oþerwhile in þe lippes of folk þat taken colde in þe wynter tyme. Congelacioun of blode is
when þe blode is congelede, i. when þe blode is colde-byten, i. taken wiþ
colde; and be cause þerof leseth his kynde colour and waxeþ wan & blo
and blak and þik & clomprede [**f. 24va**] and euyl disposede. What be þe   25
extremytes of þe body, se in the ferst boke, þe 3 c., lef {*om.*}. Be cause[9] of
chaungeyng of humores þat þe body haþ, it befalleþ often tyme þat when
þe blode or elles oþer humores changen and turnen into melancolie, which
melancoly siþen þat it is blak of kynd, it behoueþ þat þe vryn þat is causede þerof be Blake. Item,[10] be cause of brusur or of hurtyng or of blemis-   30
shyng of som noble membre in þe body, þat when blode comeþ þerto, þe
blode cacheþ a discolouryng and a blakhede, and so þe vryn in as mykel
os it comeþ þerof.

Isaac in þe 4 boke *De febribus* seiþ þat noble membres[11] of man ar þe
veynes and þe arteries of mannes body, which be cause of her noblete and   35
her worþihede, kynd is wonte oþerwhile for to meuen and fleten awaie
fro hem materies of maladies and sikenesses to oþer membres and to oþer
places of þe body. Of veynes: se in c. *de liuido colore*, lef {25}. Of arteries
þou haste aforne in the j chapitre, lef 18. Item,[12] be cause of mixtioun, i.
mengyng, of some blak liquor or of som blak mater wiþ þe vryn, as often   40
befalleþ when þat *sanguis menstruus* (*anglice*: þe blode of þe vile mater of
[**f. 24vb**] womannes sekenes that þai calle here floures) seweþ & sweteþ
and drilliþ to þe reynes and so to þe vesie and enfecteþ þe vryn and so
comeþ forþ þerwiþ. (Þise termes *sanguis menstruus* & *menstruum* is al on:
se in ca. *de liuido colore*, lef 34.)   45

Som saye þat Blak colour in vryn is caused but of 3 þingz: þat is, be
cause of adustion, be cause of mortificacioun, or be cause of mixtioun of
blak humour, s. of melancolie þat is callede *niger humor*. *Niger humor*
for it is blak be waie of kynde,[13] for it haþ most kyndely of e[rþ]e[14] and
moste is answeryng to þat element, as þou haste in þe firste boke, 4 c., 9   50
condicioun.

And vnderstonde þat Blak vryn hath euermore a þik body or þikkissh,
and for þise skiles: for þer blakhede is, þere is swarthede, derkehede, &

---

8 Item] *marg.*: 3 maner
9 Be cause] *marg.*: 4 maner
10 Item] *marg.*: 5 maner
11 noble membres] *marg.*: which ben noble membris
12 Item] *marg.*: 6 maner
13 blak ... kynde] *foll. by* for it is blak be waie of kynde *canc.* R
14 erþe] (the GSc) erthe CgHGSc, eyre RM7

dymhede and droublehede, or elles of vnkynd hete scaldand and brennand
and sleand þe kynde hete, and boþe þo causen swarthede and þikhede in   55
þe vryn.

Item, Blak vryn or it seiþ consumpcioun, i. wastyng of þe substancial
humidite in þe body, i. insencioun, brennyng, and sco[l]keryng[15] of þe
blode þat is causede of vnkynd hete, or it seiþ mortificacioun, i. quenchyng
and fordoyng of kynde hete þorgh exces of colde takyng, [f. 25ra] or elles   60
it seiþ purgacioun of wickede humores of melancolie agayn warschyng.
And in alle þise poyntes, þe body of þe vryn is þik or þikissh. For euermore incensioun of blode causeþ þikhede in þe vryn, be resoun of boyling
and walmyng of þe blode aboute in þe veyns of þe body. Also in mortificacioun the vryn is þik, be resoun þat frigidite clompreþ it & cruddeþ it   65
togeder. & also in purgacioun of melancolie, þe vryn is þik be cause þat þe
terrestre, i. þe erþihede, of melancoly is mixte, i. menke, wiþ þe vryn. And
for alle þise skiles, Blak colour in vryn euermore scheweþ him wiþ a þik
or elles wiþ a þikisshe body.

No3tforþan, *per accidens*, i. vnpropurly, and be oþer enchesoun, as often   70
befalleþ, as I saide in þe j boke,[16] lef {9}, Blak coloure may schewe hym wiþ
a þenne body, no3tforþan no3t ful þenne. And þat befalleþ when materies
narowen and streyten þe waies of þe vryn and þan passeþ and scapeþ þere-
awaie parties þat ar smale & suptil as poudre or duste. Which smale suptil
parties, in alse myche as þai ben blak, þai causen a blakhed in þe vryn;   75
and also in alse [mykel][17] as þai bene a partie þik, þai þikken þe vryn, but
no3tforþan, lesse þan half þik.

Þan vnderstond for a reule þat Blak vryn mykel in quantite, wiþ a body
inequal, seiþ warisshyng of a [f. 25rb] febre quarteyn. Which quarteyn is
causede þorgh exces of melancolie mixte wiþ þe humores and ouergoand   80
hem. Þat þe vryn is mykel in quantite, it is tokne of purgacion of mater of
þe malady and warsshing of þe sekenes: þat is for to seyn, it is token þat
kynde is my3ty in himselfe for to maistre þat wickede destemperur of þe
humoure and purge himself þerof. For be cause of purgacioun of þe mater
of þe maladie, the vryn oweþ for to multiplien, i. bene mykel in quantite.   85
Materia morbi, þe mater of þe maladye,[18] euermore is þat humour þat
causith þe sekenesse.

Item, þat þe vryn is þik and inequal, it seiþe euermore in euery maner
vryn roryng and rulyng & hurling, destourblyng and destemperour of

---

15   scolkeryng] scolkryng CgH, scokkeryng RM7, *om*. GSc
16   j boke] M7, fyrst book CgH, j° li° (*in marg.*) G, li° i° (*in marg.*) Sc, j ferst boke R
17   mykel] CgH, myche GSc, *om*. RM7
18   mater of þe maladye] *marg.*: þe mater of þe sekenesse

humores in þe body. And euermore in swiche party of þe vryn as þou seest   90
moste thikhede and moste droblyhede and moste squalpryng, in swiche
parti of þe body is moste destemperure of humours and in þat place is
him werst. And if oueral in þe vryn, ouer al þe body eke. But take hede
þat vryn mai be spisse, i. þik, in 3 wise.[19] Somtyme[20] it is spisse be cause of
noble digestioun, but þan it is but litil spisse, wiþ a clerehede & [f. 25va]   95
a liȝtnesse in colour. And þat is noble tokne, for it seiþ myȝt in kynde.
Item,[21] sometyme is þe vryn spisse be cause of largehede of þe waies of þe
vryn. And þat is oþerwhile be cause of febelnes of kynde and þat is perilouse, for it is tokne þat kynde is noȝt of power in himselfe to wiþholde ne
for to kepe þe humores[22] in þe body. Item,[23] somtyme it is spisse be cause   100
of multitude and distemperur of som humor or of humores. But in boþe
þise tuo laste poyntz is þe vryn more spisse and more ded in colour þan
when it is spisse be cause of gode digestioun.

    And þan vppon þat it is equal or inequale, so is þe distemperure in
þe body equale, i. euene or oueral alike, as we seyn "euen alike mykel,"   105
"oueral alike þicke," "oueral alike þenne," and swich maner speche. Item,
Blak vryn, be it equal, be it inequal, if it be wiþ a litil body, i. litil in quantite, þat vryn is suspecte, for it is wel perilouse.

    Item, vryn mykel derke and dymme and swart and mykel toward
blachede seyth mortificacioun. Þis terme mortificacioun I exponed in þe j   110
chapitre, lef 17. And vnderstonde þat when Blak vryn seith mortificacioun,
it is more blake þan when it [f. 25vb] seiþ warschyng of þe quarteyn. And
also vnderstonde þat when Blak vryn seiþ mortificacioun, þan went Blo
vryn byforne þat Blak vryn. Þat is þus mykel for to mene: þe vryn þat he
made nexte bifor þat þis vryn bicom Blak was Blo, þogh it be many daies   115
syth it bicom Blak. And in þis wise vnderstond, as often as Y saie swiche
vryn or swiche went bifore swich or swiche.

    Item, vryn Blak like an horne glyronde and schynand, lyke a rauens
feþer, or like þe visage of a man of Ethiop, þat be cause of hete and brennyng of þe sone is blak in the face, seiþ adustioun complete. And þan was   120
þe nex vryn bifore Grene. Adustioun & adustioun comple[t]:[24] in þe j c.,
lef {18}.

    Item, vryn Blak and þenne abouen and þik donward, wiþ a foule swart
residens in þe botume after þat þe vryn haþ his kynd residence, if it be

---

19   3 wise] *marg.*: vryn is þikkede by 3 causes
20   Somtyme] *marg.*: j cause
21   Item] *marg.*: 2 cause
22   þe humores] M7CgHGSc, þe humores þe humores R
23   Item] *marg.*: 3 cause
24   complet] CgHG, comple RM7, *om.* Sc

a womannes water, it seiþ purgacioun of hir floures þat comeþ of filþe   125
and corupcioun of melancolie, and so warschyng. If suche an vryn be of a
man, saue þat it is noȝt fully so swart, ne þe residence in þe botume is noȝt
fully so blak as when it is of a woman, it saiþ as I saide in þe firste reule,
warshyng of a quarteyn or elles of a febre þat haþ som spice of a quarteyn,
hauand reward to þe quantite of þe [f. 26ra] vryn, as Y saide.   130

Vnderstonde þat þis terme "residence" is taken 2 wise[25] in phisik:
And as þou mayste se in þis forsaid reule, sumtyme[26] it is taken for kynd
restyng in the vessel after þat þe vryn is made, <u>as I taght in þe firste boke,</u>
<u>þe 4 chapitre.</u> And somtyme[27] it is taken[28] for euery maner þik mater in þe
vryn þat draweþ doun into þe botume of þe vryn, þat we calle "seggend   135
mater," þe drestes and þe gronde-soppes. *Menstrua mulieris (anglice:*
<u>women sekenesse or womannes floures), se in þe c. of Blo coloure, lef</u>
<u>{34}.</u> *Melancolia* <u>in þe first boke, 4 c., lef {10}. And in c. of White colour,[29]</u>
<u>lef {12}.</u>

Item, þe same vryn, saue more white and ble[ike][30] and wanne, and þe   140
þik residence þerin is more whitisshe þan whan it is of þe floures after þat
it haþe restede, seiþ sekenes in þe body and principaly aboute þe reyns or
þe vesie or elles boþe. And þan and þer come vpon him an acue, i. a sharp
hote febre, þat vryn is suspecte. For þat vryn may be swich be cause of
þe febre or elles be cause of sekenes in þe reyns. If it be of þe febre, be it   145
man, be it woman, it is tokne of deþ. If it be de depressioun of þe reyns, no
drede. *Renes & lumbi:* <u>in c. de karopos, lef 59.</u>

Blak vryn and fat abouen, and wiþ an euel sauour, and wiþ þat he haue
no sekenes ne no peyn in þe lendes ne in the vesie, wiþ an acue, [f. 26rb] it
seiþ deþ. Þe blakhede bytokeneþ as I said, s. adustioun of þe blode and of   150
þe humores in þe body, i. þat the blode and þe humores ar forskalkerede
in the body and forbrenned. Þe Fathode euermore seiþ melting and wast-
ying awaie of kynde. *Fetor,* i. stynk in vryn, euermore seyþ rotyng and
fordoyng of kynde. <u>Of</u> *fetor* <u>and of Fathede in vryn, se in þe 3 boke in</u>
<u>her propre chapitlez.</u> If it haue no sauour but as vryn schulde haue, þer is   155
hope. If he haue þerwiþ peyn aboute þe lendes, þer is hope. What vryn it
be þat stinkeþ from fer, s. or it be putt to þe nose, he is but dede.

Item, Blak vryn or elles blakisshe, mykel in quantite, wiþ a blak cloude
houand in þe myddes of þe vryn in an acue, and his peyn be so huge þat

---

25 2 wise] *marg.*: residence is in 2 wise
26 sumtyme] *marg.*: j maner
27 somtyme] *marg.*: 2 maner
28 is taken] M7CgHGSc, is [*line end*] is taken R
29 colour] colourl *with second* l *underpuncted* R
30 bleike] GSc, bleyt RM7CgH

he may not slepe, and eke it letteþ his hereyng: if alle þise poyntz *in die* 160
cretica, i. in þe dai of creticacioun, and þerwiþ þou sest eny gode tokenes,
it seiþ þat he schal haue bledyng at þe nose and þerwiþ warsching. But if
wickede tokenes, it is deþ.

Vnderstonde be Blak vryn in þis reule not only swych vryn os is verreily Blake or elles blakisshe, but also þat vryn þat haþ in him **[f. 26va]** a 165
blak Skye, a swarte cloude þat makeþ al þe vryn to seme blak or blakisshe, and also for vryn þat is *rubecunda* and for purpre vryn and Ynopos
& Kyanos. Þat þe vryn is mykel in quantite, it seith þat kynde is of myȝt
and of power to helpe himselfe and for to purge and delyuer him of þe
malady, and principaly if þe vryn schewe himself mykel in *die cretica*. Þat 170
þe cloude is houand in þe myddys, it is tokne þat *materia morbi*, þe mater
of þe sekenes, is obedient to kynde, i. þat þe humour & þe humores þat
causen þe malady is schaply and able and disposede for to be ouercomen
& ouermaist[r]iede³¹ of þe kynde. What is *materia morbi*, Y seide biforn.

Þat he mai noȝt slepe & þat he is lettede of his hering for peyne is be 175
cause of feruour and of scharphede of þe mater, þe whiche mater is resoluede into fumosite, i. into a smeke, a smoþer, flyand, walmand vpward
into þe hede and þere causeþ wakyng and akyng & onreste & stoppyng
of þe eyre in his eeres. And so it makeþ him of wicke eyre and lettyng of
heryng. And þan þat ilke mater þat stieþ so vp to þe heuede, be cause þat 180
he is so **[f. 26vb]** scharp & so violent & so penitratif, i. pirsonde and per-
shonde, he bresteþ a certeyn veyne þat is in a small web, i. smal skyn, in
þe hede. And þan it haþ none oþer issue, but bristeþ out by þe noseþirle.

Dies creticus, or *dies cretica*, is calde "þe day of creticacioun." *Creticus*
is saide of þis word *crisis*. *Crisis*, i. *iudicium*, i. dome or elles *determinacio*, 185
i. a determinacioun (*anglice*: a certeyn-settyng), and it is comunely taken
for cessyng of þe febre. *Dies creticus*³² þus is descryuede comunly of phisi-
sciens: *die[s]*³³ *creticus est dies euasionis ab infirmitate febris siue ad vitam*
siue ad mortem (*anglice*: day of creticacioun is þat day þat þe maladi of þe
febre leueþ þe seke, or to lif oþer to deþ).   190

Now take god hede þat, os Ysaac techeþ in þe 4 boke *Of þe Febre*, þat
þise ar god daies of creticacioun: þe 4 dai, þe 5 dai, þe 7 dai, þe 9 dai, þe
11 dai, þe 14 dai, þe 17 dai, þe 19 dai, þe 20 dai, þe 21 dai. And þise ar þe
daies of wickede creticacioun, i. of perilouse warsching: þe 6, þe 8, þe 10,
þe 16, and þe 18. If *crisis* come in eny of þis daies, it is wicked tokne. For it 195
seiþ þat þer is fiȝt and bataile bitwene þe kynde and þe maladie, & þat þe

---

31 ouermaistriede] M7CgHGSc, ouermaistiede R
32 Dies creticus] *marg.*: Crisis
33 dies] M7CgHGSc, die R

maladie haþ more defense þan þe kynde, as it is in hem þat liȝten aȝeyns
deþ. [f. 27ra] Wherfore if þo tokenes þat scheweþ in þis waie in þe seke be
wickede tokenes, he leueþ noȝt longe; but if þe tokenes be gode, it seyn þat
þe malady wil come agayn and longe lasten.   200

The mene dais of creticacioun bitwene gode & wicke are þe 13 and þe
15. Vnderstonde þat of þe forsaide daies of gode creticacion, som ar *dies*
cretici and sum ar *dies nunciatiui* (*anglice*: som ar daies of warshing and
som ar daies of tokenyng toward warshing). Þo þat be proprely *dies cre-*
tici, þo ar alwaie gode and most certayn, s. þe 7 and þe 14, þe 20 & 21. 205
Þo þat are propur and most certeyn nunciatif, i. þe moste certeyn tokne
toward: þe 4 in rewarde of þe 7 and þe 11 in regarde of þe 14; after þo, þe
5 and þe 9 & þe 17; after þo, þe 13 and þe 19. & somtyme it befalleþ þat
nunciatif cometh in cretik and somtyme cretik in nunciatif. And þe cause
is for þe mater of þe malady is gros & hard and heuy for to defiei and wil 210
noȝt gladely be ouercomen. And while it is so, it most be þe longer or þe
malady stonde. And þerfor it passeth þe cretike daie & falleþ in þe nunciatif day after þe cretik day.

If þe mater be suptil & liȝt & eþe for to maistri, þan stant þe malady
þat is nunciatif on þe [f. 27rb] cretik. *Verbi gratia*, i. se by example: the 215
terme and þe stonding of a kinde febre tercien is þe 14 dai, but if it so
be þat þe mater of þe tercien be more subtile and more liȝt, as Y saide
riȝt now, þan is it sone ripe and redy and þan is his terme, i. he stant in
þe 11 daye. If it so be þat þat mater be mykel more subtil & as I saide,
þan þe malady hasteþ him faste and crisis falleþ on þe 9 daie or on þe 7 220
day. But if it so be þat þe mater be sumdel mixte wiþ a mater of anoþer
maladi, þan his determinacioun, i. his terme, abideþ til þe 17 or til þe 21
day. If it be myȝty, wiþ huge and grete mater and greuance of som oþer
sekenes or of myskepyng, lenger abideþ his terme. Tak gode hede þat
Isaac vseth þise termes al for on in þis mater: "stonding of þe sekenes," i. 225
when þe malady is at þe hieste, & "terme" & "determinacioun" and *crisis*
and *dies creticus*. And alle is no more for to saie but cessing and endyng
of þe malady.

Item, vnderstonde þat of wicked and perilouse cretik daies, þe 2 is þe
worste of alle; after þat, þe 6; next þat, þe 8; þan þe 10; after þise, þe 12 230
and þe 14, þe 16 & þe 18. Than þe skil whie þe [f. 27va] 2 day is wickede
is be cause þat þe mater of þe maladie is ȝit crude and indigest and kind
is noȝt ȝit of myȝt for to wirken ne maken decoccioun and digestioun of
þe mater or þe 4 daye; and so of alle þe remenaunt. And þerfor when
signes & tokenes of warsshing apere in eny of þe forsaide wickede daies 235
and warsshyng come noȝt þerwiþ, wete wel þat kynde is al fortrauailede
and astonyede and dismaiede, þorȝ violence and strengh ouergoand and
maistriand þe kinde. *Et* þat is þe skil whie Ypocras blameþ bledyng att þe

nose in þe 2 dai of an acue. & þerfor þe ferre þat the perilouse dai be fro þe
2 dai of creticacioun, þe lesse drede is.   240

Item, þe 6 day betokeneþ myȝtyed of þe malady and feblenesse of kynde.

If þou wilt aske whi od daies ar more couenant & able to creticacioun
þan euen daies, þus answereþ Isaac: odde daies ar bettre & more couenable
to creticacioun propurly and kyndely, but noȝtforþan euen ar more co-
[u]enable[34] *per accidens*, i. vnpropurly. For if it be so þat crisis begynne in þe   245
3 dai and fulfilleþ his wirkyng in þe 4 dai, wherfor crisis is to be acomptede
on þe 14 dai, for in þat 14 dai scheweþ kynde his ful wirkingz. [f. 27vb]
And on þe þrid day kind begynneþ for to wirk and in þe 4 he finissheþ and
endeþ his wirkyng.

And þerfor wise men here biforn, when þai sawe þat euen daies was   250
noȝt cretik propurly by wirkyng of þe kynde, but onely *per accidence*, i.
vnpropurly, and by oþer enchesoun þan be wirkyng of kynde, þai saide
þat odde daies ar more verreie and more able and more siker þan euen
daies. And þerfor seiþ Ypocras in his *Empidijs*: *Impares paribus sunt
forciores* (*anglice*: odde daies ar more siker for to demen warshing of þan   255
euen daies).

Alle þise poyntz seiþ Isaac nerhand worde for worde. Per I saide þis
terme *per accidence*, se in þe j bok, þe 4 c.,[35] and also in þis boke, 7 c. *de
colore karopos*, lef {54}. And vnderstande þat it is callede *dies*[36] *creticus*
noȝt onely for alse mykel as *crisis* falleþ comunely in swich dai, but for   260
alse mykel as *crisis* comunly comeþ in swich day, falleþ & eke in tokne of
sauacioun.

Item, þat odde daies ar bettre and more siker for to hopen and vnbynd-
en after *crisis* mai be by tuo skiles: or for alse mykel as þe more del of
cretik daies ben odde[37] or elles for alse mykel as þe best of [f. 28ra] alle þe   265
cretike daies is odde, s. þe 7 day.

And if þou wilt wete and knowen what day or what nyȝt[38] crisis schal
be, þus techeþ Isaac in þe same boke anone after: þou moste speren and
weten þe begynnyng of þe maladie, so þat þou be certeyn boþe of þe
nunciatif dai and of þe cretik day, and when þou art siker þerof, þou   270
moste knowen also what signes apere in euery nunciatif dai. For if gode
signes schew him in þe nunciatif dai, alle gode or elles fewe or 2 or mo &
þerwiþ þou se þat kynde wirketh (þow it litil be), and it be os Y saie in þe
nunciatif dai, *crisis* schal be in þe nexte cretik dai. After þat ilk nunciatif

---

34   couenable] Cg, conuenable H, comenable RM7, *om. (eyeskip)* GSc
35   4 c.] *foll. by* lef *canc.* R
36   dies] *prec. by* dies *at line end, canc.* R
37   odde] *foll. by* or for alse myche as þe more dole of cretik daies bene odde *canc.* R
38   nyȝt] *foll. by* schal *canc.* R

dai, as in þe 7 dai when þe 4 daie goþ aforn, & in þe 14 dai when þe 7 goþ   275
bifor, & namely if þe malady be at þe hiest, *crisis* comeþ þat sam dai, and
principali if it come to gode, i. to helþe. Wikede *crisis* ofte tyme comeþ
on þe same & somtyme on anoþer day; somtyme in þe bygynnyng of þe
malady, & sometyme at þe higheste of þe malady, i. att þe stondyng of
þe sekenes.   280

Þan stant þe malady when it is moste my3ty and moste[39] in his malice.
Wherfor vnderstond þat þe febre haþ 4 tymes,[40] i. *inicium, augmentum,
statum, & declinacionem (anglice:* þe begyn- **[f. 28rb]** nyng, þe waxing,
the stondyng, and þe fallyng, or elles þe vanysshing). *Inicium*[41] is when
þe malady and tokenes þerof come litil and litil, til þai aperen alle or elles   285
þe more party of hem. *Augmentum*[42] is when the verrei tokenes ar alle
comen and bigyn for to be wode and turment, til þe kynd and þe malady
fi3ten togeder. *Status*[43] is when þe kynd & þe malady repugnen and fei3ten
togeder, til þe tone haþ þe maistrie and þe victorie. Declinacioun,[44] i. swagyng of þe malady, þat is fro þe firste begynnyng of warisshyng, fro þe first   290
tyme þat gode tokenes bygynne, i. þat wicked tokenes bygyn to lessen,
as þe febre to feynten, þirst to lessen, and swych oþer poyntz til he be
scapede.

Item,[45] if þou wil weten in what houre of þe dai or in what houre of þe
ny3t *crisis* schal be, stodie and wete in what houre cam þe firste acces, i. þe   295
firste hache of þe febre, i. when þe febre firste turmentede him, and in þat
same houre schal *crisis* comen. And som saie wiþin þe 2 houre afore þat
hour þat it come, som saie wiþin 2 hours, and some saie by þe 2 hour or
elles by þe 2 hour byforne.

Item,[46] if þou wilt wete wheþer *crisis* **[f. 28va]** schal be gode or euel, i.   300
to lif or to deþ, or elles if after warsching he schal falle ageyn, þou most
know parfitely þe my3tes of þe pacient & tokenes þerwiþ. For þowh his
peyn be strong & huge, if his mi3tes be gode, if his onde be no3t ouerdone
streite, if he may smelle, if his poucis be skilful, and if eny tokne of decoccioun apere in his vryn, say him certeynly warschyng and þat gode. If *e*   305
contrario, it is doute & drede. Alle þise poyntz nerhand word for word
techeþ Isaac in þe forsaide boke.

---

39 moste] *foll. by* moste *canc.* R
40 4 tymes] *marg.:* 4 tymes of febris
41 Inicium] *marg.:* begynnyng
42 Augmentum] *marg.:* Augmentyng
43 Status] *marg.:* standyng
44 Declinacioun] *marg.:* Declinacioun
45 Item] *marg.:* What hour on þe nyght or dai shal be crisis
46 Item] *marg.:* Wheþer crisis schal be gode or euel

Gode tokenes in seke man[47] ar þise: myȝtihede in kynde (and þat is þe moste noble signe & tokne þat may be in a seke man); gode mynde; skilful slepe; appetit to som fode; noȝt ouerstreyt onde; smellyng at nose 310 (and namely of stynkyng thingz); liȝthede in body, i. if he mai steren and bywelden and turnen hymself; god colour in face, in þe lippes, in þe nase, & abouten the temples, i. þe thonewenges; egestioun, if it be vpon þe quantite of his ingestioun and noȝt blak in coloure ne wel swart, but more toward citrin colour, and if it stinke foule. Egestioun is schityng; inges- 315 tioun is etyng; and digestioun is defying, os seiþ þis verse: *Qui* [f. 28vb] *bene digerit ingerit egerit est bene sanus* (*anglice*: He þat wel ete, defieþ, and schite, / He is heil and hole wiþouten fit).

Swet ouer al þe body, hote or colde – but bettre is hote or elles an hote swete in þe heuede alone. But colde swete in þe heuede alone is perilouse, 320 as Isaac seiþ, þe 4 bok *De febribus*. If he fele in himself eny allegeance after þe swete, or elles if þe febre swage out þerwiþ, gode tokne and siker. Also if him þink þat his egestioun do hym gode, noble tokne. Bleding at þe nose *in die cretico*, and it be noȝt in exces but as he may godly suffre and bere, and principali if he fele eny alegeance or eny liȝtsomnessc in him þerafter. 325 Spatel white in colour and hongand wel togeder, and if he mai delyuer him þerof at onys or twies or 3 at þe most, and if he caste it wel fro him (of spatle: se in þe 13 c. *de ynopos and kyanos,* lef {81}); and brakyng wiþ eny allegance.

Wickede tokenes[48] ar þe contrarie to þise, and namely if þe ey-liddes 330 wax blo; and his nose waxe scharp & þenne & wronge; and þe noseþirle narow and gon togeder; and þe ende of þe nose colde; and his browes fallen and ar heuy; if teres of water come out at his on ey, & na- [f. 29ra] mely at his riȝt ey or at boþe agayn his wil; if þat one ey waxe lesse þan þat oþer; if his ey wax holwe and derk and dym and gastly lokand: alle þise ar 335 tokenes of deþ. And take gode hede þat þogh þer be mo wicked tokenes þan gode tokenes, ȝitt he may couer. And þogh þer be mo gode tokenes þan wicked tokenes, ȝit is no sikernes of warsshing. For þer is more dere dere in som one wicked þan helpe in 5 or 6 gode, and *e contrario*.

Et þerfor þou moste take hede at godenes and wickednes of[49] þe 340 tokenes and noȝt only at þe nombre of hem. Galien seiþ *Vppon Empidijs* þat þogh a seke body make Blak vryn in þe bigynnyng of þe malady and inward in þe malady eke, noȝtforþan he schal scape it, if þat he haue myȝt of kynde and skilful onde. Item, Galienus: when ferst in þe bigynnyng of

---

47   seke man] *marg.*: Gode tokenes in seke man
48   Wickede tokenes] *marg.*: Euel tokenes in seke man
49   of] M7CgHGSc, of of R

þe maladi come a Blake vryn, & þogh it leste so meny day and afterward   345
come into White wiþ a white *ypostasis*, if it so be þat he haue wiþin him
[mayn of kynde],[50] it seiþ sesyng and warshing. *Et* vnderstonde in this
2 reules þat Galien techeþ by Blak colour os Y saide in þe nexte reule
biforn þis 2.[51]

Þis worde *ypostasis* [f. 29rb] is somtyme taken[52] in special and somtyme   350
in general.[53] When it is taken in special, it is only in þe botume, in þe
gronde of þe vryn, and euermore when it is so, þan is it propurly *ypostasis*. Bot when it is in myddes of þe vryn, it is propurly called *eneorima*,
and when it is abouen, i. in þe ouer partie of þe vryn, it is callede *nephilis*
propurlik: *nephilis*, i. *nubes*, a skye. When it is taken generally, be it in   355
þe botume, be it in þe middis, or be it abouen, it [is][54] callede *ypostasis*
vnpropurlik; propurlik onely when it is in þe ouer partie of þe vryn. But
be it propurly, be it vnpropurly, it is euermore moste like a roke, a myste, a
cloude, a skye in þe vryn. And þe hier þat *ypostasis* halt him in þe vryn, þe
more ventosite, i. wynd, it seiþ in þe body. *Ypostasis* and al his propurtes: 360
se in þe 3 boke, þe 19 c., lef {110}.

Theophilus in his *Boke of Vryns* seiþ þat if a blak *ypostasis* or elles a
blak *eneorima* apere in þe vryn in a febre causoun, it seiþ þat þat ilk febre
causon[55] wil turne into a febre quarteyn.

Be blakhede in þe vryn is betokenede adustion of þe mater; by þe   365
[f. 29va] rok, ventosite. And also þat þat ilk adustioun is no3t so mykil þat
it ne haþ of humidite, which humidite is resoluede into a ventosite & þat
ventosite put vp the ypostasi and bereþ him alofte in þe vryn. And þan
is þe mater cacchede and dryuen aboute into þe veyns, and þere it rotteþ
and draweþ to filþe and corrupcioun & so causeþ a febre quarteyn. Of   370
þe quarteyn, se in þe next c. folwand, lef {29}. *Causonides* in þe 12 c. *de
rubicundo colore*, lef {79}. Vnderstonde þat euery Blak vryn in a febre,
what febre so it be, if þe vryn be þenner vpward þan dounward, seiþ lif.
& *e contrario*, deþ. Mo rewles of Bla[k][56] colour, se in þe laste chapitre of
þis boke, lef {om.}[57]   375

---

50   mayn of kynde] CgGSc, many of kende H, maner of a sonde RM7
51   2] M7HGSc, two Cg, tuo 2 R
52   taken] *marg.*: ypostasis is taken in 2 maneres
53   general] *foll. by* whan it is taken in special and some tyme in general *canc.* R
54   is] M7CgHGSc, *om.* R
55   causoun ... causon] M7, causon ... causon *foll. by erasure of* ides R; causon ... cau-
     sonides GSc; casonide ... causonides CgH
56   blak] M7CgH, bla R, *om.* GSc
57   Mo reules ... lef] GSc *replace this sentence with a series of appx. 9–10 regule for black
     urine.*

[2.3]

Here bigynneþ þe 3 chapitre, *de liuido coloure*, i. Blo colour

Blo colour in vryn is moste betwene White colour and Blak colour, hau-
and vnneþes more of Blak þan of White vppon ymaginacioun. And þerfor
alle auctours treten þerof next after Blak, be resoun þat it acordiþ moste
to Blak.   5
   The body of þe Blo vryn is kyndely White, but be cause of mixtioun of
partiez þat ar terrestre, i. erþisshe, and wiþ oþer parties þat bene aquose,
i. waterisshe, is þe blohede or elles blak- [f. 29vb] hede causede, for þe
parties þat bene terrestre bene kyndly blakisshe. And in þis wise is Blo
colour in vryn causede of White colour & of Blak colour. But nyh alle   10
auctours techen þat blohede in vryn is causede in 5 wise,[1] os be cause[2]
of turbacioun of humores in þe body, as it is in þe wombe flux. For in
euery flux, fleume, be resoun of his liquidite, i. of his meltandhede and
his nesshehede, he mengeþ and medeleþ him; and be resoun þerof he is
euermore principal medler and instrument in euery flux. And when he   15
renneþ and floweth aboute in þe body, þan ar þe humores al desturblede
and destemprede and in rore in þe body & in þe [v]eyns.[3] & be cause þerof
is gendrid a maner of blohede in þe vryn, i. a swarthede and a dymhede,
somdel toward blakhede.
   Item,[4] be cause of flux of humores, os in reume. In reume þe humores 20
ar desturbede and þe spiritz ar enfecte, i. dymhede and dulhede & al dismaihede, and so þe vryn takeþ a maner of blohede, for alse mykel as þe
humores in þe body haue loste here kynde brightnes, or elles haue noȝt al
here kynde brightnesse as þai schulde haue kyndely.
   Item,[5] be cause of defaute[6] [f. 30ra] of þe secunde digestioun, os it is in 25
ydropisi. For þan *epar* is distempred & biten wiþ frigidite, þe blod is noȝt
depurede ne defiede ne haþ noȝt his kynde norisshing as it schulde haue,
and þerfor þe blode comeþ to þe veyns and oþer membres & parties of þe
body. But neuerþeles, for alse mykel as it haþ noȝt his kyndly wirching *in*
epate as he schulde haue hade, & þerfor he is noȝt so kynde ne so myȝty 30
for to norsche and fode þe membres and þe parties of þe body, þe membres and þe parties of þe body take to hem of þat blode alle þat þai se able

---

1 5 wise] *marg.*: blohed in vryn is in 5 wise
2 be cause] *marg.*: j maner
3 veyns] CgHGSc, reyns RM7
4 Item] *marg.*: 2 maner
5 Item] *marg.*: 3 maner>
6 defaute] *catchword*: of þe secunde

and couenant to hem and answerant to here kynde. And þe remenant þei forsak and sende it agayn to *epar*. And þan syn þat it is v[n]pur[7] and crud & dym in colour, it causeþ swiche colour in þe vryn. And in þis wise is[8]   35 þe colde ydropisi gendrede.[9] How fele spices of ydropisi & which: 4 c. *de albo colore*, lef {38}. Of þe hote ydropisi: þe 10 chapitre *de rufo colore*, lef {57}. *Epar: 7 c. de colore karopos*, lef {1} & in þe j boke, þe 2 c., lef 3; þe 2 digestioun: in þe j bok, þe 3 c., lef {18}.

Item,[10] be cause of vnkynd hete menkede wiþ kynd hete, quenchand &   40 fordoand þe kynd hete and drawand out fro þe kynd hete þo parties þat be more subtile, which subtil parties made þe humores liȝt & bright. & so be cause þerof, þe vryn is dymish [**f. 30rb**] and bloissch. It ferþ be kynde hete & vnkynd hete in þe body of man os fire & water: mikel fyre fordoþ litil water & mykel water quencheþ a litil fire. Riȝt so it is bitwene kynd hete   45 & vnkynd hete[11] in mannes body.

Item,[12] be cause of enfeccioun and dymmyng & dullyng of þe spiritz in þe hert & in þe lyuer, & in þe arterijs & in þe veyns, & in oþer parties of þe body. *Cor*, þe hert: se in þe 7 c. *de karopos*, lef {57}. *Epar*, þe lyuer: se in þe same c. and in þe j bok, þe 2 c., lef {1}. Þe arteries: se in þe j c. of þis   50 boke, lef {18}.

Vnderstonde þat al þe veynes of mannes body bygynne at þe lyuer, os al þe synowes of þe body bygyn at þe hede, in þe hatrel byhynd in þe neþer party.

In þe lyuer bigynneþ a veyn þat is clepede *vena ramosa*,[13] the braun-   55 che veyn, for fro him sprediþ all oþer veyns. Þis *vena ramosa* is also calde *porta lactis* or *lactea porta*, mylk ȝate, for it receyueþ & vnder-fongeþ fro þe stomac a mater as white as mylk (which white mater is callede *tisanaria*, þe tisanarie[14]), be 8 veyns þat be clepede *meseraice*, þe miseraices. Of þe which miseraices, se in þe j boke, 3 c., lef 2. *Lactea*   60 *porta*[15] also is callede þat ilk rope, þat ilk gut, þat is callede *longaoun*. Of which *longaoun* þou haste in þe j bok, [**f. 30va**] 3 c., lef {3}. & þan it is called[e][16] so, s. mylk ȝate, for it is moste white of alle þe guttes in

---

7   vnpur] vnpure CgG, onpoure H, onripe Sc, vppur RM7
8   is] M7CgHGSc, it is R
9   gendrede] *marg.*: How þe colde ydropisie is gendrede
10 Item] *marg.*: 4 maner
11 & vnkynd hete] CgHGSc, & & vnkynd hete R, & (*eyeskip*) M7
12 Item] *marg.*: 5 (*overwritten with paraph*) maner
13 vena ramosa] *marg.*: vena ramosa
14 tisanarie] *marg.*: tisanarie
15 Lactea porta] *marg.*: lactea porta i. mylk ȝate
16 callede] M7CgHGSc, calledo R

þe body. Or elles it is callede mylk 3ate *per contrarium*, be contrarie, for of mylk, 3ate is him no3t, but for al þe filþe of þe wombe goþ þro3 him oute att tayle ende. <u>Also, *l[a]ctea*[17] *porta* is anoþer þing, as Y saide, þe j boke, þe þrid c.</u>   65

Item, þe forsaid braunche veyn is callede *arteria magna*,[18] þe greter arterie, for alse mykil os it is grettest of þe arteries and fro him com alle oþer arteries, and also be cause þat by hym principaly cometh kynde moystour and freschyng to al þe arteriez. <u>Arterijs: se in þis 2 bok, c. j, lef</u> {18}. Þan þis forsaide *vena ramosa*, anone it is diuised into 5 veyns þat diuisen hem anone into diuerse parties of þe lyuer,[19] and on of þo 5 veyns goþ to þe rigebone & þere he diuiseþ him into a flok of veyns þat arn calde *vene capillares*,[20] <u>of which I spake in þe j bok, þe 3 c., lef</u> {2}.   70   75

Þan þere is a veyn þat comeþ out of hem is called *kilis*, þe kile. *Kilis* is said of þis word of Grew *kilos*, i. *succus*, "iouse," for he & *vene capillares* þat ar tiede and knyt to þe rigebone bere þe iouse, i. þe vryn, fro þe lyuer into þe [**f. 30vb**] reyns, <u>os I saide in þe j bok, 3 c., lef.</u> {2}. Þan fro him sprede meny veyns aboute into þe lendes & in[21] diuerse parties, to þe hepes, to þe þies, to þe legges, fete, & toos. Of þe whiche, on[22] goþ in þe fote vnder þe knokel, & þeron is gode bledyng agayn malady of þe reyns & þe vesie & þe matrice & agayn apostemes & boches. & it is called *sophena*, "þe sophene."   80

Item, fro *vena ramosa* comen oþer veyns þat arn called *vrythides*[23] or elles *vrithides pori*, <u>os I seide in þe j boke, þe 3 c., lef</u> {3}.   85

Item, fro *vena ramosa* comen certeyn veyns þat arn callede *emoraide*[24] or *emoroides*, of this worde *ema* or *emak*, i. *sanguis*, "blode," & of þis worde *roys*, i. *fluxus*, "þe flux." For by þo veyns & in þo veyns, meny men hauen þe flux of blode, wiþ scharpe & huge peyn. & þat is callede in Englisshe "þe emoroys." Þis terme *emoroide* or *emoroides* is taken boþe for þe veyns and for þat maladi eke. And vnderstonde þat men haue here purgacions by þe emorais, as haue women by her floures. <u>Þe emorais & how fele spices be þerof: se in þe 3 boke, 18 c., lef</u> {109}.   90

---

17 lactea] CgHGSc, lectea RM7
18 arteria magna] *marg.*: arteria magna
19 lyuer] *foll. by* and on of þo 5 veyns þat diuise hem anone into diuerse parties of þe lyuer *canc.* R
20 vene capillares] *marg.*: vene capillares
21 & in] M7CgH, in G, to Sc, & into & in R
22 on] *marg.*: Sophena
23 vrythides] *marg.*: vritides
24 emoraide] *marg.*: emoroide

Item, fro *vena ramosa* com meny wonder smale veyns & come al into on   95
in þe bak of þe lyuer, and þat is called *vena concaua*,²⁵ þe holwe veyne, for
he is grete & holwe. & he is anone diuisede **[f. 31ra]** into 2 branches. Þat on
branch, os Galien seiþ, goþ inne by þe myddes of *diafragma*, þe mydrede,
and entreþ into þe left syde of þe hert, & of þat artarye cum alle þat oþer
arteries & veyns þat gon vpward in þe body: to þe þrote, þe nek, þe heuede,   100
þe armes, handes, and fyngres. <u>*Diafragma: 7 c. de karopos,* lef</u> {57}. Þan by
þis artery, þis branch þat comeþ þus vp to þe hert, is þe hert tiede & knet
to þe lunges & draweþ to him eire by þe pipes of þe lunges, by whiche eyr
þe hert is refresshede, i. colide & temperede. And þis artarie þus at þe hert
is called *adortus*, "adort." *Adortus*, i. *ad cor ortus* (*anglice*: spryngond at þe   105
hert), for at þe hert he diuiseþ him into 2 braunches: on goþ to þe lunges &
fro þe lunges forth to þe riȝt honde, noȝt euen streiȝt but awrang; þe toþer
branche goþ euen streiȝt to þe lefte hande, and þat is þe skil whie þe pouce
is more certeyn to deme of in þe lefte wirste þan in þe riȝt wirste.²⁶

Þat veyn þat comeþ fro þe lunges to þe riȝt hand, os I saide, when he   110
comeþ at þe riȝt scholder, þere he diuiseþ him like a crokede fork and his
on braunche goþ to þe heuede; & þat oþer, as Y saide, to þe riȝt arme, and
þat is called *vena cephalica*,²⁷ þe heuede **[f. 31rb]** veyn. Bledyng of þis veyn
is helpyng agayn þe sephalarge, agayn þe falland euyl, agayn sekenes of þe
eyȝen os bolnyng o þe eyȝen & blod fallyng into þe eyȝen and swyche oþer   115
poyntz. *Cephalargia*, þe cephalarge, is taken for euery maner malady in þe
heuede comand fro wiþinward.

Vnder *cephalica vena* liþ a veyn þat is called *mediana*,²⁸ þe myd veyn.
Blodlast in þis veyn is agayn *dis[ma]*²⁹ & *asma* & *octomia* & *peripulmonia*,
& principaly agayn al ma[la]dies³⁰ of þe spirituales. <u>*Disma* is said in þe j</u>   120
<u>bok, þe 4 c.,</u> lef {om.}. *Asma* &<u> *octomia* & *peripulmonia*: se inward,</u> lef
{om.}. Þe spiritual membres: se in þe 7 c. <u>*de colore karopos,* lef</u> {56}. Ȝit
vnder þis veyn, s. vnder þe myd veyn, is anoþer veyn þat is callede *vena*
*epatica*³¹ (*anglice*: þe lyuer veyn). And also it is calde *vena basilica*, þe baas
veyn. & minucioun, i. blodelast, on þis veyn, is principaly agayn sekenes   125
of þe lyuer and of þe stomac & agayn þe pleuresy & agayn sekenes of
þe nutrityues. Sekenes <u>of þe lyuer is callede *epatica passio*: se inward.</u>³²

---

25   vena concaua] *marg.*: vena concaua
26   riȝt wirste] *marg.*: þe pulse is more certeyn in þe riȝt side þan in þe lefte
27   vena cephalica] *marg.*: Cephalica
28   mediana] *marg.*: Mediana
29   disma] GSc, dissuria RM7CgH
30   maladies] M7CgH, passiouns G, passion Sc, madies R
31   vena epatica] *marg.*: epatica and basilica
32   inward] *foll. by* lef *canc.* R

Pleuresis, þe pleuresy: se inward.[33] *Membra nutritiua,* membres nutrityues: 7 c. *de colore karopos,* lef {58}.

Item, fro *vena concaua* comeþ veyns to þe stomac, & fro the **[f. 31va]** 130
stomac come certeyn veyns vp to þe nek & into þe þrote & serue vnto þe
voys & ar callede *fibre,* þe fibres. *Fibra,*[34] i. os *vibrans,* i. brayand out wiþ
my3t, for vp þat þe fibres ar stronge & my3ty, so is þe voys. Item, vnder þe
baas veyn, faste by þe albowe, is a veyn þat comeþ fro þe *splen,* þe mylt,
& goþ into þe litil fynger. & bledyng of þat veyn, whereuer on may haue 135
hym, fordoþ sekenes of þe splene & mykel abateþ wikede humores of
melancolie & mykel liteþ man. & þis veyn is callede *sp[l]enetica*[35] *vena,*[36]
þe splene veyn. And as is of eny of þise 4 veyns in þat on arme, s. þe heuede veyn, þe spiritual veyn or elles þe myd veyn, þe lyuer veyn, þe splene
veyne, ri3t so it is in þat oþer arme.   140

Item, in woman is a veyn þat is calde *kynirz,*[37] þe kyner, & bigynneþ at
þe lyuer, as alle veyns don, & diuiseth him into 2 braunchez. Þat on goþ to
þe lefte syde & þat oþer to þe ri3t; and eiþer of hem ar diuised in diuerse
branches, of which branches som go to þe matrice, berand wiþ hem of
blode to þe norisshing and fodyng of þe matrice and also for to gendre þe 145
floures. And þe remanant of þe braunches go to þe pappis, beronde wiþ
hem eke of þe blode, for to make it white and turne it into mylk **[f. 31vb]**
and into fode of þe childe.

And [as] alle[38] þe veyns bygyn at þe lyuer, ri3t so alle þe synowes[39] bigyn
at þe cerebre, i. þe brayn in þe heuede, and alle þe bones atte þe hede 150
panne. First come 2 synowes fro þe braynes into þe forparty of þe heuede
and anone diuisen hem in þe myd forheuede. And þat one goþ to þe ri3t
eye, þat oþer to þe lefte eye; and eþer of hem is callede *opticus*[40] or elles
vena visibilis, optik or þe veyn of si3t, for by hym þe spiritz & þe my3tes
of þe sight ar born fro þe cerebre to þe eyen, for to cause and 3if sight. 155

Þan oþere two synowes come fro þe same party of þe cerebre but more
outwarde, s. at þe endys of þe front, gon to þe eeris, berand eke wiþ ham
spiritz and my3tz for to forme þe heryng. And þerfor eyþer of hem is calde
neruus audibilis,[41] þe synow of heryng. And eke it is callede *posticius,* for

---

33 inward] *foll. by* lef *canc.* R
34 fibra] *marg.*: Fibra
35 splenetica] CgHSc, splenatica G, spenetica R, spenitica M7
36 splenetica vena] *marg.*: splenetica
37 kynirz] *marg.*: kyneris
38 And as alle] CgHG, And as Sc, And alle RM7
39 synowes] *marg.*: Nerue
40 opticus] *marg.*: opticus or nerf visible
41 neruus audibilis] *marg.*: Nerf audible

þai begyn byhynde and go bakward. Item, þai ar callede *ossa petrosa*, ston   160
bone, and also *nerui petrosi*, synowy ston, for here hardnes. For þai ben
hard be waie of kynde, þat þe aire may þe bettre smyten & bere þe bettre
stroke & þe heryng [be][42] þe more my3ty. For þe more harde & þe more
sad þat a þing be, þe bettre it souneþ, as a belle of sad meta[l][43] souneþ bettre þan a bel of lede.   165

Item, fro[44] the same partie of þe cerebre com **[f. 32ra]** 2 herd gristeles
in þe nose and ar callede *nerui odorabiles*,[45] þe smellyng synowez. Oþer
tuo to þe tunge þat ar callede *nerui gustabiles*,[46] þe s[walw]yng synowes.[47]
Oþer tuo eke cum fro þe same party of þe cerebre, of which on þat riseþ on
þe ri3t half goþ to þe ri3t schulder, and þer he is crokede, and his on braun-   170
che passeþ into þe ri3t honde & þat oþer to þe ri3t fote. But no3tforþan
þai boþe ar diuisede into 5 braunches and þo 5 go to þe 5 fyngres, euerych
to his; on þe same wise, his felawe þat ryseþ on þe lefte halfe passeþ to þe
lefte schuldur, and ry3t so is crokede in þe lefte schulder, and goþ so forþ
as his felow in þe ri3t halfe. And þis arne called *nerui tangibiles*,[48] þe felyng   175
synowes. For in hem & by hem and by þe branche þat comeþ of hem is
þe toching and þe felyng in man, and principaly in þe handes & in þe fete.
& alle þise forsaide synowes in mannes body arn callede *nerui sensibiles*,
synowes of wytte and of felyng, for þai ar as it were þe instrumentz of
mannes wyttz & felynges.   180

Alle oþer synowes in man arn called *nerui motiui*,[49] synowes of movyng
& of stering. For in hem & þro3 hem principaly is þe meuyng & stering of
best. And þise synowes motiues begin at þe cerebre in þe ha- **[f. 32rb]** trel,
i. in þe hynner party of þe heuede, as þe toþer begynne beforn, as Y saide.
But sum bigyn at þe hatrel *immediate* & som *mediate*. Þis 2 termes *medi-*   185
ate & immediate: þe j boke, þe 3 c., lef {3}. Þo synowes begynne in þe hatrel
immediate þat rechen to þe next placis, as to þe nek; *mediate* þat rechen
and spreden to þe ferþer placis of þe body, be mene of þe nuk. *Nuca*,[50] þe
nuk, is þe marowe of þe rigebon & it bygynneþ in þe hynder party of þe
cerebre byhynde, & lasteþ doun to þe laste ende of þe bak, lyand alonge   190

---

42 be] may be GSc, *om.* RM7CgH
43 metal] M7CgHG, mater and metal hit Sc, metak R
44 fro] M7CgHGSc, fro (*line end*) fro R
45 nerui odorabiles] *marg.*: Neruez odorables
46 nerui gustabiles] *marg.*: Neruez gustablez
47 swalwyng synowes] senewes of swologh (swologht Sc) GSc, smellyng synowes RM7,
    (smelling *canc.*) \tastyng (*in later hand*)/ senewys H, *om.* Gc
48 nerui tangibiles] *marg.*: Neruez tangiblez
49 nerui motiui] *marg.*: Nervez motiues
50 Nuca] *marg.*: Nuca

in þe bak, white os mylk and wapped in 2 þenne skynnes þat ben of þe
materie of *pia mater* & *dura mater*. And by þo two þen skynnes is *nuca*
defendede and kepede fro þe hardnes and fro hurtyng of þe iountours of
þe ryge. What ar *pia mater* & *dura mater, se in þe 7 c. de karopos, lef* {56}.

Þe rigebone is of 18 ioyntours. 6 bene accomptede for þe nek & 12 for   195
þe bak. Þise[51] 12 ioyntoures ar callede *spondilia dorsi*,[52] þe ioyntours of þe
bak. Þan bytwene euerych of þe tuo ioyntours ris tuo synowes, þat in a
man gone doune and maken þe ʒerde. And þe ʒerde is þe ende of þe synowes, for in him al þe sinowes endiþ. In a woman, þo 2 **[f. 32va]** synowes
go to þe ouer mouth of þe matrice, and wiþ hem somtyme þe matrice   200
mouþe speriþ hym and somtyme openyth hym, for to vnderfonge þe sede
and þe kynde of generacioun \of man/, as þou schal se inward, þer I speke
of þe matrice of woman.

Item, fro þe hynder partie of þe heuede come 2 synowes and gon to
þe ouer chauel, & þan forth to þe neþer chauelle, & þere it is eftesones   205
reflecte, i. bowede agayn, to þe ouer chauel. And þis is þe skil whi þe neþer
chauel moueth & þe ouer chauel noʒt.[53]

Item, þere come 2 synowes fro þe[ny]sward,[54] and go to þe tunge. And
by hem þe tunge moueþ þe fode when on etiþ.

Item, o[þ]er[55] tuo synowes com fro þenward and go to þe lunges and   210
ar reflecte agayn[56] to þe tunge, & þai ar callede *nerui vocales*,[57] þe speche
synowes, for vppon þe disposicioun of hem is sounyng of speche in þe
tunge.[58] For somtyme þise synowes bene ouer large and þan mow þai noʒt
soune þis letter "S." And þis[59] synow is called *psidius*, þe psidi or elles
wlisper. *Psidius* also is he þat wlispeþ & it oweþ to be writen *psi-*. And   215
somtyme þise synow endeþ in þe myddes of þe tunge, & þan he mai noght
wel bring forth þis letter, "I." And þan is **[f. 32vb]** eyþer of þo synowes
callede *stancus*, þe stanccy, or elles þe stamerer. And *stancus* is he þat sta-
mereþ and þerof comeþ *stancitare*, stameryn, os *psidiare* is to wlispe.

Of þise forsaid þinges it semeþ wel what arterijs bene, and also þe dif-   220
ference atwene arterijs and veyns. For euery artarie is a veyn, but noʒt *e*

---

51 Þise] *foll. by* þis *canc.* R
52 spondilia dorsi] *marg.*: spondiles of þe bak
53 ouer chauel noʒt] *marg.*: Whi þe ouer chauel moueþ noʒt
54 þenysward] M7, theneward CgHG, þens Sc, þeyns (*line end*) inward (*with in under-
    puncted*) R
55 oþer] CgHGSc, ouer RM7
56 and ar reflecte agayn] *foll. by* & ar reflecte agay *canc.* R
57 nerui vocales] *marg.*: Neruez vocales
58 speche in þe tunge] *marg.*: Whi lisper and stamerer
59 and þis] *prec. by* and þis *canc.* R

contrario. For *vena* is as mykil for to saie os *viema* (*anglice*: þe waie of blode), of þis worde *via*, "a waie," and of þis worde *ema* or *emac*, "blode." For þe veyns ar þe places & þe waies of blode. Or elles *vena*, as who seith *viema*, i. *vasa sanguinis*, þe vesseles of blode,[60] for þe blode is contenede in   225 þe veyns as liquour in a vessel. And þerfor in þis faculte, veyns ar callede þe waie of blode & þe vesseiles of blode. What arterijs bene and wherof saide, <u>se in þis boke, þe j chapitre, lef</u> {18}.

Þe forsaide pipes of the lunges ar callede *fistule pulmonis* & *canales pulmonis* (*anglice*: þe lunge pipes). <u>*Pulmo*, os I saide, is þe lunge of a beste: se in</u>   230 <u>þe 7 c. *de colore karopos*, lef</u> {57}. *Fistula* & *canalis*, a pype. Wiþin þis pipes of þe lunges is oþerwhile gaderede & gendred, be cause of wickede humores & of vnhelþe, foule corrupt mater, and þat causeth a maladie [**f. 33ra**] þat is callede *sansugium*:[61] sumtyme wiþoute þe pipes, fast by aboute hem, & þan it causeth sekenes þat is callede *disma*[62] and sometyme a sekenes þat is   235 callede *asma*;[63] & somtyme boþe wiþin and wiþoute & þan a sekenes þat is callede *octomia*.[64] Alle þise 4 maladyes are sekenes of þe lunges.

Þan for to know þise 4 sekenes of þe lunges, tak hede þat *sansugium* is when þe onde is large inward and streite outward. *Disma* is when þe onde is streit inward and harde for to aperceyue fro wiþou[t]ward,[65] þat is to saie,   240 to oþer mennes heryng. *Asma* is when it is streit outward and esie for to here, for when on haþe þe *asma*, he ratelith & rikelith in his ondyng. *Octomia* is when it is boþe *disma* & *asma*, so þat boþe *asmaticus* and *octomicus* make rikelyng in her ondyng, lik to as when on smyteþ tuo strawes þat on to þat oþer. *Asmaticus* & *octomicus*, *sansugenicus* and *dismaticus* ar þai þat   245 haue þo maladies. *Pulmonicus*[66] is he þat haþe sekenes of þe lunges.

But þogh blohede in vryn be causede in 5 wise, os Y saide and os ny3 alle auctours techen, no3tforþan Gilbert seiþ expressely þat it is causede but [**f. 33rb**] in on maner, os when tuo bodies ny3 togeder, of which þat on is bright and clere & þat oþer schadoweþ and dymmeþ & derkeþ. If þe   250 derkenes of þat on be more þan þe brightnes of þat oþer, þan when þai neihen togeder, þe clerenes & þe brightnes of þat on is menusede, i. is þe lesse, be cause[67] of ny3hede of þat oþer. And so is caused a maner of dymhede & derkehede þat is mykel toward blohede or blakishede. Example he geuyþ

---

60   vesseles of blode] *marg.*: What be veyns
61   sansugium] *marg.*: sansugium
62   disma] *marg.*: disma
63   asma] *marg.*: asma
64   octomia] *marg.*: octomia
65   wiþoutward] M7CgHG, owtwarde Sc, wiþouward R
66   Pulmonicus] *marg.*: pulmonicus
67   be cause] *foll. by* by cause *canc.* R

by a stikk when it begynnes for to brenne, and eke example by a candel os   255
when on liȝtes it, and also be example of þe reynbowe, which reynbowe is
but a refleccioun of liȝt in a hol cloude, I passe be cause of prolixte.

  Et þerfor, os he seyth, blohede in vryn is a schadowyng and a dymmyng, ouercomend and ouergoand þe *spiritus* & þe kynde hete & þe
humores, and so is caused dymhede & blohede in vryn. And vnderstonde   260
þat blakhede & blohede ar al on in significacioun, saue þat blakhede is
more maliciouse þan Blo.

  Item, vnderstonde þat þer is tuo maner of blohede[68] in þe vryn: somtyme þe
vryn is Blo mykel like a draght of lede wiþ a plum in papir or in a perchemyne
lef, and swich **[f. 33va]** blohed euermor seiþ mortificacioun; & somtyme it is   265
os it wer a maner of dymhede, a dirkhede acordand mykel toward blakhed, &
swich maner blohede somtyme seiþe mortificacioun and somtyme adustioun.
But þus schalt þou wete & knowe when þat on & when þat oþer: if it so be
þat þer apere in þe vryn a maner of grenehede, or elles if vryn aforn þat vryn
aperede wiþ a maner of grenehede, it seiþ adustioun. If no grenehede, morti-   270
ficacioun. <u>Adustion & mortificacioun in þis bok, j c., lef</u> {18}.

  Item, tak hede þat blohed in vryn sumetyme it is total, i. oueral Blo,
and sometyme particuler, i. Blo but on party. If þe blohede be total, i.
þorghoute Blo, it seiþ on of þise 2 poyntz: oþer it seiþ mortificacioun of
blode and noȝt of þe lyuer, or elles it seiþ mortificacion boþe of blode &   275
of þe lyuer. But when þat on & when þat oþer, þus schalt þou know: late
þe vryn haue his residence & if it afterward schewe him wiþ no blohede,
it[69] seiþ mortificacioun of þe blode and noȝt of þe lyuer; if it so be þat þe
vryn afterwarde, þat it haue his kynde residence apere blo, it seiþ mortificacioun of boþe, s. of blode & of þe lyuer eke.   280

  When þe vryn is but parti- **[f. 33vb]** culer Blo, i. but on place þerof, þat
is euermore abouen in þe ouer party of þe vryn, or elles fro þe myddes
vpward. And þis is þe philosophie: for þe spiritz þat ar sent oute wiþ þe
vryn ar, or þai com oute, vmbrede & dirkede & dymhede be cause of vanysshyng and lessyng of kynde in þe body. & þe propurte and þe myȝght & þe   285
vertue of þe hete and þe spiritz is for to drawe vpward kyndely, and þerfor
þorgh wirkyng of ham, þe blohede halt him abouen in þe vryn. And þerfor
euery maner of blohede in vryn betokeneþ mortificacioun, os it befalleþ
comunely in þe emytrices.

  An emitrice is as mykel for to saie os a menket febre. And þerfor tak   290
hede þat þere be 3 emytrices:[70] þe lesse and þe more and þe myd. The lesse

---

68 of blohede] *foll. by* of blohede *canc.* R, *marg.*: 2 manerz of blohede
69 it] M7CgHGSc, it it R
70 emytrices] *marg.*: spices of þe emytrices

emitrice is a febre þat is componede of a febre cotidien continuel & of a
febre terciane interpollate; the more emitrice of a febre quarteyn continuel & of a febre tercien interpollate; the mydde emytrice of a febre tercien
continuel & of a cotidiane interpollate. *Febris cotidiana*,[71] a febre cotid- 295
ian, is þat turmenteþ euery day. *Febris continua*, a febre contynuel, þat
turmenteþ continuely, i. alwaie, and seseth no3t til he part, or to deþ or to
lif. *Febris terciana*, a febre tercien, is þat **[f. 34ra]** turmentes euery 3 daye,
for to saie on wiþ þe first axces, and tuo wiþ þe nexte dai after, & 3 wiþ þat
oþer day þat he takeþ agayn. And þis maner of febre tercien is callede *sim-* 300
plex terciana, a simple terciene, for euermore a simple terciene hath but
on day reste bytwene 2 axces. Of þe febre tercien be dyuerse spices,[72] os
terciana vera & *terciana non vera, terciana naturalis* & *terciana non natu-*
ralis, duplex terciana & *duoterciana*. *Terciana vera*, a verraie tercyene, is
þat lastiþ but 7 axces, as Ypocras seiþ. *Terciana non vera*, 9 or 11 daies, or 305
elles mo. *Terciana naturalis* & *terciana non naturalis*, a kynd tercien and
an vnkynde tercien, ar þe same as *vera* & *non vera*. *Duplex terciana*, a
double tercien, is þat turmenteþ euery day, but strenger, i. more scharply,
fro þe 3 dai to þe 3 day. *Duoterciana*, a deutercien, þat haþ þe first daie
of interpollacioun, i. of restyng betwene, os *simplex terciana* hath, but it 310
turmentith twise on þe þrid daie, i. it hath 2 exces on þe þrid day.

Febris interpolata, a febre interpolate, is in 3 maner: on þat is callede
simplex interpolata, a simple interpolate, þat turmenteþ bo[t]e[73] onis on
þe day, i. þat hath but on axces on **[f. 34rb]** þe daye. *Bina interpolata*, or
duplex interpolata, a double interpolate, twies on þe day. *Trina interpolata*, 315
or *triplex interpolata*, a treble interpolate, þrise on þe daye.

Febris quartana,[74] þe febre quarteyn, is eke in meny wise: *simplex quar-*
tana, qua[r]tana[75] *vera* al on; *quartana non vera, bina quartana, duplex*
quartana & *duoquartana*. *Simplex quartana* & *quartana vera* al on: þat
turmenteþ euery 4 day & 24 houres, & hauand 2 daies betuene of interpo- 320
lacioun, os *simplex terciana* haþ one day atwene.[76] *Qua[r]tana*[77] *non vera*,
a false quarteyn or elles a faws quarteyn, is þat turmenteþ more or lesse
þan 24 houres. *Bina quartana* or *duplex quartana*, a twey quarteyn or a
dubul quarteyn, al on: þat turmentz þe 4 day & þe 2 day after þe 4 day.

---

71 Febris cotidiana] *marg.*: spice of cotidiens
72 spices] *marg.*: spices of þe tercien
73 bote] but CgHGSc, boþe RM7
74 Febris quartana] *marg.*: spices of þe quarteyn
75 quartana] M7CgHGSc, quatana R
76 day atwene] day hatwene (*with* ha *canc., in error for* h *canc.*) R
77 Quartana] M7CgHGSc, Quatana R

Duoquartana, þe deuquarteyn, haþ 2 axces in þe 4 day, os deuterciene haþ   325
on[78] þe þr[i]d[79] day 2 acces.

Item, þer is a maner of febre þat is callede *epiala*.[80] *Epiala* is saide
of þis worde *epy*, i. *supra*, abouen, and of þis word *algor*, colde. For
in *epiala*, i. in þe colde febres, he is colde abouen; þat is to seyn, in þe
owter partyes of his body, and hote wiþin þe body. And þis febre is   330
euermore causede **[f. 34va]** of fleume and melancolie gros and corrupt
and gaderede in þe stomak. For of wickede humores gaderand into filþe
and corrupcioun in þe stomac, þer is resoluede fro hem, i. þer comeþ[81]
of hem a fumosite and þat greueþ & distemperiþ þe hert. And so is þere
causede an vnkynde hete wiþin þe body. And þan som of þat fumosite   335
smyt out and bresteþ out to þe vtter places of þe body. And þere it
diffundiþ and disparpliþ þe fleume vitre þat is vnder þe hide, and of
þat is causede cold. *Fleuma vitrium*, *fleuma album*, *and fleuma naturale*
(fleu[m][82] vitre, fleume blank, & fleume naturel): *in capitulo de g[l]auco*[83]
colore, *lef* {43}.   340

Item, anoþer febre þat is callede *lipparia*, þe hote febre, but noȝt þat
þat þai calle þe brennand febre. And is *e contrario* in þe lippiarie to þat
it is in þe epial. *Lipparia*[84] is caused of corupt colre vnder þe hyde. While
colre gadereþ into corrupcioun, þere comeþ a fumosite smytand aboute
þe hert, & þere causeþ a distemperure of hete. & þan þat colre þat is so   345
distemperede diffundiþ and dilateþ him by þe inder parties of þe body and
causeþ vnkynde hete in þo parties. And some of þat þat it draweþ to þe
inder parties of þe body and þere he diffundeþ **[f. 34vb]** and disperpleþ þe
fleume vitre þat he fyndeþ þere. And be cause of diffusioun and disperplyng of þe fleume is causing of [vn]kynd[85] colde in þe body. And þise 2   350
febres, s. *epiola* & *lipparia*, ar febres interpolates, i. ar called so.

Item, þer is a febre þat is cleped *effimerina*,[86] effimeryne, and þis is þe
lest greuand febre þat is. For þe same dai it comeþ, þe same day it goþ. And
þerfor it bereþ þe name of a worme þat is calde *effimera*, which worme þe
same day þat it is genderede, þe same dai it dieþ. Sum saie þat it is saide   355
of þis word of Gru *effimeron*, litil & subtil, for þis[87] febre is of a mater þat

---

78 on] *foll. by* one *canc.* R
79 þrid] M7, 3 CgHGSc, þrd R
80 epiala] *marg.*: epiala
81 comeþ] M7CgHGSc, co (*line end*) comeþ R
82 fleum] CgHG, flewma Sc, fleu. M7, fleu R
83 glauco] CgH, ȝolowe G, þelo Sc, g auco M7, gauco R
84 Lipparia] *marg.*: lipparia
85 vnkynd] GSc, kynd RM7CgH (*see note*)
86 effimerina] *marg.*: effimerina
87 for þis] *foll. by* fe for þis *canc.* R

is[88] simple & subtil, þat is to saie in spirit, for þe *spiritus* ar but a litil fadede
and feyntede, and anone it passeth awaie.

A cotidien continuel comeþ[89] of fleume þat is corrupte in þe vesseiles
of þe blode (vesseiles of blode ar þe veynes). And þis febre is knowen be   360
continuel akyng of þe heuede and by hete first lent, by schronkkelyng of
þe browes, & redehede in þe eyen, and bolnyng in þe face, and coloure lik
askes, euyl sauour in þe mouthe, bolne wombe and brakyng, & by astony-
ing and maseing of mynde & of þe wittes. For grete asstonying in þe febre
is verrai tokne [f. 35ra] þat fleume is cause of þat febre. If he speke mykel,   365
colre is[90] in þe cause. If he spek noȝt, melancolie.

Febris terciana cometh[91] of colre corrupte in þe vesseiles. And þou
mayst know it by akyng of the heuede, & mykel wakyng, and dasowyng
in þe eiȝen, and emty brayn, rede eyȝen, & now here now ȝonde, drie
mouþ (and namely þe palate), blak tunge be cause of brennyng of vnkynd   370
hete, & also by quakyng at þe hert.

Febris quartana cometh[92] of corrupte melancolie in þe vesseiles. & þis
is comunely þe manner þerof: first gonyng, þan þe lippes wax ded & wan,
þan stifhede and starkehede; after þat huge colde & quakyng and reysyng,
as al þe body schulde tobristen; and at þe laste comeþ a lent hete & litil   375
swete or none. And tak þis for a reule: þat þer oweþ no medycyn to be
ȝeuen in þe quarteyn byfore þe 7 acces. Item, þat no stronge medicyne
oweþ be ȝeuen hem. Item, þat his medycyn oweþ be ȝeuen him noȝt only
at o tyme but often tyme.

Þan vnderstond for a reule: þat Blo vryn wiþ a litil body and wiþ a maner   380
of Fathede abouen, in maner of gres or oyle, & [f. 35rb] wiþ a droublihede,
seiþ a wombe flux or elles flux of þe emoraies, saue þat in þe flux is þe vryn
more whitisshe, in þe emorays more bloisshe. And vnderstond here and
nerhand alwaie, when I speke of Blo vryn (noȝt only for vryn pure Blo
but also for a maner of dirkehede and dymhede moste accordyng toward   385
blakhede, as Y saide aboute þe firste ende of þis chapitre), þat þe vryn is
Blo is for þis skyl: for in euery wombe flux, þe humores in þe body & in þe
veyns ar distempred and distourblede, and renne and hurle togedre in þe
vesseiles, i. in þe veyns, and in þe body. And þan medelith fleume wiþ þat
oþer humores, for fleume is euermore principal cause & instrume[nt][93] of   390

---

88   þat is] *foll. by* þat is *canc.* R
89   cotidien continuel comeþ] *marg.*: Whereof comeþ þe cotidien continuel
90   is] *foll. by* is *canc.* R
91   Febris terciana cometh] *marg.*: Wherof tercien comeþ
92   Febris quartana cometh] *marg.*: Wherof comeþ febre quarteyn
93   instrument] CgHGSc, instrumei RM7

flux. And so vnder hem alle, þai cause þe flux and gendre vnkynde colour in þe vryn.

Þat þe vryn is litil is be cause þat al þe moystour in þe body renneþ and seweth to þe guttes. Þat it is gresie and fatte seiþ þat kynde meltiþ and wasteþ & vanyssheþ awai. Þat it is þikkisshe and droublisshe it seith þat 395 þe humores in þe body ar al distemprede & distourbled, [**f. 35va**] and þat is by cause [þat]⁹⁴ terrestretes and aquosites of þe humores in þe body ar myxt togeder, and þerof it is caused.

Item, vryn Blo & fat abouen and wonder litil in quantite seiþ deþ, and namely if þer come an acue vpon hym þerwiþ. That it is Blo is be cause þat 400 þe humores and þe kynde ar nerhand consumte, i. wasted and fordon, as it falliþ comunely in þe etik. Þat it is fat, as I saide in þe nexte reule aforne. What is etik: se inward, lef {23}. Þat it is wonder litil, it seiþ þat þe passyng places, i. þe waies of þe vryn, ar deppede and stoppede, þat þe vryn may no3t haue his ful course oute os he schulde haue. 405

Item, vryn Blo and litil & often tyme made, i. now a drylle and now a drylle, seiþ *stranguiriam*, þe stranguyrie. Se stranguyrie, þe j boke, þe 4 chapitre, lef {7}. *Stranguiria*⁹⁵ is causede þorgh oppilacioun, i. stoppyng, of þe nek of þe vesye, or of þe stone, or of sum vnkynd humor, or elles þorgh stoppyng of som aposteme bredand þerabouten. By alle þise 4 causes may 410 superfluites of wiked humores wiþholden and letten þe vryn. And by cause of swyche poyntes ar oþerwhile þe spirites and þe kynd hete dirked & dymhede & enfecte & feblis- [**f. 35vb**] schede, and so is blohede in vryn oþerwhile causede, & namely in þe stranguirie.

Item, vryn Blo and litil, wiþ smale Greyns aboute in þe body of þe 415 vryn, and þe blohede be particuler, s. aboue, it seiþ *malum spirituale*, os *pthisica* or *ethica* or *pulmonica passio*. But þe same maner vryn wiþ total blohede, i. throghoute Blo, seiþ *pleuresis*, or *passio epatica*, or *catarrus*, or elles passioun of þe matrice, i. sekenes of þe modur. Now for to know parfitely þise 2 forsaide reules and al þe termes þat bene menged þerin, 420 vnderstond þat *malum spirituale* (*anglice*: sekenes of þe spirituales, i. of þe spiritual membres). Whiche be þe spiritual membres, and also nerhand al þe membres of mannes body, se in. c. *de karopos* {57}. And whie þai ar callede þe spiritual membres is by resoun of þe *spiritus*, i. of ondyng and of drawyng of þe wynde, for in þo membres and by þo membres, s. þe 425 hert, þe lunges, þe mydrede, þe tracheartarie, and þe epiglote, is drawyng of wynd and ondyng and meuyng of lif. *Liuiditas particularis* and *liuiditas totalis* is expounede in þis same c., lef {28}.

---

94 by cause þat] CgHG, by cause of RM7, cause þat Sc
95 Stranguiria] *marg.*: Wherof cometh þe stranguirie

Pthisica[96] is a malady, a sekenes, þat is called þe pthisik. *Pthisicus* is he þat haþ þe pthisik. Þis terme *pthisica* or *pthisis*, **[f. 36ra]** þat al on is to 430 saye, is often tyme [take][97] propurly and often tyme vnpropurly. When it is taken propurly, it is noþing but *vlceracio pulmonis*, i. blemysshyng and wastyng and dwynyng awaie of þe lungz. Vnpropurly: or elles largely, as Y saide ry3t now, or elles for consumpcioun of alle þe body. And as þe comentour, i. expositour, seiþ vppon Ypocras *Afforismys*, in þe 5 particule: 435 *pthisica* is principally bytwene þe 18 3ere and þe 25 3ere. *Et* þai þat ben taken þerwiþ wiþin 25 3ere, þai scape no3t comunely þe 35 3ere; and þogh þai do, þai leue no3t longe after.

And þai ar disposede to þe pthisik[98] þat haue longe bodyes and swong wronge legges, longe & smale neckes, & smale and streit brestes. And as 440 Auicen seiþ, o skil is for swiche folk ete mykel and defie litil, wherfor þe veyns be replete, i. fillede, wiþ foule corrupte mater of blode. For feble digestioun euermore causeth wicked blode, and þorgh defaute of gode blode, þe membres of þe body may no3t haue here kynde norisshing ne fodyng as þai schulde haue. And þan bygynneþ her kynd for to wasten and vanysshyn 445 and dwynen awaie. And whie more in þat age þan in oþer, þis he saiþ is þe skil: for in þat age and in þo 3eris, **[f. 36rb]** þe blode is more plentouse and more habundant in hem þan in eny oþer age, and in þo 3eres 3onge men fonden and assaie here strenghes in doyng of meny þinges þat genderith and causith corrupcioun of blode & hendryng & drying and apeyryng of kynde. 450

And forþermore seiþ þe same comentour þat he þat hath þe pthisik, if it be so þat his spotel be layde on an hote coole of fire, or in the colis, and it haue a wicked or stynkyng sauour, it seiþ corrupcioun and wastyng of kynd. And if it be so þat he moute þerwiþ, i. if his here falle awai, it seith deþ. For stynk of spotel betokeneth euermore wastyng and any[n]tissh- 455 ing[99] of kynde, and heres falleyng, myslikyng & failyng of kynde, which kynd schulde com fro þe lyuer. Þise þinges seith he.

Þan if þou wilt weten of hym þat haþ þe pthisik, wheþer he schal longe leue or no3t, tak þis for a certeyn experiment[100] and a certeyn reule: do hym spit in a disscheful of water and if it houe, it is tokne þat he schal longe 460 leue þerwiþ or ellis scape. For þat seyþ þat þere is my3t and kynde in his lyuer. Noghforþan, al hole þerof may he no3t be. For who so be rotede in þe pthisik, he may **[f. 36va]** holpen[101] but he is incurable.

---

96 Pthisica] *marg.*: pthisica
97 take] GSc, seyne H, *om.* RM7Cg
98 disposede to þe pthisik] *marg.*: Which ben disposed to þe pthisik
99 anyntisshing] CgH, anentesyng G, aventing Sc, anytisshing RM7
100 experiment] *marg.*: Experiment of þe pthisik
101 holpen] RM7, ben holpynn CgH, not be holpen GSc

Item, tak þis for a reule: þat who so haþe þe pthisik, and he moute on his
heued, and þerwiþ com vpon hym a dyarie[102] or a dissentarie, þer is noȝt   465
but deth. *Diaria est simplex fluxus ventris* (*anglice*: a dyary is a wombe flux
wiþoute eny oþer peyne or sekenes). *Dissenteria*[103] *est fluxus ventris cum
corrosione intestinorum & egestione sanguinis*: a dissentarie is a wombe
flux wiþ peyn of fretyng and knawyng in the wombe and in þe guttes and
wiþ blody egestioun. *Egestio*: se aforne, c. 3, lef {*om.*}.   470

Item, if on spit blode and it come noȝt of bresour, as phisiscens sai, it is
of þe lunges. And oþerwhile þogh it come þorogh bresure, it may come
of þe lunges [as wel as of oþer parties of þe body].[104] Item, *etica* or *ethisis*
is a spise of þe pthisik þat is callede þe etik. *Eticus* is he þat haþ it. *Ethica*
is propurly consumpcioun of al þe body, & þe same is *pthisis* when it is   475
taken vnproperly, os Y saide while er, so þat *ethi*[*ca*][105] propurly & *pthisica*
vnpropurly ar al on. And þerfor þis is a gode argument: þis man is *pthisicus*
vnpropurly, *ergo* he is *ethicus* propurly, & *e contrario*, *ethicus* propurly,
ergo pthisicus vnpropurly.

Ethicus or *etica* is no more for to saye but a lent [**f. 36vb**] febre forwast-   480
and al þe body. And is saide of þis worde of Gru *ethis*, i. a duellyng or elles
root, for after þat it makeþ duellyng and is comen in root, it passeth neuer
awaie. And it is caused þorgh defaute of membres of þe body, late takand
her immutacioun, i. chaungeyng, and when þai take here chaungeyng, it
is long or þai letten it. And often tyme *ethisis* is causid of[106] passioun of   485
þe soule, os of lastand wraþ, longe & grete besynes, longe and grete studie
and care and druryhede, and of swych oþer poyntz. But raþeste it cometh
by passioun of þe body, as of longe trauail, longe sekenes, mykel fastyng,
mykel wakyng, continuel studying, hasty etyng, wicked fying, complexioun hote & drye, of potacions þat bene hote and dry, þorough exces in   490
lechery principalli, and if he haue noȝt his diete as kynd wolde haue, and
swyche oþer poyntz.

Et þis be þe veray tokenes of disposicioun to þe etik:[107] mykel hete in
þe hondes, and namely wiþin in þe paumes, [more][108] þan wonte was (but
first it is but litil and siþen more and more by proces of tyme), and also   495
grete hete in þe soles of þe fete. And þis hete – þus in þe hondes and in þe

---

102 dyarie] *marg.*: diaria
103 Dissenteria] *marg.*: dissenteria
104 it may come … of þe body] GSc, it maye comyn eke of the lungis CgH, it may come
    of þe lunges RM7
105 ethica] CgHSc, etica G, ethi RM7
106 causid of] *marg.*: Etik wherf it comeþ
107 disposicioun to þe etik] *marg.*: signis of þe etik
108 more] G, *om.* RM7CgHSc

fete – is causede þorgh hote fumositees þat comen of þe spirituales [f. 37ra]
by cause of vexacioun, i. of trauaylyng, þat þai haue & suffre by resoun
of distemperure of vnkynde hete þat þai taken, and þat it is so consumptif
to hem. *Et* þo hote fumositees smyten f[or]th[109] and briste aboute and   500
enflamme dyuerse partyes of the body. And so is rudyhede in þe chekes
by þe same skyl and anguisshe in þe lefte spawd. For þat party of þe body
is nygh þe spirituales, and namely nygh þe hert þat lith in þe lefte halfe of
man and principal of þe spirituales, for by cause of hete and dryhed þat
þe spirituales han þorgh vexacioun of vnkynde hete, os Y sayde ry3t now,   505
þo membres and partyes þat be annex to hem, i. nygh hem, ar smyten and
astonyede and distemperede be cause þerof.

 Et diuerse cowh, somtyme dry and somtym moyste:[110] drye cowh by
cause of siccite of þe spirituales þat cometh os Y saide. *Tussis humida*,
moyste cowh, be cause of superfluytes of materies þat ar conteynede in þe   510
spirituales and lenehede of body þat is causede of vnkynde hete, smet &
disperpliþ about in þe membres of þe body wiþinne, and dissoluand and
wastand þe kynde humores in þe body and anyntisshond þe spirituales.
And tak gode he- [f. 37rb] de: þat þogh þus mykil vnkynd hete be in þe
body and in þe spirituales, noghtforþan comunely in þis malady, it is but   515
litil or elles onneþes to his þinkyng. For comunely þai þat ar moste disposede þerto, þai ar disposede to so mykel colde þat þai fele but litil of þat
hete, but if it be in grete hete os in somer. And 3it mow þai comunely worse
suffer grete hete þan oþer folk. But nerþeles þai suffer grete straythede and
dryhede & disese at þe brest. Company of woman distroyeþ him moste.   520

 And vnderstonde þat þer be 3 spices,[111] i. 3 diuerse kyndes, of etik. Þe
firste spice[112] of þe etik mayst þou know by grete dryhede of þe body
and by vnkynde hete, alwaie somdel more þan kynde hete; by vnkynd
hete in þe hondes and in þe fete; and by þe powse, when þai ar often distemprede, somtyme more and somtyme lesse; and by mykel þerste, and   525
namely if þirste ouergo hym more bifore mete þan after; if his vryn be
high Citrine and longe tyme lastand so; and if rede Grayuel[113] schewe him
in þe botume.

 The secunde spice[114] is knowen by exces of hete in þe body, for þe body
is more trauayled wiþ hete in þe 2 spice þan in þe firste; and by le- [f. 37va]   530

---

109 forth] CgH, froth RM7, out GSc
110 somtym moyste] *marg.*: Cowh hote or drie
111 3 spices] *marg.*: þre spices of þe etik
112 firste spice] *marg.*: j spice
113 Grayuel] grauell CgHGSc, grayuel *or* graynel (l *in lighter ink at line end*) R, graynes
  M7
114 secunde spice] *marg.*: 2 spice

nehede and apayryng & myslikyng and dwynyng of body (and so in þe first spice, but more alwaie in þe 2); & by þirst and if he be more hote after mete þan aforne, s. in exces, for by resoun comuly euery body is more hote after mete þan biforne; and if his vryn be redysshe and laste so longe tyme and with mykel Grauel in þe botum.   535

In þe 3 spice[115] of þe etik, þe body is so mykel feblisshede and so consu[m]pte[116] and fordwynede awaie, os Auicen seith, that if on lyfte vp his skyn, it goþ noȝt pleyn doun aȝeyn but it be put doune agayn; and he is peynede alse wel bifore mete as after. Þe j spice is curable; þe 2 nerhand incurable; þe 3 is incurable.   540

Passio pulmonica[117] is conuertible wiþ þis 2 termes: *pulmonia* & *peripulmonia*. *Pulmonica passio* is generally euery maner passioun and sekenes of þe lunges. *Pulmonia*[118] and *peripulmonia* ar al day taken for on, and vnneþes schalt þou fynde eny distinccioun bytwene þat on and þat oþer, and neyþer þere is grete difference bytwene. *Pulmonia* is saide of þis word 545 *pulmo*, þe lunge (*anglice*: þe pulmonie or elles sekenes of þe lunges). *Pulmonia* is aposteme on the **[f. 37vb]** lunges and *pulmonia* is sekenes of þe lunges wiþ grete peyn and streythede of onde att þe breste. Item, *pulmonia* is when þe lunge melten and wasten and dwynen awaie.

Peripulmonia[119] is saide of þis worde *pery*, i. *iuxta*, byh or nyh, and 550 *pulmo*, as who saie, a sekenes bredand by or nyh aboute þe lunges, os in þe pipes of þe lunges or in places þernyh and about, as Y saide afornhande, in þis same chapitre, lef {30}, þer I saide what be *fistule, canales pulmonis.*

And vnderstond þat *sansugium* & *disma* and *asma* & *octomia*, of which 555 I spak in þe same place, ar 4 spices of pulmonie or of peripulmonie, and mowe be saide *pulmonia* or *peripulmonia*. And vnderstond þat in þis malady, s. in *pulmonia*, þe vryn may be Blo in 3 wise:[120] somtyme[121] by cause of replecioun, sometyme by cause of compressioun, and somtyme by cause of consumpcioun and wastyng of þe lunges. If þe vryn in *pulmo-* 560 *nia* be Blo be cause of replecioun, þa[n][122] he feleþ peyn & heuynes, os it were a pays aboute hese[123] spirituales, and somdel more o þe lefte half. If

---

115 3 spice] *marg.*: 3 spice
116 consumpte] M7CgHGSc, consupte R
117 Passio pulmonica] *marg.*: passio pulmonica
118 Pulmonia] *marg.*: pulmonia
119 Peripulmonia] *marg.*: peripulmonia
120 3 wise] *marg.*: 3 maners is þe vryn blo in pulmo<nie>
121 somtyme] *marg.*: j maner
122 þan] M7CgH, thenne GSc, þam R
123 hese] RM7, the CgHGSc

it be by cause of compressioun[124] – os when þe lunges bene ouerlayde and ouerwalmede or croden or schouyn wiþ some oþere membre, os wiþ þe stomak or wiþ þe[125] **[f. 38ra]** splene or ellis wiþ þe matrice – when it is so, 565 he may knowe it and wite it by felyng boþe of þe membre þat presseþ and of þat membre þat is pressede. If it be by cause of wastyng[126] and anyntisshyng of þe lunges, þan þere scheweþ hem smale Greynes in þe vryn, wiþ mykel Froþ abouen, and þe vryn wannysshe, dedisshe, & bloisshe. And þat is perilouse vryn. And whan it is so, he felith huge peyn on his 570 spirituales, for þan þe lunges ar consumpte and here substance fallyþ and dropith and dwyneþ awaie, and passeth forþ by þe lyuer, and so forth by *venas capillares* into þe vesie and enfecteþ þe vryn. *Vene capillares* in þe j bok, c. 3, lef {3}.

Pleuresis[127] is a malady wiþ stronge peyn and scharpe ake vnder þe rib- 575 bis, and þerwiþ comunely a febre, and somtyme wiþ spittyng of blode. Schortly to vnderstonde: *pleuresis* is an apostume o þe ribbis, and is said of þis 2 wordes: *pleura* or *pleuris*, i. *costa*, & *herere*, to cleue & hongen. *Pleura* & *pleuris* & *costa* ar al on, saue þat *pleura* & *pleuris* is þe ribbe of a man & *costa* is þe ribbe boþe of man & best. Now in pleuresi & *pulmonia* ek 580 is gret colleccioun of superfluites of vile corrupte materes, ouergoand and chekeand þe spirituales. Whiche col- **[f. 38rb]** leccioun, when þe kynde ne þe kynde hete be noȝt of myȝt for to defien it, ne for to deneyin it ne cachyn it awaie, it gadereth into materes contagiouse, i. attri and venymouse. And so þat mater contagiouse bredith into aposteme, sometyme of 585 þe lunges and somtyme of þe ribbes, cla[m]mand[128] and cleueand þeron.

When it is on þe ribbis, it is called *pleuresis* or *pleuresia* or *pleumonia* or *perip[leu]monia*[129] or elles *pleuria*, þat alle ar on to say (*anglice*: aposteme of þe rybbis). *Pleumo* & *pleura* & *pleuris* al on. And when it is on þe lunges, it is callede *pulmonia* or *peripulmonia*, os Y saide while er. And 590 vnderstonde þise termes *pleuresis* & *peripleuresis*, *pleuria* and *peripleuria* & *peripleuresia*, *pleumoniasis* & *pleumonia* in regard of þe ribbes, riȝt os Y saide while er of *pulmonia* and of *peripulmonia* in regard of þe lunges. Se more of þis mater in c. *de rufo colore*, lef {71}, & in c. *de inopos* and *kyanos*.[130] Þan of þe forsaid vile mater, passeth forþ by *vena concaua* (of 595 which it is saide in þe lef) to þe lyuer and þere enfecteth and envenymyth

---

124 compressioun] *marg.*: 2 maner
125 wiþ þe] *catchword*: splene or
126 wastyng] *marg.*: 3 maner
127 Pleuresis] *marg.*: pleuresis
128 clammand] claumand RM7, clamming CgSc, clammende H, cammyng G
129 peripleumonia] CgHGSc, peripulmonia RM7
130 kyanos] *foll. by* lef *canc.* R

þe blode. For in þe lyuer is þe pryncipal se and þe principal place of þe blode, after þat [f. 38va] in þe veyns, and þer it corumpeþ and fordoþ þe *spiritus*. And so by cause of enfeccioun, boþe of þe spiritz and also of þe blode, is blohede causede in vryn.   600

Epatica passio is sekenes of þe lyuer. Of *epar*, þe lyuer, it is callede *epatica passio*. *Epatica passio* mai be caused in 3 maneres:[131] or by cause of feblenes of þe lyuer, i. whan it is colde-biten; or by cause of oppilacioun, i. stoppyng; or elles by cause of replecioun. Þan if þe vryn apere bloisshe wiþ a maner of whitishede, it seiþ þat þe lyuer is colde-byten, and by cause 605
þerof þe lyuer is febil & vnmyȝty. Of whiche feblehede and vnmyȝtyhede ar wicked humores and wickede fumositees of humores in poynt for to gadren & gendren in þe ypicondres. And so it is comunely in þe colde ydropisie. <u>Of ydropisy and of his spices, se in þe chapitre *de albo colore*, lef {38}</u>. *Ypocondria*, þe ypocondres, ar þe places vnder þe lyuer and þe 610
splene. If by cause of oppilacioun þe lyuer be distemprede, þan is þe vryn menely þik & high in colour. If þe lyuer be replete, þan is þe vryn bloyshe and þikkish wiþ a dymhede and wiþ ake and peyn vnder þe riȝt ypocondre.

Catarrus,[132] as auc- [f. 38vb] tours of phisik seyn & techen, is a comune flux fro o member to annoþer. *Et catarrus* is saide of þis worde *cattha*, 615
i. *commune*, comune, and of þis *roys*, i. *fluxus*, a flux or a rennyng, os wo seiþ, *catarrus* is a comune flu[x].[133] And vnderstonde þat *catarrus* is propurly reume in þe hede alone, as whan it is abouen in þe hede, os in[134] þe brayn whan it is taken wiþ colde and smyt into þe former party of þe heuede, and at þe nose it comeþ out.   620

But *reuma*,[135] þe reume, is generaly euery maner of flux of humores comand fro þe hed to þe neþer partyes of þe body, os to þe eyȝen, to þe nose, to þe chokes and iowys, þe þrote, and þe breste. If it passe þe ouer partyes of þe hede, i. if it come to þe gomes or to þe chokes or to þe þrote or þo partyes, it is noȝt *catarrus*, but it is *reuma* propurly, for *catarrus* is 625
no more to say but *capiterus* or elles *capitarrus*, i. reume flowend and rynnyng abouen in þe heuede. And *reuma* is said of þis worde *roys* and of þis worde *manacio* (*anglice*: swymyng and flowyng), for *reuma* swymmeth and floweþ aboute in dyuerse parties of þe body. But *catarrus* is when it is only abouen in þe heuede, þat is callede in Englisshe þe snyke, os *rupia* 630
[f. 39ra] is þe pose. But vnderstonde þat differens is bitwene *catarrus* and

---

131 3 maneres] *marg.*: epatica passio on 3 maners
132 Catarrus] *marg.*: Catarrus
133 flux] CgHGSc, flus RM7
134 in] *prec. by* in (*at line end*) *canc.* R
135 reuma] *marg.*: Reuma

rupia, þow þai be boþe abouen in þe heuede. For in *catarrus* he nesith amonge, but in *rupia* it is so stronge þat he may noȝt nesen for peyn.

Matrix[136] is a membre in woman þat is callede þe matrice, þe moder. *Et* it is called *sentina corporis mulieris* (*anglice*: þe sentyne of a womannes 635 body), <u>for þe skil þat I saide in þe j, þe 4 c., þe 10 *condicio*, lef</u> {12}. It is called *receptrix* and *scista seminis maris* (*anglice*: þe receyuour and þe cofre of þe sede of man), for þerin is þe sperme, þat is callede þe sede of þe male & femal, receyuede and kepte til tyme of formyng cometh. Þis matrice is villouse, i. wolly and rogh, wiþin, þat it may þe bettre holde and kepen 640 þe sede vnderfongede. *Et* þat is þe skyl often tyme whie som women þat bene so often knowen of man mow noȝt conceyue: for þe wolle of her matrice wiþin is so rubbyd and frotede and wered awai wiþ mannes ȝerde, by cause of exces in þat synful crafte.

Item, Ypocras seiþ summe woman may noȝt conceyue be cause of ouer- 645 don sclenderhede and lenehede, *et* som for ouerdone fathed, for þe mouthe of here ma- **[f. 39rb]** trice is so streyt and so narow þat þe sede may noȝt entre. And some womannes matrice is so lymouse, i. so slypir & so slippy, þat þe matrices be noȝt of powere for to kepe ne wiþholde þe seede. Item, somtym þe seede of man and somtyme of boþe is so þenne þat it mai noȝt 650 be kept. Some men ar so colde and dry in complexioun þat þay may neuer-more gendren, for þe sede of swyche folk is noȝt able to generaccioun. Þan wheþer it be defaute in þe man of elles in þe woman þat sche noȝt conceyueth, þis is þe experyment for to wite, os techeþ *Liber geneciarum*, the *Bok of Genecyis*: fille 2 clene pottes, on wiþ þe mannes vryn and put 655 þerto a gode porcioun of brenne, and þat oþer wiþ þe womannes vryn and brenne also; late it stond 17 daies or 15 daies and in him þat þe defaute is, his vryn schal stynke and be ful of wormes.

Item, þe matrice haþe wiþin him 7 smale chaumbres, 7 smale kawates or elles 7 smale halkes, after þe figure of þe infaunt. And þat is þe skil whie 660 woman may conceyue and bere 7 childer at onys and no mo. <u>Now as Y saide, þe j boke, þe 4 c., lef</u> {12}, ryȝt as the drestes[137] **[f. 39va]** & þe filþe in a vesseil draweþ doun to þe botume, ryȝt so al þe corrupcioun and al þe vile materies of superfluites of foule humores in mannes body (of whiche þai alle be ful) gader hem þider kyndly, for to haue here issue and here 665 purgacioun out of þe body awaie by þe neþer membre. And þat byfalleþ woman comunely euery monyth onys; and som woman onys in 5 or 6 or 7 wekes þat ar most clene; and som ar moste vnclene, onys in 3 wekes. And þat vile mater is þe superfluyte of alle þe 4 humores. *Et* it cometh fro hem,

---

136 Matrix] *marg.*: matrix
137 drestes] *foll. (on next page) by* tes *canc.* R

i. fro woman, by here neþer membre fro þe matrice, os grut and filþe out 670
of a kychyne goter, like attre and blode menket togedir. *Et* it stant most
by here sperme and here vile corrupte matier, and it stynkeþ & þai also.

We calle þis sekenes *menstruum*[138] (*anglice*: þe moneth euyl or womannes malady). Þat vile mater is callede *sanguis menstruus* (*anglice*: monyth
blode), for os I saide, it cometh hem onis in þe monyth and comunely 675
about þe ful mone. Þai, s. women, calle þat sekenes and þat ilk mater boþe
þat cometh fro hem in þat sekenes her floures. And if a man [**f. 39vb**]
knewe a woman while sche haþe þat malady – and þan sche had leuer þan
eny gode, for þan is here moste[139] appetite to lecherie. And if þai had helpe
of man þat tyme, þai schulde be hole þow sche were in poynt of deþ. For 680
but he hadde þe bettre helpe, his membre forfareþ and rotith awaie, or
elles he is lepre. For þat tyme, þai ar so hote and þat mater is so venymouse
and so corosif, i. so bitand and fretand & maliciouse, þat it sleiþ þer it
comeþ, in so mykel þat if it be laide bitwene þe barke and þe body of a tre
þat is growand, it groweþ neuer after. And also if it be caste in an hondes 685
mouth or on his tunge, he turneþ wode.

Þan þis matrice is open and clouen on þe former ende, as þou seste þe
membre of litil ȝong mayden childe or like þe fishe of a muscle or elles lik a
whete kirnel. And þat is callede *orificium matricis*, þe mouth of þe matrice.
Þan when man schal sow his sede in þe felde of his kynd, i. in woman, þis 690
matrice takeþ þe mannes ȝerdes ende in here mouth and draweþ it in and
sokeþ o þe ende of þe ȝerde, riȝt as þe water leche sokeþ þe blode of a man
or as þe lampraye o þe stone, [**f. 40ra**] for to haue his kynde fode til sche
hath out þerof fro þe man þat she axceþ.

Þis matrice, os Galien seiþ in his *Bok of Anathomyes*, liþ on þe guttes; 695
and on þe nek of þe matrice is þe vesie, and vnder þe vesie is longaon, & al
byneþe is *uulua*, i. *ualua ventris* (*anglice*: þe wombe ȝate). *Valua* is a ȝate or
a ȝate wiþ 2 sperynges. Þan wiþin þe mouþe of þe forsaide matrice ar two
stones schapen like ballok stones of a man, and þai [ar][140] callede *testiculi
matricis*, or *testiculi mulieris* (*anglice*: þe moder ballokes stones). By þise 2 700
testicules passeþ þe womannes seede wiþ þe mannes seede forth vp into þe
matrice, for to formen and maken a body of hem boþe, if þe sede be able
to generacioun. For if it be ouerdone hote in kynde or ouerdone colde,
ouerdon moyste or ouerdone drye, it is vnable.

Þan when þe sperme is þus receyuede in þe matrice, þe mouþe of þe 705
matrice closeth & spereth him togeder so faste and so harde and so streyt,

---

138 menstruum] *marg.*: Menstruum
139 moste] M7CgHGSc, moste moste R
140 þai ar] M7, thoo are GSc, tho arn CgH, þai R

as Ypocras seiþ, þat a nedeles poynt schulde noȝt go bitwene, & so is concepcioun. If þe sede be vnable to generacioun, as Y saide, or elles her spermes accord noȝt in kynd of complexion, þe matrice haþ no deynte þerof, and þerfor lateþ it passe oute **[f. 40rb]** agayne þer it come in by her   710 wombe ȝate.

Euery woman is kyndly *frigida* & *humida,* and þe moste hote woman of þe worlde is more colde þan þe moste colde man of þe worlde. And þat is þe skil whye þai ar more ful of corrupcions & filþes of superfluytes of humores þan men. When co[nce]pcioun is þus [done],[141] as Y saide, þan by   715 cause þat þe matrice hath þat it wolde haue and þat it ȝernede so beforn, and also be resoun þat þe kynde of þe sparme is warme by waie of kynde and fulfilliþ þe warmehede of þe matrice and of þe woman, kynde hete is mored and encresede in her matrice and in her body. Wherfor þer gadereþ noȝt so fele superfluytes and corrupcions as bifornhand. And eke þe childe   720 is norisshede and foded wiþ þat blode of þe matrice, wherfore þat þe matrice hath noȝt so mykel nede[142] of purgacions os it hadde biforne. And þis is þe skil whi þat comuly al oþer bestes, alse sone as þai ar borne, or elles sone after, gone or crepe & man noght, for he is[143] fostredde and fod-ede in his modres wombe wiþ blode of þe matrice, and oþer bestes noȝt so.   725

Item, þe skyl whie **[f. 40va]** woman seseþ noght of lechery after þat sche haþ conceyuede os vnskilful bestes doþ, is boþe by cause of mynde þat sche haþ of þe grete likyng þat sche hade in ȝyuyng of here sperme and resceyuyng of þe mannes sperme and þe maner of doyng, and also by resoun þat sche is euermore colde in complexioun, as I saide, & her   730 matrice eke. & man & his sede is hote in complexioun. For riȝt as þe cold-est man þat is, is hoter þan þe hotest woman þat [is],[144] riȝt so her spermes haue hem in complexioun.

Sperma is white blode, þe sede of beste, comand fro him by þe instru-mentz, i. by þe membres of generacioun, decisede, i. wroght, and broght   735 fro þe pure substance of alle þe membres & lymes of hym. Of whiche cometh kindly swyche os þat is whos it is. *Et* þat is þe cause þat if þe fader haue a malady þat is incurable, os gowte, þe podagre, þe falland euyl, or lepre, þe childe hath þe same and in þe same place. Sperme of þe man is *cal-ida* & *humida*; of þe woman *frigida* & *humida*; *matrix frigida* & *humida.*   740 Þan when þe seede is taken and resceyuede in þe matrice and þe matrice is closede and shete, os Y saide, if it so be þat þe sede duelle on þe ryȝt half

---

141   concepcioun is þus done] CgHSc, concepcioun is this doon G, corrupcioun is þus gadrede RM7 (*see note*)

142   so mykel nede] *foll. by* so mykel nede *canc.* R

143   for he is] *foll. by* fos he is *canc.* R

144   is] CgHGSc, *om.* RM7

of þe matrice, hit haþ þe more & þe bettre norisshyng and fodyng of þe blode, by resoun [**f. 40vb**] þat *epar* liþ on þe ryȝt halfe, fast by þe matrice, and þan it is formed into a male. If it rest in þe left halfe of þe matrice, by 745 cause þat it is fer fro þe welle of kynde hete, i. fro þe hert, & also for it is fer fro þe principal see and place of blode, þat is *epar*, þerfor it turneþ into a femal.

If it byleue in þe lefte halfe, hauand somdel more [on þe ryȝt],[145] it shal be a male feminyne, i. a womannysshe man and feynt hertede. If it reste 750 in þe lifte half of þe matrice, somdel toward þe riȝt half, a bolde sturdy woman.

Item, wiþin þis matrice is a þenne webbe,[146] a þen skyn þat is called *secunda* or *secundina*, þe secundyn, or elles *saccus infantis*, þe childes sak. In þis secundyne is þe childe wappede and þis secundyn waxeþ as þe child 755 waxeþ and it is tyed to þe matrice and to þe childe. And when þe childe draweþ to his birþe, þe secundyne brekeþ and comeþ forþ oute wiþ þe childe at þe wombe ȝate, hongand on þe childe, knet to nauel.

When it is þus conceyuede in þe matrice, þan os seiþ Seynt Austyn in a pistel þat he writ to Seynt Jerom, þe firste 6 daies, it is as it were mylk; 9 760 daies after þat, it is blode; 12 after þat, it is a sadde body, s. a litil gobat of fleisshe; 18 daies, it takeþ [**f. 41ra**] his formes of membres and lymes þat it shulde haue; and al þe remanant of tyme til þe birþe, it is in waxing.

Conceptum semen sex primis crede diebus
Fit quasi lac reliquisque nouem fit sanguis & inde 765
Consolidat duodena dies, bis noua deinceps
Effigiat tempusque sequens producit ad ortum.

Aristotel, in þe *Boke of Kynd of Bestes*, þe 9 boke, þe 2 c., seiþ þat if it be a male, it haþ his forme and lif and meueþ at þe 40 daye, a femal at þe 80 day or þerabouten. Wiþ þis accordiþ somdel Seynt Gregorie in þe glose 770 vpon þe 3 boke of Holy Write, s. vppon *Leuiticus*, þe [1]2[147] c.

Þan sekenesse of þe matrice is in þis wise: somtyme þe matrice of woman passeþ out of þe kynde[148] place donward so mykel þat it is in poynt to bresten oute at þe neþer membre, i. at wombe ȝate. *Et* þat is by cause of colde, os of colde complexioun or of colde takyng fro abouen or of 775

---

145 hauand somdel more on þe ryȝt] havyng (hauende H) sumdel more on (of HGSc) the ryȝht half CgHGSc, hauand somdele more M7, hauand somdel (<...>yng on þe ryȝt somdel *canc.*) more R
146 webbe] *foll. by* webbe *canc.* R
147 12] CgH, 2 RM7GSc
148 kynde] M7CgHGSc, knynde R

trauaile or of childe birþe, or elles by cause þat sche is more colde abouen þan byne[þ]en.[149] And whan it is so,[150] s. þat it goþ so donward in woman, it [is][151] callede propurly *depressio matricis* or *oppressio matricis* or *precipitacio matricis*. *Depressio, oppressio* & *precipitacio* al on to sai in þis purpos (*anglice:* schouyng **[f. 41rb]** doune, crowdyng doun, and beryng doun).   780

Somtyme þe matrice shouyt so hyh vpward in þe body þat it presseth and croudeth so þe mydrede þat þe woman þenketh þat sche schulde tobresten, and oþerwhile so it falliþ. And when it styeþ þus vp to þe mydred, þe spirituales ar so crusshede and pressede and trauailede þerof þat sche is in poynt to dyen. And þis is callede *suffocacio matricis*,[152] suffo-   785 cacioun of þe matrice. Suffocacioun is strangelyng, chekyng, & it cometh of colde entreand beneþe by þe wombe ʒate, and somtyme of colde sittyng & somtyme of colde baþing, sometyme þorgh trauaile of childeberyng, and somtyme by cause þat þai ar wyde benethe and colde liʒtly entreþ þere into þe body, and somtyme for þai haue no company of man, and   790 for swiche oþer poyntes. And whie it goþ so vp to þe mydredde is for þe spirituales ar warme kyndely and þe matrice wolde haue hete, for it is colde of kynde and woman eke. And þerfor, alse mykel os it may, it fleyþ colde and seweþ hete.

Item, somtyme þe matrice draweþ to þe ryʒt side *et* somtyme to þe lefte   795 side, and þan it is **[f. 41va]** callede propurly *distencio matricis*,[153] distencioun of þe modur (*anglice:* strekyng oute and racheyng out). And þorghoute al phisik, vnneþes shalt þou fynde eny distinccioun betwene þise termes *depressio matricis, oppressio,* and *precipitacio, suffocacio,* and *distencio,* þat þai ne ar taken indifferently. But if þou take gode hede to þise   800 poyntz þat Y haue saide, when þou spekest wiþ eny seke woman, þou schalt wet & know when it is þat one & when þat oþer, if þou be wyse & sliʒh.

Som say þat *distencio matricis* is when þe matrice dilateþ here, i. sprediþ & racheþ out herselfe, and goþ ferþer oute abrode oute of þe kynd place   805 þan it schulde done, & so it is. And þat it doþ so is bi cause of exces of humidite. *Et* þan þe parties of þe matrice þat ar so distent, when þai neihen & tochen perauenture oþer parties of oþer membres þat ar more hote and more warme, þer more hete is, þer comunly it draweþ raþeste. *Et* whensoeuer eny of þise poyntz befalle, woman haue huge sekenes & peyne &   810 gendereþ in hem reume & colleccioun of superfluytes and vile mater.

---

149 byneþen] bynethynn CgH, bynethe GSc, bynenen RM7
150 so] *marg.:* precipitacio matricis
151 is] CgHGSc, *om.* RM7
152 suffocacio matricis] *marg.:* Suffocacio matricis
153 distencio matricis] *marg.:* distencio matricis

Et þan often tym þai lese appetit & comeþ a colde aboute þe hert & þe spirituales, & þis colde is callede **[f. 41vb]** *syncopis*[154] (*anglice*: þe co[ghe],[155] in som contre þe cothe). And þan her powcis die and þai mai noȝt, or elles vnneþe, be perceyued. And somtyme in þis sekenes þai waxen so contract, 815 i. so clongen & schronkelede togeder, & here myȝtes ar so benomen hem, þat here hed & knees gon togeder, and þai lese speche, and grosshyng wiþ þe tethe, and þe breste bolnyth, and þai seme as þai schulde die, and often so don. And þis bifalleth mykel in wydowes þat were wont biforne for to haue company of man & haue noȝt as þai were wont, for þai ar ful of 820 sperme & it turneþ into corrupcions & venymouse materijs, and may noȝt awaie as it was wonte.

Item, wifes haue it – some, but fewe, as þo þat be mykel colde in kynde or for her men be fro hem, & þai þat ar noȝt myȝty in kynde for to dyly- uere out here sperme and filþes þat ar gendrede in hem, but by cause of 825 colde & of feblenesse in kynde it rotyþ in hem, and somtyme sleith hem.

Item, maydenes haue þis passioun oþerwhile, for when þai come to age, as aboute 14 ȝere or a litil byforne, here fleisshe wolde haue company of man, for þan be þai wonder ful of mater of sperme. Which plente of sperme, **[f. 42ra]** but if it be so þat sche may delyuere it oute þorogh felyship of man 830 or elles on oþer halfe, os destroie it by trauaile or penance or þorgh swete by þe porus, it gaderiþ into filþe and corrupcioun. & þan colde fumositees styen vp about þe hert & þe lunges and þe instrumentz of þe voys and to þe arterijs, and þerof is causede *sincopis* & impediment, i. lettyng of speche and of þe spiritus. <u>Instrumentz of þe voys ar þe fibris, of which I spake in</u> 835 <u>þis same chapitre.</u>[156] <u>Which are þe arterijs: in þe first c., lef</u> {18}.

And when here floures cessen & faylen, þat þai haue hem no more (& þat is comunely aboute þe 50 ȝer if sche be a lene woman, & somtyme aboute þe 60 ȝer; if sche be[157] menely fat, about þe 40 ȝere, and if she be riȝt fat, aboute 35 ȝere), þan I say, when here floures cessen and fayle hem, 840 þan namely bigynneþ *distencio matricis*, distencioun of þe moder. & þan but if it be so þat þai loue & trusten wel of a man, or elles þai be syker þat he canne þeron,[158] meny women dye raþer þeron þan telle it eny man for schame. Women knowe it wel ynow ychon on oþer.

Of alle þis **[f. 42rb]** forsaide materijs, s. of the matrice & of al þat longeþ 845 þerto, techeþ Aristotil to þe fulle in þe *Boke of Kynde of Bestes*, by al þe 9 bok & þe 10 eke, which I passe be cause of prolixite. And in alle þis

---

154 syncopis] *marg.*: syncopis
155 coghe] cowgh GSc, cothe RM7, *om.* CgH
156 chapitre] *foll. by* lef *canc.* R
157 be] *foll. by* a *canc.* R
158 þeron] *foll. by* And *canc.* R

forsaide sekenesses of þe matrice, kynde hete & þe spiritz ar smyten &
taken and enfecte and feblisshede, & so causith blohede in þe vryn, os I
said. Of þe forsaide Greyns & also of Cercle of þe vryn, and what þai be   850
and what þai saie & howe þat þou schal knowe hem, se in þe 3 boke.

Item, vryn wiþ a Cercle blo os lede, or elles mykel toward, seiþ *epilencia*
(*anglice:* þe falland euyl). Þis are þe names of þe fallend euyl:[159] *Epilen-*
cia, morbus caducus, morbus comicialis, pedicoun, ierariolon, ira dei. In
þis malady alwaie þe membres of lif ar enfecte þorgh colde, & dul & feynt   855
and feble, & þat bitokeneþ euermore þe blo Cercle. And whosoeuer haue
þe falland euyl, his vryn apereþ so. Which bene membres of lif, se in c. *de*
karopos.

Item, þe same maner vryn wiþ smale Greyns seiþ a maner of sekenes
þat is called *alchites*. *Alchites* is þe þrid spice of ydropisi, and it is said of   860
þis word in Gru, *alchi*, i. *vter* (*anglice:* a costrel) & of þis **[f. 42va]** Latyn
worde *tonus* (*anglice:* tewn or sounde). For whoso haue þat malady, and
one gif him a litil stroke o þe bely, his wombe souneþ lik a costrel or botel
þat were but half ful. Of þe 3 spices of ydropisy, se in þe next chapitle
folwend.   865

[2.4]

De albo colore, of White coloure: c. 4

At þe first begynnyng of þis chapitle, tak hede þer is two maner of
White colour in vryn: on þat is mykel toward mylk or chalk, and anoþer
þat is whitisshe & wannyssh & waterisshe, most like water or glas. And
vryn in þis last wise White is euermore propurly callede *vrina aquosa*   5
(*anglice:* watrie vryn). & in þis wise vnderstonde White colour by al þis
chapitre.

And swych maner White vryn euermore seiþ indigestioun of humores
in þe body. Þan vnderstond þat vryn White, os I saie, and þen & wiþ bright
verges, i. if it seme as it hade bryght raies & stremes, shinand and glyrand   10
as glas when þe sonne schyneþ þerin, it is a euydent signe, i. apert tokne,
of sekenes of þe splene. Splene is þe mylt; sekenes of þe sp[l]ene[1] & *sple-*
netica passio, al on. Se *splen*, in c. **[f. 42vb]** *de karopos*, lef {59}.

---

159 fallend euyl] *marg.:* fallyng euel

---

 1 splene] CgHGSc, spene RM7

Þat þe vryn is White in þis malady is by cause þat þe kynde hete is
feblysshede and lessed þorgh exces of melancoly and þerfor is þe vryn   15
cru[de]² & indigest. Þat it is þenne is by cause þat superfluytes of melancoly defendeþ þe euesyng of þe splene and houeth and baggeþ ouer þe nek
of þe vesie and þirsteþ and constreyneþ þe wayes of þe vryn. And whe[n]³
þo be so pressede and þristede, þe vryn is subtile & þenne by cause þerof.
Þat [it is]⁴ bryȝt and wiþ shynand bemys, os I saide, it is by cause of mykel   20
siccite of melancoly. And þerfor swych vryn is callede *vryna virgulata*,
verged, i. ȝerded, vryn; also *vryna fenestrata*, wyndowede vryn; and also
vrina radiata or *vrina radiosa*, rayede vryn or vryn ful of bright raies. And
al is for þe same skyl, os Y saide.

Item, vryn first White at begynnyng and longe tyme lastand so, & wiþ a   25
maner of bloohede or dymhede in þe ouer party of þe vryn, it seiþ a sekenes þat is callede *leucofleuma*, a leucofleume. Leucofleume is þe 2 spice of
þe yposark. *Yposarca*⁵ & *ydropisis* Ypocras calleþ al on. Vnderstonde þat
þer ar 3 spices of *ydropisis*:⁶ one þat is causede of aquosite,⁷ **[M7, f. 25v]**
watrihede, which aquosite haþ in hem a saltishede, þe which saltishede   30
causeþ exces in drynk. & þis salt waterishede is causede & gendred ner
abouten þer *syfac* is. (Vnderstond þat, as techeþ Galien in his *Anatomyes*,
epar, þe lyuer of man, is wounden & wappede in 2 [þ]enne⁸ skynnes, 2
þenne webbes, or 2 þenne rymes, riȝt os it war in 2 smale nettys. & þise 2
rymes kepen & defenden *epar* fro hurtyng & blemysshyng. Þe ouermest   35
of þise 2 rymes is called *zirbus*, & þe nederest, s. þat is next *epar*, is cald
syfac. And by þise 2 rymes, *zirbus* & *sifac*, passen certeyn veyns fro þe
lyuer to þe splen, berand wiþ hem melancoly fro *epar* to þe splen.) & þis
spice of *ydropisis* is callede *alchites*,⁹ & euermore it cometh of a feble lyuer,
i. of a colde lyuer, & so is euery spice of þe colde *ydropisis*, as þe most dele   40
of auctours techen. Ypocras calleþ þis spice of *ydropisis* only *ydropisis*.
Whie is it called *alchites*, I saide in þe next c. biforn, in þe last ende. *Ypo-*
sarchicus & *ydropicus* is he þat haþ þe sekenes.

Þe 2 spice¹⁰ of yposarc is mykel caused of þe tysanare. *Tysanaria* in þe
next c. aforn, lef {*om.*}. And as þai sai, þis spice of *ydropisis* is gendrede in   45

---

2   crude] CgHGSc, cru RM7
3   when] M7CgHGSc, whe R
4   it is] M7CgHGSc, is it R
5   Yposarca] *marg.*: yposar<ca>
6   3 spices of ypdropisis] *marg.*: 3 spices <of y>dropisie
7   R *wants five leaves here; text supplied from* M7
8   þenne] thynne CgHGSc, ȝenne M7, *wanting* R
9   alchites] *marg.*: þe j maner is alchites
10 þe 2 spice] *marg.*: þe 2 spice leucofleume

empty & voide places of þe guttes, & it is callede *leucofleuma* or *leuco-fleumancia*, þe leucofleume, as I saide. Ypocras calleþ it *fleuma album*, þe white *fleuma*.

Þe 3 spice[11] of *ydropisis* is causede þrogh ventosite in þe body. And his 3 spice is called *tympanites*, of þis Latyn worde *timpanum* (*anglice*: a taw-bre), for who so haue þis spice of *ydropisis*, ȝif him a litil stroke on þe wombe & it sounneþ like a taubre. Ypocras calleþ þis ma[n]er[12] of *ydro-pisis sicca*, þe dry ydropisy. Of þe drye ydropisi, se in c. *de rufo colore*, lef {*om.*} Item, how þe colde ydropisis is gendrede & causede, se in þe next c. aforne, lef {*om.*}.

Þan when I saide firste, i. in þe bygynnyng of þe sekenes, for if þat malady be longe tyme lastand þe mater of þe sekenes is multipliede & strenghede by proces of tyme, & þan is þe vryn White & þik. Þe forsaid blohede, or elles dymhede, i[s][13] caused þrogh enfeccioun & of vnpure-hede & distemperur of humores in þe body.

Item, vryn White & þinne & mykel in quantite seiþ exces of mete or of drynk or elles of boþe, for riȝt os mykel oyle quenches liȝt in þe laumpe and os grete quantite of water cheketh & strangeleþ a litil fire, riȝt so exces of mete & of drynk qwencheþ & fordoþ þe kynde hete in body of man, þat it may noȝt haue his office of digestioun os he schulde. & why it is mykel in quantite may sewe of þe same skil.

Item, vryn White & þinne wiþ smale Grauel, as it were smale chesel,[14] & þe next vryn bifor þat were White & þik, i[t][15] seiþ a malady þat is called *nefrisis*,[16] þe nefresie, i. þe stone in þe reyns, i. þe lendes. Now vnderstond þis rewle in þis wise schortly: if it be so þat ane vryn schewe hym White & þik, & after þat com an vryn White & þenne wiþ smale chesel in þe botume, it seiþ þe ston in þe reyns, noȝt in bredyng but þat it is brede.

And þerfor seiþ Ypocras in his *Afforismis* þat shir vryn, i. White & clere, & namely in hem þat ar frenetik or nefretik ([frenetik is][17] he þat haþ þe frene[s]y,[18] se inward). *Nefresis* & *nefresia* is propurly when on haþ þe ston in þe reyns, i. in þe lendes, os *calculus* is when þe stone is in þe vesie. But *lapis* is taken generaly for þe stone, boþe in þe reyns & in þe vesie

---

11 3 spice] *marg.*: 3 Spice is tympanites
12 maner] CgHGSc, mater M7, *wanting* R
13 is] CgHGSc, it M7, *wanting* R
14 chesel] e[1] *written over* i M7
15 þik it] CgH, þik is M7, thikkyssh GSc, *wanting* R
16 nefrisis] ri *poorly formed*
17 frenetik is] CgHGSc, if M7, *wanting* R
18 frenesy] CgHGSc, frenely M7, *wanting* R

ek. *Nefresis*[19] or *nefresia* is saide of þis worde in Gru *nefresim*, i. reyn, þe
lende. *Ren* in Latyn, *reyns* in Franche, lendes in Englisshe or þe nere is   80
somtyme **[M7, f. 26r]** taken for þe menbres þat we calle þe neres, & somtyme for þat place of þe bodi þere neres lyen in, s. þat place betwene þe
bak & þe tayl end þat we callen aboue þe croupe or þe neþer pece or þe
leny pece.

Reyns propurly ar two menbres in best, ny rounde & auelong & som-   85
dele hole, lyand in þe first ende of þe lendes, s. in þe ouer party of þe
lendes, s. in þe lonye. How *lapis is gendred, se in c. de karopos.* Whie
þe vryn is White in þe nefresie is by resoun þat alle þe accion, i. al þe
wirkyng, of þe kynde hete is occupiede & besie aboute þat place þer þe
mater of þe malady is. & by resoun þerof, þe 2 digestioun is impotent, i.   90
vnmyȝty, for to make & wirke digestioun os it schulde done, & so is þe
vryn White.

Item, it is thenne be cause þat þe rynes ar so constreynede & so wiþ-
stode wiþ þe ston þat þe vryn is spolied [and][20] refte of his kynde coloure
þat he schuld haue, wherfor neþer haþ he þe kynd body þat it schuld haue   95
ne þe kynde colour þat it schulde haue. Grauel & chesel: se in þe 3 bok,
11 c., lef {*om.*}.

Item, if it so be þat on be in an acue & his vryn appere rubie or *subrubea*,
rubecunda or *subrubecunda*, & þerwiþ no certeyn token of creticacioun,
os no swete, ne bledyng at þe nose, ne none solucioun of wombe, ne none   100
oþer gode tokne, os I saide in c. *de nigro colore,* lef {*om.*}, if his vryn turne
into White & þenne, it seiþ a malady þat is callede *frenesis*,[21] þe frenesy.
Frenesis is a disturblyng of þe soule, wiþ haraioushede & rauyng. & it is
euermore causede þorgh exces of colre, walmand & styond vp into þe
brayn of þe heude, for þe mater þat schuld be in þe body & in þe lyuer for   105
to coloure þe vryn, be cause of exces of hete & eke for þe mater in himself
is hote, os I saide in þe j bok, þe 4 c., lef {*om.*}.

And by cause þat he is hote & dry, he is so liȝt of kynde þat he stieþ vp
to þe heuede & wirkeþ in þe heuede & scaldeþ & brenneþ þe brayn, & so
fordoþ wyt & mynde. And vnderstand a reule þat Þeophil ȝeueþ in his   110
Boke of Vryns, in þe c. of White & þenne coloure, which reule neuermore
faileþ: White vryn o þe forsaid wise in a frenesy, & þogh þe vryn kepe him
in swich colour longe tyme, & þer hapen to come a bledyng at þe nose or
a swete, & namelik in þe heuede, or elles som gode tokne of creticacioun,
he scapeþ þe frenesie. & *e contrario* he is but ded.   115

---

19 Nefresis] *marg.*: Nefresis or þe stone
20 and] CgHGSc, of M7, *wanting* R
21 frenesis] *marg.*: frenesis

Whie þe vryn is White in þe frenesie is by cause þat þe kynde hete is
hent vp to þe braines of þe heuede, & so i[s]²² þe lyuer depriuede & refte of
his kynd hete, þat he may noȝt defie þe vryn as he schulde. It is also þenne
for þe same skil.

Item, vryn White & þenne & mykel in quantite & wiþ smale & longe   120
resolucions, os it falleþ oþerwhile in water þat fleisshe is wasshen [in],²³
it seith a passioun þat is callede *diabetes, est immoderata vrine effusio.*
Diabet²⁴ is out of course makyng of vryn. & þis malady somtyme cometh
of distemperure of þe hete in þe reyns, *et* somtyme it is causede þrogh
exces in lecherye, & somtyme þrogh traiuail or of rennying or skippyng   125
or swich maner of poyntz. Þe cause whie þe vryn is White & þenne &
also mykel in quantite in þe diabeth, is be cause þat þe humidite of þe 2
digestioun is soken & drawen awaie anone fro hym into þe reyns by *venas*
capillares, of which þou hast in þe j bok, þe 3 c., lef {om.}.

And so be cause of hasty passyng awaie of þe vryn to þe reyns, it may   130
noȝt haue his kynde restyng & kynde dwellyng in the lyuer, to he tak
his kynde digestioun & his ful colour, but passeth so forth to þe reyns al
rawe. & when he comeþ to þe reyns, þer may he noȝt tak his kynd colour,
for neyþer is he scaply þerto, by cause þat he had noȝt aforhand his kynd
disposicioun in þe lyuer, & eke for alse mykel as he makeþ no residence,   135
i. no dwellyng, in þe reyns, but anon swy[mm]eþ²⁵ forth to þe vesie be
vrithides, **[M7, f. 26v]** *of which it is seide in þe j bok, þe 3 c., lef* {3}.

Þe forsaid fleshy resolucions²⁶ ar riȝt noȝt but wastyng, meltyng, & fallyng awaie of þe self substance of þe reyns & of þe neres causede þorgh
violence of hete, which violence of hete is causede þrogh vexacioun, i.   140
þorgh mystrauailyng, os þai þat ȝeue hem ouer mykel to lecherye & to
foule spices þerof. Wherfor meny take here deþ, & nyh al ende þerof or
þan þai schulden.

Item, vryn White & þenne & wiþ resolucions as smale as Motes in þe
sonne, & white & ronde, seiþ *arteticam passionem. Artetica passio* is cau-   145
sede of mater reumatik falland fro þe cerebre doun to þe neþer parties of
þe body, & namely to þe parties þat ar more noble & more worþi, as to þe
spirituales. *Of which spirituales, se²⁷ in c. de karopos.* Which parties, in as
mykel as þai be more noble, here draught is þe more myȝty. *Also which be*
þe noble menbres, I saide in c. de nigro colore, lef {19}. Item, *artetica passio*   150

---

22   is] CgHGSc, it M7, *wanting* R
23   in] CgHGSc, & M7, *wanting* R
24   Diabet] *marg.*: Dyabetes
25   swymmeth] CgHGSc, swyenneþ M7, *wanting* R
26   fleshy resolucions] *marg.*: fleishie resolucions
27   se] CgH, se (*line end*) se M7, as thow schalt have GSc, *wanting* R

somtyme comeþ of colde & somtym of gret siccite, os seiþ Gilbert, & also
it comeþ of meny oþer cause[s],²⁸ as I saide in þe next c. aforn, lef {om.},
þer I spake of þis worde *ethica. Et* wet wele þat euery sekenes of þe spirituales, in as mykel os o þe spirituales, it may be callede *artetica passio.*²⁹
Also *artetica passio* & *gutta artetica* al on. Se in þe 3 bok, 16 c. de attomis.   155
    Whie þe vryn is White & þenne in *artetica passione* is bi cause of defaute
of kynd hete in þe 2 digestioun. For in *artetica passione* is grete hete, but
þe hete & þe spiritz renne to þat place þer þe peyn & þe sekenes is, for to
help hem kyndely, as mykel os in him is. & by cause þerof, þe lyuer & þe
veyns be empty & voyde.   160
    And vnderstond þat þe Comentour vpon Giles seyth þat by 3 skiles
comunly is þe vryn White.³⁰ Se in þe begynnyng of þis chapitre. Som-
tym³¹ by cause of stoppyng & stuffyng³² of humores in þe body, &
namely of colre, þat þe body is no3t euentede for to lete out þe wickede
humores & þe exces of hem, & namely of colre. Item, be cause of huge   165
ake & preking & peyn in þe body, os it falleth in *colica passione* euermore
when on haþ it.
    And for alse mykel os but few folk knowe what *colica passio*³³ is propur-
lik, & mykel folk haue it & wene it be þe stone, vnderstonde þat *coloun* is a
gutt liand fast by þe nek of þe vesie; into which *colon* passeþ þe þik mater   170
out of þe ylions, forth into *longaoun*, as auctours techeþ & os I saide in þe
j bok, þe 3 c., lef {3}. & of þis menbre *coloun* is saide *colica* or *colica passio,*
þat al on is for to saye, & it is caused in þis wise: oþerwhile þe vesie, &
somtym þe nekke of þe vesie, & somtyme boþe ar stuffed & distemperede
þorgh exces of vnkynd hete, & þan þat ilke distemperure of vnkynd hete   175
distempreþ & distourbleþ *colon* & dryes þe *feces*, i. þe drestes þat ar in
coloun, & þan is þare ake & peyn a litil aboue þe schar, somtyme a[s]³⁴
þogh he shuld deie. And somtyme it comeþ þorgh exces of colre. & mykel
folk & also many entermetours of lechecrafte wene & deme it for þe ston.
And here motif is for hem þenkeþ it [is on]³⁵ þe vesie, but þis is þe dif-   180
ferens atwene: When o[n]³⁶ haþe þe stone in þe vesie, it is callede *calculus*

---

28 causes] CgHGSc, causeþ M7, *wanting* R
29 artetica passio] *marg.*: Artetica passio
30 3 skiles ... White] *marg.*: 3 cause of white vryn
31 Somtym] *marg.*: 1
32 stuffyng] CgHGSc, stufflyng M7, *wanting* R
33 colica passio] *marg.*: Colica passio
34 as] CgGSc, as (*line end*) as H, a M7, *wanting* R
35 is on] CgGSc, is o H, as of (*with poorly formed* a, *somewhat like* i *with small loop on
    left side*) M7, *wanting* R
36 on] CgHGSc, os M7, *wanting* R

propurly, & þan is huge peyn & prichyng in þe schore, wiþ a maner of
yche & grete difficulte in pyssyng, & as it were a brennyng in þe ȝerde,
& wiþ herd wombe by cause of pressyng & þristing & constreinyng of
longaoun. And þerwiþ also cometh often tyme *ylica passio.* Longaoun: in 185
þe j bok, þe 3 c., lef {3}. *Ylioun & ylica passio:* in c. de karopos, lef {5 < 3>}.

But when it is *colica passio*,[37] þan is þe peyn byfore þe vesie somdele,
for *colica passio* is bytwene þe reyns & vesie. *Et* þat peyn is fer more þan
in þe stone or in *artetica passione* oyþer, & his pissyng is noȝt so lettede
as in þe stone, & it turmentz and [M7, f. 27r] bryngeþ on more doun, & 190
more leseþ his appetit, & more anyntissheþ hem þan þe stone. Of þe stone
& how it is gendred, in c. *de karapos.* Item, *colon* in Grue tunge is anoþer
þing: se in þe nexte rewle folewyng.

Et þerfor who so haue *colicam passionem* & his vryn be White & þenne,
it is stronge peril, & namely if þe vryn kepe him so longe tyme, s. 5 daies 195
or 7 or 9 or more. & þerfor seiþ Ypocras þat White vryn in *colica* is þe
werst tokne þat may be in þat sekenes. Ypocras sawh a woman haue *colicam passionem* & here vryn waterissh & scherissh, & he saide of hire þat
sche shulde noȝt skape 7 daies; & þe 7 day sche diede, as Galien & Ysaac
rehersen. 200

But if þe vryn apere wele colourede in *colica*, it is a noble tokne, os Auicen & Gilbert sein. For it seiþ þat þe mater þerof, which may be in 2 wise,
os I said riȝt now, is broken & disperplede & discaterede, & þat kynde
bygynneþ for to ouercomen & ouermaistrien þe malady. Why þe vryn
is Whit & þenne in *colica*, for þe same skil þat I saide in *artetica*, & in þis 205
same reule. Of þe forsaide resoluciouns, se in þe 3 bok.

Þe 3[38] skyl whi þe vryn is watrisshe & wannysshe is by cause of feblisshede of digestioun of þe humores, by resoun þat þe humores mow noȝt
be defiede ne depurede os þai schulde if digestioun were gode. Wherefor
þe humores ar mixte wiþ þe vryn & so þe vryn scheweþ him in suche 210
wise, & so it is comunely in þe ydropisi. & þis is euermore a general significacioun of vryn waterisshe & wannyssh, & also coldehede of þe lyuer,
be cause of which coldehede digestioun is lettede & þat causeth rawe &
watery humores in þe body. & þat is þe principal cause whie þe vryn is
whitissh & waterisshe. 215

Item, vryn White & þenne wiþowten eny oþer condicions seiþ *nigra
colera:* [*nigra colera*][39] is noþing but exces of melancolie & it is saide of þis

---

37 colica passio] *marg.*: differentie betwene þe stone & colica passioun
38 þe 3] *marg.*: 3
39 nigra colera] In englysh a blak colre Nigra colera Cg, Anglica a blak colour Nigra
    colera H, a blak Colre GSc, *om.* M7, *wanting* R

worde in Gru *colon*, i. *fel*, þe galle, & of þis worde *roys*, i. as *fluxus*, a flux of þe galle. Þan is *nigra colera*, a blak colre, þus mykel for to say: a flode & exces of þe galle.   220

Also *melancolia* is saide of þis worde in Grew *melan*, i. *niger*, blak, and of þis worde in Grew *colon*, i. þe galle, os who saie a blak galle or blak humor. & so *nigra colera* & *excessus melancolie* & *niger humor* (*anglice*: þe blak colre & exces of melancolie & blak humor) ar as who saie al on. <u>Of þis proces & of þat I saide in þe j bok, þe 4 c., lef {6}, þer I expounede þise</u>   225 <u>2 termes *regnat* & *dominatur*; & ek of þat I spak in þe j c. of þis bok, lef {18}. Þeras I speke of þis worde *melancolia*, þou mayst wete what is exces of melancolie.</u>

Et vnderstond þat melancoly disposeth þe vryn, i. causeth colour in vryn, in 2 wise: be cause of his owen self, i. of his owen kynde, & also by   230 cause of his qualites. By cause of hymself, he maketh þe vryn blakissh, as it falleth comuly in warschyng of a quarteyn. Item, by kynde of his qualites, þe qualites of melancoly, as *frigiditas & siccitas*, for *melancolia* is *frigida* & *sicca*, <u>os þou haste in þe j bok, 4 c., lef {om.}</u>. By cause of his coldhede, he causeth whithede in þe vryn, for þe propurte of coldehede is for to make   235 Whit vryn or elles ȝelow. And þerfor auctoures seyn þat *albedo in vryna est filia frigiditatis* (*anglice*: whitehede in vryn is þe childe of coldhede). Be cause of drihede he makeþ þe vryn þenne, for þat is þe propurte of dryhede, for to cause in þe vryn thynhede & clerehede.

Item, vryn White & þenne, wiþ a blohede or a grete dymhede abouen   240 [M7, f. 27v] or elles wiþ a blo Cercle (þat al on is to seyn), it seiþ *epilencia*, þe epilence. <u>*Epilencia:* in þe next c. aforn, lef {37}</u>. The dym Cercle is by cause of passioun in þe menbres of lif, & principaly of þe cerebre þat is principal of þe menbres <u>of life. (Se in c. *de karopos* & *li.* 3, c. 2)</u>. Þat þe vryn is wannissh & watrisshe in þe epilence is bi cause þat kynde haþ so grete   245 compassion o þe menbres of lif, þat kynd & kynd hete are noȝt tentif ne besie about þe lyuer for to haunten & vsen here office of digestioun, but þai ar so besie for to h[el]p[40] him þat [is][41] rote & wel of lif, s. þe brayn, þat þe body, & namely þe lyuer, is destitute. & so is þe vryn discolorede þrogh defaute of digestioun.   250

Item, vryn White & thenne, wiþ a maner of ȝalowhede & grenishede & bryght & clere, saiþ a malady þat is callede *scotomia*, þe scotomie. *Scotomia* & *vertigo*[42] al on in þis faculte, os when on þenkes þat þe house or al þe worlde turneþ vp-so-doun or turneth aboute hym (*anglice*: þe dase or

---

40 help] GSc, helpyn CgH, hlep M7, *wanting* R
41 is] CgGSc, his M7H, *wanting* R
42 Scotomia & vertigo] *marg.*: scotomie & vertigo

þe daswe). *Et* þis malady is often tyme causede of melancolye in þis wise: 255
fumosites gros & blak styen vp into þe cerrebre & þer dimmen & dullen
& distempre þe spiritz of þe sight & þe *spiritus* of lif, & þat is þe daswie
in þe heuede. Þe whithede cometh of þe grete frigidite; þe clerehede & þe
brighthede of grete siccite.

Item, if þe vryn apere White & þenne in an acue, it seiþ deþ. But vnder- 260
stond þis reule in diuerse wise: for þe vryn, or it apere so in þe bigynnyng
of þe acue, or in þe waxing, or at þe stonding, or elles at þe wanisshyng
þerof, for þise ar callede þe 4 tymes of þe malady, os I saide in þe c. of Blak
colour, lef {23}. If an vryn schew him White & þenne in þe byginnyng of
an acu, i. of a scharp febre, it seiþ crudite of þe mater & feblehede in kynde, 265
& þat þe malady wil longe lasten, & þat kynd & þe malady schulde haue
strong fiȝit togeder & þat þe malady wil haue þe maistri – & principally if
þer be wickede toknes, os I spake of gode toknes & wickede toknes in þe
c. of Blak colour, lef {om.}.

And þerfor þat seke man or woman is noȝt for to take on honde, but if it 270
be so þer apere gode signes, & namely miȝt of kynd, & þan it seiþ scapyng
& warschyng of þe sekenes, & þat an emposteme is for to brede vnder þe
mydrede. If þe vryn apere suche in þe waxing or in þe stondyng of þe malady, & bifore þat vryn went *rubea* or *subrubia, rubicunda,* or *subrubicunda,*
oyþer it seiþ þe frenesy or it seiþ mortificacioun of kynd hete be cause þat þe 275
substancial humidite is consumpte & dwynede awaye. & þat is bi cause þat
he haþ noȝt his kynd norisshyng, os he wolde & os he schulde haue, & þat þe
pacient is anentisshede þerof. And boþe þise poyntz sein deþ. *Frenesis þou*
hast aforne, lef {39}. Mortificacioun: þe j c., lef {17}. Vryn rubea & subrubea,
rubecunda & subrubecunda: inwart in here propre chapitles. Þe substancial 280
humidite is þe blode of þe lyuer, & his kynd fode & norisshing is kynd hete.

If þe vryn schew him so in wanysshyng of an acue, & aforn þat vryn
aperede eny signes of creticacioun, it is tokne of sa[f].[43] Þus seiþ Giles.
Noȝtforþan, Gilbert seiþ þat if þe vryn schew him White & þenne in þe
wanesshyng of þe malady, it seiþ þat þe sekenes wil begynne agayn, for it 285
seiþ þat þe kynd & þe malady haue had here feiȝit togeder, & þat kynde
ouercome þe remanant of þe malady & so faileþ & sekenes maystre. And
þow Gilbert seiþ þus & Giles, as I saide riȝt now, noȝtforþan þai ar no
contrarie. What is creticacioun & toknes of creticacioun, þou hast in c. of
Blak colour, lef {23}. 290

Item, vryn White & þenne in olde folk seiþ feblehede of digestioun &
þat is be cause of age & defaute of kynd hete. Item, vryn White & þenne in
a child seiþ colde of þe lyuer.

---

43   saf] CgHG, soft Sc, sak M7, *wanting* R

Item, vryn White & þenne, wiþ ake & [**M7, f. 28r**] pricking & heuynes
aboute þe spaudes & þe schuldres & þe nek, seiþ a malady þat is callede   295
lippotomia, þe lippotomie. *Lipotomia* & *sincopis*, al one. <u>*Sincopis* in next</u>
<u>c. aforne.</u> And when on feliþ on þis wise in þe forsaide places, it is tokne
þat *lipitomia* is for to comen. & þus it is caused: when kynd hete lesseth
& faileþ, gros fumosites styen vp aboute to places, & so riste sodeynly þat
peyn. & when þo wicked fumosites neȝhen þe hert, þan of hem comeþ a   300
colde aboute þe hert & þe spirituales, & þat menbre þat is *radix wite*, þe
rote of lif, s. þe hert, is at mischeif & disese. & þan lesseþ þe meuyng & þe
myȝtz of þe soule, & so is þe body half dedisshe & made. & þat is þe cothe
or þe swounyng, <u>os I saide in þe next c. byforne, lef</u> {*om.*}.

Item, if a vryn apere White & þenne in þat day þat þe pacient haþ his   305
axces, it seyþ a verray quarteyn caused of a kynd melancolie. But þan on
þe next day after þe acces, þe vryn owe for to be *pallida* or *subpallida*, Pale
or elles Palesshe; & in þe 3 day or in þe 4 daye or elles in boþe, it oweþ for
to be White or elles ȝelowe.

Item, if þe vryn apere *rubea* or *subrubea*, *rufa* or *subrufa*, or elles *citrina*   310
in þe day of acces, [it][44] seiþ *quartanam notham*, & þis wise comunly þe
vryn sheweþ him swche in quarteyns. Þat þe vryn scheweþ him of bettre
coloure in þe dai after þe dai of þe acces þan in þe dai of þe acces, þis is
þe philosophie: for melancolie is so heuy & crude & compacte & indigest, i. so vnshaply & so rawe & so clabbed, clammede, & so [vna]ble[45] to   315
digestioun, þat he may noȝt so sone be diterminede, but wil last so longe
tyme. <u>*Quartana vera*, a verraie quartayn, in þe next c. aforne, lef</u> {*om.*}.
<u>*Quartana notha* & *quartana non vera* al one; se in þe same c. Þai called</u>
<u>a false quarteyn as *terciana non vera*, a false tercien. It schuld be said a</u>
<u>false quarteyn & a false terciane. What is *fleuma naturale* (*anglice:* a kynde</u>   320
<u>*fluma*): in c. *de glauco colore*. *Vrina pallida* or *subpallida*, also *vryna alba*</u>
<u>or *glauca* & *vrina rubea* & *subrubea*, *rufa* & *subrufa*, & *vrina citrina*, in</u>
<u>here propre c.</u>

If an vryn schewe him White & þenne or elles ȝelowe [and][46] þenne, &
litil in quantite, & þik & drobly in þe botume, & after þat com an vryn   325
mykel in quantite & þenne, it seiþ warsshyng of a febre *cotidien* causede
of a *fleuma vitre*. <u>*Fleuma vitrium*, a fleume vitre, in c. *de citrino colore*, in</u>
<u>þe last ende.</u>

And take hede þat euerych of þe 4 humores, outtake *fleuma vitrium*
al one: when indigestede, he causeþ þennehede in þe vryn; digestede,   330

---

44 it] CgHGSc, is (*line end*) is M7, *wanting* R
45 vnable] CgHGSc, wamble M7, *wanting* R
46 and] CgHGSc, *om.* M7, *wanting* R

þikhede. But *fleuma vitreum*, þe fleume vitre, doþ *e contrario*. *Et* þer-for *fleuma vitre*, ȝit w\h/il he is crude & indigest, he makeþ resistence & wiþstant þ[e]⁴⁷ kynde, þe which kynde wolde delyuer out þe vryn & may noȝt, by cause of hym. But afterward, whan digestioun is comforted & miȝted þrogh kynd hete, þa[n]⁴⁸ þat ilke vitre, or elles what humour þat   335
it be þat is in þe cause in þis wise, is resolued & disgregate, i. suptilide & vnclat & discaterede & dis[per]plede,⁴⁹ & so is þe vryn multipliede & þenned. Herewiþ acordes Theophile in his *Vryns* & Ypocras eke in his *Affurmis*, þe 4 particule.

Item, if an vryn schew him White & þenne, wiþ resolucions like fisshes   340
scale[s],⁵⁰ blakis & swartisshe, it seiþ a sekenes of þe matrice caused þorgh exces of melancolie, þe which mel[ancoly]⁵¹ is swarte & blake of kynde. For [of]⁵² alle þe 4 humores it is most terrestre, i. it is most erþissh, & most haþ of þe kynde of þe erþe. Þo Scalis, os seith þe Comentour vpon Giles, ar of þe wommanes sperme. Of Scalis of vryn, se in þe 3 bok, [c.]⁵³ 15;   345
[of]⁵⁴ þe matrice & sekenes þerof, in þe next ca. aforn, lef {*om.*}.

Item, vryn White & þenne, wi[th]⁵⁵ smale & blak resolucions in þe bot-ume of þe vryn, seiþ *emeraidas* or elles *condilomata*. Of þise smale reso-lucions, se in þe 3 bok; also emoraide & *condilomata* in þe 3 bok, 18 c., lef {*om.*}, **[M7, f. 28v]** *De sineribus*.   350

And vnderstonde generally þat by vryn White & þenne, os I saide & as al þis chapitre spekeþ of White vryn: vnderstond euermore principaly indigestioun & defaute of kynde hete, & also swich poyntz os be causede of hem, [a]s⁵⁶ enclusioun of wynde in þe body; & extencioun, i. rachyng & bolnyng, in þe ypocondres; & bolnyng in þe wombe & in þe sides &   355
about þe rybbis; & slowhede & erkhed & dulhede & heuynes in þe body & in þe armes & in þe legges & in al þe body, boþe anentys þe wittes & eke anentes þe meuyngges of þe soule; & euyl dispocisioun in þe heued, & namely in þe left half. What ar þe ypicondres, se in þe next c. aforn, lef {*om.*}.   360

---

47 þe] CgHGSc, þ M7, *wanting* R
48 þan] then CgHGSc, þam M7, *wanting* R
49 disperplede] CgHG, disperlid Sc, disipled M7, *wanting* R
50 scales] CgHGSc, scaleþ M7, *wanting* R
51 melancoly] CgHGSc, melien M7, *wanting* R
52 of] CgHGSc, *om.* M7, *wanting* R
53 c.] GSc, *om.* M7CgH, *wanting* R
54 of] CgGSc, *om.* H, in M7, *wanting* R
55 with] CgHGSc, wi M7, *wanting* R
56 as] CgHGSc, is M7, *wanting* R

Inclusioun of wynd[57] is causede o[n][58] þis wise: kynde hete is feble & litil, & þerfor vnmiȝty for to resoluen, i. breke & vndo & waste awaie, þe wiked humores; wherfor, by cause of emptihede in parties in þe body, gadrith & gendrith eyre & wynde in þe voyde places. & þan þat ilke wynd distendiþ, i. racheþ & bosmyth & b[o]lnyth,[59] þe places & aggreueþ al þe   365 body. *Et* þus is inflacioun, i. bolnyng, of wynde causede. For þe spiritz of whos vertu is causede þe meuyng & þe liȝtsomnes & þe miȝt of þe menbres & lymes of þe body ar feyntede[60] & feblisshede, by cause of þe qualmysh & þe rokish fumosite comande of þe humores þat ar so crude & indigest by cause of defaute of kynd hete. & þan þe superfluytes of þe humores, þat   370 be also causede þrogh defaute of kynde hete, be resoun þat þai be heuy by waie of kynde & **[R, f. 43ra]** al þorgh defaute of kynd hete, os I saide, þai descende doun into the braune of þe armes & of þe thies & þe legges. & þan him þinkeþ to his felyng al heuy & [er]kesom[61] and al dedishe.

And also þe forsaide fumosite passeþ forþ about to the instrumentez of   375 þe 5 wyttes,[62] s. to þe eris, to þe eyȝen, & al þat oþer, & dulleþ & hendreþ & distempereþ and indisposeþ hem, and the spirites also. & so it causith impediment of al þe wittes & þe *spiritus* also, of þe meuyngz & of þe miȝtes & þe wirkyngz of þe soule. Item, þat same fumosite, or fumosites, which stieþ þus vp into þe heuede and entriþ the cerebre, it causeþ wicked   380 disposicioun & ake in þe heuede, & namely in the lefte half, for þer, s. in þe lefte half of þe heuede, is þe principal se, i. the principal place, of melancolie. For þer he regneþ more þan in eny oþer place of þe body, saue in þe splene. *Et* þerfor, syn þat ilk fumosites comeþ, os I saide, þorgh feblehede of kynde hete, it draweþ kyndly into þat place þat is more answerand and   385 accordyng to him in kynde in þe hede.

And vnderstond þat euerych of þe 4 humores haþ 2 principal sees,[63] i. 2 principal places to him in þe body of man, in which propur places he regnyth & is lord & sire and maystre, and most power haþ: o place abouen in þe heued and anoþer bineþe in the body. Blode in the **[f. 43rb]** forme partie   390 of þe heuede, in the body in the lyuer, and þo ar his principal sees. *Colera* hath the riȝt side of þe heued & þe galle in þe body. Melancolie þe lefte half of þe hed & þe splen. Flume þe hyndur partie of þe hede & þe lunges.

57 Inclusioun of wynd] *marg.*: how wynde is genderd in mannes body
58 on] Sc, in CgH, of G, os M7, *wanting* R
59 bolnyth] CgSc, bolmyth G, bonyth H, belnyth M7, *wanting* R
60 feyntede] CgHGSc, feteynde M7, *wanting* R
61 erkesom] CgH, irkefull GSc, sekesom RM7
62 instrumentez of þe 5 wyttes] *marg.*: Instrumentz of 5 wittes
63 principal sees] *marg.*: eche of þe 4 humoures haue 2 principal sees

[2.5]

De glauco colore, of Ʒelow colour: c. 5

Glauca vrina, Ʒelow vryn, os alle auctoures techen, is moste lik a bright horne, whitisshe & ʒelowisshe. And alle þai saie þat Ʒelow vryn may noght be þik propurly, for Ʒelowe vryn is euermore bright, and if þikhede were medelede þerwiþ, þe þikhede schulde fordo þe brighede, for wiþoute 5 brighthede is no ʒelowhed. & þat is þe skyl whi auctoures trete of Ʒelow vryn next after whitisshe vryn, for it is next by waie of kynde, boþe in colour and eke in significacioun.

In colour, for it is but os White vryn, saue þat it is a litil more intense, i. a litil more dep in colour, and þat is by cause of þe ʒelowhede. Also in 10 significacioun, for it signifieþ riʒt as doþ vryn þat þe next c. aforn treteþ of, saue þat it seiþ lesse indigestioun þan doþ vryn whitish & watrish. And so his colour is white propurly, & his significacion is indigestioun, i. feble digestion, os it is of vryn whitissh & þennysh, outtake os Y sai. & also þat Ʒelow vryn seiþ þat *melancolia dominatur* in þe body, as watrish vryn seiþ 15 þat *fleuma dominatur* in þe body. Þis terme *dominatur:* see in [f. 43va] þe j boke, 4 c., lef {6}.

And vnderstonde þat euery of þe 4 humores[1] diuisiþ and turnyth & chaungeþ þe colour in vryn vppon diuerse tymes of þe malady. *Verbi gratia: melancolia* fi[r]st[2] in þe bigynnyng of þe sekenes, fro alse mykil os it 20 is ʒit but indigest and noþing of his grose parties is ʒit myxt with þe vryn, it makeþ þe vryn ʒelowissh. But aft[e]rward,[3] when þe malady accreseþ & is in his state, and kynde haþ more wroght and maystried þat humour & disperpleþ him wel about, þan it makeþ þe vryn Blak & grose, i. swartisshe & þikisshe. 25

Item, *fleuma* first while he is indigest, þan he makeþ þe vryn White or whitisshe & menely þenne, but inward in encresyng of þe malady or in stondyng of þe malady, when kynde begynneþ to myʒten & haue þe maistrie ouer him, and skatereþ and disperpleþ him abrode þorgh helpe of hete, it mathe þe vryn Pale or Palisshe and gros. 30

Item, colre first he makeþ the vryn þenne, but when he is mixte wiþ fleume, it is engrossede, i. þikked, & so *fleuma* grosseþ þe vryn & mathe him more depe in colour þan he was first. For os I said in þe next c. aforne,

---

1 4 humores] *marg.*: Euery humour chaungeth þe colour after dyuerse tymes of þe sekenes
2 first] M7CgHGSc, fist R
3 afterward] M7CgHG, after Sc, aftrward R

euery humor indigest causeth thenne vryn, digestede þicked, saue the
fleuma vitre, þat doþ *e contrario. Et* þerfor, os **[f. 43vb]** I saide, þer is no   35
difference bitwen vryn þat is White & þenne & ʒelow vryn, saue os Y said,
þat ʒelow vryn is noʒt so maliciouse. For in as mykel as it is more deep of
colour⁴ þan White, it seiþ more kynd he[t]e⁵ & lesse perille þan in White.
And þerfor saue þise 2 poyntz, os Y saide while er, þou schalt deme of
ʒelowe vryn riʒt os of whitisshe vryn, and alle þe same þinges þat ar said   40
in þe next c. aforn.

Ferþermore vnderstond þat ʒelowish vryn wiþ menly thichede seiþ a
melancolik man or woman (wheþer it be) hole. *Item*, vryn ʒelowe & more
thik þan thenne seiþ exces of an egre fleume. Now take hede þat, as techeþ
Johannicius in his *Ysigogis*, j c., þer ar 5 maner of fleumes.⁶ O maner of   45
fleume⁷ þer is þat is propurly callede *fleuma*, for it haþ no maner mixtioun
of oþer humores ne of oþer humor, but he kepiþ his kynde qualites, s.
frigidite & humidite. For *fleuma* is kyndly *frigidum* & *humidum*, & þat is
fleuma naturale, the kynde fleume.

Anoþer maner of fleume⁸ þer is þat is callede *fleuma dulce* (*anglice*: a   50
freisshe fleume), & þat is mixte wiþ pur blode. & þerfor of al fleumes,
fleuma dulce haþ most of calidite & humidite, & þerfor it is beste of alle
fleumes after *fleuma naturale*.

Þe þrid spice⁹ **[f. 44ra]** is *fleuma salsum* (*anglice*: þe salse fleume) þat þai
calle comuly þe sawsefleume. *Salsum fleuma* is enfecte wiþ colre, i. myxt   55
& maystriede and ouercomyn wiþ colre. And by cause þerof, he is moste
calidum & *siccum*, for þe qualites of colre ar *calidus* & siccite.

The 4 spice¹⁰ is *fleuma acetosum* or *fleuma acrum*, þat al on is to mene:
a fleume acetouse or elles egre fleume or sharp fleume, a sowre fleume.
Acetosum & *acrum* is scharp & soure¹¹ & egre os soure ale or scharp vine-   60
gre or eysel. And þis maner of fleume haþ moste of melancolie & þerfor it
haþe moste of his qualites, s. of frigidite & siccite, for *melancolia* is *frigida*
& *sicca*.

þe 5 spice¹² of fleume is *fleuma vitreum* or *fleuma aqueum*, a fleume
vitre, an ewe fleume, or a wattry fleume. And þis fleume is caused þorgh   65

---

4   deep of colour] *foll. by* depe of colour *canc.* R
5   hete] CgHGSc, hete *corr. from* hede M7, hede R
6   5 maner of fleumez] *marg.*: 5 spices of fleume
7   O maner of fleume] *marg.*: j fleuma naturale
8   Anoþer maner of fleume] *marg.*: 2 fleuma dulce
9   þrid spice] *marg.*: 3 fleuma sal<sum>
10   4 spice] *marg.*: 4 fleuma acetosum
11   & soure] M7CgHSc, sowre & stoure G, (& soure ?*lightly canc.*) & soure R
12   5 spice] *marg.*: 5 fleuma vitrium

grete frigidite & of coagulacioun, i. þorgh coldehed and cluddyng of blode, os it is comuly in olde folk þat faile kynde hete be cause of age.

But vnderstond þat suche maner of vryn, s. ȝelowe & more þik þan thenne, os vpon þat I said while er & eke os autoures seyne, it oweþ raþer for to be callede Whit vryn[13] þan ȝelow vryn, for it was more of whitehed   70 þan of ȝelowhede,[14] **[f. 44rb]** who so deme wil þe vryn þerof. *Et* þerfor tak hede þat þer be 3 maner[15] of White vryn: on[16] þat is bright and clere, acordyng mykil toward grenehede, & swich maner of vryn euermore seiþ *dominium* of melancolie. *Dominium* is no more for to saie but lor[d]ship[17] & maistre. Þan is it þus mykil for to saie þat melancolie regneþ & is maistre   75 in þe body, <u>os Y saide in þe j boke, þe 4 c., lef {om.}. Vnderstond melancolie, os Y saide þe j c., lef {18}.</u>

Anoþer maner[18] of whitehede þer is þat is somdel briȝt, but þat is but litil goand o partie toward redished. & in as mykel as it is lesse briȝt, þe body þerof haþ þe more of þikhede. And wiþout faile swich maner of   80 vryn euermore seiþ a colre drenchede in fleume, and ouergon wiþ exces of fleume.

Þe 3 maner[19] of White vryn is þat haþ right none of al þis condicions, s. neyþer of grenehede ne of redishede, & þat seiþ euermor fleume, <u>os it is said in þe nexte c.</u> biforne.   85

[2.6]

De lacteo colore, of Mylk-white colour: c. 6

Lactea vrina, Mylk-whit vryn. Now tak hede þat[1] White vryn, os þe nexte c. afore saue one spekeþ of, is noȝt propurly White vryn for it is noȝt propurly ne parfitely whit **[f. 44va]** but whitisshe, wannysshe, and waterisshe, os Y saide. And þerfor it is but a mene coloure atwene Whit & oþer   5 coloures, able for to vnderfongen and receyuen al coloures. Þer ar but 2 coloures þat propurly ar callede, s. white & blak; & alle oþer coloures ar

---

13 vryn] M7CgHGSc, vryn (vryn *poss. canc.*) R
14 ȝelowhede] *foll. by* vryn for it hath more of whitehede þan of ȝelouhede *canc.* R
15 3 maner] *marg.:* 3 maner of whitnesse in vryn
16 on] *marg.:* 1
17 lordship] CgHGSc, lorship R, lorspit M7
18 Anoþer maner] *marg.:* 2
19 3 maner] *marg.:* 3

---

1 þat] *foll. by* mylk *canc.* R

called but mene coloures bitwene hem two, for all oþer coloures ar mixte
& compownde of hem two.

But whit colour of which al þis c. treteþ of, is propurly white coloure,   10
for \of/ alle coloures in vryn, it is most contrarie to Blak colour, and so is
none oþer colour but þis. *Et* it [is][2] callede *lactea*, i. Mylk-white, noȝt for
þat it is white os mylk – for so white is none vryn – but for it goþ most
toward Mylk-white. Þerfor þai liken it moste to whei in coloure.

Vnderstond also þat *vrina lactea* is wiþ a white & þennyshe body. *Et*   15
for to know how Y tak þis term "thenysshe," tak hede þat þer is differens
bytwene "þenne" and "thennysshe":[3] for "thenne" is propurly when it is
mykel thenne, s. right thenne; "thennysh" when it is but o partie thenne,
or elles menely thenne. *Et* on þe same wise, vnderstond "thik" and "thikis-
she," "white" & "whitisshe," "blak" & "blakisshe," "blo" & "bloish,"   20
"citrine" & "citrinyssh," & so of alle oþer. Thus techen auctoures.

Et þis colour in vryn is euermore causede of frigidite ouergoand humidite, os Auicen techeþ. For when colde wirkeþ into moyst, þe colde[4]
ma- [f. 44vb] keþ þe moystour white; & colde wirkeand into dry causeth
blak. For riȝt os when hete wirkeþ into moist it causeth blakhede, & when   25
hete wirkeþ into dry it causeth whithede, on þe same wise colde doþ *e*
contrario.

Þan if an vryn schewe him *lactea* and *subtenuis*, os Y saide riȝt now, in
the bygynnyng of an acu wiþ wicked tokenes, it seiþ deth. Þat þe vryn
is *lactea* & *subtenuis*, i. Mylk-white & þennysshe, it seiþ þat þe mater is   30
compacte, i. crude & indigeste, & þat þe lyuer is ouercomen wiþ colde &
reyuede of his kynd hete, by cause þat þe kynde hete wil stien vp into þe
cerebre. & þat is a tokne þat he is disposede to a frenesi, & þat is more
perile, for it seiþ wasting and enyntisshing of his cerebre.

Mannes brayn is a membre, as phisik techeþ, þat it is wonder softe &   35
nesshe & tendre in kynde. *Et* syn þat his owen kynde hete is but litle &
feble, as þou schalt se in þe nexte c. folwand, it may noȝt wel suffre exces
of hete. *Et* þerfor when it is trauaillede by ouerdone hete, it is ouercomen
and schent. *Et* þerfor if a frenesie come in an acue, it is but deth, but þe
more grace be.   40

Þat þe vryn is *subtenuis* is by resoun of compaccioun of þe humor or of
þe humores, & also þat þe kynde hete is hent vp & stieþ vp to the cerebre,
and eke by cause þat þe lyuer is reft of his kynde hete, so my- [f. 45ra] kel
þat þer is no resolucioun, i. no brekyng ne no disperplyng of þe humour, &

2 is] M7CgHGSc, *om.* R
3 þenne & thennyssh] *marg.*: difference bytwene þenne & þennysh
4 þe colde] *marg.*: coldenes and hotenesse ben cause of diuerse coloures

so þer is none inspissacioun, i. no thikhede in the vryn, for os I said in þe   45
2 last chapitres aforne, euermore humor indigest þenneþ þe vryn, digeste
thikkeþ þe vryn. Compaccioun of þe mater is when þe vryn is clabbede &
clammede and clumprid togeder & rawe & indigest, i. hard for to defien.
And os I saide, swich vryn wiþ [y]lle[5] tokenes is tokne of deþ. But if þe
forsaid maner be wiþ gode tokenes, it seiþ warshing of þe malady. *Et* þat   50
noȝt be resoun of swyche maner of vryn, for swich maner of colourede
vryn is euermor in hymself suspecte & wicked & perilouse, but be cause
of þe goode tokenes þat somtyme apere þerwiþ.

Item, vnderstond anoþer poynt: þat þogh an vryn apere swiche & wiþ
gode tokenes, noȝtforþan þe malady wil noȝt sone sesen,[6] but þat it wil[7]   55
longe lasten, & þat þe malady in himself is stronge and myȝty be cause of
compaccioun of mater of the malady, os I saide riȝt now. For þe mater is
so herd clabbed and clammyd & so onid togeder & fortifiede, be resoun of
his crudite & of his indigestioun, þat he wiþstant & feiȝteþ herde wiþ þe
kynde & wil noght be obedient to kynde, i. wil noȝt be ouercom ne ouer-   60
maistried of kynd, ne resoluede ne digestede. And þerfor gode to- **[f. 45rb]**
kenes tellen & schew wheþer he wille ouercomen or noght. & so gode
tokenes telle how it shal be. <u>Which ar gode & which wickede tokenes, I
said in c. of Blak colour, lef {23}</u>.

And os I saide, þogh þer be meny gode tokenes & fewe wiked, or meny   65
wicked and fewe gode, or elles euen of bothe, þe more myȝty tokenes wil
haue þe maistri. But þe best tokne þat may be in seke man is myȝt of kynd,
& þe contrarie is werst. *Et* þat is þe skil whie often tyme ȝonge folk may
bettre be holpen, & also þat medicyn takeþ rather þe effecte in hem þan
in olde folk, & also þat often tyme ȝonge folk seme so dede þat her pitte   70
is made & al þingz redy – & ȝitt þai couer to leue. & þat is be resoun þat
in þe fiȝt betwene þe kynd & þe malady,[8] þe maladie ouercometh kynde,
al saue þat þe kynd hade a sparcle of myȝt more þan he, but in olde folk
comuly it is noȝt so.

Item, þe same maner of vryn in þe encresyng, i. in þe waxing of þe mal-   75
ady, i. after þat it haue longe holden him (os after þe 2 or þe 3 acces; som
sai after þe 5), it saiþ[9] þe same þing. And on þe same maner schalt thow
deme þerof.

---

5 ylle] CgH, evill GSc, alle RM7
6 sesen] *foll. by* but þat it wilt noȝt sone sesen *canc.* R
7 wil] *foll. by* noȝt *canc.* R
8 þe kynd & þe malady] CgH, kynd *and* malady *transposed* GSc, þe kynd & þe malady
   & RM7
9 after þe 5 it saiþ] after þe 5 & it saiþ RM7, aftir the 4 it sayth GSc, after the 4 day it
   seyth CgH

Item, the same maner of vryn in þe stondyng of þe maladie: deme in þe
same wise.   80
Item, þe same maner of vryn in the fallyng of the malady & mykel in
quantite [f. 45va] seith þat the kynde hete & þe malady haue hade here fiȝt,
& þat kynd bigynneth for to go aboue & haue þe maistrie, & bytokenyth
warshyng if he haue gode tendyng to.

Þat þe vryn is *lactea*, it saiþ þat þe vnkynd hete is gon or elles is goond.   85
Þat it is *subtenuis*, it seiþ þat þe materies þat afornhand were so gros &
so compacte, now þai ar so subtilede & thennede & broght to reule &
to recleym. Þat it is mikel in quantite, it seiþ þat þere is sufficient purgacioun of þe mater of the malady, i. of þat humour þat þe malady was
causede of; but if the vryn be lesse in quantite þan it was biforn, i. þan in   90
the stondyng or þan in þe encresing or helles þan in þe biginnyng of þe
acue, it seiþ deþ. *Et* þerfor if on make White vryn in a brennand febre,
and namely to þe 4 daye & in þe 4 dai, he dieþ þe 7 day elles þerabouten.
Þe bygynnyng of a febre & þe waxing & þe stondyng & the fallyng: in c.
of Blak colour, lef {23}.   95
Item, *vryna lactea* & *subtenuis* in þe begynnyng of a typik febre seiþ
crudite & compaccioun of þe mater & þat the malady wil longe laste. The
whitehede seiþ þat þe materijs of þe malady ar humores flumatik[10] & þai
ar so compacte þat þai ar wel herde to breken & for to resoluen. The þen-
[f. 45vb] nyshede seiþ also compaccioun of þe mater. *Pthiphis* & *pthiphia*   100
& *pthphica febris*, *febris interpolata*, *febris planetica*, and *febris erratica*
al on: an errant febre.[11] *Febris erratica* þus is des[cribet][12] in phisik: an
errant febre þat al the while þat one hath it, vncerteyn tymes it turmenteþ
& vncerteyn tymes it seseþ. & somtyme it is causede boþe of colre & of
fleume & of melancolie. And of alse fele humores os he is causede of, alse   105
fele siþes he turmentiþ o þe day. & somtyme it haþ on[13] day betwene, somtyme 2, somtyme 3, sumtym 4, somtyme 5, & somtyme mo. It is said *pthiphus*, i. *reuolucio* (*anglice*: a turnyng agayn), for it turneþ agayn, i. comeþ
agayn, but noȝt at certeyn tyme. *Et* be cause þat he kepeþ no certeyn tyme,
it is callede *febris erratica*, a febre errant.   110
Et when I saide *pthipica febris* & *febris interpolata* ar al [on],[14] vnderstonde þat I take a febre interpolate for *interpolata non vera*, i. for an vnueray interpolate. *Interpolata vera*, a veray interpolate, is þat turmenteþ at

---

10 flumatik] fliumatik *with first* i *underpuncted* R
11 errant febre] *marg.*: Errant febre
12 describet] M7, discryved G, discernyd Sc, discryed CgH, des (*line end with hyphen*) R
13 on] j Cg, a HGSc, on þe RM7
14 on] CgHGSc, *om.* RM7

certeyn tymes[15] or at certeyn daies & resteþ a certeyn tymes, os it doþ in
terciens & quarteyns, <u>os I said in þe c. of Blak colour, lef</u> {*om.*}. *Interpolata* 115
non vera, an vnverraie interpolate: þat **[f. 46ra]** turmenteþ at vncerteyn
tyme and resteþ at vncerteyn tyme.

And whi it is callede *febris planetica*,[16] a febre planetik, j skil[17] may
be þis: *planeta* is as mykel for to saie os errant, or elles vnstedfast and
wandrand, riȝt so it is of febre errant. For riȝt os alle oþer sterres haue on 120
certeyn, riȝt, and euen course, and þe planetz haue j maner of course þat
is contrarious and errond and wandrawnt and vnstedfast, riȝt so al oþer
febres haue certeyn course, i. here accesses comen at certeyn; but the febre
errant kepeþ no certeyn. Anoþer cause[18] whi it is callede *febris planetica*
may be þis: for it hath his course, i. it turmenteþ by his accesses, vppon 125
þe course of þe humour or of þe humores of which he is caused, which
humores regnen & ar most prest & habundant in mannes body vppon the
course of þe planetz, i. in þo houres þat her planetz regne in. And so may
euery febre be called *planetica febris*.

Now[19] for alse mykel os Y speke of planetz[20] and of here courses, and a 130
wise leche owe for to know dyuerse þinges, vnderstond þat þer be 7 planetz.
Þe firste & þe most negh vs is Luna of alle, þe 2 is Mercurius, þe 3 Venus, þe
4 Sol, þe 5 Mars, þe 6 Jubitre, þe 7 is Saturnus. Þise 7 planetz renne euermore
[f. 46rb] continuely agayn þe firmament fro þe west to þe est, and þat is called
proprius cursus planetarum, þe propre course of planetz.[21] It is also calde 135
motus erraticus and *motus contrarius*, here course errant and here contrarie
course, for it errith & is contrariouse to þe firmament. For þe firmament
& alle his sterres, saue þe 7 planetz, turneth euermore continuely wiþout
cessing fro þe est into þe weste, more swiftely þan eny þing þat we see wiþ
eye, & wiþ more hurre & noyse þan bodily ere mai here. And [but] þise[22] 140
7 planetz letteþ the violence & tempreþ þe huge course of þe firmament,
alle þinges here beneþe were fordone þorgh þe violence þerof. Noȝtforþan,
þorgh violence of þe course of þe firmament, þe planetz ar movede fro þe
est to þe west, & þis course[23] is callede *motus violentus* & *motus improprius*
planetarum, þe violente course & þe vnpropre course of the planetes. 145

---

15 at certeyn tymes] *foll. by* or at certeyn tymes *canc.* R
16 febris planetica] *marg.*: For 2 skiles it is called febre errant
17 j skil] *marg.*: 1
· 18 Anoþer cause] *marg.*: 2
19 Now] *initial* N *slightly enlarged and ornamented*
20 planetz] *marg.*: 7 planetes
21 propre course of planetz] *marg.*: þe propre course of planetes
22 but þise] but the CgH, but þo Sc, but yf thoo G, þise RM7
23 þis course] *marg.*: violente course of planetes

Now vnderstond þat Luna,[24] the mone, is *frigida* & *humida*, a planete more god þan wik, hauand more effecte, i. more myȝt, in creatures here beneþe[25] þan eny oþer planete, os seiþ Ptholomeus in his bok þat is callede *Almagisti*, boþe by cause þat it is neer to vs of al the 7 planetz & eke by resoun [f. 46va] þat it is most swifte in course of all þe planetz. For in 27   150 daies & nygh[26] 8 houres, he fulfilleþ his course, i. passeþ al þe Zodiac,[27] i. al þe 12 signes of þe firmament, duellond in euerych of þe 12 signez 2 daies naturel & 8 houres & 13 degres & 10 minutes. Þe Zodiac is þe cercle of þe 12 signis of þe firmament, as þou schalt se inward, lef {*om*.}.

A signe of þe firmament is þe 12 part of þe firmament. Þis be þe 12   155 signes:[28] Aries, Taurus, Gemini, Cancer, Leo, Virgo, Libra, Scorpio, Sagittarius, Capricorn[u]s,[29] Aquarius, Pisces. Of þis Zodiac, i. of þe cercle of þe firmament, how it is departede into 12 signes, and of þe 7 planetz & here speres, & of þe 4 elementz & here speres: se anone in a figure, lef {49}.

A dai naturel[30] is 24 houres longe, s. fro mydnyȝt to mydnyght, or fro none   160 to none, or fro sonset to sonset, or wher þou wilt bigynne. Day of comune vse,[31] i. os the comune calleth the dai, is fro þe son rysyng to þe son setting. Cristen men bygynne þe dai naturel fro mydnyght, bothe be cause þat Criste þat is our liȝt was born of a m[ay]den[32] at mydnyght of þe Sonday, & also by resoun þat þe sone þat causeþ and makeþ þe day is at mydnyght at his fer-   165 rest poynt & bygynneþ for to com vp agayn for to make þe dai. Jewes by- [f. 46vb] gynne her dai naturel at euen, for the first boke of Holy Writte seiþ *factum est vespere & mane dies vnus* (*anglice*: euen & morn was made o day). Sarasynes bigynne at myddai, for þai sai þat the sone was made at mydday.

Vpon this faculte, i. vpon phisik, *dies naturalis* is þus diuisede, s. into 4   170 quadres, i. into 4 quarteres. Þe first quadre bygynneþ at þe 9 hour of þe nyght exclusif, i. þe 9 houre noght tolde, to þe 3 houre of þe day artificial inclusif, i. þat 3 hour tolde. & þat quarter is *calida* & *humida*, & in þat regneþ *sanguis*. Þe 2 quadre bygynneþ at þe 3 houre of þe day artificial exclusif & endiþ at þe 9 oure of þe same day inclusif. For in þat tyme reg-   175 neþ colre, for þat tyme is *calida* & *sicca*. (Vnderstond þat *dies artificialis* & *dies vsualis* & *dies vulgaris*, dai artificial & day vsual & day as þe commune

---

24 Luna] *marg.*: Luna
25 beneþe] GSc, benethynn CgH, in beneþe RM7 (be *poss. canc.* R)
26 nygh] *foll. by* & *canc.* R
27 Zodiac] *marg.*: Zodiac
28 12 signes] *marg.*: 12 signes
29 Capricornus] CgHGSc, Capricornes RM7
30 dai naturel] *marg.*: dai naturel
31 Day of comune vse] *marg.*: dai vsuale
32 mayden] myaden *with* y *and* a *overpuncted*

takeþ þe day, ar al on for to saie.) Þe 3 quadre is fro þe 9 houre of þe dai
vsual exclusif til þe 3 oure of þe ny3t inclusif. & þat quadre is *frigida* &
sicca, & in þat quadre regneþ melancolie. Þe 4 quadre is fro þe 3 houre of   180
þe nyght exclusif to þe 9 houre of þe same ny3t inclusif. & þat quadre is
frigida & *humida, et* þat tyme is fleume in his my3t. And þise ar the skiles
whi meny sekenesses & maladies ar more scharpe & somtyme more leþi in
som quadre of þe day or of þe **[f. 47ra]** nyght þan in som. *Arabes meridie,*
Romani media nocte / Gens Judea sero, wlgus quoque solis ab ortu.[33]   185

Day natural is departede in many parties:[34] in quarteres or in *quadra*, in
hora, in *punctus*, in *momentum*, in *vncia*, & in *thomus* (*anglice*: [in][35] quar-
teris or into quadris, þat al on is for to saie;[36] in oure; in poynt; in moment;
in vnce or in vnche; & in thome, i. in an indiuisible, i. into a þing þat may
no3t be departede). *Quadrans* or elles *quadra* is þe 4 part of a day natural,   190
þe space of 6 hours. An houre is þe 24 part of a dai naturel. *Punctus*, a
poynt, is þe 4 part of an houre. *Momentum* is þe 10 part of a poynt. *Vncia*,
an ownce or elles an vnche, is þe 12 part of a moment. *Thomus* is þe [4]7[37]
part of an vnche, & it is saide of þis worde in Gru *thomus*, i. wiþouten
diuisioun, for it is so litle þat[38] it may no3t be dyuysede, i. departed.   195

Þe forsaide 12 signes astronomyens parten[39] into gres, gres into minutz,
& minutz into secundes, secundes into terces, & terces into quartes,
quartes into quintes, & quintz into sextes. A gre is þe 30 porcioun of a
signe. (What is a signe, I sayde.) *Minuta*, a mynute, is þe 60 part or elles
porcioun of a gre. *Et* vnderstond þat in a mynut-while, þou mayst say ren-   200
ably a *pater* & an *ave*. A secunde is þe 60 part of a mynute; a terce þe 60
part **[f. 47rb]** of a secunde; a quarte þe 60 part of a terce; a quynt þe 60 part
of a quart. *Et* a sexte, þe 60 part of a quint. And lowere is no nombri[n]g[40]
in astrono[m]ye.[41]

The next planete after þe mone fro vs is Mercure:[42] *frigidus* & *humidus*,   205
tempre, gode wiþ gode planetz & sterres, & wik wiþ wik. He fulfilleþ his
course in 338 daies, i. in so fele daies he passeþ al þe Zodiac, i. al þe 12
signes of þe firmament. Mercure goþ euermore wiþ þe sone, for when he
is ferrest fro þe sonne, he is but 30 degres. He is wonder white in coloure

---

33 ab ortu] M7CgHGSc, ab or ortu R
34 Day naturel ... parties] *marg.*: diuisioun of day naturel
35 in] CgH, *om.* M7GSc, an *plus partal char.* (?g), *canc.* R
36 for to saie] *marg.*: after compot
37 47] CgHGSc, 17 RM7
38 þat] M7CgHGSc, þat þat R
39 astronomyens parten] *marg.*: After astronomy
40 nombring] nowmbryng CgH, nombrig RM7, nombre GSc
41 astronomye] M7CgHGSc, astrononye R
42 Mercure] *marg.*: Mercure

and ful of ra[y]es⁴³ and bemes, but for he goþ so ny3h þe sone, vneþes or   210
elles but selden may he be seyn. He disposeth man to faire speche. He is
lorde of watres, os Luna is lady of wateres. He is also lorde of seedes, os
is Luna lady whil she is newe. Also Mercurie is lord of marchandise, for
he þat is born in þe houre þat he regneþ, he is schaply to þat craft. In what
houre what planete regneþ, se inward. Also, þe quantite of þe planetz &   215
here fernesse & quantite of þe sterres: se afterward.

Þe nexte planete after Mercure is Venus:⁴⁴ *calidus* & *humidus*, a gode
planete. Gode planete or wicked planete, vnderstonde in effecte. He fulfilleþ his course in 348 daies. He trempeþ & slakeþ þe malice of Mars. He
is neuermore ferrer fro þe sone þan 2 de- **[f. 47va]** gres at þe moste. When   220
he folweþ þe sone, þan is he callede *Vesper* & *Hesperus* (*anglice*: þe euen
sterre). When he goþ afore þe sone, he is callede *Lucifer* & *stella matutina*,
þe day sterre & þe morn sterre. He is þe moste bright sterre of heuen.

Sol,⁴⁵ þe sone, is noblist of alle planetz & þerfor he is in þe myddes of
alle þe planetz, os a lord amonge his meny, or kyng in mydward of his   225
oste. He is *calidus* & *siccus*, tempre. He 3eueþ my3t & vertue to alle erthely
creatures þat bereþ lif. Þe more nyh he be to vs, þe more allegeance is in
sores and in maladies, & more ferre, the more *e contrario*. He fulfilleþ his
corse in 365 daies & 6 hours & 13 mynutz & 45 secundes, and þat makeþ a
3ere hole. He dwelleþ in euery of þe 12 signes 30 daies & 10 houres.   230

Now of þe forsaid 6 houres þat byleue in þe 3ere,⁴⁶ in þe 4 3ere ar gadrede
24 hours, s. a dai naturel, & þat ilk dai in þe 4 3ere is euermore ymped in and
sett in Februarie in þe vj of þe kalends of Marche, s. on Seint Mathies dai, þat
falleþ euermore on F lettre. & þan þat 3ere euermore, F stant for 2 daies, &
þan it schal be 2 saide sexte kalends of Marche. *Et* þat is þe skil whie þe 4 3ere   235
is euermore callede *bisextus*, bysexte, i. twise sex, for þat dai is twise seyde, s.
2 dayes togedre, þe vj kalends of March. The peple calleþ it lepe 3ere.

& bi cause of fulfillyng of a dai naturel of þo 6 **[f. 47vb]** houres in þe 4
3ere, os I saie, euermore þat bisexte 3ere, i. þat 4 3ere, haþ 366 daies & 13
mynutz & 45 secundes þerin. And anoþer 3ere ar but, os I sai, 365 daies &   240
6 hours & 13 mynutz & 45 secundes. Also it is saide *bis sexte*, i. 2 sexe, and
þat is for to wete, for þat dai þat Seynt Mathies day falleþ on is euermore
þe 12 dai of þe kalends of Marche when it is lep 3ere; and when it is no3t
lepe 3ere, þan Seint Mathiez dai is but þe 11 dai of þe kalends of Marche.
And take hede þat when lep 3ere falleth, Seynt Mathies dai schal be holden   245
o þe laste day o þe fest.

---

43   rayes] CgHGSc, raþes R; y *and* þ *indistinguishable in* M7
44   Venus] *marg.*: Venus
45   Sol] *marg.*: Sol
46   3ere] *marg.*: bisext

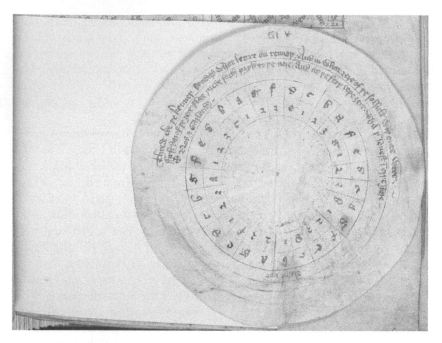

Plate 2. Dominical Letters and Leap Years. © The British Library Board: London, British Library, Royal MS 17 D.i, f. 51*.

    Than if þou wilt sikerly wete when schal þe lep ȝer be, tak þis for a reule þat neuer schal faile: euermore when þe lesse nombre of þe ȝere of our Lord may be diuisede into 4 parties euen alike, þe nexte Seynt Mathies day folwend schal be bisexte, þogh þe course of Rome & on ȝonde-half 250 bigynne þe ȝere of our Lord at þe natiuite of oure Lorde. Noȝtforþan, we þat ar in þe west partie of þe world, we bygynne þe ȝer of Criste at þe incarnacioun of Criste. Also, þe lesse nombre of þe ȝeres of Criste I take for þe last 10, or elles for al þe nombre þat comeþ after þe last 10. *Verbi gratia.* <u>We ar now in þe 1378 ȝere</u> of Criste: þe lesse noumbre here is 8. 255 And when þe ȝeres of Criste <u>com to 1380, þan schal</u> **[f. 48ra]** þe laste 10 be þe lesse noumbre. So þat þe lesse noumbre, os I tak here, is euermore fro þe laste[47] j inclusif to his 10 inclusif. Þan þou maiste noȝt depart j into 4 euen, ne 2 mowe noȝht be diuisede into 4 euen, ne 3 neyþer, but 4 mow be twynnede into 4 parties, ilk alike mykil. And þerfor euermore þe nexte 260 Seynt Mathies day after is bisexte. Item, 5 mow noȝt be twynnede into 4 euen, ne 6, ne 7, but 8 mowe, and þerfor þe next Seynt Mathis dai after is

---

47   fro þe laste] *foll. by* fro þe laste *canc.* R

Plate 2 (*continued*). © The British Library Board: London, British Library, Royal MS 17 D.i, f. 52 (verso of f. 51*, folded over).

bisexte. Item, 9 mow noght, ne 10, ne 1[1] neyþer,[48] and so euermore whil þe world lasteþ.

Et ne were þis dai þat is þus caused of þise 6 houres at þe 4 ȝeres ende   265
kepte & sette in at his certeyn, we schulde erre foule, seond a day comand in þe ȝere & noȝt conteynede in eny of alle þe moneþes of þe ȝere, & so schulde þe kalender be defectif. And eke þer schulde no feste in þe ȝere be stedfaste ne certeyne. And also, but it wer kepte os I sai, ȝole day schulde wiþin 364 ȝere falle in as longe daies & in þe same tyme of the ȝere os   270
þe Annunciacioun doþ, or elles werre, þat ȝol schuld falle þer mydsomer day falleþ, as þe Maistre of þe Compote preueþ in his ferst *Boke of Compote*, þe 4 c. *Et* meny oþer causes schulde elles bifalle, in so mykel þat we schulde neuer we- **[f. 48rb]** ten ne knowen what day wer what dai. I passe mykel be cause of prolixite.   275

And for to haue þe lep ȝere euermore wiþout eny studye or wiþout eny acontyng, and euermore þe Sonday lettre wiþout eny kalender, & also in what ȝere of þe sol-cicle we ar, se by þis figure þat stant on þe pacche. *Ciclus solaris* (*anglice*: þe sol-cicle) is a reuolucioun of tyme, i. comyng or

---

48   ne 11 neyþer] M7, ne 10 neyþer R, neyther CgH, *om.* GSc

wending aboute of a tyme, in whiche reuolucion ar fulfillede al þe vari-   280
ance & al þe diuersetees þat befalle in þe ȝere, by þe concurrant & by þe
bisexte. And þis space of tyme is fulfillede in 28 ȝere, for in so mykel space
al þe forsaide variances ar complet, i. fulfillede. For euery fest in þe ȝere[49]
haþ had his course by euery dai in þe weke, and also bysexte haþ had his
course by euery dai in the weke. & so in al þe sol-cicle riste an hole weke   285
of þe bisextes.

[f. 51*/52, *inserted volvelle; Plate 2*][50]

+ Nos & Garlandus ||
First dai of þe ȝere, flite þrede forth, pryk to þe nere,
and at þe ferþ, lepe ȝere, whil þou leuest in erþe here. ||
Threde eke þe kenneþ, Sonday what lettre on renneþ   290
And in what ȝere of þe sol-sicle, wiþoute were. ||
[*at bottom of diagram:*] Nascitur Christus

[f. 48rb] What ar þe concurrantz Y passe. But tak hede on what lettre
Sondai[51] goþ, os I teche in þe verse. & by þis verse þou shalt weten euermore on what nombre þi concurrant goþ. F E D C B A G are concurrantz: 295
when þe Sonday goþ on F, þe concurrantz goþ þat ȝere on j. When þe
Sonday goth on E, þe concurrant goþ on 2. When on D, on 3, & so of alle
þat oþer.

For to knowe & for to wirke by þe forsaide figure, the verses þat I haue
writen abou[t]e[52] techeþ [f. 48va] expressly anogh. And if þis forsaid fig-   300
ure be loste or fordon, by þise verse [þ]ow[53] mayst make it aȝein; and þou
mayste konne it on þi fyngres:

Fons . est . dans . bis . a . gro . fun . dum . ci . bat . au . fer . e . da . cem ;
Au . gens . [blank] . [blank] . cas bos . an . gens . e . di . ci . bus . glans.

In þise 2 verses ar comprehendede & sett euermore þe first lettre of þe   305
first sillabe in þe figure, of þe first lettre of þe 2 sillabe in þe 2 space, and
so þow schalt wete where þou schalt sett þi lep ȝere. Se by þis verse: B C;
D E; [F G; A B];[54] C D; E F; G A. Vndur B, s. vndur þe 4 lettre, þe 4 lettre

---

49 ȝere] M7CgHGSc, ȝeȝere (*first ȝe poss. canc.*) R
50 *Diagram and text on inserted leaf 51*/52 are given here, for ease of reference to Dan-*
    iel's discussion in the main text on f. 48ra–vb.
51 Sondai] *foll. by* Sonday *canc.* R
52 aboute] GSc, abowtyn CgH, aboue RM7 (*see note*)
53 þow] M7CgHGSc, tow R
54 F G; A B] CgHGSc, *two blank spaces separated by points* R, *blank space* M7

fro F, is acompted C; & E vnder D, s. in þe 4 space fro B exclusif; and so
of al þat oþer.   310

If þou wilt knowen the sol-cicle & þe lep ȝere in þi fingeres, do þus: tak
28 sillablis, of which 28 sillablis, þe ferst lettres ar fonden for þe Sonday of
28 wynter. And accompte hem by the ioyntz of þi 4 fyngres. (I speke noȝt
of þe þombe.) Set þe first ȝere of þe sol-cicle in the grond of þi lik-pot in
þi lefte hande, þe 2 ȝere in þe 2 ioynt, þe 3 ȝere in þe 3 ioynt, þe 4 in þe lik- 315
pot ende, þe 5 in the grounde of mykel-man, & so forth thoroghoute til þe
cicle come oute. & euermore in þi fingris endis falleþ lep ȝere.

As often as þou seest 2 lettres togeder, þe ton vndur the toder, þat lettre
þat is put out of þe waie, s. that [f. 48vb] lettre þat stant byneþe, schal be
Sondai lettre by Januari & Februarie, to Seynt Mathies dai come, & þat 320
lettre þat stant abouen him, stille in his ordre, schal be Sondai lettre forth
þorghout al þe ȝere. & so forþ by al þe cicle while þe worlde lasteþ.

Also þe sone, as I saide, dwelleþ or elles woneþ in euerych of þe 12
signes 30 daies & 10 houres, which 10 houres gader hem togeder, i. into
[12]⁵⁵ siþes 10 houres, and þai make in the ȝere 5 daies, of which 5 daies, 325
on is set in Januari, þe 2 in Marche, þe 3 in May, þe 4 in Octobre, þe 5 in
Decembre. And ne were þo 10 hours þat bleue so ouer, euery monyth in
the ȝere schulde haue euen 30 daies, mo ne lesse.

Ne haue no wondur of Februarie þat haþ but 28 daies, ne of Jul þat haþ
31 daies, & August 31 daies eke. For þow Julius Cesar þe emperoure of 330
Rome dede take 2 daies out of Februarie & put hem into a monyth þat he
callede Julius after his owen name, and also Augustus Cesar, emperour of
Rome, made his monyth for to haue 31 daies eke, & callede it August after
him, noȝtforþan þe sonne dwelleþ neþer þe more ne the lesse in a signe þan
in anoþre, for þai had no power in þe planetz ne in þe firmament.   335

Item þe forsaide 13 minutes & 45 2ᵉ in a 100 ȝere cause a day, & þat dai
is ympede in Decembre. And þat ȝere haþ euermore⁵⁶ [f. 49ra] when he
comeþ aboute 367 dais, and it is callede *magnus bisextus* (*anglice*: þe grete
bisext or elles þe grete lep ȝere).

Mars⁵⁷ is *calidus* & *siccus* in exces, & þerfor he is a noyouse planete, for 340
he disposeþ to werres, batelles, and⁵⁸ fiȝtes, & sleyng of folk, & to bryn-
nyngis of houses. But be cause of temprure þorgh þe godenes of Venus and
Jupitre, often tymes his malice is refreynede & wiþstant. He is rede os fyur
colour & sparkelond. (And al þe planetz sparcle, but þogh oþer sterris do

---

55   12] 30 RCgHGSc, 13 M7 (*see note*)
56   euermore] *catchword*: when he
57   Mars] *marg.*: Mars
58   and] M7CgHSc, G *damaged*, and (*line end*) & R

so to our sight, it is noȝt but by cause of meuyng of eyre bytwene hem &   345
our sight. Som saie þat planetes sparcle noȝt.) Mars fulfilliþ his course in
2 ȝere, dwelland in euery of þe 12 signes 60 daies, & in euery gre aboute 2
daies natu[r]el.[59]

Jupitre[60] is *calidus* & *humidus*, tempre. In alle his myȝtes & wirkingz,
he is gode & neuermore wicked: Jupitre, i. a helply fader. He is bytwene   350
Mars & Saturnus: þe hender partie of him slakeþ and trempeþ þe malice
of Mars, and þe ȝonder party of Jupitre releseth & trempeþ þe malice of
Saturnus, so þat ne wor he, þe malice of Mars & of Saturnus scholde fordo
þe more del of creatures in erþe. He is faire and bright in colour, white os
mylk. But when he goþ hie vp, þat he nygheþ to- **[f. 49rb]** ward þe cercle of   355
Saturne, þogh he be kyndly white & bright, noȝtforþan he takeþ a dymhed
& a palehede þorgh þe presence & þe nerhede of Saturne. He fulfilleþ hes
course in 12 ȝer, dwellond in euery of þe 12 signes j ȝere & in a gre aboute
[a 7] daies.[61]

Saturnus[62] is *frigidus* & *siccus* (vnderstond alwaie in effecte, for oþerwise   360
is noght he hote ne colde). Saturnus is ferrest fro vs of al þe 7 planetz,
[wikedest of] al[63] in effecte. And when he regneþ, & þat is euermore when
he is in Capricorn or *in Aquario*, þan ar grete flodes or grete droghtes of
which al de[r]this[64] & hungres, or elles general sores & sekenes & pestilence in man comeþ. When he nygheþ þe sone so, or þe sone him, of his   365
malice he dymmeþ þe liȝt of þe sone & þe myȝt and þe vertue of þe sones
[hete].[65] & so when he nygheþ Jupitre or Jupitre him, it letteþ mykel of his
malice, but he noȝt Jupitre saue in liȝt, for when he comeþ nygh Jupitre,
he takeþ liȝt & brightnes of Jupitre, for his kynde colour is pale & wan.
Saturnus filfilleþ his course in 30 ȝere, dwellond in euery of þe 12 signes 2   370
ȝere & a half. *Et* syn þat euery of[66] þe 12 signes is departede in 30 degrees,
it semeþ wel þa[t] he[67] goþ euery monyþ a gre.

This [12][68] signes, i. parties of þe firmament **[f. 49va]** in whiche þe firmament is departed, & þe speres of þe 7 planetz, & þe speres of þe 4 elementz,
& in what signe what planet regneþ, se in þis figure [Plate 3]:   375

---

59   naturel] M7CgHGSc, natuel R
60   Jupitre] *marg.*: Jupitre
61   aboute a 7 daies] abowtyn a 7 dayes CgH, abowten his cours 7 dayes GSc, aboute
       [*blank space*] daies RM7 (*see note*)
62   Saturnus] *marg.*: Saturnus
63   wikedest of al] & wickeddest G, and wickid Sc, and werst of all CgH, proued soþ al
       RM7
64   derthis] CgHGSc, dethis RM7
65   hete] CgHGSc, *om.* RM7
66   of] M7CgHGSc, of of R
67   þat he] CgHGSc, þat she M7, þa she R
68   12] M7CgHGSc, 21 *with* 2 *underpuncted, poss. to indicate transposition* R

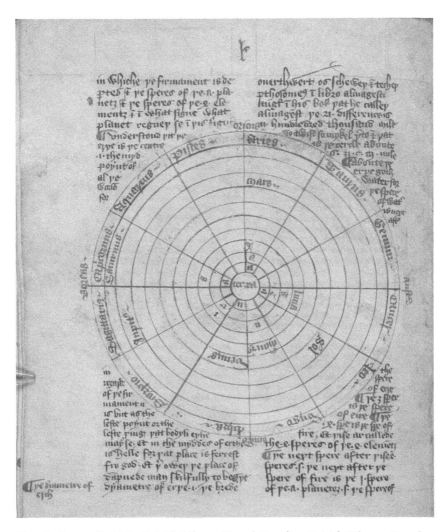

Plate 3. *Rota celi*. © The British Library Board: London, British Library, Royal MS 17 D.i, f. 49v.

Vnderstond þit þe erþe is þe centre, i. the mydpoynt, of al þe world. For in regarde of þe firmament, it is but as the leste poynt or the leste þing þat bodyli eyhe may se. *Et* in the myddes of erthe is helle, for þat place is ferrest fro God. *Et* þer oweþ þe place of dampnede man skilfully to be.

Þe dyametre of erþe,[69] i. þe brede [**f. 49vb**] ouerthwert, os scheweþ &   380 techeþ Ptholomeus *in libro Almagesti* (*anglice*: in his bok þat he calleþ

---

69   Þe dyametre of erþe] *marg.*: þe diametre of erth

Almagest), þe 21 difference, is 11 hundred[70] thousand mile. Do twise so mykel þerto & þat is þe cercle aboute, s. 33 c. M. mile.

Aboute þe erþe goth water, for þe spere of water is next after the spere of erþe. Þe 3 spere[71] is þe spere of eire. Þe 4 spere is þe spere of fire. *Et þise* 385 ar callede the 4 speres of þe 4 elementz.

Þe next spere after þise 4 speres, s. þe next after þe spere of fire, is þe j spere of þe 7 planetez, s. þe spere of **[f. 50ra]** þe mone.

Luna,[72] as techeþ Ptholomeus, is as mykel as þe 39 part of al erþe. *Et* fro erþe to þe mone, i. to þe hidder partie of the spere of þe mone, is an 390 100,000 & 9,000 & 36 myle. And fro þe mone to Mercure,[73] i. fro þe hidder partie of þe spere of þe mone to þe hidder partie of þe spere of Mercurie, 700,000 & 42,000 mile.

Mercure is nerhande as mykel os þe 22,000 part of þe erþe. And fro him to Venus[74] is 500,000 & 28,000 & 750 myle.　　　　　　　　　　　　　　395

Venus is as mykel as þe 37 part of erþe. And fro Venus to Sol[75] is 3000,000 & 700 & 40 myle.

Sol is 166 siþes alse mykel as al erþe & a litle more. Fro him to Mars[76] is 1000,000 & 800,000 & 65,000 myle.

Mars is alse mykel os al erþe & half erþe þerto & þe 8 part of erþe. Fro 400 him to Jupitre[77] is 28,000 M, 800,000 & 47,000 mile.

Jupitre is os 95 siþes as mykel os erþe. Þe space fro him to Saturne[78] is 46,000 M, 800,000 & 16,000 & 250 myle.

Saturnus is 91 syþes as mykel os al erþe. And fro him to þe sterres,[79] i. to þe firmament þer þe sterres ar fix, is 65,000 M & 300,000 & 57,000 & 405 half a þousand myle.

Þis firmament wiþ his sterres Ptholomeus diuiseþ [into][80] 6 ordres, i. into 6 speres. *Et* al þe sterres in þe firmament ar called *stelle fixe* (*anglice*: stedefast sterres). Þo sterres þat ar callede planetes, þat gone in here propre speres euermore **[f. 50rb]** agayne the firmament fro the west to þe est, os I 410

70　hundred] M7CgHSc, c. G, hundredred R
71　spere] M7CgHGSc, sp*erere* R
72　Luna] *marg.*: þe quantit & distance of þe mone
73　Mercure] *marg.*: Mercure
74　Venus] *marg.*: Venus
75　Sol] *marg.*: Sol
76　Mars] *marg.*: Mars
77　Jupitre] *marg.*: Jupitre
78　Saturne] *marg.*: Saturnus
79　þe sterres] *marg.*: þe sterres
80　into] Sc, it yn to G, *om.* RM7CgH

saide, ar callede *stelle arratice*, or *stelle retrograde* (*anglice*: errond sterres
or elles bach sterres). *Et* euery grete sterre fix of þe firste ordre, i. of þe 1
spere of þe firmament, for to bigynne at þe ȝondrast ferst, is 97 siþes as
mykel os al erþe. *Et* euery grete sterre fix of þe 2 spere of þe firmament is
90 siþes as mykel os al erþe. Of þe 3 spere, 72 siþes os erþe. Of þe 4, 54 as   415
erþe. Of þe 5, 36 os al erþe. Of þe 6 ordre, þe leste sterre þat we se is 18
siþes as mykel os al erþe.

Þan herby it semeth wel þat þe most body[81] of al þe worlde is þe son;
next after him þe 15 sterres; after hem Jupitre; after him Saturnus; and after
him al þe sterres fix; after hem Mars; after him erþe; after erþe, Venus; after   420
Venus, Luna; after Luna, Mercurius.

Now þis heuen wiþ his sterres & þe firmament is þe 12 spere & it is
called in Latyn *primum mobile vel primus motus* (*anglice*: þe ferst þing
þat stereþ, or elles þe first þat maketh to stere). And for þis skil, for it is
þe principal þing þat stereþ & makeþ[82] al other þinges vnder him, i. al þat   425
is here benethe stirred, for aboue him is noþing sterede, but he meueth &
stereth alle þe sterres & planetes and speres vnder him, and her [f. 50va]
meuyng is meuyng of al þinges here byneþe. Þe 13 spere (þat Ptholome
calleþ þe 10 spere) is callede *celum imperium*, i. þe set of God, & dwellyng
& resting place of angeles & blissed soules. *Et* þat heuen is noȝt moeble   430
ne sterede, but stable & stedefaste & quiete wiþouten ende. And al þise 11
speres, s. fro erþe exclusif to þe firmament inclusif, ar callede heuenis. *Et*
byȝonde *celum*, i. biȝonde þat heuen þat is ouer al heuenes, i. *celum impe-*
rium, is riȝt noght.

And for I spak of regnyng of planetz,[83] vnderstonde þat þan regne þe   435
planetes & ar in her moste myȝt when þai ar in here principal houses.
For when a planete is in his house, he is as a man in his owen propur
place. Þe principal house of þe mone is Cancer; Virgo of Mercure; Libra
of Venus; Leo of Sol; Aries of Mars; Sagittare of Jupitre; Capricorn of
Saturn.   440

Now whie a signe is called þe house of a planete is for þis skil: for þat
plane[te][84] was ferst made in þat signe, or for as mykel os þat planete ferst
apered in þat signe to man on erþe, or elles for alse mykel os þat signe most
acordeþ to þat planete. Also þer is difference bitwene þe principal houses
of planetis & þe secundarie houses. Þe principal house of a planete, i. þat   445

---

81 þe most body] *marg.*: þe gretnes of þe bodies of planetez
82 makeþ] M7CgHSc, *om.* G, ma(*line end*)makeþ R
83 planetz] *marg.*: of houses of planetz principales
84 planete] CgHGSc, plane RM7

signe þat is principal house to a planete, accordeþ in both qualites to that pla- **[f. 50vb]** net to whom he is signe & principal house.

Þe secundarie house of a planete[85] is þat signe of þe firmament þat accordiþ to hym, bot in o qualite alone. And so is Geminis house to Mercure; Taurus to Venus; Scorpio to Mars; Pisces to Jupitre, and Aquarie to   450 Saturn. But noȝtforþan Sol & Luna, eþer of hem haþ only o house, i. Sol haþ Leo & Luna haþe Cancer.

Þe qualites of other signes & of planetz, se in þis wise: Aries, Leo, and Sagittare: *ignea, colerica, masculina,* & *orientalia* (Est). Taurus, Virgo, & Capricorn: *terrea, melancolica, feminina,* [*bori*]*alia* (North).[86] Gemini,   455 Libra, & Aquarius: *aerea, sanguinea, masculina,* & *occidentalia* (West). Cancer, Scorpio, & Pisces: *aquea, fleumatica, feminina, meridionalia* (South).

And euerych of þis 12 signes haþ principal part & maistri in mannes body. Aries principaly haþ þe hed of man; Taurus þe neke & þe þrote;   460 Gemini þe schuldres & þe armes & þe hondes; Cancer þe brest & þe longes & þe spirituale membrez; Leo þe stomac & þe hert; Virgo þe wombe & þe lyuer & þe guttes; Libra þe reyns & þe schere & þe vesie; Scorpio þe taile ende & þe priue membris; Sagittarius þe hipes & þe þies; Capricorn þe knees & þe hames; Aquarius þe ligges & þe calues of þe ligges and þe   465 ancles; **[f. 51ra]** Pisces the fete.

And os astromyens teche, if eny membre of man be hugely hurte, do no lechecraft þerto while þe mone is in þe signe of þat membre. & if þou wilt weten in what[87] signe & in what gre of what signe euermore þe mone is (for as Y said, þe lune haþ most effecte in bodies heer byneþe), se by þis   470 table þat folweþ:

Tabula lune [Plate 4; Table 2]

Tak þe age of þe mone in þe first side of þis table, s. in þe lefte halfe, & tak hede in what **[f. 51rb]** monyth þou art, and in þe same signe is þe lune, & in þe same gre as þe nombre in þe riȝt side, euene ouer anentes þe age   475 of þe mone, telleþ.

Item, if þou wil wete what planet in what oure of þe day regneþ, se euermore by þis next table sewand.

---

85   secundarie house of a planete] *marg.*: houses secundari<e> o planet<z>
86   borialia North] CgH, australia north RM7, australia GSc
87   in what] M7CgHG, in what in what R, in what degree of what Sc

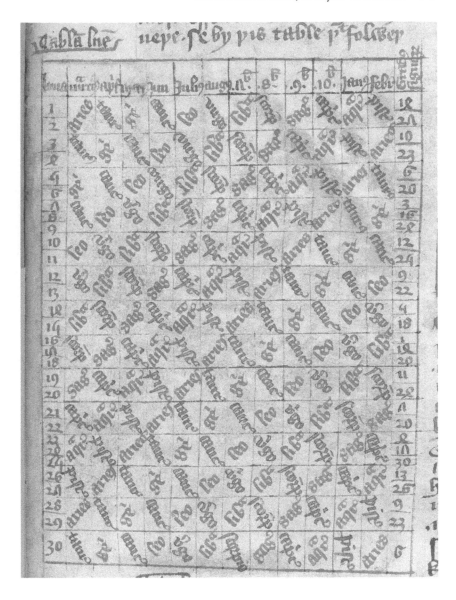

Plate 4. *Tabula lune.* Cf. Table 2. © The British Library Board: London, British Library, Royal MS 17 D.i, f. 51ra (detail).

Table 2. *Tabula lune* (f. 51ra)†

Day of the Moon	March	April	May	June	July	Aug.	Sept.	Oct.	Nov.	Dec.	Jan.	Feb.	Degrees of the Signs
1	Aries	Taur	Gem	Canc	Leo	Virgo	Libra	Scorp	Sagit	Capri	Aquar	Pisc	14
2													27
3	Taur	Gem	Canc	Leo	Virgo	Libra	Scorp	Sagit	Capri	Aquar	Pisc	Aries	10
4													23
5	Gem	Canc	Leo	Virgo	Libra	Scorp	Sagit	Capri	Aquar	Pisc	Aries	Taur	6
6													20
7	Canc	Leo	Virgo	Libra	Scorp	Sagit	Capri	Aquar	Pisc	Aries	Taur	Gem	3
8													16
9													24 [for 29]
10	Leo	Virgo	Libra	Scorp	Sagit	Capri	Aquar	Pisc	Aries	Taur	Gem	Canc	12
11													25
12	Virgo	Libra	Scorp	Sagit	Capri	Aquar	Pisc	Aries	Taur	Gem	Canc	Leo	9
13													22
14	Libra	Scorp	Sagit	Capri	Aquar	Pisc	Aries	Taur	Gem	Canc	Leo	Virgo	5
15													18
16	Scorp	Sagit	Capri	Aquar	Pisc	Aries	Taur	Gem	Canc	Leo	Virgo	Libra	1
17													14
18													20 [for 27]

#													
19	Sagit	Capri	Aquar	Pisc	Aries	Taur	Gem	Canc	Leo	Virgo	Libra	Scorp	11
20													24
21	Capri	Aquar	Pisc	Aries	Taur	Gem	Canc	Leo	Virgo	Libra	Scorp	Sagit	7
22													20
23	Aquar	Pisc	Aries	Taur	Gem	Canc	Leo	Virgo	Libra	Scorp	Sagit	Capri	4
24													17
25													30
26	Pisc	Aries	Taur	Gem	Canc	Leo	Virgo	Libra	Scorp	Sagit	Capri	Aquar	13
27													26
28	Aries	Taur	Gem	Canc	Leo	Virgo	Libra	Scorp	Sagit	Capri	Aquar	Pisc	9
29													23
30	Taur	Gem	Canc	Leo	Virgo	Libra	Scorp	Sagit	Capri	Aquar	Pisc	Aries	6

† Latin terms in Tables 2 and 3 are translated or modernized from the original tables.

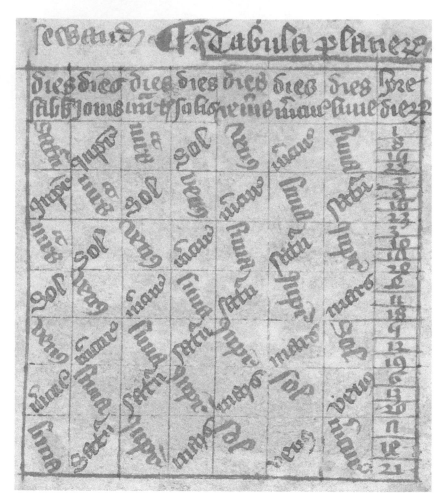

Plate 5. *Tabula planetarum*. Cf. Table 3. © The British Library Board: London, British Library, Royal MS 17 D.i, f. 51rb (detail).

Tabula plane[t]arum[88] [Plate 5; Table 3]

Suppose þat þis day be Sonday, þan Sol hath þe first houre, i. regneþ & is   480
mayster and haþ most might in þat houre of al þe planetz. Venus haþ þe
2 houre; Mercure þe 3; Luna þe 4; Saturnus þe 5; Jupitre 6; & Mars 7. Þan
comeþ Sol agayn and haþ þe 8 houre; Venus þe 9; Mercure þe 10; Luna 11;
Saturnus 12; Jupitre 13; Mars 14. Eftesones comeþ Sol agayn, & takeþ þe

---

88   planetarum] M7, planearum R, *om.* CgHGSc

Table 3. *Tabula planetarum* (**f. 51rb**)

Saturday	Thursday	Tuesday	Sunday	Friday	Wednesday	Monday	Hours of the Day
Saturn	Jupiter	Mars	Sun	Venus	Mercury	Moon	1
							8
							15
							22
Jupiter	Mars	Sun	Venus	Mercury	Moon	Saturn	2
							9
							16
							23
Mars	Sun	Venus	Mercury	Moon	Saturn	Jupiter	3
							10
							17
							24
Sun	Venus	Mercury	Moon	Saturn	Jupiter	Mars	4
							11
							18
Venus	Mercury	Moon	Saturn	Jupiter	Mars	Sun	5
							12
							19
Mercury	Moon	Saturn	Jupiter	Mars	Sun	Venus	6
							13
							20
Moon	Saturn	Jupiter	Mars	Sun	Venus	Mercury	7
							14
							21

15; Venus 16; Mercure 17; Luna þe 18; Saturn 19; Jupitre 20; Mars 21. Þan   485
comeþ Sol agayn þe 3 tyme & haþ þe 22; Venus þe 23; [**f. 51va**] Mercure
þe 24. And so endiþ þe dai naturel. Þan comeþ Luna and haþ þe j houre
on þe Mononday, Saturne þe 2, Jupitre þe 3, Mars þe 4, Sol þe 5, Venus
the 6, Mercurie þe 7. Þan comeþ Luna agayn, os Sol dede on his dai, and
takeþ þe 8 houre, Saturne þe 9, and so til þou come to 24. And so is þe   490
Monondai don. And þan comeþ Mars and takeþ þe j hour of Tywesdaie,
Sol þe 2, Venus 3.

And so þe daie bigynneþ euermore at mydnyght, os I saide biforn, os al Cristen men vse, outetaken Eluenden in his *Kalender*, þat he bigynneþ his dai at midday after þe Sarasenis (& in þat he is for to blame). Þogh I haue 495 gone out of my waie, i. a litil fro my purpos, I þonk God I haue noȝt erryd.

Item, *vrina lactea*[89] & *subtenuis* & mykel in quantite in þe ende of a febre pthisik, os I saide, or in the ende of a febre interpolate, it is noble tokne, for þe whithede seiþ vanissching & wanysyng awaie of vnkynd hete. Þat it is *subtenuis*, it seiþ subtiliacioun of þe mater of þe malady. 500 What is subtiliacioun of þe mater of þe sekenes, þou mayst wel wete by þe proces þat Y saide biforn in þis same chapitle, þer I spak of compaccioun of humores and also in the nexte chapitre aforne þis, lef {*om.*}. Þat [f. 51vb] it is mykel in quantite, it seiþ sufficient purgacioun of humores þat were cause of sekenesse. But if it be *lactea* & *subtenuis* & litil in quantite in þe 505 ende, os Y saide, it seiþ comyng agayn of þe malady, & but wonder be, deþ or elles boþe.

Item, *vrina lactea, subtenuis* & wiþout febre, is wik, for it seiþ þat þe body is disposed to ydropisi. In swich febre interpolate comunely falleþ *frigus* (*anglice*: colde). Auicen seiþ þat *frigus* is causede of mater, i. of 510 humor, noȝt corrupte. *Calor*, hete, of mater corupte. When mater þat is cause of febre is gadred wiþout his vesselles, i. wiþoute veyns, þat þat kynd maystrieþ and ouercomeþ þerof, kynde schoffeþ & cacheþ him oute to þe otter parties of þe body as fer as he may, for to mundefie[n][90] þe body, i. for to purge & make clene þe body. Which mater causand febre, if it be 515 fleumatik, ferst it causeþ *frigus*.[91] If it be colrik, it causeþ *rigor* (*anglice*: starkyng or rasking for colde). If it be melancolik, it causeþ *oripilacio*[92] (*anglice*: tethe grussling). In interpolates & in cotidiens, comunly is *frigus*; in terciens *rigor*;[93] in quarteyns, *oripilacio*. And take hede þat as auctoures of phisik techeþ, difference is bitwene *rigor* & *frigus*, as seiþ Haly in his 520 *Persectif* & al auctours. For *rigor* is wiþ prichyng &[94] [f. 53ra][95] peyn in *membris animatis* (*anglice*: in þe membres of lif), and somtyme os þer wer priching wiþ a thorne. And þat is bi cause of fumosites hote & scarp stiand vp to þe heuede. Which bene *membra animata*, þe membres of lif, se in

---

89 vrina lactea] *marg.*: Item de vrina lactea
90 mundefien] Cg, mundyfie GSc, mundefieþ RM7, *om.* H
91 frigus] *marg.*: frigus
92 oripilacio] *marg.*: horripilacio
93 rigor] *marg.*: rigor
94 prichyng &] M7CgHGSc, prichyng & [*new leaf (f. 53)*] & R
95 *The volvelle now numbered 51* and inserted between ff. 50 and 51 was originally numbered 52 (still visible on the blank back side) and attached to a leaf between ff. 51 and 53 (Plate 2 above). For the verses on the volvelle, see above, 2.6.287–92.*

þe next c. folwend. When it is but *frigus*, þan is colde in membris, os it 525
wer snowe or yse, & þat is be cause of fumosites þat ar heuy & slowe in
comyng.

Item, ȝit in anoþer þere is difference atwene *rigor* & *frigus*. For when
it is *rigor*, þer is more quakyng & chyueryng þan when it is but *frigus*, &
þat is bi cause of scharphede of colre perschond and prickand þe membres 530
of lif. Whan it is but *frigus*, þer is noȝt so mykel quakyng & chyuering
os when it is *rigor*, & þat is be cause of dulhede & dedehede of fleume
corupte. Item, when it is *rigor*, þer is ferste stronge colde & chyuering
& afterward strong hete, be cause of smerthede & wodehed of colre. But
when it is *frigus*, lent chyuering and afterward lent hete, be resoun of dul- 535
hede of fleume.

Item, *oripilacio* is different fro boþe, s. fro *frigus* & *rigor*, for in oripilacioun is more huge rasyng & schaking þan when it is *frigus* or *rigor*. Item,
in oripilacioun is cold be resoun of coldhede & *rigor* be reson of siccite.
And as þe rigebon schul- **[f. 53rb]** de tobreste an[d]⁹⁶ þat is by cause of 540
terrestrete of melancolie.

[2.7]

De colore karopos: cap. 7

Color karopos, for as mykel os it is moste nere towarde White colour &
ȝelow colour in vryn, boþe in kynde and in likenes, & moste acordand in
significacioun, þerfor auctoures teche of Karopos next after hem.

Now for to knowe colour Karopos,¹ vnderstond þat os auctours teche, it 5
haþ somdel of white colour & somdele of ȝelowe colour & somdele of blac
colour, bot more of white,² os a cloþe made of white & blak stondand by
þe white. And þerfor auctours likene it to þe heres of a camel skyn.

And euermore colour Karopos seiþ þat fleume gleymouse & byndand
& melancolie g[r]os³ and indigest maistre in þe body. If it haue more of 10
white þan of ȝelowe, it seiþ þat fleume & melancolie maistre in þe body,
but fleume more. If it haue more of ȝelowe⁴ þan of white – which ȝelow

---

96 and] CgHGSc, & M7, an R

---

1 Karopos] *marg.*: 3 maner of karopos
2 more of white] *marg.*: j
3 gros] CgHGSc, goos RM7
4 more of ȝelowe] *marg.*: 2 (*no marg. number for the third "maner" in* RM7, *but included in* CgHGSc)

coloure is euermore whitisshe, but kyn[d]ly⁵ more toward mylk-white
þan white, <u>os it is saide in þe 3 c. biforne</u>, for euery vryn þat is ȝelow stant
moste by whithede with a maner of brighthede goand toward rudihede   15
kyndly – it seiþ that flume & melancoly maistrieþ, but more melancolie. If
it haue euenly of bothe, s. of whithede & ȝelowhede, it seiþ of bothe alik,
s. of *fleuma* & of melancolie. And þan when it haþ euen alike of boþe, s.
of whithed & ȝelowe- **[f. 53va]** hede, it is propurly Karopos. Þus speken
auctoures.   20

Et if þis be soþ, þan is Karopos a mene colour bitwene white & ȝelow, os
we se in þis ȝonge bachileres heuedes þat norisshe here longe lockes, which
colour is callede in Latyn *flauus* (*anglice*: white-ȝelow or elles ȝelowisshe).
Þe Comentour vppon Giles in þis same place seiþ þus: *color karopos*, seiþ
he, is flauouse like a kamel skyn, or elles þe onych stone. And I haue ler-   25
ede of hem þat haue seyn þousandes of kamayles in þe contrees of Rome
& beȝonde, þat alle kamailes, or þai be gray or dunne or elles white-gray.
And we se at eye þat white-grey & white-ȝelow ar noȝt al on. But take
hede þat, os I saide riȝt nowe, þer is 3 maner of Karopos.

And vnderstonde þat þogh al þis four coloures, s. *alba* & *glauca*, *lactea*   30
& *karopos*, bitokne feblenes of digestioun in þe lyuer, noȝtforþan Karopos leste. Wherfor it is bettre coloure þan eny of þise oþer 3. And þerfor
auctoures callen it *colorem gaudiosum* (*anglice*: ioyouse colour, or elles a
ioyful coloure), for it seiþ þat kynde is schaply and disposed for to haue
þe maystrie & þe victorie in þe duel, i. in þe fiȝt, atwene þe kynde & þe   35
sekenes. <u>Os I saide in þe c. of Blak colour</u>, *duellum*, a duel, is a fiȝt bitwene
[f. 53vb] twyne. And þerfor, if it so be þat a seke mannis water apere ferst
White & þan ȝelow & þan *lactea* & þan Karopos (or elles which of al 3
it apere, so þat þe laste be Karopos), it is a blissede tokne, for it seiþ þat
kynde schapeþ him for to wirke and ouercome þe maladye (þogh it so be   40
þat colour Karopos euermor signifieþ fleume viscouse & malancolie gros,
os Y saide while ere).

Et tak gode hede þat Whit vryn & ȝelowe vryn & Mylk-white vryn, as
þe 3 c. biforne speken, ar euermore wiþ a þenne body, or elles thennysshe, but Karopos is euermore wiþ a þik body. *Et* þerfor diuerse auctoures   45
make no distinccioun, i. no dyuerste, bytwene Karopos & Whit & Ȝelow
& Mylk-whit, saue Karopos is, os Y saie, euermore wiþ a þicke body & þe
toþer wiþ thenne or thennysshe.

It befel in þe toun of Stawnford in þe grete hostiel, þat a man of 30
or 35 ȝere age ȝede long tyme wiþ a grete sekenesse. & when he made   50
water, it steynede þe wawis like ȝelow brunstoun or pagil floure þat

---

5   kyndly] M7CgHGSc, kynly R

groweþ in mede, & thike as eny horse pisse, in so mykel þat 7 daies
after were þe wawes dyede of his vryn. At þe laste, þe malady keste
him doun. Euery man him dempte no bet þan dede. Dyuerse leches
seyne his water, þat alwaie was on: deye he schulde. [f. 54ra] The kyng-   55
es leche, makand his iourne thorogh þe town, saw his water: leue he
schulde noȝt after þe 3 day.

Þat herd he in mustryng as he myȝt and fast þoght on þat word. When
þai were al gone, he dede his wif make him a coppe ful of myes, of half a
quart, for al metes him wlatede saue myes alone. & in 13 daies hadde no   60
mete comen in his mouþe, hauand þe jawnys & þe ydropisy ek wonder
stronge and a stronge cotidien þerwiþ. When he hadde eten þise myes
agayn [n]yght,[6] he wapede hem warme & slepte & swette, til he myȝt no
longer suffre for stink of swete. Eftesones he ete myes as fele and on þe
same wise swette. & þan him þoght þat he was hole, but vneþes myȝt he   65
meue himself, ne speke myȝt he noȝt for feynt and feble. But as he myȝt,
he askede mete. And as sone as he was comforted wiþ met, he dronk euery
day, morwe & euen, centorie, i. peti bugle, as he was taght agayn þe jawnys
(for grete bugle knewe þai noȝt). And so he curede.

Now som saide þat þe forsaide vryn was ȝelow, as it semede wel at   70
eye. Et som saide þat it was noȝt ȝelow vryn propurly, for vryn propurly
ȝelow is euermore thenne & clere or elles þennysshe & clerisshe [f. 54rb]
naturaliter, i. be waie of kynd. But it was Karopos propurly, þat is euermore þik naturaliter & somtyme white-graye, moste lik a colour þat þai
callen a kenet, somtyme whit-ȝelow, & somtyme ȝelow, & somtyme euen   75
bitwene boþe whit-ȝelow [& ȝelow],[7] bot euermore þik. And þerfore
Karopos is wel likenede to þe stone þat is called onyx, os Y said biforne,
for if þou loke wel þe 5 boke of Albert Of Preciouse Stones and also þe
coment vppon þe Lapidarie, þou schalt se þat þe onix stone is of þe same
maner coloures os Y said ryght now of Karopos.   80

Þan vnderstond for a reule þat vryn Karopos, i. Whit vryn or ȝelow
vryn or Mylk-whit vryn or elles whit-graye vryn wiþ a þik body, if it
haue a maner of dymhede abouen (which dymhede may noȝt wele be perceyuede, but if þou put þi hond to þe vrynal), it seiþ a leucofleume. Leucofleuma in c. de albo colore, lef {38}. In þe leucofleu[me],[8] comunely þe   85
stomac bolneþ after mete, & eyȝen bolne & fade & wax dymmysshe &
bloisshe and þe face also, & þe feet blouten. But tak hede þat swych maner
vryn seiþ þe leucofleuma noȝt in as mykel os Karopos, but in as mykel os

6 nyght] HGSc, myght RM7Cg
7 & ȝelow] CgHG, om. M7Sc, & ȝelow canc. R
8 leucofleume] M7CgHGSc, leucofleu (line end) R

it is whitisshe. & þerfor Whit vryn seiþ more ve- **[f. 54va]** reye þe leucofleume þan doþ Karopos.   90

Item, vryn Karopos, wiþ a maner of small Grauel or chysel in þe
ground, seiþ *colicam passionem* or *iliacam passionem*. If it be *colica passio*, þan he haþe grete peyne vnder þe nauele. If it be *iliaca passio*, þan in
þe lefte side. If it be bothe *colica passio* & *iliaca passio*, þan he feleþ grete
peyn in boþe þo places. What it is, *colica passio*, Y saide in *capitulo de albo*   95
colore, lef {40}.

Ylica passio[9] is causede in þis wise: *ylion* is a small gut, a small rope,
lyand in þe body a litil aboue þe reyns. Which ylioun semeþ to þe sight os
it were a grete hepe or a grete barouful (and þow it is but on if it be rachede
oute), þat we calle þe smale guttes, þe smale ropes, be it of a man, be it of   100
a beste. In þise *yliones* ar somtym gendred & gaderede wicked humores
fleumati[k][10] & viscouse. *Et* þan by resoun of ventosite & also by reson
of litilhede of colre, which colre be cause of his hete & his clerehede & his
brighthed schulde put & cachen and delyuer oute awaie þe drestes & þe
wickede viscouse humores out of þe ylions, þat vile viscouse mater gaderet   105
& clumpreþ togeder in þe *yliones*, i. in þe guttes, and stuffeþ & wiþstoppeþ
hem. *Et* be cause þerof, wynd in þe *yliones*, for þai ar neuermore wiþout
wynde & is stof- **[f. 54vb]** fede and may noȝt oute.

And so be cause þat kynde is noght of myght for to cache oute þat wynd
& þat wicked mater betyme,[11] ne also kynde hete is noȝt myȝty on his   110
partie for to helpe to defien it ne delyuer it oute, þer he halt him stille &
causeþ swich peyn & anguisshe þat him þenkeþ os on thirlede him wiþ a
wymble or a persour. And þus is *ylica passio*.

And in þis reule & also in al þe reules be þis chapitle, vnderstond Karopos os I saide in þe reule bifore þis.   115

Item, vryn Karopos & litil in quantite, wiþ sond or chesel in þe botome,
seiþ *c[a]lculus*.[12] *Calculus* is þe ston[13] in þe vesie, os *nefresia* or *nefresis* is þe
ston in þe reyns. *Lapis* is for bothe. *Nefresis* & *nefresia* in c. *de albo colore*,
lef {38}. Vnderstond þat *calculus* is caused in 3 wise: or of grete plente of
superfluytes of som vnkynd humoure, or humores þat ar gros & viscouse,   120
or of st[r]eythede[14] of þe waies of þe vryn fro þe lendes to þe vesie. Or elles
by cause þat kynd hete is noght myghty for to maistri ne for to cache out

---

9 Ylica passio] *marg.*: yliaca passio
10 fleumatik] CgHGSc, fleumatil RM7
11 betyme] *foll. by* ne also kynd hete is noght of myȝt for to cache oute þat wynde & þat
    wickede mater betyme *canc.* R
12 calculus] CgH, calculum GSc, culculus RM7
13 ston] *marg.*: þe stone is gendrede in 3 wise
14 streythede] CgH, streytnes Sc, steythede RM7, *om.* G

þat mater þat gadreþ & clompreþ in þe vesie. *Et* when it is so þat þorgh
eny of þise causes or þorgh dyuerse of hem or elles þorgh al (as comuly it
bifalleþ in þis [**f. 55ra**] malady), þat swich humor or humores mak duell- 125
yng in þe vesie or in þe reynes lenger þan þai schulden, þo parties þat ar
more moist wasten & swelten awaie, & þo partes þat ar more terrestre &
dry beleue stille. And so þat mater drieþ and hardeþ, and so is gendrede
into a maner grauel. & þan, but if kynd and kynd hete be of mygh for to
cache and dylyuer it forth out of þe body betymes, þat grauel gadreþ and 130
clatiþ togeder & so groweþ into a stone. And þan is kynd noght of mygh
for to defien it, ne for to delyuer him þerof, but if it so be þat he be mykel
more fortifiede and myghtede þan he was in gendryng þerof, riȝt as þou
seeste at eye in vesseiles when þer cleueþ of mater to þe botome or to þe
sides, and so be proces of tyme. 135

And þan it falleþ often tyme þat his fete ar colde & slepand,[15] and
his heryng feblissheþ. And þe cause of al þise poyntez is for þe sinowes
by whiche þe spiritz & þe myȝtes of kynde hete passen aboute to þe
extremytes of þe body, os to þe fete, to þe handes, & to þe eres, & so of al
oþer, ar so constrit & so astonyede and distemprede throgh violence of þe 140
malady þat þe myȝtes of þe spiritz and of þe kynde mow noght be sent,
ne haue here kynde course to her instrumentz, for to haue & to do here
office os þai schulde.

& also *yliaca passio* often tyme co- [**f. 55rb**] meþ þerwiþ, for comunli in
þe stone, the tharmes þat we calle *yliones* ar pressede and thirstede be cause 145
of þe stone in þe reyns. & by cause þerof, þe superfluites of þe j digestioun
ar wiþstant & wiþset in þe *yliones* and so causeþ inflacioun, i. bos[m]yng[16]
& bolnyng, & þerwiþ huge peyne. And þis is also *yliaca passio*.

Item, *yliaca passio* comeþ oþerwhile *in calculo* alse wel as *in nefresia* &
by þe same cause os Y saide riȝt nowe. *Calculus & nefresia* in c. de albo 150
colore, lef {36} Item, *ylica passio* is callede aposteme in þe reynes. Se in c.
de ynopos, lef {77}.

To hem þat haue þe stone or ar disposede to þe stone ar nocyf, i.
noyouse:[17] alle metes & drynkes þat cause grose humores, os boef &
pork, waterfoule, al maner bonys, and al friede metes, al salt metes; & 155
mylk & euery maner chese, & namely þat þai calle freisshe chese (oute-
taken gotes chese, for it is *calidus* & *humidus*); hard eyren; stokfissh;
notz & walnotz; peskes and euery frute til it is loyn & meluede to þe ful;
thik wyne, thik water, and rawe water; þik ale, new ale, feble ale, and if it

---

15 slepand] *marg.*: <c>ause of slepyng of fete
16 bosmyng] CgH, bosynyng RM7, swellyng Sc, *leaves wanting* G
17 noyouse] *marg.*: which þinges noyeþ þe stone

be ouer olde or go ouer lowe, & longe stondand ale, or euyl boliede ale;　160
& al swiche maner þinges.

Item, alle þo þat cause viscouse humours, os poddynges and sawcestres,
and euery mete þat is made of þe inward of beste (of schepes inward, is lest
wicked); and skynnes [f. 55va] of bestes and eles and euery ponde-fisshe;
rys & floure & pankakes and therfe brede and euyl baken brede and all　165
swyche.

Item, alle þinges þat let digestioun, os reyn water and snowe water,
watri fruyt, mykel etyng, often etyng, mykel drynk, mykel baþing, mykel
wachyng, & exces in lechery.

Item, vryn Karopos if it haue longe tyme so, s. 2 watres or 3 or mo, it　170
seiþ ake & peyn in the heuede. If it apere so newely, it seiþ þat it is for to
comen. And þis is þe philosophie: when *fleuma* haþ longe tyme holden
himself in þe body & regnede þerin, þe hete þat haþ wroght into þat
fleume, now at þe laste he haþ maistriede þat fleume and resoluede him,
or elles þe more party of him, into fumosite thik and vaporouse. Which　175
fumosites stien vp to þe cerebre, and when þai haue þer none issue, þai
cause ake and peyn in the heuede. Bot if it so be þat *fleuma* bigyn newely
for to regnen in þe body, or elles late bigan, þe kynd suffiseth noȝt ȝit nor
may noȝt ȝit maystry ne resoluen him, but abydeþ til he mai. And þerfor
when þe vryn apereþ so, it seiþ þat ake wil comen. Þis also techeþ Ypocras　180
in þe laste ende of þe 4 boke of *Afforismis*.

Item, *vryna karopos* inequal, i. more þik in som place þan in some,
and drobly, seyth exces and destemperure of a fleume [f. 55vb] naturel[18]
wiþouten febre, & þerwiþ feble digestioun and ake in þe hede, and namely
in þe hendre partie, for þer is þe se of fleume (os Y saide in þe laste ende　185
de albo colore), & bolnyng & rising aboute þe sydes & in þe chokes, &
wicked taste in þe mouthe and mykel spitting, dulhede of þe wittes, slowhede and slombrihede & grete heuynes. And al þise poyntz ar causede
þorogh resolucioun of humores gros & crude mater, of whiche mater
comeþ a fumosite. And when þat fumosite may noght be consumpte ne　190
maistriede of kynde hete, be cause þat kynd hete is but feble, it passed
forth to dyuerse parties of þe body & agreueþ hem and noyeþ hem. And
þat fumosite spredeþ aboute to þe ypicondres and þer causeþ inflacioun.
<u>Ypocondria</u> in c. <u>de liuido colore, lef</u> {27}. Also þat fumosite stieþ vp by
ysophagus to þe tunge and þere it is inspissede, i. thikkede, aboute þe　195
tunge, and þer causeþ wicked tast & mykel spotel. <u>Ysophagus, se inward,</u>
<u>lef</u> {57}. And þan it stieþ so vp to þe hede and þere causeþ peyne and
ake, and so spredeþ aboute by þe synowes of þe body and dulleþ and

---

18　naturel] M7CgH, natuerel R, kind Sc, *wanting* G

feblissheþ þe mewyng & þe wittes and þe myȝtes of þe body and of þe
soule. And so is al þe body distemprede. 200

Þe whitehed is be cause of frigidite & by cause of fleume, for fleume is
kyndly colde and white, & þerfor he cau- **[f. 56ra]** seþ whitehede[19] in the
vryn. Þat it is spis is bi cause of humidite of fleume, for humidite thickeþ
þe vryn, <u>os Y saide in c. *de albo colore*, lef</u>[20] {*om.*}. Þat it is inequal is bi
cause of turbacion and disturblyng of humores in þe body, <u>os Y saide in 205
c. *de nigro colore*, lef</u> {19}. Þat þe bodi of þe vryn is vnpur, i. thickesh and
droblissh, it seiþ defaute & feblehede of kynde hete, in þat it is noȝt of
myght for to purge ne to clense þe substaunce of þe blode.

Item, vryn Karopos litil & drubli, and wiþ smal long resolucions or
elles wiþ smale Greynes, seiþ a course and a gadring of wicked & colde 210
humores in the body, for to gader and gendre into aposteme. Item, þe
same maner vryn seiþ þe wome flux. Þis is þe philosophie: in þe wombe
flux þe blode is mykel priued and refte fro his spiritz & his kynde and
his myȝtes. And by cause þerof þe 2 digestioun, s. *epar*, is feyntede &
feblede and haþ noȝt his kynde myght for to drawe to him his succosite, 215
i. humidite. And by cause þerof ar the humores but litil & fewe & feble.
And þat is þe skyl whie þe vryn is litle & þe egestioun mykel, s. often. *Et*
þerfor seiþ Ypocras þat mykil vryn made by nyght seiþ litle egestioun; &
mykel egestioun, litle vryn. Egestioun is lyueraunce behynde, os ingestioun is etyng. 220

Þe forsaide re- **[f. 56rb]** solucions come of mater of fleume, descendant
fro þe stomac into þe ylions, <u>of whiche ylions it is saide biforne</u>.[21] Þat þe
vryn is desturblede & droubli is bi cause of myxtion & distemperur of
humores in þe body. But tak gode hede þat þogh þise 2 forsaide vryns ar
os who saie al on, noghtforþan þis is þe difference atwene: for whan swich 225
maner of vryn seiþ colleccioun of wicked mater drawand toward an eposteme, þan is þe sorehede & ake and peyn and greuance þer it gadereth or
þere it wolde gedre in þe body, wheresoeuer it be. And also a[s][22] Theophilus techeþ, it hath a maner of Fathede abouen, & noȝt so when it seiþ
þe wombe flux. But when it seiþ þe wombe flux, þan is al þe peyn in þe 230
wombe & in þe þerme.

Item, tak god hed þat al þise forsaide reules moste be vnderstonden riȝt
os I saide in þe j reule sa[ue][23] on, s. noȝt alse mykel os Karopos, but in as
mykel os white.

---

19 whitehede] *foll. by* whithede *canc.* R
20 lef] *poss. canc.* R
21 biforne] *foll. by* lef *canc.* R
22 as] CgHSc, a RM7, *wanting* G
23 saue] CgHSc, sa RM7, *wanting* G

Item, if it be so þat after þe forsaide maner vryn þat seiþ colleccioun of 235
aposteme come an vryn Karopos, & mykel in quantite, it seiþ solucioun, i.
ondoyng and wastyng & waneshing & vanysshyng awaie, of þat mater þat
so wold haue bredde into aposteme. In 3 wise is vryn spisse, <u>os þou haste
in c. *de nigro colore,* lef</u> {19}.

Now vnderstond þat mannes body is distincte in 4 parties,[24] which 240
4 parties ar callede in þis fa- **[f. 56va]** culte *4 regiones corporis humani*
(*anglice*: þe 4 regions or elles þe 4 principal partes or placis of mannes
body).

Þe first region[25] conteyneþ *membra animata,* þe membres of[26] lif. And
þis regioun bigynneþ at þe epiglot exclusif & lasteþ vpward. Membres of 245
lif ar þise: þe cerebre, *pia mater* & *dura mater,* & alle þo synowes þat ar
þerabouten þo parties. Which synowes bring þe *spiritus* of lif to þe cerebre, for to 3eue witt and maken & formen stering and my3t & vertu of þe
soule and of þe lif, and be cause þerof ar callede *membra animata* (*anglice*:
þe membres of lif). 250

Of þe membres of lif, *cerebrum,* þe cerebre[27] or elles þe brayn, is most
principal and most noble, & for þis skil: for þogh it so be þat þe soule
(which is lif to al þe body)[28] be oueral in þe body and in euery partie of þe
body alike (for alse wel is þe soule in þe litle fyngres ende as in eny oþer
place of þe body), no3tforþan þe soule is more principaly in þe cerebre, be 255
cause þat þe soule haþ his principal mi3tes and vertues of wirkyng more
þer þan ower elles, os ymaginacioun & resoun and mynde, as þou schalt
se afterward.

Þus is *cerebrum* descryuede in þe *Boke of Anathomyes,* i. in þe *Boke of
þe Exposisioun of þe Inder* **[f. 56vb]** *Parties of Mannes Body*: þe cerebre is 260
a membre *calidus* & *humidus per se,* saue he is *frigidus* & *humidus per accidens,* rounde & neysshe and softe and tendre in his[29] substance, and white
in colour, & distincte in 3 celles, in 3 kawates. No3tforþan some sai þat it is
frigidus and *humidus per se,* but al saie þat it is *humidus.* And for þis skil it
is *humidus*: þat it schulde be bettre & þe more redilik tak and vnderfonge 265
impressiones and formes of witte and of vnderstondyng in seing and hering
and in demyng & in auisementes. Þise termes, *calidus* and *humidus,* <u>þe j
boke, 4 c., lef</u> {6}. Þis terme *per se* is as mykel for to saie as propurly, in his
owen kynd. *Per accidens* <u>in þe j bok, þe 2 c., lef</u> {7}.

---

24 4 parties] *marg.*: þe 4 regions of mannes body
25 Þe first region] *marg.*: þe first regioun
26 of] *foll. by* of *canc.* R
27 cerebre] *marg.*: cerebre
28 lif to al þe body] *foll. by* for wiþouten þe soule *canc.* R (*see note*)
29 his] *foll. by* sub *canc.* R

Gilbert, in his Coment vpon Giles, seiþ þat *cerebrum* is *frigidum* & 270
humidum per se, & for þe sam skil þat it is *humidus*, for þe same skil it is
nesche. It is rounde for þis skil, os seiþ Constantyn in his coment: þat it
schulde haue no anglis, i. none hernes ne corners, in whiche schulde superfluytes gaderen for to gendre or cause eny malady, & also for þe more
round a þing is, þe bettre it is kepte and sauede fro strokes & fro hurtinges. 275

It is white coloure, for of al coloures þat be, whit coloure is moste able for
vnderfonge & resceyue formes and impressions. Item, it is distincte, i. diuisede, in 3 plies,[30] i. in 3 foldynges or in 3 ka- [f. 57ra] wates. Which 3 plyes ar
callede 3 celles by cause of 3 diuerse maner of operacioun, i. of wirking, þat
he haþ. Þe firste[31] of þe 3 celles is callede by þise 3 names: *fantastica, ymagi-* 280
natiua, and *visualis* (*anglice*: þe fantastik, ymaginatif, and þe place of mannes
sight). *Et* þis is þe forparty of þe heuede, ouer þe eyen, & it bereþ þo names
by reson þat in þat place of þe hede is mannes fantasie & his ymaginacioun
of casting & of vnderstondyng, and þe myght and þe vertue & þe inder siȝt
of wit & of demyng in man. *Et* þis ymaginatif[32] is *calida* & *sicca in complex-* 285
ione, and for þis skil: þat by þo qualites it schulde kyndely be depurede and
purgede fro superfluytes, and also þat it schulde the bettre drawe and tak
þe coloures and þe formes of þinges in casting & demyng fro wiþoutwarde.

The myd plie[33] or þe myd celle is callede *racionatiua*, þe racionatif, for
þer is myȝt & vertu of di[s]cresioun[34] and of resoun.[35] And[36] it is *calida* 290
and *humida*, þat by þo qualites it schulde þe better conformen him to þe
propurtes of þinges in knowyng and in demyng, i. in chesing þe gode and
leuing þe wicked.

Þe 3 plie,[37] i. þe 3 partie, of the brayn is callede *memoratiua* or *memo-*
ralis, þe memoratif[38] or þe memorial, i. the place [f. 57rb] of memore & of 295
mynde in man, þat we calle in Englisshe þe hender party of þe heuede or
elles þe hatrel or þe iolle. *Et* it is *frigida* & *sicca*, þat by cause of þo qualites it schulde be god retentif, i. god holdyng & keping, of þinges þat ar
receyued & laide þere vp. For colde & drye const[r]eyneþ[39] & holdeþ and
byndeþ and kepeþ togeder. 300

---

30 3 plies] *marg.*: 3 distinccio<uns> of þe cerebre
31 firste] *marg.*: j
32 ymaginatif] *marg.*: ymaginatif
33 myd plie] *marg.*: 2
34 discresioun] M7CgHSc, dicresioun R, *wanting* G
35 resoun] *marg.*: racionatif
36 And] M7CgHSc, & and R, *wanting* G
37 3 plie] *marg.*: 3
38 memoratif] *marg.*: memoratif
39 constreyneþ] CgHSc, consteyneþ RM7, *wanting* G

Þan in þis wise, operacioun, i. wirkyng, of þe cerebre: al þe first, ymaginatif perceyueth and comprehendiþ þinges fro wiþouteward, be þe instrumentz of þe 5 wittes (os by þe ey3en, by þe eres, and by al þe manant).
And anone in a thoght, he sendiþ þo þinges so perceyuede & conceyuede
by certeyn synowes þat ar callede *nerui sensibiles*, þo synowes of witt or 305
elles þe wytte synowes, to þe soule & presentiþ & scheweþ & telleþ to þe
soule þo þinges, he for to deme þerof os him þinkeþ. Þan anone þe soule
draweþ him to his se, s. to þe myd party of þe heuede þat is callede racionatif, for þere is þe principal sete & dwelling place of þe soule. & þan þer
in the myddes, os a kyng or a iustice in his se, auyseth hym and demeth 310
of þo þingz þat afornhand were fantasiede and ymagynede & cast, wheder
þai be honest or inhonest, faire or fowle, gode or wickede, to done or to
leue, and **[f. 57va]** for what ende. And þus demen ymaginacioun and skil
and reson togeder.

Þen after al þis, whan þe soule haþ þus descernede, i. dempte & iuggede, 315
what is for to done and what for to leue, what to kepe & what to refuse,
þo þinges þat ar for to done and for to kepe þe soule sendeþ hem forthe to
þe memoratif, & þer he leyth hem & putteþ hem vp for to kepe in tresour.
And þan if it be so þat þat party of þe heuede be wel tempred and proporcionede in his qualites, swich þinges ar wel kepte & longe tyme. And þan 320
þai come at wil or elles noght.

Ymaginatif haþ mykel of þe spirit, be reson þat þe spirit shulde sufficiently renne and haue her course to and fro þe instrumentz of þe 5 wittes,
and swiftly and smertly bere bode, and telle to þe soule his conceytes þat he
takeþ fro wiþoutward. & also he haþ litil of marrow, i. of kynd of marow, 325
& þat is be resoun þat þe course of þe spirites schulde haue no letting
þerby. The racionatif haþ mykel of þe spirit, þat by reson þerof þe soule
mai sufficiently wirk and fulfille his spiritual operacions for þe wirkynges
of þe soule ar spiritual, i. gostly. Item, it haþ mykel of þe marowe, þat þe
spirite schulde be wel comfortede & myghted þerby. *Memoratiua* haþ but 330
litle of þe spirit, þat þo þing þat ar laide vp þer in store schuld **[f. 57vb]**
noght lightly slyde awaie be cause of plente and multitude of spiritz. And
it haþe litle also of marowe, for marowe is kyndely *humida* & þat þat is
put & sette in moyste, it slit li3tly awaie. Of þise þinges afornesaide, þou
maist concluden þe skil whie som folk[40] tak more sone þan some folk, and 335
some of better dome þan some, & some more for3etel þan some.

Pia mater and *dura mater*[41] ar tweie smale þenne skynnes, or tweie
þenne webbes, or elles tuo þenne rymes, in which þe cerebris ar wrappede

---

40 folk] M7CgHSc, forlk R, *wanting* G
41 Pia mater and dura mater] *marg.*: pia mat\<er\> & dura m\<ater\>

& hylde. Þe first is nexte þe brayn, & þat is callede *pia mater* (*anglice*: þe
tendre moder, or elles þe softe moder). If þat be perchede, þer is but deth.   340
Þe toþer is callede *dura mater* (*anglice*: þe hard modir). Þou *dura mater* be
pershede, þere is lif ynogh, if hert and age be gode. Ouer þe cerebre & þise
2 thenne webbes is *craneum*, þe heued pan, hylonde & defendant hem al.

Þe 2 regioun[42] conteyneþ þe spiritual membres, i. *ysophagus, trachearteria, epiglotum, arterie, canalis pulmonis, pulmo, cor*, & *diafragma*. &   345
so þise 2 region bigynnyþ at *epiglotum*[43] inclusif & endiþ at *diafragma*
inclusif.

Epiglotum is þe þrote bolle, or elles þe þrot golle, vnder the chynne. In
some contre, it is callede þe strowpe. Galienus in *Libro anathomiarum
suarum*[44] [**f. 58ra**] calleþ it *cartilago gutturis* (*anglice*: þe þrote crushil or   350
þe þrote crushilbone). *Cartilago* is a crushilbone. *Epiglotum* is also callede,
nyh alwaie in phisik and in gramer eke, *vua* or *vuula* (*anglice*: þe vuel or
elles sekenes of þe þrote golle). *Et os* þe trachearterie lieþ o þe wesand, riȝt
so þe strowpe liþ o þe trachearterie, as þou shalt se anone. It is *frigidum*
& *siccum* & it serueþ in 3 þinges: it serueþ to þe membres of lif, cachand   355
& defendant þe superfluytes of fleume, þat þai be noȝt choked ne stuffede
þerwiþ; and it serueþ to þe spirituales in þe same þing. Also wickede eyre
& duste and poudre þat entreþ by þe noseþirles & oþerwhile by þe mouþ,
he letteþ it and kepeþ it fro þe spirituales. In þis membre falleþ somtyme a
sekenesse þat is callede also in phisik *vua* or *vuula*, or elles *casus vuule*, þat   360
is no more for to saie but sekenes of þe vuul, i. of þe þrote golle. *Et* as þe
auctour of *Anathomyes* techeþ, þis sekenes is somtyme causede of blode,
somtyme of colre, somtyme of fleume, and somtyme þorgh melancolie. If
it come be cause of exces of blode, þan þe vue scheweþ him rode. If be of
colre, citrine or citrinysshe. If be cause of fleume, more white or whitisshe.   365
If it be thorogh exces of melancolie, bloish or blakische.

Ysophagus[45] is þe wesonde; [**f. 58rb**] by hym passeþ the fode into þe
stomac. It bigynnyth at þe rote of þe tunge in þe þrote and endiþ at þe hert
colk, i. att þe mouthe of þe stomac. & hit is hol & playn wiþin, þat þe fode
schulde noȝt be lettede; & it is *frigida* & *sicca* in complexioun.   370

Trachearteria,[46] þe trachearterie, or elles þe trachel (oþer Englisshe
fynde Y none). Þerfor it is a membre *frigida* & *sicca in complexione*, and
hol & pleyn, lyand on the wesonde bitwene þe wesand and þe strowp,
begynnand in þe neþer ende of þe stroup, os seiþ some. But as Galien

---

42 2 regioun] *marg.*: 2 regioun
43 epiglotum] *marg.*: epiglotum
44 suarum] *catchword*: calleþ it cartilago
45 Ysophagus] *marg.*: ysophagus
46 Trachearteria] *marg.*: trachearterie

seiþ, bigynnande in þe rote, s. in þe neþer ende, of þe tunge, and lyonde   375
on þe wesande bitwene þe wesonde & þe stroup. And þis is his office: he
draweþ & bereþ air and spiritz to þe lungez. Þat it is holle is be cause þat
þe aire mai esely entre & passe þerby. It is pleyn, þat þe voys schulde noght
be lettede in speking, os *ysophagus* is hol & pleyn þat þe fode schulde no
lettyng haue in swolwyng of þe fode. *Et* tak hede þat when on eteþ, tra-   380
chearterie spereþ him and *ysophagus* openyþ him. And when on spekeþ,
ysophagus closeþ & *trachearteria* openyþ. And þis is þe cause whie: when
on eteþ spekand, somtyme a crom of brede entreþ þe trachiartery and may
no3t aweie but by koghing or smyting betwene þe schuldres. By þis trachiarterie comeþ eire to þe lun- **[f. 58va]** ges and by þe lunges to þe hert.   385
Trachearterie is as mykel for to saie os arterie drowonde & ledand þe spirit
of eire. <u>Arterie in þe j c. of þis boke, lef</u> {18}.

Þe place atwene trachearterie and *ysophagus* is callede *ismon*. In which
place somtyme gendreþ and gadereth an humor þat turneþ into aposteme
þat is callede *squynancia*, þe squynancy.[47] Somtyme it gadereþ in þat ilk   390
place and somtyme wiþoute, aboute þat ilk place. When it is only wiþin,
or elles bothe wiþin and wiþout, it is called *squynancia* propurly. But if it
be onely wiþouten, þan is it propurly *synancya*, þe synacy. Þus seieþ Galienus in his *Boke of Anathomyes*. And boþe þise maladies ar called *ismonia*;
ysmonicus is he that haþ it.   395

Canales pulmonis[48] & *fistule pulmonis*, al on (*anglice*: þe lunge pipes),
<u>as þou hast in c. *de liuido colore,* lef</u> {32}. *Pulmo* (*anglice*: þe lunge) is a
membre softe and tendre, *frigidus* and *humidus* in complexioun, and hau-
and 3 wenges, i. 3 lappates, & 2 mewynges, i. 2 maner of steryng. Item, it
is softe and tendre þat it schulde be þe more able to vnderfonge eyre. Þat   400
it is *frigidus* & *humidus*, it serueþ wel, for þere ar wonte to brede colde[49]
apostemes, os *pulmonia* and *peripulmonia*, <u>os Y saide in c. *de liuido colore*,</u>
<u>lef</u> {32}. It is wengede þat it schulde þe **[f. 58vb]** bettre gif eire and coling to
the hert. It is mewyng in 2 wise os is þe hert, s. speronde & openand. Sper-
and, he delyuereth & cacheþ fro him superfluytes; & openand, he draweþ   405
eire for [to][50] refreisshe þe hert & for to slake & tempre þe hete of þe hert.

Cor,[51] þe hert, is principal of al þe membres spirituale. Wherfor vnderstonde þat 4 membris in man ar principal membres in man, s. *cerebrum*,
cor, *epar*, and *testiculy*. For wiþouten hem may mankynd no3t be. And
eke for also mykel as \if/ eny of þo 4 be hurt, man leueþ noght. It hath þe   410

---

47   squynancy] *marg.*: Squynancie
48   Canales pulmonis] *marg.*: canales pulmonis
49   colde] *foll. by* colde *canc.* R
50   for to] CgH, to Sc, for RM7, *wanting* G
51   Cor] *marg.*: Cor

qualites of fire, i. it is *calidum* & *siccum*, and schap of þe lowe of fire or elles like a pere, & a sadde body, brode abouen & narwe beneþen, & haþ 2 maner of meuynges. It is *calidum* & *siccum* for it is welle & gronde of al þe kynd hete in mannes body, os <u>þou haste in þe j boke, þe 3 c., lef</u> {3}. It is formede like a flamme of fire or elles like a pere or a pynote. *Contra*, mayst 415 þou seyne: a pere is narwe aboue & brode beneþe, but *cor* is *e contrario*. Wherfor take hede þat man is callede *arbor euersa*[52] (*anglice*: a tre turned vp-so-doun), for he hath al his rotes & his sp[r]inginges[53] fro vpwarde, for alle þe synowes of þe body haue here bigynnyng of springing fro þe cerebre, al þe bones at þe hede panne, al þe arteries in whiche ar þe spiritz 420 of life atte þe hert, & **[f. 59ra]** alle þe veynes at þe lyuer, as <u>þou hast in c.</u> <u>de liuido colore, lef</u> {33}. And so *cor* conformeth him to disposi[ci]oun[54] & schapyng of kynde. And þat is þe cause whie it is brode benethe and narwe aboue. And þerfor Grekes calle man *antropos*, i. *arbor euersa*.

It [is][55] sad in himself þat he schulde noȝt liȝtly be dissoluede be cause 425 of his hete. Item, he is euermore mevyng in 2 wise, s. opnand & sperand: openand to hale into him eire to tempryng and refresshing of his hete; closande for to cache & dryue awaie and purge himself fro wickede humores & superfluytes of wicked humoures. Vnderstond þat *cor* standeþ propurly in þe lefte half of man, vnder þe ribbes. And noȝtforþan þe riȝt half hathe 430 more noble kynde hete fro þe hert þan þe lefte halfe, for þe hert opennyþ him euermore toward þe right half more þan towarde þe[56] lift halfe. And also by reson þat *epar* liþ more on þe riȝt half þan o the lefte halfe, os <u>I</u> <u>saide þe j bok, 3 c., lef</u> {4}. And þis is þe philosophie whi þe riȝt halfe of man is more warme & more able to steryng & meuyng & wirking þan þe 435 lifte halfe.

Diafragma[57] is þe mydrede. It is also callede *mappa ventris*, þe bely borde-cloþe, & *mappa spiritualis*, þe spiritual borde-cloþe, for þe *spirituales* membris, as who saie, lyen þeron, riȝt as þe borde-cloþe bereþ þat liþ þeron. *Diafragma* is seide of þis worde **[f. 59rb]** *dia*, i. 2, and of þis 440 worde *fragma*, i. [b]rekyng[58] & diuising, for it diuiseþ and departeþ & bereth vp þe spirituales fro þe toþer membres þat ar vnderneþen, s. the pawnche and þe guttes. & þerfor it is strawght & rawght oute, os it were a celoure of cloþe or of a skyn, and is tyede al aboute to þe sides of þe

---

52 arbor euersa] *marg.*: Arbor euersa
53 springinges] CgH, springyng G, springes Sc, spinginges RM7
54 disposicioun] M7CgHGSc, disposioun R
55 is] CgHGSc, *om.* RM7
56 more þan towarde þe] *foll. by* more þan toward the *canc.* R
57 Diafragma] *marg.*: diafragma
58 brekyng] M7CgHGSc, krekyng R

body. *Diafragma* is *frigidum* & *siccum*, os some seyne, & some seyn þat   445
it is *frigidum* & *humidum*.

The 3 region[59] lesteth fro *diafragma* exclusif to þe reynes & þe lendes
exclusif. What ar *renes*, it is saide in *capitulo de albo colore*, lef {39}.
Lumby, þe lendes, ar þe nedrerest places donwarde, as þe hepes, þe þies,
& þe botokes. *Lumbi* ar *calidi* & *sicci*. *Renes* ar *frigidi* & *sicci*. Sometyme   450
ar *lumbi* taken for þe reynes, & also for þo parties aboute þe neþer ende.
And þis regioun conteyneth *membra nutritiua*, þe membres nutritiues.[60]
Membra nutritiua ar þise: *epar, stomachus, splen, fel, intestina, zirbus,* and
syfac, & al þat oþer þermes þat ar þere.

Epar is þe principal membre of al þe nutritiues, os *cerebrum* of þe mem-   455
bres of lif, *cor* of þe spirituales, and *renes* of þe generatiues. (Som saie þat
testiculi ar principal of þe generatiues.) *Epar* is *calidum* & *humidum* in
complexioun, softe & tendre, purpre in colour, hol wiþin and baggand
wiþoute, & hauand 7 wenges, 7 flabbes, 7 [f. 59va] lappates. It is *calidum*
& *humidum* þat it schuld be of gode digestioun, for þe colder lyuer, þe   460
werr digestioun in þe lyuer & þe schorter. It is softe & tendre & nesche &
purpre colour most toward blode, for it is noȝt but *massa sanguinis*, os I
saide in þe j bok, þe 2 c., lef {j}. It is holwe wiþin & baggond & lapped þat
it schulde þe more liȝtly touche þe stomac wiþ his lappates. Of *epar*, þou
hast in þe ferst boke, þe 2 c., lef {j}, and in þe 3 c., lef {om.}.   465

Stomacus, þe stomac of man, os *jecur* is þe mawe of euery oþer best.
Stomacus is *frigidus* & *siccus* in complexioun, rounde & auelong, rowh
wiþinne, & synowy abouen & fleishi beneþe, and hauyng two mouthes:
one aboue, openand towarde þe hert, and another bynethe, openand
toward þe lyuer. It is *frigidus* & *siccus* be cause þat it schulde be of gode   470
retencioun, i. schulde holde & kepe þat comeþ þider in, for þo qualites ar
kindly retentif, i. holdand & byndand. It is rogh & wolly by þe same skyl;
rounde & auelong þat it schulde be þe more able for to receyue plente of
fode. Narow abouen, þat it schulde be of gode appetit & scharpe; charnouse beneþe, þat þe fode schulde be bettre defie whan it comeþ into þe   475
botume of þe stomac. Opnand vpwerde to þe hert and donward to þe
lyuer, þat he may make sufficient digesti- [f. 59vb] oun thorow benefice
of kynde hete of boþin. When þe fode is vnderfongede in þe grownd of þe
stomac, þer it is a party decocte, & þan kynde sendiþ it fourth to *epar* by
8 veyns þat ar called *meseraice*. And þan al þat is pure, þer it is eftesones   480
decocte & defiede, as þou haste pleynerly in þe j boke, þe 3 c. Sum saie
þat *stomacus* is *frigidus* & *siccus naturaliter*, & some saie þat it is *frigidus*

---

59   3 region] *marg.*: 3 regioun
60   membres nutritiues] *marg.*: Membres nutrityues

naturaliter & *calidus accidentaliter*, & sum seyn þat it is *frigidus* & *siccus per se*, but it is *calidus* & *humidus per accidence*, and þai saie soþe.

Vnderstond þat þise 3 wordes ar al on to saie: *naturaliter, proprie* & 485 *per se*, i. kyndly, propurly, & of his owen kynde, i. by waie of kynde and complexioun of þo elementz by which it stant most by, os Y saide in þe j boke, 4 c., 9 condicioun, thorowhoute. *Et* þise 3 wordes ar al on to seye: *accidentaliter, per accidence*, & *improprie*, i. as vnpropurly, and by oþer skil, & by oþer encheson þan of himself or of his owen kynd, os Y haue 490 saide oftyme biforne.

Verbi gratia, i. se by example: þe stomac is colde *per se*, i. of his owen kynde, but he haþ *epar* euen vnder him, in so mykel þat he is nyh closed in him os a pot ouer þe fire, and þat geueþ him hete fro beneþe. *Et* he haþ *cor* abouen him, noȝt euen abouen, but somdel more on þe lifte half. *Et* þat 495 *cor* geueþ hym hete fro abouen, but som- [f. 60ra] dele more on the lifte half.[61] And so þorogh benefitz of boþen, s. þorogh benefice of þe herte abouen and of þe lyuer fro byneþe, he haþe his hete and his myȝt for to wirke & defien þe fode & elles noght. And so þou seest wel þat þe stomac is hote *per accidence* & noght *per se*. 500

Splen,[62] þe mylt, os Galien seiþ, is an euelong membre, lyond more toward þe lifte side. And it is callede *splen* of þis word in Latyn *splendere* (*anglice*: bene bright & schyne). *Et* it is callede so *per contrarium* (*anglice*: by þe con-trarie), for it is neuer bright ne schynand, but euermore swart & dym & blackish or bloishe or atwene boþe. & þis is þe philosophie: for it haþ mykel 505 of kynde of þe erþe, for erþe is kyndly blackishe, & þerfor *splen* is principal se of melancolie, os þou haste in þe laste ende *de albo colore*. For os þou haste by þe proces in þe j boke, þe 4 c., þe 9 condicion, *splen* & melancolie ar al of on complexioun, wherfor it semeþ wel þat *splen* is *frigidus* & *siccus*.

Fel[63] we calle þe galle. Wherfor take hede þat on þe lyuer hongeþ os it 510 were a bledder or a thenne ryme, wonder eþe for to breste for tendre. & þis ryme is callede *sista fellis*, or *sistis fellis*. Þe wete mater þat is wiþin þis ryme is callede *fel*. Often tyme *fel* is taken for al & it is *calidum* & *siccum*.

Intestina[64] of- [f. 60rb] ten tyme ar taken for *yliones*, of which Y spak biforne in þe lef {59}. But propurly, *intestina* ar euery maner guttes of 515 man & beste while þai er in þe body, *exta*[65] when þai ar oute of þe body. *Intestina* ar *frigida* & *humida*. Of al þat oþer guttes in man, þou haste in þe 3 c., lef {19}.

---

61 half] *foll. by* Et þat cor geueþ him hete fro abouen *canc.* R
62 Splen] *marg.*: Splen
63 Fel] *marg.*: fel
64 Intestina] *marg.*: Intestina
65 exta] *marg.*: exta

Zirbus & *sifac* ar 2 smale webbes, 2 small rymes, bewapande þe lyuer, os I saide in c. *de albo colore, lef {j}*. Þe qualites of *zirbus* & *sifac* rede Y   520
noght. Item, þer is a webbe, a ryme, in which al þe ylions and al þe guttes saue *longaon* ar biclosede in. And Galienus, in his *Bok of Anathomyes*, calleþ it *epigozontaymenon*. Þis *epigozontaymenon* somtyme bresteþ & þan þe ylions, i. som of þe smale ropes, falle down into *osceum*. And often tyme suche folk ar callede brusten-coddede, os þise plectoric men. *Plec-*   525
toricus is he þat is[66] fat and corciouse. *Osceum* and *bursa testiculorum*, al on (in Englisshe, þe ballok codde or þe ballok purse). *Longaoun* in þe j bok, þe 3 c., lef {3}. O þe forsaide *ypigozontamen* is grees þat Galienus calleþ *omentum*. *Omentum* is comunly taken for euery maner talow or gres hauand of þe guttes or of the membres wiþinne bestes body. *Omen-*   530
tum also is a maner of mete þat we calle poddynges.

[f. 60va] The 4 regioun[67] of mannes body conteyneþ þe membres gen-eratiues, s. *renes, lumbi, vesica, osceum, testiculi, virga vi[rilis],*[68] *matrix, testiculi matricis, vulua,* & *tentigo. Renes* & *lumby,* Y saide riȝt nowe beforne.   535

Vesica, þe bledder, is a membre rymmyshe & skynnysshe & rounde & hol, þe schap of an vrynal. Into which bledder þe vryn falliþ down fro þe reynes by 2 smal waies, os it were 2 smale veynes þat ar callede *vrichides,* or elles *vrichides pori,* os Y saide in þe j boke, þe 4 chapitle, lef {om.}. *Vesica* is *frigida* & *sicca.* Which by sekenes of þe vesie, þou hast in þe j boke, 4   540
c., lef {om.}.

Osceum, I said biforne. *Testiculi,* þe ballok stones, *calidi* & *sicci. Virga virilis,* þe mannes ȝerde, *frigida* & *sicca. Matrix* & *testiculi matricis,* þe moder and þe moder ballok stones, in c. *de liuido colore,* lef {34}. *Wlua* is the wombe ȝate of woman. It is *frigida* & *humida.*   545

As Holy Writ witnesseth & telleþ,
3 þinges schulde neuer be fulfillede:
Helle is þe first, il woman myd,
Couetouse man, þat is þe 3;
The laste 2 schal neuer be ful   550
Til helle hathe hem in his gulle,
Couetouse folk & lecheures al.
Holy Writ neuer lyn schal.
Sely him þat þise wil fle:
Þe pyne of helle schal he noȝt se.   555

---

66 is he þat is] M7CgH, he þat is (*line end*) he þat is R, thoo (þey Sc) that are GSc
67 4 regioun] *marg.*: 4 regioun
68 virilis] CgHGSc, vi (*line end*) R, *om.* M7

Tentigo is callede *paries vulue* (*anglice*: þe wombe-ȝate wawh), or elles *lingula* [**f. 60vb**] *vulue* (*anglice*: þe wome-ȝate tunge). In som contre it is callede þe kiker in þe cunt. And it is called *tentigo* by cause þat in ȝonge women it wiþstant & wiþholt the mannes ȝerde, þat he mai noȝt comunly haue entre at wil, til þe woman be often defoulede. 560

Þe toþer lyms of man, s. þe armes and þe þies & þe legges, ar but as bowes and braunches of a tre. Þe hed here is þe rotes of þe body, for os I saide, man is callede *arbor euersa* (*anglice*: þe tre went vp-so-down).

Now to þise forsaid 4 regions of þe body ar answerande 4 regions of þe vryn.[69] 565

Þe j regioun[70] of þe vryn is callede *circulus vrine*, þe Cercle of þe vryn. Þe Cercle of þe vryn is þe ouer parti of þe vryn, þat euermore telliþ & scheweþ þe disposicioun of þe membres of lif and of here place, s. of þe heuede, as þou schalt se in þe 3 boke, þe 2 c., lef {87}. *Membra animata*, þe membres of lif, Y saide toforne. 570

Þe 2 regioun[71] of þe vryn is þe place nexte þe Cercle donwarde, s. þe place atwene þe Cercle & þe myddis of þe vryn, & þat is nerehond[72] al on wiþ þe Cercle. *Et* by þis regioun, by þis place of þe vryn, is euermore knowen þe disposicioun & þe state of spirituales and of her places. For if it be derke & dymme, or þick and drobly, or elles al, it seiþ sekenes & 575 distemperure of þe spirituales, causede þrogh[73] superfluytes of wickede humiditez, [**f. 61ra**] & namely & it be fulle of smale Greynes,[74] it seith *asma* & *disma* & *empima* & colleccioun of wickede mater aboute the spirituales. And tokenyng of þise poyntz is þat he is st\r/eyte at þe breste and schorte ondede. Þe spiritual membres hauen mykel of þe aire to here 580 fodyng kyndly & þerfor kyndely þai spiren, i. þai sende oute eire & hale into hem aire, & þat is þe skil whie þai ar callede spiritual membres. And þerfor auctoures calle þis 2 regioun *corpus aereum* (*anglice*: an airisshe body), or *regio spiritualis* (*anglice*: þe spiritual place). *Asma & disma* in c. *de liuido colore*, lef {28}. *Empima* is a malady when on blediþ at þe 585 mouþ. *Empima, emothois, emothoia, emathasis,* & *emathasia*: al on sekenes. & ar saide of þis worde *emath* or *emoys* (*anglice*: blode) & of þis worde *emothois*, pouryng or rennyng att þe mouþe, os who saie a course of blode at þe mouþe.

---

69 4 regions of þe vryn] *marg.*: Of 4 regions of vryn
70 j regioun] *marg.*: j
71 2 regioun] *marg.*: 2
72 nerehond] M7CgHGSc, nereh(*line end*)hond R
73 þrogh] *foll. by an extraneous minim or beginning of some other letter* R
74 Greynes] M7CgHGSc, g(*line end*)greynes R

Þe 3 regioun[75] is þe myddes of þe vryn, and þat serueþ for þe membres 590
nutritiues. For if it apere nebulouse, i. mystisshe and rokisshe, skyisshe
and cloudisshe & þickishe, it se[i]th[76] sekenes and wickede disposisioun
o þe nutritiues, as wombe ake, inflacioun, feble digestioun, & wlatyng, &
swich oþer sekenes os comen by cause of replecioun o þe stomac and o þe
entrailes.   595

The 4[77] regi- **[f. 61rb]** oun of þe vryn is þe founde of þe vryn, þe neþer
partie þerof, and þat euermore telleþ þe disposicioun of þe membres generatyues, s. of þe neþer regioun of þe body, for if it be ʒisty, i. d[r]esty[78]
& þik & droubly & grauely, it seiþ distemperance and vnhelþe of þe generatiues, os it is in þe nefresi, in þe litiasy, & in þe stranguirie, & in oþer 600
sekenes o þe vesie & o þe reyns and o þe lendes. *Nefresis* and *nefresia:* in c.
de albo colore, lef {38}. *Litiasis* & *stranguyria,* þe j boke, [4] c.,[79] lef {*om.*}.

Et if þou tak gode hede at þise 4 forsaide regions of vryn, answerond
to þe 4 parties of mannes body, wiþ reules þat ar saide and wiþ reules þat
folweþ, wiþouten doute when þou seest an vryn, þou schalt verayly se & 605
knowe where & whe[r]of[80] is sekenesse in þe body of man.

[2.8]

De colore pallido, of Pale color: c. 8

Affter þat we haue tretede of coloures in vryn þat signifieþ mortificacioun,
os Blac colour & of Blo coloure, & eke of þo coloures þat signifieþ priuacioun of digestioun, os White coloure, [ʒ]elow[1] colour, Mylk-white
colour, and Karopos, now pursue we forthe of þo colours þat bitokne   5
bigynnyng of digestioun, s. Pale coloure & Palisshe coloure & Subcitrin
coloure, os al **[f. 61va]** autoures of þis faculte speken and techen. For *alba
vrina* and *glauca vrina* & *lactea* & *karopos*, of whiche it is saide nexte
biforne, seyn wanyshyng and failing of digestioun, saue *karopos* lesse.

Pallida & *subpallida* seyn bigynnyng of digestioun, s. of humores.   10
Citrina & *subcitrina*, meine digestioun; *rufa* & *subrufa* & *rubea* &

---

75 3 regioun] *marg.:* 3
76 seith] M7CgHGSc, semeth *with two minims overpuncted* R
77 4] *marg.:* 4
78 dresty] CgHGSc, desty RM7
79 4 c.] CgHSc, c. 4 G, 2 c. RM7
80 wherof] M7CgHGSc, wheof R

---

1 ʒelow] *first letter poorly shaped, like an incomplete* d?

subrubea, complete digestioun; *rubicunda* & *subrubicunda*, exces of digestioun. *Inopos* & *kyanos*, destruccioun of digestioun; *nigra, liuida,* & *viridis*, mortificacion & adustioun, and al vpon intencioun and remission. Intencion, i. depnes in colour; remissioun, i. lachede in colour.   15

Now in þis wise teche auctoures for to knowe Pale or Palisshe colour in *vrina*: suppose þat a litle of galle of a nete were menket wiþ a gode quantite of water, þan þe colour þat comeþ of bothe is *pallidus* or *subpallidus* (*anglice*: Pale or Palisshe). Riȝt so, when a litle of colre is menkt wiþ a gode porcioun of fleume, þan is þe colour in þe vryn Pale or Palissh. And   20 so is colour *pallidus* or *subpallidus* in *vrina* euermor causede of colre and of fleume. But vnderstonde þat þe quantite neþer of þat on humour ne of þat oþer in þis mixtioun, i. neþer of þe colre ne of þe fleume, is noght comprehendede ne vnderstonden of vs, but only by estimacion, i. by [f. 61vb] gessing, riȝt os if on tak a certeyne porcioun of wyne and menge it   25 wiþ a god porcion of water þat þou seest noȝt, and þan schew þe þat mixtioun, þou wost neþer þe quantite of þat one ne of þat oþer, but by gesse. And þerfor ne were þat ilk litle quantite of colre þat causeth, os Y saie, þat palehede in the vryn, elles were þe vryn *alba* or *glauca* or *lactea* or *karopos*.

And þerfor take þis for a reule: þat if on make an vryn White or Ȝelow   30 or Mylk-white or Karopos, & afterward come an vryn Pale, it is verray tokne þat þan at arste kynde bigynneth for to myȝten himself & for to wirke & for to skateryn & sparplyn þe wickede humores, & first colre, for he is more subtile and more able for to be sparplede.

Vryn Pale or Subpale þroghoute spis, i. oueral þicke, seiþ a febre cotid-   35 ian causede of a kynde fleume. Þat it is remys, i. lache & feynt in coloure, for euery Pale coloure may wel be saide remys, is by cause of coldehede of fleume. For fleume is kyndly colde; and al þat haþ of fleume, in as mykel as fleume, it is kindely colde. Þat it is spis is be cause of humidite of fleume, for *fleuma* is *frigidum* & *humidum*, & humidite euermore þickeþ þe vryn   40 kyndely. What is a kynde fleume & how meny spices of fleume þer ar, I saide in *capitulo de glauco colore*, lef {43}.

Item, vryn Pale or Sub- [f. 62ra] pale þoroghoute thenne, & wiþ a maner of grenyshede, seiþ *dominium* of a colre aduste (*anglice*: a brent colre; adust, i. brente). A colre adust is þus mykel for to saie, a colre distemprede   45 þorogh onkynd hete. What is *dominium*, I saide in þe j bok, þe 4 c.,[2] þer I spake of þise 2 wordes: *regnat* & *dominatur*. Þan is þis reule þus mykel for to mene: when an vryn scheweþ him so, it seiþ a febre, which febre is caused þorogh exces of melancolie innatural. Which melancoly innatural is causede þorgh adustioun of colre & þis is þe skil: for colre aduste is lesse   50

---

2 4 c.] *foll. by* lef *canc.* R

hote & dry þan is a naturel colre, and þerfor by cause of his feynte hete,
he makeþ þe vryn Pale, and by resoun of his siccite, he makeþ þe vryn
thenne. And þerfor vnderstonde þat *colra adusta* & *melancolia innaturalis*
(*anglice*: a brent colre & an vnkynd melancolie) ar al on.

   Et riȝt os *colra adusta* & *melancolia innaturalis*, þat ar al on, euermore   55
makeþ³ þe vryn Pale & thenne wiþ a maner of grenehede, riȝt so *sanguis adustus* makeþ þe vryn Whit and þenne wiþ a maner of rudihede or
redishede. *Et fleuma adustum*, menely thik wiþ a whitehed. And take gode
hede to þise poyntz þat ar saide in þis reule, for oþer reules þat folwe.

   Vnderstond also þat, os seiþ Johannicius in his *Boke of Ysagogis*, þe j   60
c., þat þer is 4 maner⁴ [**f. 62rb**] of colre: *colera rubea, colra citrina, colera
nigra,* & *colera viridis* (*anglice*: a rede colre, a colre citrine, a blak colre, &
a grene colre).

   Colera rubea & *colera naturalis*: al on. He is kyndely rede & clere &
pure in himself, and he is noȝt ouergone ne myxte wiþ none oþer humor   65
ne humores. & þerfor he is *colera naturalis*, a kynde colre.

   Colera citrina stant by *colra r[u]bea*⁵ & by fleume, but more by *colra
rubea* þan by fleume. & þerfor it is lesse hote þan *colra rubea*. *Et* þis spyce
of colre is leste noyouse & leste wicked of al colres. & þis spice of *colra* is
callede also *colra vitellina*, for it is most like in colour to þe ȝolke of an eye.   70
Vitellinus is like þe ȝolk of an aye in colour.

   Colera nigra is in 2 wise: on þat is causede þorgh exces of melancolie,
& þat is blake like drestes of blode, & þis maner of *colra* is propurly *nigra
colra*, for it stant moste by blak humor, i. by melancolie. And it is ferre
worse þan *colra citrina*, for it is *frigida* & *sicca*, as þe humoure þat he most   75
hath of. Þise 2 spice⁶ of blake colre is causede thorowh grete adustioun
of colre, and þis spice of colre is ouerdone hote & it is werse & more
noyouse.

   Colera viridis is also in 2 wise: þe first is callede *colera* [**f. 62va**] *prassina* (*anglice*: þe colre prassyn).⁷ *Et* it is seide so of an herbe þat is callede   80
prassius, & also *marubium* (*anglice*: prassyn, or elle horhow, for a collre
prassyn is grene & bitter as þat herbe). And þis colre is gendrede comuly
in þe stomac of hem þat ar wont for to vse herbes which ar ouerdone
hote in complexioun, os cresses, poritz, lekes, garlik, & oynons & such
maner þingz. For by cause of grenehede & rawehede of such maner þingz,   85
oftym colre caccheþ scharphed & sourhede & rawhede and grenehede,

---

3 makeþ] G, make Sc, makyn CgH, makeþ make RM7
4 maner] *marg.*: spice of colre
5 rubea] M7CgHGSc, rebea R
6 Þise 2 spice] GSc, The 2 spece CgH, þise 2 spices RM7
7 colre prassyn] *marg.*: Colre prassyn

and so is al distemprede & oute of his owen kynde, & þerafter scheweþ
him þe vryn. Galienus seiþ þat *colera prassyn* is gendrede of a colre vitellyn: when colre vitellyn is hugely scalt & brent, þat ilke adustioun causeth a blakhede, which blakhede, syn it is mixte wiþ citrinehede, causeth a   90
grenehede. And þerafter apereþ þe vryn.

   Anoþer maner þer is of grene colour, þat is grene os ruste of bras or
copur.[8] & þis is causede þorgh ȝitt more adustioun of a colre prassyn, os
when a colre prassyn is so mykel aduste þat his humidite is al fully wastede
& fordon. & þis *colera*[9] is callede *colera eruginosa* (*anglice*: a rousty colre).   95
& þis colre bit & frete os venym, and it is werste of alle colres. And þerfor
when an vryn scheweþ him in swiche colour, he scapeþ noȝt deþe [f. 62vb]
be waie of kynde.

   Item *vrina pallida* or *subpallida*, menely thenne, seiþ a cotidien causede
of a fleume acetouse. *Febris cotidiana*, a febre cotidiane: in c. *de liuido*   100
colore, lef {28}. *Fleuma acetosum* & *fleuma acrum*: al on (*anglice*: an egre
fleume). 5 spices of fleume: se in c. *de glauco colore*, lef {43}.

   Item, vryn *pallida* or *subpallida* menely thyke seith *fleumaticum sanum*
(*anglice*: a fleumatik hol). Vnderstonde þis reule in þis wise: vryn Pale or
Palisshe & menely þik seiþ *dominium fleumatis naturalis* wiþouten eny   105
febre. *Fleuma naturale*, a kynd fleume, in c. *de glauco colore*, lef {43}.

   Item, if so be þat on be discrasede, i. euyl disposede & seke in þe body,
& his vryn apere *alba* or *glauca* or *lactea* or *karopos*, and sone after (or þe
next vryn after) aper Pale or Palisshe, it is noble tokne, for it seiþ þat kynde
& kynde hete begynneþ for to risen & comen agayne, & take ageyne here   110
myȝte, & wirke toward digestioun, & maistrie the malady, & hemself for
to be maistres & reulers in þe body.

   And þerfor for to haue more declaring of þis reule & eke of al reules þat
ar saide, vnderstonde a poynt þat is ful nedeful in þis faculte: þer is 2 maner
of demyng[10] in vryn: on þat is callede *judicium simplex* (*anglice*: a simple   115
[f. 63ra] dome or an ofolde demeng), os when one demeþ of an vryn onely
os the vryn scheweþ him for þe tyme, hauand no maner regard to oþer cir-
cumstancis, but onely os þe vryn scheweþ him for þe tyme. Anoþer maner
demyng in vryn þer is þat is callede *iudicium curealium*, i. a dome hauand
regarde & consideracion toward mo poyntes & condicions þan on: as if   120
þou deme of an vryn hauande regarde & consideracioun to þe state þat he
is nowe in, and to þe state þat he was in langer or ȝisterday or tonyght, also
hauand consideracioun to his myȝtes, to his age, to his complexioun, what

---

8 ruste of bras or copur] *marg.*: Colre erugynos
9 colera] *marg.*: Colre
10 2 maner of demyng] *marg.*: 2 maner of domes

his vryn was þat he made nexte aforne, or þe next nyght aforn, & to swich
oþer poyntes and condicions. And þis last maner of demyng is euer more   125
certeyne & more siker.

Verbi gratia: if it so be þat an vryn of a body þat is discrasede schew
him Pale or Palissh, and his vryn were beforn *alba* or *glauca* or *lactea*, or
elles *karopos*, it seiþ þat kynde encreseþ & couerith agayn, & digestion
begynneth for to strengþe. *Et* also euen agaynwarde, if þe vryn schew him   130
e contrario. Also a vryn Ruf or *subrufa* or elles *subrubea* in a hote body,
& also in a hote mater, seiþ digestion complete; but in a body þat is of
colde complexioun and eke in colde mater, it seiþ exces of digestion. And
[f. 63rb] also þe same vryn þat seiþ mene digestioun in a hote body seiþ
complete digestioun in a colde body. Also, when vryn scheweþ him ferst   135
thenne or thennysshe, and after þat þer come an vryn a party myxte, more
& droubli þan it was biforne, be it neuer so litle, it is verray tokne of bigynnyng of digestioun.

And if it be so þat after þat apere *nubes* or *eneorima*, it seiþ gode digestioun, or elles mene, and þe skil is þis: for first when kynd bigynneþ for to   140
wirke into þe humores, & þe kynde hete is ȝit but litle & feble, wherfore
kynde hete may noȝt ȝitt comprehende to þe ful þat þat passeþ wiþ þe
vryn. And by cause þat þe kynde hete is ȝit but litle, os Y saie, it wirkeþ but
litle in þe vryn. Afterwarde by proces of tyme, when kynde hete gadereth
more myght to him and maistrieþ & ouercomeþ þe wickede humores &   145
haþ his course wiþ þe vryn, þan kynde hete comprehendiþ & aggregeþ to
him þe humidite & so wirkeþ into þe vryn. For þat is þe kynde of hete:
for to aggregen, i. for to gader, to him moysthede. And when it is so, þan
scheweþ him in þe vryn *nubes* or elles *eneorima*: if kynde hete be litle &
mykel ventosite in þe body, *nubes*; if more of kynde hete & lesse of[11]   150
[f. 63va] ventosite, *eneorima*.

And afterward, when kynde is more myȝty, s. when kynde and kynde
hete haþ suptilede and maistriede þe mater, þan apereþ *ypostasis*. And þat is
tokne þat kynde haþ foȝten & haþ þe maistrie & is of myȝt for to ouercome
þe remenant & is at his abouen. And þerfor seiþ Ysodre in þe 4 boke of   155
Ethimologies, 10 c.: it bihoueþ him þat schal be a leche for to knowe þinges
þat ar passede & wete þinges þat now ar & for to se tofore þinges þat ar
for to come. Nubes & eneorima & ypostasis in þe first bok, 3 c., lef {4}; &
in þis boke, in c. de nigro colore, lef {24}; & in þe 3 boke in his propre c.

Item, vryn Pale or Subpale & thenne & clere, wiþ a[12] continuel febre or   160
in a lente febre wiþ god tokenes, & namely with som appetit & wiþ myȝt

---

11   of] M7CgH, of (*page break*) of R, *om.* GSc
12   a] M7CgHGSc, a (*line end*) a R

of kynde, seiþ bredyng of aposteme vndre þe myddred in þe riȝt ypicondre. Þat þe vryn is Pale or elles Palisshe is by cause of frigidite of þe mater,
and þe myȝt[ys][13] of kynde ar al fortrauailede be cause of[14] maystriing of
þat wicked mater. What is *materia morbi, þe mater of þe maladye: in c.*   165
de nigro colore, lef {20}. That it is thenne & clere is by cause of crudite;
& of compaccioun of þe mater, þe malady is scharpe & longe lastande.
Et [f. 63vb] þerfor when kynde is so trauailede & tormentede o þis wise,
he seþ þat he may noȝt haue his purpos for to purge þe mater ne delyuer
him þerof, neyþer by bledyng att þe nose, ne by swete, ne by none oþer   170
maner weie of purgacioun. He doþ þe beste wise þat he may and fondiþ
litle & litle for to helpe himselfe, for to cache & dry[u]e[15] þe mater fro þe
membres þat ar more noble and more worþi (of which I spake in c. *de*
nigro colore) to þo membris þat ar lesse noble & lesse worþi, and namely
to þe riȝt ypicondre. For þer is more vertue & more myȝt of drawyng þan   175
in þe lifte ypocondre, for it is more nere þe lyuer, as Y saide in þe j bok, 3
c., lef {*om.*}. And þerfor suche maner of vryn wiþ swiche signes seiþ warisshing, be bredyng of aposteme o þis wise. And if þer be no gode tokenes,
& namely if kynde bc wonder feble & no maner appetit, raþer deme deþ
þan lif.   180
   Whet is compaccion of þe mater, I saide in c. *de lacteo colore;*[16] *ypo-*
condria, þe ypocondres: in c. de liuido colore.[17] *Febris continua & febris*
lenta: in c. *de liuido colore,* lef {28}. *Bona signa,* gode tokenes: in *capitulo*
de nigro colore, lef {23}. *Materia morbi, þe mater of þe malady, in c. de*
nigro colore, lef {20}.   185
   But wel mai be þou seiste þat þe forsaide mater of apostem oweþ raþer
for to draw to þe lefte side þan to þe riȝt side, for þe mater is colde kyndly
& þe liȝfte halfe is more cold [f. 64ra] kyndely þan þe riȝt halfe. For Aristotel seiþ þat þo þinges þat ar answering in qualitees of kynde, raþer þai
draw þat on to þat oþer, þan þo þinges þat ar contrariouse in qualite. *Ergo,*   190
syn þe lift side is more colde – for Saturnus haþ his propurte & his myȝt
& his vertu ouer þe splen, and þai answere togedre in qualite; & Sol & *cor,*
Jupitre & *epar,* Mars & *fel,* Venus & *pulmo,* Mercure & *diafragma,* Luna
& *intestina* – it semeþ wel þat it oweþ for to drawen more to þe lefte halfe.
   I answer þat if it were so þat þe forsaide mater of aposteme mew[e]d him   195
& dr[o]we[18] him vpon þe proporcion & vppon þe kynde of frigidite, &

---

13   myȝtys] CgH, myȝt RM7GSc
14   of] *foll. by* frigidite *of canc.* R
15   dryue] M7CgHGSc, drye R
16   colore] *foll. by* lef *canc.* R
17   colore] *foll. by* lef *canc.* R
18   mewed him & drowe] CgHGSc, mewand him & drawe RM7

also that kynde were so feble þat he myȝt noght wirke into þat ilke mater, þan were it soþe & þe skil were gode. But now it is so þat kynde, os seiþ þe vryn, is myȝty & kynde hete on his side eke. *Et*[19] þerfor helpande þe myȝt of kynde, kynde hete comprehendeþ & concludiþ him in his place, and so   200 meveþ him and fleteþ & cacheþ him & dryueþ him to þat party or to þat place þer moste is of hete, þat he may þe bettre be defiede & ryped. *Et* whi hete meveþ it more towarde þe riȝt half þan towarde þe lefte is by cause of hete answerond to hete. And also for alse mykel os þat party is more moiste þan the lifte side & humidite is more helpand toward maturacion,   205 i. to ripinge. [**f. 64rb**] For þe riȝt half of man is *calidus* & *humidus*, & by resoun þerof more myȝty. It is *calidus* be cause of hete of þe lyuer, for þe lyuer is more o þe riȝt half, os I saide in þe j boke, 3 c., lef {2}, & also for þe hert hath his aspecte, i. is openonde þiderwarde. Þe hert, os I saide in þe nexte c. aforne,[20] lith more on þe lifte half, but he openeþ him toward þe   210 riȝt side. And by cause þat he openeþ him þidirward, he ȝeueþ more kynde myȝt & vertu of hete to þe riȝt side þan to þe lefte. And þat is þe skil whi man is more stronge & myȝty, & also whie mykel folk is more large, on þe riȝt half þan o þe lifte. Of þis also þou maist haue a gode answere & gode lernyng eke.   215

If a febre come in a spasme, it is tokne of warshing, but so is it noght þogh a febre come in ydropisi, & noȝtforþan boþe þo maladies ar caus- ede of wickede humidite in body & of inspissacioun of wickede humours repleisshynd, i. fulfilland, & stoppand þe veyns. Now seyn fesiciens þat in ydropisie is more of wickede humydite. For when ydropisie is rotede &   220 maystriede, it may noȝt be driede, & þerfor raþer comeþ deþ þan ydropisi falliþ. But in þe spasme is more of gode matere þan of wik, & þerfor kynd hete turneþ him raþer to þe humidite þat causeþ replecioun of humores in þe spasme, þan to the wicked, waterouse humidite in ydropisi. Þis is [**f. 64va**] skil whie kynde hete rather wasteþ & fordoþ þe spasme þan   225 ydropisi. What is *spasmus*, se in þe c. of Grene coloure, lef {84}.

Gi[l]bert[21] seiþ þus: þer be 2 principal membres of lif[22] in man: on þat is callede *membrum formale vite hominis* (*anglice*: þe formal membre in man), s. *cor*. And it is callede þe formal membre of lif be cause of kynd het, whiche kynde hete is callede *instrumentum* of myȝt & vertu & of   230 wirkyng of kynde in man. And by cause þerof, þe hert is callede þe wel of hete in man.

---

19 eke Et] M7, eke And CgB, eke and Et R, also And GSc
20 aforne] *foll. by* lef *canc.* R
21 Gilbert] M7, Gilbertus CgHGSc, Gibert R
22 2 principal membres of lif] *marg.*: 2 principalez membrez of lif

Anoþer²³ membre þer is, þat is callede *membrum materiale vite humane*
(*anglice*: material membre of lif), s. *epar*. And it is called so be resoun of
humidite, nurishonde & sustenande þe lif. Which nurishand humidite is   235
callede *pabulum caloris naturalis* (*anglice*: fode & fedyng of kynde hete),
for in hote & moiste stant þe lif of al þat beriþ lif in erþe.

But now is it so þat þe ydropisy corupteþ & wasteþ & fordoþ þe lyuer,
for þe lyuer in on þat is smyt wiþ an ydropisie, propurly is no lyuer. And
þerfor if on haue þe ydropisie & þere come vppon him a febre þerwiþ (for   240
febre is a passioun of þe hert, for os Constantinus seiþ in his *Boke of Vryns*
þat a febre is a passion propurly of þe hert, ry3t os *ydropisis* is passioun of
þe lyuer), and syn it is so þat lif stant no3t [f. 64vb] but in temperure of þo
two membres, nedes lif most faile in swich cas.

Item, þowh wilte axen how it is þat a febre comande in a spasme is   245
tokne of warshing, but þogh a febre come in þe pallesie, it is no3t so, &
no3tforþan boþe þe spasme & eke þe palsie comen of wickede humidite
in þe synowes. Þis is þe philosophie: þat ilk mater þat causeþ þe spasme is
more gros & more compacte þan þat mater þat causeth þe pallesie. And by
cause þerof, it halt himself abouen in þe pores of þe synowes. But þe mater   250
of þe palsie is more fleumatik & more nesche & flowande, and be cause
þerof, it nessheþ & sokeþ & perseþ & þirleþ & entreþ þe synowes. & so
by cause þerof, þe synowes ar more appert, more bloute, & more ful in þe
palsie þan in þe spasme.

Now febre is a distemperure of vnkynd hete & þe febre halt him in þe   255
ouer partie of þe membres in þe body, so þat he persheþ no3t þe membrez
vpon al her parties as doþ þe fleumatik mater in þe palsi. And by resoun
þerof, þe febre drieþ vp þe superficial humidite, but no3t þe substancial
humidite wiþin in þe body. *Et* for þis skil, þe febre fordoþ þe spasme and
no3t þe palsi.   260

Item, vryn Pale or Subpale, & froþi abouen, & wiþ a maner of dymhede or bloishede, & fattisshe, & as [þ]ow²⁴ askes were drenchede in þe
vryn, & þerwiþ þe vryn be litle in quanti[te]²⁵ [f. 65ra] and he þat made þe
vryn haue no wombe flux, [it seiþ *pthisicam*, þe pthisik. Sum tyme þe vryn
scheweth hym nerhand swich in the wombe flux,]²⁶ & þat is by cause of   265

---

23 Anoþer] M7CgHG, And a noþer Sc, Another (*line end*) noþer R
24 þow] thogh G, þow3 Sc, thowhe Cg, *om.* H, yow R, you M7 (*letter* y = *both* þ *and* y
    in M7)
25 quantite] M7CgHGSc, quanti (*page end*) R
26 it seiþ pthisicam ... wombe flux] it seyth Thisicam the thisyk Sumtyme the vryn shew-
    eyth hym nerhande suche in the wombe flux CgH, it sayth ptysichim the ptisike ptisica
    in ca de liuido colore Sum tyme þe vryn scheweth hym nerhande in the wombe fluxe
    GSc, *om.* RM7

perturbacion of þe humores in þe body, & also be cause þat þer comeþ but litle humidite to þe lyuer, for it passeth waie wiþ egestion. But þan is noȝt þe vryn so froþi ne so asky os it is in þe pthisik. *Pthisica, þe pthisik: in c. de liuido colore,* lef {31}.

Þat þe vryn is Pale or Palisshe is by cause of sekenes of kynde[27] hete 270 aboute þe nutrityues. [The nutrityues kyndly han compassyoun on the spirituales, and therfore when the spirituales ar seke, the nutrityues][28] ar desisede kyndly and gretly desolat. Þat it is[29] spumouse, i. f[r]oþi,[30] is bi cause of passioun of þe lunges. Which f[ro]þihed[31] of þe lunges may be caused in 3 wise:[32] or be cause of grete mocion of þe lunges, or by cause 275 of distencioun, i. of rysing and bolnyng of þe lunges, or elles by cause of ventosite aboute þe lungez.

Þat it is dym or elles bloisshe, it seiþ enfeccion of þe spirituales & also of þe lyuer, which infeccioun is causede of wickede mater, thike and dresty & venymouse, þat renneþ by *vena concaua* to þe lyuer & þer enfectiþ, 280 i. coruptiþ & envenymeth, þe blode, & fadiþ & dymmeth & dulleth þe *spiritus. Vena concaua* in c. *de liuido colore,* lef {26}. The fathede seith os Y saide in c. *de nigro colore,* lef {21}.

Þat it is synerouse, i. asky, it seiþ meltyng and wasting of the lunges, for [f. 65rb] *pulmo,* of which I spake in the nexte c. aforne, is in colour mykel 285 toward askes. And when it is so þat þe humores ar harde agitate, i. sterede & rollyede & trauailede and renne & hurle, in here vesseiles, i. in þe veyns of þe body, þai tak & bere wiþ hem þo poudres, þo askes, þat cleue o þe vesseilles. Which poudres & askes ar noȝt but resolucions, i. meltingz & wastinges & bleuynges awaie, of þe lunges. 290

That the vryn is but litle in quantite, it seiþ consumpsioun of þe sub-stancial humidite of þe indre membres in þe body, for þe substancial humidite of þe inder membres in þe body draweþ hem to þe lunges; & þat þat beleueth stille in þo membres, vnkynde hete & distemperoure of þe febre drieþ it vp and wasteþ it awaie. & þat is þe skil whie litil vryn comeþ 295 oute of þe bodi. And vnderstonde *pthisica,* or *etica,* of wiche þou hast sufficiently in c. *de liuido colore,* is but a lent febre wastand & destroy-and þe body. And noȝtforþan þe febre is noȝt mykel felte, noȝt mykel

---

27 of kynde] *foll. by* of kynde *canc.* R
28 The nutrityues kyndly han ... nutrityues] CgH, kyndely have compassioun of the spirituales And therfore when the spirituales are seke the nutritiuis GSc, *om.* RM7 (*eyeskip*)
29 is] *foll. by* is *canc.* R
30 froþi] M7CgGSc, forthi H, foþi R
31 froþihed] M7CgHSc, frothed G, forþihed *with* r *underpuncted* R
32 3 wise] *marg.*: 3 causez of froth

perceyuede, þogh it anyntisshe him gretely wiþin þe body. And þe skil
whie it is but litle perceyuede fro wiþoutward is by cause þat it halt him   300
mykel in þe sad membres, s. in þe bones & in þo þat ar bony. & passioun
of þo membres ar noȝt alse mykel³³ [f. 65va] felt as of oþer membres. And
þat is by resoun þat þai ar more sad & haue more quiete & stedfast þan
oþer membres.

   Item, in þis malady, in þis febre, þe membres in þe body ar ful drie, &   305
þan [is] hete feynt³⁴ & litle humidite into which he may wirk in, he halt
him abouen in þe ouer parties of þe membres. & þerof meny vaporez stie
vp & walme forth aboute to þe vtter parties of þe body. & þis is þe cause
whi þat febre is noȝt mykel sene outward, þogh it be huge & grete inwarde.

   Now tak hede þat þer ar 7 skyles of litilhede of vryn.³⁵ On³⁶ mai be by   310
cause of litil mete & litil drynk. Anoþer³⁷ may be *enfrasis*, i. oppilacioun,
stoppyng of þe veynes of þe vryne, os it is in *stranguiria* & in *litiasi*, of
whiche Y saide in þe j bok, þe 4 c., lef {7}. Item,³⁸ scharphede and fretyng &
bitinge in water-makyng, os it is comunely in sekenes of þe vesie, of which
maner sekenes it is saide in þe j boke, þe 4 c., lef {7}. Item,³⁹ þorogh mortifi-   315
cacioun o þe vesie, i. whan þe vesie is so contracte, i. so cronclide & shronkelide & cropen togeder os a schronclid purse, & þat is by cause of defaute
of kynde hete & of kynde humidite. Wherfor he is noȝt of myght for to
kepe ne wiþholde þe water wiþin hym til tyme. Item,⁴⁰ [f. 65vb] be cause
of þe palsy of þe vesie, os it falleþ often tyme in folk þat is elde & feble, &   320
also in folk þat is plectoric, i. fat folke, & in folk þat ar mykel fleumatic and
disposede to þe palsi and to þe ydropisi. For in swich folk ar þe synowes
so mollisshede, i. so neisshede, be cause of myche humidite, þat þai mowe
noght conteyne ne wiþholde þe vryn to þe tyme. Item,⁴¹ þorogh exces of
vnkynde hete in þe body, wastande þe kynde humidite of þe body, os it is   325
in acuis & also in continuel febre, os in þe pthisik. For þe kynde humidite,
þat shulde dilate & sprede & sprai him into multiplicacioun of þe vryn,
throgh violence of vnkynd hete it is wasted, distroiede, & fordone. And
þat is þe skil whie litil vryn in acuis and in continuel febre is tokne of deþ,
for grete desiccacioun & consumpcioun of þe membres in þe body cause   330

---

33   alse mykel] *added in lighter ink after the end of the line and column*
34   þan is hete feynt] CgH, þan hete feynt RM7GSc
35   7 skyles of litilhede of vryn] *marg.*: 7 causes of litil vryn
36   On] *marg.*: j
37   Anoþer] *marg.*: 2
38   Item] *marg.*: 3
39   Item] *marg.*: 4
40   Item] *marg.*: 5
41   Item] *marg.*: 6

litle vryn. Item,[42] vryn is oþerwhile litle be cause of mykel egestioun &
of oþer superfluytes, os in þe wombe flux & in grete swete & swich oþer.

And *e contrario*, 7 causes þer ben whie vryn is mykel in quantite.[43] Be
cause[44] of mykel mete & mykel drynk. Item,[45] be cause of rawe humores
in the nutritiues. Item,[46] be cause of superfluytes of humores. Item,[47] be   335
cause of consumpcioun of[48] **[f. 66ra]** al þe body, os in hem þat ar taken
wiþ þe etik and ar consumpte. For consumpcion of al þe body o party
multiplieþ þe vryn. Item,[49] in hem þat be constipat, i. sad-wombede, os
when þe lyuer is of god[e] myght[50] for to drawen & gete to him þe moysthede of þe fode, and þat is principaly when þe lyuer is *calidum & siccum*.   340
& so is it comuly in hem þat ar diabetic. Diabetik is he þat haþ *diabetes*,
þe diabete. What is *diabetes* Y saide in c. *de albo colore*, lef {39}. Item,[51]
when þer is none *emfraxis*, but kynd is myȝty for to delyuer oute þe vryn
myȝtely, os it is in hem þat ar myghty and fryke in kynde, & in hem that
ar *calidi & sicci*, and also in hem þat vse metes & drynkes þat ar diuretik.   345
Item,[52] litle egestioun and litle delyueraunce of superfluytes.

And take hede þat he þat makeþ swyche maner of vryn os Y saide in þis
reule, and þer come on him a flux, it is wickede tokne. For, os seiþ Ypocras,
who so haue þe pthisik, and þer come vpon him a diarie, it seiþ but deþ.
Diaria & discenteria, a dyarie & a discentarie: in c. *de liuido colore* lef   350
{31}. And tak hede þat þai þat haue þe pthisik, comunly agayn þe deþ hem
comeþ a flux. And þan be cause of þe febre, þe kynde hete & þe spirit and
þe myght of þe body ar **[f. 66rb]** so wanysshede and wastede & destroiede,
& þe kynde humidite is consumpte. And in þe flux is ȝit more[53] deperdicioun and more consumpcion of kynde hete and of þe *spiritus* and of   355
kynde humydite. & þerfor, thorogh bothe, kynde is so mykel consumpte
þat he is noȝt myȝt for to kepe ne wiþholde to hym of þe hete ne of þe
spiritus, for to gouerne ne for to reule. And when kynd hete & kynde
faileþ, lyf nedes moste faile, for in þo 2 stant lif of beste, as lif of þe tree in
the rote. & þerfor þer is none hope of lif þer a flux comeþ in a pthisik. Of   360

---

42 Item] *marg.*: 7
43 mykel in quantite] *marg.*: 7 causes <of> mykel vr<yn>
44 cause] *marg.*: j
45 Item] *marg.*: 2
46 Item] *marg.*: 3
47 Item] *marg.*: 4
48 consumpcioun of] *catchword*: al þe body os
49 Item] *marg.*: 5
50 of gode myght] M7CgH, myche of myght GSc, of godo myght R
51 Item] *marg.*: 6
52 Item] *marg.*: 7
53 is ȝit more] *foll. by* is ȝit more *canc.* R

þe pthisik & of þe etik and of here spices and what folk ar disposede þerto, I saide sufficiently in þe c. of Blo colour lef⁵⁴ {31}. And alle þo poyntes þat I haue saide of vryn Pale or Palisshe, þe same poyntes vnderstond of Citrin[i]sh.⁵⁵

[2.9]

De citrino colore, of Citrin colour: c. 9

Citryn colour in vryn is mene bitwene ȝelowe & rede, & Subcitrin is more bitwene ȝelow and white. Now vnderstonde: riȝt os Pale colour is causede of mykel¹ fleume & litil colre, os I saide in þe firste ende of þe nexte c. beforn, riȝt so Citrin colour *e contrario*, of mykel colre & litle   5
fleu- [f. 66va] me. Wherfor it folweth þat, os *pallida vrina* seiþ *dominium* of fleume & colre in þe body, but principaly of fleume, ryght so *vrina citrina* seiþ *dominium* of colre & of fleume but principaly of colre. What is *dominium*, often tyme haue I saide beforne. Vryn Citrin or Subcitrine euermore signifien gode digestioun & myȝtihede in kynde and of kynde   10
he[te],² but Citrin more þan Subcitrin. *Et* þerfor vryn Citrin & vryn Subcitrine euermore seiþ *dominium* of colre, but in diuerse wise. For when it is so þat colre is myxte wiþ blode, þe vryn is Citrin, mykel toward redhede. If þe colre be mixt wiþ melancolie naturale, þan is þe citrinhede of þe vryn mykel toward ȝelowhede. If colre adust be myxt wiþ a colre naturel, þe   15
vryn is Citrin, mykel toward grenehede, i. þe vryn is Citrin wiþ a maner of grenehede. *Et* if colre be myxt wiþ a fleume, þe vryn is Citrin wiþ a maner of white. *Et* in þis wise is Citrin colour diuerse in þe vrin, vpon dyuerse kyndes of diuerse humores þat he is menkt wiþ.

Þan tak þis for a reule: þat vryn Citrin or Subcitrin, wiþ a þyn body   20
þoroghoute, seiþ meny þinges. In ȝonge folk, & namely fleumatik or melancolik, it seith a simple terciene. Swiche vryn is noȝt answeronde to his complexioun, for þe kynde vryn of ȝong folk [f. 66vb] fleumatik, & þai be hole, schuld be *alba* or *lactea* or elles *pallida*, with a body menely þik or menely thenne. And þerfor, in as mykel os it is Citrin, in swiche com-   25
plexion it seiþ exces of hete & incencioun of blode, i. if his blode were

---

54 lef] *foll. by* and lef *canc.* R
55 Citrinish] M7CgHGSc, Citrinush R

---

1 of mykel] *foll. by* of mykel *canc.* R
2 hete] M7CgHGSc, he (*line end*) R

distempred þorogh exces of hete & causede a febre, þan schulde þe vryn
be depe in colour, i. more þan Citrine, and þik. If fleume, feynt coloure
and þik body. If melancolie, wan coloure, s. ȝelowe or ȝelowishe, & then
body. And þerfor swiche vryn in ȝonge folk fleumatik or elles melancolic,   30
wheþer it be, seiþ a simple tercien, saue þat in a melancolik, it is more
thenne þan in a fleumatik. For þe kynde vryn of a melancolik schulde be
ȝelow or Palisshe & thenne. *Et* so it seiþ a party exces oute of temperure, s.
exces of hete, incencion of colre, os Y saide riȝt nowe, bot noght so mykel
exces os in a fleumatik, for it is more nere his kynde þan in a fleumatik.   35

If olde folk, & namely fleumatik or elles melancolik, make swich vryn, s.
Citrin oueral thenne, seiþ *duplex terciana*, a double tercien. *Simplex terciana*
& *duplex terciana*: in c. *de liuido colore*, lef {om.}. For swich vryn acordeþ
noght wiþ þe kynde vryn of olde folke hole, for euermore in olde folk
[f. 67ra] hole, what complexion so þai be, the vryn oweþ for to be White or   40
Whitisshe & dedisshe, be cause of feblenes of kynde hete, & namely in fleumatik & melancolik; in olde folk colrik & hole, wiþ a maner of grenehede. &
þerfor Citrin vryn in olde folk seiþ grete distemp[er]ur[e][3] of complexioun.

Item, if a chylde beneþe 14 ȝere make Citrin vryn, it seiþ *febris continua*,
a continuel febre. *Febris continua* in c. *de liuido colore,* lef {29}. Childes   45
vryn in þe j boke, þe 4 c., lef {om.}. *Et* þe same vryn in on þat is colrik
seiþ þat he is hoole & fers, for þat is þe kynde vryn of colrik complexioun. *Et* if þe same maner of vryn apere so long tyme togeder, it seiþ *febris*
erretica (*anglice*: þe febre erront), & namely in autumpne and in wyntre,
for þan comuly hete goand biforn is noȝt ȝitt al fully quenchede & colde   50
comande is noȝt ȝitt fixe, i. is noȝt ȝit stedefastly satlede[4] [M7, f. 44v] so
þat neþer is ȝit parfit. & so be cause of hete byforn-goand, þe humores ar
adust, & by cause of colde comende, þai ar engrosede. & so þai be distemprede & causen planetik febres & febres quarteyns. *Et* for alse mykel os
þai ar causede þorgh distemperure of diuerse humores, þai turmenten in   55
diuerse wise, somtyme [R, f. 67rb] fro þe 3 dai to þe 3 daie, sumtyme fro
þe 4 dai to þe 4 dai, & somtym fro þe 5 daie to þe 5 daie.

But take hede þat þe vryn apereþ so principaly after þe day of acces: þe
vryn schulde be discolourede kyndely be cause of melancolie, but be cause
of þe distemperure of þe febre, þe vryn takeþ colour more high & is Citrin   60
or Subcitrin & thene. *Febris eirratica* & *febris planetica:* in c. *de lacteo*
colore.[5] *Febris quartana:* in c. *de liuido colore,* lef {29}.

---

3 distemperure] M7CgHGSc, distempur R
4 satlede] *lower third of f. 67 is cut away; text supplied from M7 (as also in next three*
   columns)
5 colore] *foll. by* lef *canc.* R

Item, vryn Citrin wiþ a þen body, mykel toward palehede and oueral
thenne, seiþ *dominium* of a melancolie naturel wiþouten eny febre. *Mel-*
ancolia naturalis þus is descryuede in phisik:[6] *melancolia* is on of þe 4   65
humores, thik and heuy & drubly, kyndly causede & gendrede of þe
drestes of þe blode. And *melancolia* is saide of þis worde in Gru [M7, f.
44v] *melan*, i. blak, & of þis word in Gru *colo*, i. humor, os who sai a blak
humour. & when þis melancoli humor is causede, os I saie, of grounde-
sopis of þikhede of þe blode, anone he diuiseþ in 2 parties. On halt him stil   70
wiþ þe blode & goþ aboute in þe body wiþ him, & þat be cause of nede
& of helpe. It [R, f. 67va] is[7] helply and noteful þat it is myxte wiþin the
blode, be cause þat it schulde lede the blode & make it schaply and auenant
to þe membres and parties in body, which membres & parties owen for to
be fedde and norisschede wiþ humor melancolie. It helpeþ also þe blode   75
gretely, for he enspisseþ him, i. thikeþ him, & halte him in temperure þat
he slide noȝt ne slyp noȝt liȝtly awaie or he haue made and wroght[8] wiþ
digestioun, os he schulde done. Þat oþer partie of melancolie is sent to þe
splene by cause of nede & of helpe, boþe for to fode & norisshe the splene
& for to mundefie, i. to clense, al þe body.   80

Item, vryn Citrin wiþ a thenne body, but more þenne aboue þan downward, & namely wiþ smale Greynes swymmand in þe vryn and Burble
houand aboue, seyth strey[t]nes[9] at þe breste and sekenesse & feblenes of
þe spirituales & disposicion to- [M7, f. 45r] ward þe p\t/hisik. Þat þe vryn
is þenne in Citrine is noȝt be cause of grete hete in þe body, for þan schuld   85
it be more tinct, i. more high in colour, for grete hete causeth depe colour,
ne by cause of frigidite, for þan schuld it be whit, for grete frigidite kyndely blecheþ þe vryn, i. makeþ white. Ne humidite makeþ noȝt thenne,
[R, f. 67vb] for humydite enspisseþ the vryn; but it is thene be cause of
gret siccite þat is in þe body, & namely in þe spirituales and þerabouten. &   90
it is Citrin be cause of distemperure of þe febre, al be it so þogh þe febre be
noȝt or vnneþes perceyuede. And þerfor, swich maner of vryn seiþ grete
distemperure of siccite in the body, & namely aboute the breste[10] & þe
spirituales.

Pectus & *thorax* (*anglice*: þe brest & the breste bone)[11] ar 2 partyes of   95
man þat bene hard & heuy, & be cause þerof, þe breste is *frigida* and *sicca*,
for bones ar *frigida* & *sicca* in complexioun. And þerfor, riȝt os þai ar

---

6   in phisik] *marg.*: What is melancolia naturalis
7   is] *foll. by* al *underpuncted* R
8   wroght] *foll. by* wiþ *canc.* R
9   streytnes] CgGSc, streynes RM7H
10 breste] *foll. by* bone *canc.* R
11 þe brest & the breste bone] *marg.*: þe brest & þe brest bone

holpen & kepte & fodit by þenges þat ar answerande to hem in kynde &
in complexion, as walkyng, desport, gode eyre, merth, metes & drynkes
þat be newe, freishe, swete, & liciouse, noȝt ouerdone trauaile, & swych   100
oþer poyntes, o þe same wise þai be noyede & greuede & blemischede be
þingz þat bene [**M7, f. 45r**] *e contrario*. Þat it is more thenne vpwarde, it
is tokne at þe body is more desiccate & more drye aboute þe brest & þe
spirituales þan in ony oþer place of þe body. Þat þe vryn is granelouse &
ampullouse, ful of Greynes & Burblis, is tokne of mykel dryhede & st[r]eyt-   105
nisse[12] at brest & sekenes of þe spirituales. Of [**R, f. 68ra**] <u>Burbles and
Greyns: in the 3 bok</u>.

Item, vryn Citrin or Subcitrine, wonder þenne & bright & clere, os it
were vergede and fenestrede, <u>os Y saide in c. *de albo colore*</u>,[13] seiþ distemperure of þe splene, i. *splenetica passio*. <u>Se [s]plen</u>[14] <u>in c. *de karopos*,</u>   110
<u>lef</u> {59}.

Item, vryn Citrin, thenne & mykel in quantite, wiþ þirst & lenehede in
body, & wombe constipat, i. harde, seiþ distemperure of þe liuer, i. *epatica*
passio.[15] & þis is causede þorgh grete siccite of þe lyuer þus: when *epar*
is gretly distemprede þorgh dryhede, os often tyme falleþ in grete hete   115
takyng, and somtyme of threste, *epar* draweþ to him al þat he may of
succosite, i. moystoure, oute fro þe ropes & þe guttes, for to helpen &
moysten & myȝtten him. And þat is cause of þe mykelhede in quantite of
þe vryn in þis malady. *Et* comunly þis is the tokne of *epatica passio*: þat he
feleþ a peyn about þe ypico[n]dres,[16] & namely in þe riȝt ypicondre, and   120
þerwiþ him þenkeþ sometyme þat as it were a flawme walmeth vp to þe
þrote. & þat is noȝt elles but a hote drye fumosite, brestand out and stiand
& walmand so vp, & þerof often tyme folk cachen here deþ. <u>*Epar* in c. *de*</u>
<u>*karopos*, lef</u> {*om.*}, [**f. 68rb**] <u>& in the j boke, þe 2 c., lef</u> {j}. <u>*Epatica passio*,</u>
<u>wherof & in howe fele wise it is causede: se in c. *de liuido colore*, lef</u> {*om.*};   125
<u>*ypocondri* þeraboute.</u>

Item, vryn Citrin & thenne & bright, wiþ Burbles abouen, seiþ myslikyng of þe lunges, but it wil sone passe awaie. But if it be ful of smale
Greyns, it seiþ os Y saide in þe 3 reule beforne.

Item, if it so be þat an vryn apere Citrin in þe first bigynnyng or aboute   130
þe bygynnyng of an acue, it seiþ crudite and compaccioun of þe mater;
prolixite, i. longe lastand, of þe sekenes; and by cause of prolixite of þe
malady, falling & failying of myȝttes; and be cause of fayling of myȝtes,

---

12 streytnisse] CgHGSc, steytnisse M7, *wanting* R
13 colore] *foll. by* lef *canc.* R
14 Se splen] M7, splen CgHGSc, se plen R
15 epatica passio] *marg.*: epatica passio
16 ypicondres] ipocondris CgHSc, epocondris G, ypicomdres RM7

failyng of kynde – and þat but he be wel kepte & holpen. <u>Crudite in com-</u>
<u>paccioun of þe mater: in c. *de lacteo colore*, lef</u> {45}.   135

Item, if þe same maner vryn apere wel inwarde in an acue, & bifore þat
vryn appere an vryn *rubea* or *subrubea*, Rubicund or Subrubicund, *et* þerwiþ be no tokne of creticacioun, it seiþ þat he schal falle in a frensy, for it
is tokne þat þe mater wil stie vp into þe brayn. But if it so be þat þer apere
eny tokne of creticacioun, & namely **[f. 68va]** swych tokne þat he fele any 140
aleggawns, be it neuer so litle, it seiþ warsshing. <u>*Vrina rubea* or *subrubea*,</u>
<u>*rubicunda* & *subrubecunda:* se inward in here propre c. Creticacioun in c.</u>
<u>*de nigro colore*, lef</u> {42}. <u>Gode tokenes in þe same c., lef</u> {43}. <u>*Frenesis* in c.</u>
<u>*de albo colore*, lef</u> {39}.

Item, if þe same maner vryn apere in þe vanysshing of an acue wiþ eny 145
gode signe, it seiþ wanysshing, for it is tokne þat kynde[17] begynneþ to
encresen & my3ten. If it so be þat wiþin [þe][18] 3 daie (som say wiþin þe 5
day, some wiþin þe 7 dai, and some sai þat wiþin þe 9 day) after þat it is
warschede of a febre, þe vryn schewe him Citrin, and wonder thenne &
clere, it seiþ recidiuacioun, i. comyng ageyn, of þe febre. *Et* in þe same cas, 150
if it apere Citryn and gros, it seiþ expulsioun, i. purgacioun, and clensing
of þe mater, s. of þe colre.

Forthermore ouer the forsaide reule, vnderstonde þat vryn Citrin and
menely thenne and equal seiþ generally a colre citrine. <u>What is colre citrin</u>
<u>& how fele spices ar of colre: in c. *de pallido colore*, lef</u> {61}. Colre citrin is 155
componede of a kene colre þat is kyndely rede & of a kene fleu- **[f. 68vb]**
me þat is kyndly *frigidum* & *humidum*. Be cause of frigidite and humidite
of þe fleume (for *fleuma* is *frigidum* & *humidum*) is þe thenhede of colre
lessede, i. þe colre hath the lesse myght for to make þe vryn thenne. For
colre, in as mykel os he is kyndely hote & drye & rede, he þenneþ & clereþ 160
& rudieþ þe vryn; but fleume, in as mykel os he is kyndly colde & moyste
& white, he thykkeþ & droubleþ & whiteþ þe vryn. And so be reson of
whithede of fleume, þe redehede of þe vryn is þe lesse. *Et* in þis wise is
colre ci[trin][19] causede, and by þis skil, vryn of a colre citrin is lesse tinct
& lesse thenne þan vryn of a colre naturel. *Colera naturalis & colra rubea*, 165
a kynde colre & a rede colre: al on.

But take gode hede þat *colera citrina* somtyme is digeste & somtyme
is indigest. When *colra citrina* is indigest, þe vryn is Subcitryn & wonder
then. And þat is by skil þat while he is indigest, he wiþstant[20] þe kynde

---

17 þat kynde] *foll. by* þat kynd *canc.* R
18 þe] M7CgHGSc, *om.* R
19 citrin] CgHGSc, ci (*poss. as an abbreviation*) RM7
20 wiþstant] *foll. at line end by* þe *canc.* R

þat wolde delyuere himself oute & may noȝt. Wherfore þere may no gros 170
humor passen out wiþ þe vryn wiþ whos myxtioun þe vryn schulde haue
his inspissacioun. Bot *colra citrina* digest causeþ vryn Citrin or Subcitrin
wiþ a mene þennehede. And þis is þe philosophie: for colre citrin digest
wiþ- **[f. 69ra]** stant noȝt the kynde in delyuering oute os when he is indigest, but þer passeþ oute some gros humour wiþ þe vryn. And by reson 175
þerof is þe vryn noȝt ouerdone thenne but menely. If *colra citrina* take
mykel distemperur of hete, os it comuly befalliþ in acues, þan is þe vryn
more intense, i. more tinct & more depe in citrinhede. And if *colra citrina*
be noȝt distemprede þrogh hete, þan is þe vryn more remis, i. lesse tinct
in citrinhed and more þenne. And þat is be cause þat fleume vitre and 180
red colre ar myxt togedre, os Y saide. *Fleuma vitrium* & *fleuma album*, a
fleume vitre & a fleume blawnch: al on. How fele spices of fleume þer be,
I saide in c. *de glauco colore*, lef {43}. Item, colre & his spices: se in þe next
c. biforne.

[2.10]

Vrina rufa, Rudy colour: c. 10

Rvfa vrina (*anglice*: rody vryn) is most like fyne golde & *subrufa* goldis-
she. Vryn Ruf or Subruf wiþ a mene body, bitwene thik & þenne, pur &
equal, seiþ *corpus eucraticum*, a body eucratik, i. þat þe body is in gode &
euen proporcioun of þe 4 qualites, i. in gode euen temperure atwene colde 5
and hete. For if þe humores in the body wer distemprede thorogh grete
exces of hete, **[f. 69rb]** þan schulde þe vryn be dep in colour, os rede or
blode-red. If þe vryn were distemprede þorogh exces of colde, it schulde
be discolourede, os Subcitrin or more lowe. *Et* þerfor, Ruf colour seiþ
gode mene atwene bothe. In as mykel as þe body of þe vryn is pur, i. noght 10
swarte ne dym[1] ne dresty ne droubli, it seiþ þat kynde hete is myghty
for to purgen & clensen þe materijs, i. þe humores. Þat it is equal, os I
saide in c. *de nigro colore*,[2] it seiþ þat þer is no temperure ne disturblyng
of humores in þe body, but þat þai be alle accordede and tempre. Þat it
is mene bitwene þik and þenne, it seiþ also gode temperure & propor- 15
cioun of þe humores in þe body. And þerfor *color rufus*, rody colour or
golden colour, in vryn is a mene colour atwene al coloures. For þer is none

---

1 ne dym] *foll. by* ne dymme *canc.* R
2 colore] *foll. by* lef *canc.* R

other coloure þat so mykel acordeþ to al coloures in kynde os he, for of
al coloures he hath somwhat kyndly. And þerfor he most acordeþ to al
þe 4 humores. But tak gode hede þat þogh swich vryn betokne os I saie,   20
noȝtforþan noght euery complexioun so, for sometyme swyche coloure
beto- [f. 69va] keneþ wik, as þou schalt se. But vnderstonde þat euermore
ryght os vryn Citrin seiþ gode temperur in a colrik, riȝt os I saide in þe
nexte c. aforne, riȝt so seiþ vryn Ruf in one þat is sanguine.

Item, vryn Ruf or Subruf and þenne in a childe seiþ a febre cotidien.   25
In ȝonge folk, a simple terciene. In olde folk fleumatik & in woman noȝt
sanguine, a double tercien. For it seiþ þat þai ar mykel oute of here kynde
temperure, and þat þorogh exces of hete, for þe kynd vryn of olde folk &
of women þat ar noȝt ful sanguine oweþ³ for to be palish, wannyshe, &
dymmysshe.   30

Item, þe same maner of vryn in some tyme of þe ȝere, os in *autumpno*
& in wynter, it seiþ a *notha*. *Notha* & *quartana non vera:* in c. *de liuido
colore,* lef {29}. Wherof þe quarteyn is causede, I saide in c. *de nigro colore,*
lef {29}, and in c. *de liuido colore,* lef {29}. Of oþer febre in þe same place.

And take gode hede þit more peril is to falle in a febre in autumpne   35
þan in wynter. For in autumpne, þe sonne goþ from vs, but in wynter
it is comyng towardes vs. And þerfor in autumpne, do on most close &
kepe þe warmest, for þe humo- [f. 69vb] res of mannes body ar taken
wiþ hete afore-goande & smyt wiþ a colde comande, & so þai engrosen
and clodden & clompren togedre and ar distemperede, and þerof ar often   40
tyme causede dyuerse febres, somtyme terciens, somtyme quarteyns, and
sometyme oþer. *Et* þerfor in autumpne is þe werst tyme of al the ȝere for
to falle in sekenes. Of autumpn and of al þat oþer parties of þe ȝere, I saide
sufficiently in þe j bok, þe 4 c., lef {14}.

Item, þe same maner of vryn, if it apere swich longe tyme togeder & no   45
febre, it seiþ calefaccioun, i. chaufyng, & vnkynd hete o þe lyuer. Whiche
chaufyng & distemperure of þe lyuer is causede thorogh exces of vnkynde
hete, and þat vnkynde hete of þe lyuer causeth þat coloure in the vryn.

Item, vryn Ruf or Subruf wiþ a mene body & wiþ a maner of dym
Sky abouen in the vryn, þe malady ȝit beande in þe bigynnyng, or elles   50
þerabouten, it seiþ an hote febre interpolat, causede of a salt fleume, þat
þe comune calleþ þe sawsfleume. Þe dym Sky is causede of meuyng and
trauaylyng of þe vnkynde hete & of resoluyng of vapoures & of fumosites.

Item, þe same maner of [f. 70ra] vryn, or elles þe same maner of vryn
wiþ no Skye abouen, wel inwarde in þe sekenes, os after þe 3 acces, it seiþ   55
a tercien. And tak hede þat euery maner of fleume is vnpur of himself, and

---

3 oweþ] CgHGSc, orweþ RM7

by cause þerof, he makeþ þe vryn skyisshe & clowdisshe & dymmysshe.
And also in þe febre ar resoluede fumosites of melancolie. Whiche fumosites of melancolie, siþen þai ar liȝt be waie of kynde, þai passe vp to þe ouer
parties of þe vryn & þer cause a maner of Skye.   60

Item, if it so be that in þe begynnyng of þe sekenes it schewe him in þe
vryn o þe same wise, saue a litil more þik þan þenne, it seiþ a febre cotidien.

Item, vryn Ruf or Subruf & menely þenne, no Skye, i. no dymhede,
abouen but with a body pur & inequal, & a party more þik abouen vpon
estimacioun, it seiþ þat his body haþ mykel of salt fleume or þat he is   65
mykel disposede þerto. And if it so be þat in swiche an vryn apere meny
smale resolucions, it is tokne of scabbe. *Et* tak þan gode hede þat if þo
ilk resolucions appere in þe ouer partie of þe vryn, it is tokne of scabbe
bredyng in þe ouer party of þe body. If in þe myddes of þe vryn, þan on þe
wombe and þerabouten. If in the **[f. 70rb]** nether partie of þe vryn, aboute   70
þe generatyues & þe þies & þe legges. If þai appere oueral aboute in þe
vryn, also þe scabbe in al þe body.

Item, vryn Ruf or Subruf somdele more þik þan thenne, or elles atwene
boþe, an no Sky, no dymhede abouen, & þe vryn apere so longe tyme in
on þat haþ ydropisie, it seiþ but deth. For it is verray tokne þat þo wi[c]k- 75
ede[4] humores þat causen þe ydropisi ar smyt & taken & scolcret wiþ
vnkynde hete of þe febre. And so he is takne wiþ an hote ydropesie. Which
wickede vnkynde humores, syn þat þai ar so fele in þe body & þe body is
so ful of hem þat þe wickede distemperur and þe vnkynde hete of þe febre
wil first destroie & fordo al þe kynde substancial humidite in the body,   80
or euer may kynde be of myght for to wiþstonde or helpen for to fordo
þe wickede humores. And þis is þe hote ydropisye,[5] & þus causede, s.
when an hote febre cometh vpon one þat is in þe ydropesie. And þerfor
as Ypocras seiþ in his *Boke of Pronostiks*, if it be so þat þer come an hote
febre in ydropisie, it is þe werst signe þat may befal, for þan he is incurable.   85

[f. 70va] The same seiþ Theophilus in his *Bok of Vryns*. Ryȝt, seiþ he, os
wattri vryn, i. White vryn,[6] is gode in ydropesy, for þan is he curable, riȝt so
vryn Ruf is wickede in ydropsi, for þan is he incurable. Constantyn & Gilbert & Thade & alle autoures seie þe same. *De ydropisie frigida,* of þe colde
ydropisie: in *capitulo de albo colore,* lef {38} & in c. *de liuido colore,* lef {25}.   90

Item, þe skil whie an hote febre comand in ydropisie fordoþ noȝt[7] þe
ydropisi: as in þe spasme, in c. *de pallido colore,* lef {63}.

---

4 wickede] M7CgHGSc, wiþkede R
5 ydropisye] *marg.*: hote ydropisie
6 vryn] *foll. by* vryn *canc.* R
7 fordoþ noȝt] CgHGSc, *foll. by* as RM7

Item, vryn Ruf or Subruf, menely þik & inequal, & cloudisshe abouen,
i. wiþ swar[t]nes[8] & dymnes in þe ouer partie, it seith a febre cotidien
causede of a fleume þat is callede *fleuma dulce*, a douce fleume (*anglice*: a   95
freish fleume). If it be noȝt fullik Ruf, but more Subruf, and haue alle þe
forsaid poyntz, it seiþ *fleuma* wiþoute febre. <u>*Fleuma dulce* & oþer spices</u>
<u>of fleume: in c. *de glauco colore*, lef</u> {43}.

Euery maner of fleume, os Y said whil er, is vnpur & vnclene in himself
kyndly, & be cause þerof, euery maner of fleume causeth a maner of dym-   100
hede & dirkehede in vryn. But *fleuma dulce* coloureþ þe vryn in 2 wise:
[f. 70vb] o wise be cause of his myxtion wiþ oþer humores, and þan be
reson þat he is kyndely white & spise, os euery maner of fleume is, he
causeth whitehede & spishede, but lesse white þan doþ *fleuma naturale*
and more þik þan *salsum fleuma*. For *fleuma dulce* is somdel lesse white   105
kyndely þan *fleuma naturale* and somdel more moyst þan *fleuma salsum*.

Also when *fleuma dulce* coloureþ þe vryn þrogh kynde of his qualites,
he makeþ þe vryn Subruf or elles Ruf, & þat is by cause of menehede þat
he hath of blode. For *fleuma dulce* haþ more of þe qualitez of blode, which
blode is kyndely *calidus* & *humidus*, þan euery oþer fleume, <u>os þou maist se</u>   110
<u>in c. *de glauco colore*</u>. Þat þe vryn is spisse, os Y saide, wiþ swich a colour,
it seiþ roryng & bollyng & hurlyng. Of humores in þe body ar causede
meny fumosites & ventosites in þe body. Þat it is inequal, it tokeneth <u>os</u>
<u>Y saide in þe c. of Blak coloure, lef</u> {20}. Þat it is but menely spisse, it seiþ
but menely hurlyng and disturblyng of humores. Þat þe body is vnpure, it   115
seiþ defaut of kynde hete & þat it is noȝt of powere ne of myght to clense
and purge þe humores. Þe dym Sky is by cause of resolucion of fumosites
of melancolie & is causede by distemperure of þe febre. Whiche fumo-
[f. 71ra] sites, in as mykel as þai be liȝt, kyndly þai drawe vpward to þe
ouer party of þe vryn and þer causen a maner of derkenes & dymnes.   120

Item, vryn Ruf or Subruf, menely thenne or menely þik, wiþ a maner of
blohede abouen, and þe vryn apere longe tyme so, it sciþ þat þe spirituales
ar greuede and trauailede wiþ plente of salt fleume or of freisshe fleume: if
it be menely thenne, wiþ a salt fleume; if menely þik, wiþ a fresshe fleume.
Et þise be þe tokenes: kogh & streit onde, disesse at breste.   125

If a woman make swich vryn, it seiþ þat sche haþ a sekenes on þe matrice,
which sekenes comeþ of exces of a salt fleume or of a freishe fleume. But
of whiche, knowe os Y saide now. But than in the womannes vryn appere
also resolucions lik fisshes skales, somtyme white & somtyme blak, &
þan þise be þe tokenes þerof: grete peyne on here moder, & namely in þe   130
lift ypicondre, wiþ gret distencion o þe matrice & grete enflawmyng &

---

8 swartnes] swartnesse CgHGSc, swarnes RM7

walmynges. *Ypicondria* in c. *de liuido colore,* lef {26}. *Matrix* & *distencio matricis:* in þe same c., lef {34}.

The matrice is of- **[f. 71rb]** ten tyme gretly ouercharged and ouerleide wiþ salt fleume and halt him þere vnkyn[d]ly[9] & turneth him into filþe and corupcioun, & swymeþ forþ by *vena concaua* to *epar* & þere enfecteþ & corrupteþ þe blode. & so forth to þe vesie by þe water ʒatz þat ar callede *vrichides* and in þe vesie causeth blohede in þe vryn in Ruf colour by þis proces. & also if þou wil vnderstonde þe chapitles of Blak colour & of Blo colour, þou maiste se and knowe wel þat a dym Sky or elles a blohede in þe vryn is for to vnderstonde a swartnesse, a dirkenesse, & a dymnes in þe vryn. And þerfore take gode hede þat þis maner of swartnes and dymnes in vryn, be resoun of þe rody colour, it may noght wel be aperceyuede, but þou put slyly þi honde to þe vrinal. *Vena concaua:* in c. *de liuido colore,* lef {26}. *Epar* þe j boke, þe 2 [c.],[10] lef {*om.*}, & in þis boke, c. *de karopos,* lef {*om.*}. *Vrichide* in þe j boke, 3 c., lef {*om.*}. Þise forsaide *vrichides* in woman ar knyt to þe matrice.

Item, vryn Ruf or Subruf, oueral þik & dymmysshe abouen, but noght Blo, i. noʒt mykel dymmyshe, seiþ a febre cotidien causede **[f. 71va]** of a fleume naturel.

Item, vryn Ruf or Subruf, oueral þik & Blo abouen, & wiþ resolucions lik Bren, and it so be þat þe vryn haue aperede so noʒt longe tyme (som say noght ouer 3 acces), it seiþ þe pety emitrice.

What is an emitrice & how fele spices of emytrices þer be, I saide in c. *de liuido colore,* lef {28}. Som auctours, os Maistre Ferare & Maistre Platearye & also Maistre Johan de Sancto Paulo, seiþ þat þe pety emytrice[11] is caused of colre in þe vesseiles and of flume wiþoute þe vesseiles. But Giles & Maistre of þe Mesondeu seyn *e contrario:* of colre corrupt wiþouten & of fleume corrupt wiþin. *Vasa humorum,* vesseiles of þe humoures, ar þe veyns in þe body. The kynde of colre is for to colour wel þe vryn & þe kynde of fleume is for to discolour þe vryn. And þerfor bi cause of bothe, þe vryn is mene in coloure, s. Ruf or Subruf. Þat it is thik is os I saide in þe 4 reule biforne, & eke in meny captres aforn. Þe blohede abouen is by cause, os I haue often tyme saide, in c. of Blak coloure & in þe c. of Blo colour and in oþer c. eke. Of þo resolucions þat ar lik Bren & **[f. 71vb]** eke of al oþer thinges þat apere in þe vryn: se by alle þe 3 bok.

And tak gode hede þat þis blohede, s. þis dymhede, abouen in þe vryn – and generaly þe blohede in euery maner of vryn of high colour – may noʒt

---

9 vnkyndly] M7CgHGSc, vnkyn(*line end*)ly R
10 þe 2 c.] M7CgH, þe 2 R, *om.* GSc
11 pety emytrice] *marg.*: pety emitrice

or elles vnneþes be aperceyuede but os I saide in þe nexte reule aforne saue
2. And in þis forsaide malady, s. in þe petit emitrice, þe pacient feleþ grete   170
colde in his extremites, and þis colde comuly bigynneþ ageyn euen, or
elles þe sone declynond. & þat is bi cause of colre þat is putrefact, i. corrupt, wiþoute þe vesseiles. Which colre, þogh it so be þat he regne fro þe
3 houre of þe daie to þe 9 houre, <u>os Y saide in *capitulo de lacteo colore*,</u>[12]
noghtforþan he is lettede of fleume þat is putrifacte in þe vesseiles & seweþ   175
the course of fleume. *Et* þan is þe pacient in huge trauaile til þe mornyng,
for in þat while he is turmentede of bothe þo wickede humores; & þan til
þe 3 houre, he is in gret trauel. For eftesones þe toþer mater, i. þe toþer
humor, is putrifacte and þe toþer mater is redy towarde putrifaccioun, i.
corrupcioun & rotyng. & þan fro þe 3 houre of þe dai til agayn euen, he   180
is in rest, for þan he is turmentede [f. 72ra] but of þat on mater. And þan
at euen comeþ þe acces eftsones. And in the acces he liþ comuly þe eyen
closede and þe browes hongand, ne he openeþ vnneþes his eyen but he be
callede or spoken to. & þat is bi cause of moyst fumosites þat ar resoluede
of þe fleume & stie vp into þe heuede, & dulle & feyntish þe eyne in þe   185
hede & þe veynes and þe synowes in þe hede, & in þe body, & in þe armes,
& in the legges. And so þai and þe trauailing of þe malady togeder cause
swich heuynes & dulhed and dismaying.

Item, vryn Ruf or Subruf, oueral þik and droubli, and bloish and dymmysh abouen, & of late tyme, os I saide riȝt nowe in þe nexte reule aforne,   190
it seith a pleuresie. <u>*Pleuresis:* in c. *de liuido colore*,</u> lef {33}.

But for it is harde for to knowe and deme when swich maner vryn seiþ
a pety emitrice & when a pleuresi, be cause of likenes of the vryn, se þe
differens bitwene:[13] in þe pleuresie is grete peyn and ake in þe side & vnder
the ribbes & cowh and grete disese of drawyng of honde & febre wiþouten   195
interpolacioun, i. wiþouten sessyng, & eke þe blohed is more esye to aperceyue. *Et* þis condicions are noȝt in þe peti emytrice, s. no peyn vnder þe
ribbes, ne kowh or elles ful litil, no streythede [f. 72rb] of onde, and also in
þe pety emytrice is interpollacioun, os I saide in þe next reule aforne. And
also in þe emitrice mai noȝ þe blohede be aperceyuede, but os I haue saide   200
in þe reule biforne. But in pleuresie, it may be seyn wel at eye.

Item, vryn Ruf or Subruf & spis & bloish abouen, and longe tyme so
schewand him, seiþ *alchitam* or elles *empimam*. <u>*Alchitam:* in c. *de liuido*
colore,</u> lef {32}; <u>*empima:* in c. *de karopos*,</u> lef {62}.

But when it seiþ *alchitam* and when *empima*, þus þou schalt knowe   205
atwyne: if his wombe be wonder boln & his fete & þe face wan and

12 colore] *foll. by* lef *canc.* R
13 differens bitwene] *marg.*: difference atwene pleurisi & emtrice

dymmysh & dedish and colourles & þe eyen eke, it seiþ the[14] alchite. If
it seye þe empime, þe face is oþerwhile whan & bleche, but noʒt so os in
alchita, ne no bolnyng, but onde streyte & spotel grose & sanyouse, i.
attri, & blody & þerwiþ huge peyn at þe breste.   210

Item, vryn Subruf and spisse, and fro þe myddes vpward Blo, and wiþ a
coloure mykel like askes & mykel Froþ abouen, seiþ þat *pleuresis* turneth
into a *peripulmonie*. *Pleuresis:* in c. *de liuido colore*, lef {33}; *peripulmonia:*
in þe same c., lef {32}.

Item, vryn Ruf or Subruf, and spis and bloyshe abouen, and [f. 72va] 215
granelouse, i. ful of smale Greynes, seiþ bredyng of aposteme aboute þe
schore & in þe armehole or aboute the priue membres. & in which of þise
places it bredeþ, þer is felt sore & peyn, & wel þe more peyn by cause of
neruosite, i. by cause þat þe place is ful of synowes.

Item, þe same maner vryn, saue wiþ mykel Froth aboue, seiþ reume & 220
grete disese at brest & sekenesse of þe lunges.

Item, vryn Ruf or Subruf, þik abouen & eke beneþe, & wiþ a blohede &
fattishede abouen, & with *crinoydes*, & longe tyme so schewand him, þe
vryn seiþ þe 3 spice of þe etik. *Etica & his spices & wherof it is causede &
tokenes of disposicion þerto: se in c. de liuido colore*, lef {32}; *crinoides* in 225
þe 3 bok, in þe 14 c.

Þat þe vryn is rody in þe etik is by cause of dryhede of vnkynde hete in
þe body, & principaly in þe spirituales, of which vnkynde hete is causede
grete bulying & hurlyng & distemperure & so in al þe inder parties &
membres in þe body. Þat it is impure & thikkish & drobly is os Y haue 230
saide in þis c. & in þe c. of Blak colour eke. Þat it is dymmysh & bloysh,
os Y saide in þe c. of Blak coloure & in þe c. of Blo colour. Also þe blak-
nesse os Y saide in *capitulo* of Blak colour, lef {19}, & os þou mayst se in
þe 3 bok.

[2.11]

De rubeo colore, of Rede colour: c. 11

Rvbeus color, Rede colour, in vryn is more high þan is *rufus color*, s.
more toward rede, i. mene bitwene rede golde & rede blode. And it is
causede of blode and colre myxt togeder. For os Y saide in þe c. of Pale
coloure, right os but a litil of netes galle myxt wiþ a gode quantite of   5

---

14 the] M7CgH, ther R, *om.* GSc

water in a vesseil causeth noȝt [f. 72vb] rede colour, but Pale colour or
elles Subcitrin, & mykel galle menket wiþ a litil quantite of water causeþ
a Citrin coloure or elles a Ruf coloure, riȝt in þe same wise, litle colre
myxt wiþ þe vryn causith but a feynt colour in þe vryn, os Pale or Subcitrin. But if mykel of colre be myxt wiþ the vryn, þan is þe colour in þe   10
vryn wel tinct, os a depe Citrin or Subruf or Ruf. & þe more of colre, þe
more goþ þe vryn toward Rede coloure. And by resoun þat colre kyndly in himself is thenne & bright & clere, þerfor he causeþ vryn þenne
& bright & clere, but whan it is so þat blode & colre ar myxt togedre,
þai cause Rede colour in þe vryn. And if be more þickish & droblysh, it   15
stant by blode; if it be more bright & clere,[1] be colre. *Et* þe skyles are by
cause of þe qualites of blode and of colre, os Y haue often tyme saide in
meny c. biforn.

   Vrina rubea or *subrubea* & clere seiþ a febre tercien. *Febris terciana*
in c. *de liuido colore*, lef {*om.*}. And tokne of þis is þat þer is ake in his   20
heuede, & namely in þe riȝt half, for þer regneþ colre. And his mouthe is
byttre and his eres syngen. Þat it is swiche colour, it seiþe grete brynnyng
of vnkynd hete & grete distemperur of colre. That it is thenne & bright
[f. 73ra] a[nd][2] clere, it is tokne of grete siccite.

   Item, *vrina rubea* or *subrubea*, & more þenne abouen þan beneþe, &   25
wiþ a dymhede abouen, haþ diuerse significa[cioun],[3] vppon diuerse age
and diuerse complexioun, os doþ vryn Citrin. For in a childe, it seiþ a
febre cotidien. In ȝonge folk, and namely of colrik complexioun, a tercien.
In olde folk, and namely fleumatik or melancolik & also in woman, & þat
principaly if þe malady haue noȝt longe tyme lastede (os but o day or 2 or 3),   30
it seiþ a double tercien.

   If þe vryn schewe him so long tyme, and þe pacient haue no febre, it seiþ
calefaccioun of the lyuer. But þan hath the vryn a maner of dymmyshede,
os I saide abouen, and þerwiþ a maner of ȝelowhede or grenehede & also a
party froþi. If þe vryn aper so, s. *rubea* or *subrubea* & more thenne abouen   35
þan bineþen, & dymmysh abouen & þat in a febre, þan or it hath aperede
so longe tyme or but a schorte tyme. If longe tyme, it seiþ *quartana nota*,
a nothe quarteyn. *Notha* in þe next c. aforne, lef {69}, & in þe c. *de liuido
colore*, lef {*om.*}, and in c. *de albo colore*, lef {43}.

   If þe vryn haue lastede so no while, as but 3 daies at þe moste, it seiþ a   40
tercien. But *in estate*, it seiþ bothe a terciene & chaufyng of the lyuer. In
autumpne & in yeme, [f. 73rb] a quarteyne.

---

1 bright & clere] CgHGSc, clere & bright & clere RM7
2 and] M7CgHGSc, a R
3 significacioun] M7, significaciouns CgHGSc, significa (*line end*) R

Item, *vrina rubea* or *subrubea* menely þik, and vnpur and inequal
and oueral droubly, seiþ a tercien continuel. Constantyn seiþ þat a febre
contynuel is in 2 wise: for oyþer it is causede of colre corrupt wiþout þe   45
veseiles or elles of corrupte vapoures flawmand continuely vp aboute the
hert. Also a febre interpolate in 2 wise: for oyþer it comeþ of corrupt
mater wiþout þe vesseiles or elles of corrupt vapores enflammand þe hert
now & nowe by þrowes. Þus seiþ he. Þat þe vryn is *rubea* or *subrubea*
betokeneþ os I saide in þe j reule; þat it is þik & vnpure & inequal and   50
oueral drubly, os I haue often tyme saide.

Item, the same vryn or elles menely thik, & it haue a grenyshede abouen,
seiþ þe mydde emytrice. <u>Of which emytrice þou hast in þe c. of Blo colour,
lef</u> {28}. In þe myddes emytrice is huge brennyng, bi cause þat colre is continuely bullyede, os a plawand pot and hurlond aboute in þe vesseiles, and   55
fleume wiþout þe vesseiles. *Et* þerfor colre, sin þat he is liȝt of kynde, &
when he is brent & purede by resoun þerof riȝt more liȝt, he stieþ vp & halt
him abouen in þe **[f. 73va]** vryn, and so causeþ þer a maner of grenehede.
But þat ilk grenehede is so litle þat it is noȝt perceyuede but þou put þerto
þi honde, <u>os I saide in þe next c. aforn of blohede</u>. Item, þe same maner   60
vryn, saue wiþ a maner of blohede abouen, seiþ *pleuresim*. <u>*Pleuresis:* in c.
de liuido colore, lef</u> {33}.

For alse mykel os colleccion of mater wickede is in þe membres, s. vnder
þo ribbis, which ribbes ar hote kyndly and liȝtly fele peyn & anguishe
anone as þai be oght bot wel, & also bi cause þat þai ar euermore meuyng   65
& stiring, þat ilk mater so collecte þer it boileþ & hurlith & brenneþ, & so
causeþ malady hote & scharpe, s. þe hote febre. And by cause[4] þat colre in
grete quantite is hugely aduste & made liȝt by resoun of hete & of brennyng, it draweþ vpwarde in þe vryn. And þat is þat semes os it were a
grenehede abouen in þe vryn *et* somtyme a dymhede, which dymhede is   70
comunly callede a blohede abouen in þe vryn.[5] But whan it appereþ more
toward grenehede, þan is þere more incensioun, i. more brennyng, of
humores in the body þan whenne it semeþ **[f. 73vb]** more toward blohede,
i. dymhede.

Item, þe same vryn, saue wiþ a maner of grenehede abouen, seiþ þe same   75
þing, s. þe pleuresi. And if it so be þat a dirk Ski, a dymhede þat comunly
is callede a blohede, apere so abouen apertly in þe vryn, wiþouten eny
laying to of þi honde, or elles a maner of grenyshede, wete wel þat þat is
noȝt but by cause of fumosites and of vapoures þat ar resolued of colre, &

---

4 And by cause] *marg.*: how grenehede & blohed is gendred
5 et somtyme ... in þe vryn] *foll. by* and sometyme a dymhede which dymhede is
   comunly called a blohede abouen in þe vryn *canc.* R

bi cause of liȝthede ar stiede vp to þe ouer parties of þe vryn, & þere cause   80
a dymhede or a grenehede or bothe, os Y haue saide beforn. Ypocras in
his *Bok of Pronostikes* teches þat grete routoures ar noȝt mykel pleuretik:
acide ructantes non valde pleuretici sunt.

[2.12]

De vrina rubicunda, of Blode-rede vryn: c. 12

Urina rubicunda is the moste high vryn in coloure þat is or may be. And
it is moste like fyne rede or elles blode when it is most fyne & moste
pure bright, i. blode-rede, & *subrubicunda* is most lyke wattri blode. *Et*
meny auctoures treten of *rubea* & *subrubea*, *rubicunda* & *subrubicunda* al   5
vnder on, outetak, os þai al sein, þat Rubecund & Subrubecund euermore
bitokne more[1] insensioun, i. more brennyng[2] [f. 74ra] and more scaldyng,
of the humores in þe body bi cause of more exces of vnkynde hete þan
rubea or *subrubea*.[3] And sum trete of Rubicunde by himself & of *subrubi-*
cunda & *rubea* vnder on, and *subrubea* and *citrina* vnder on, and of Sub-   10
citrin and Pale al vnder on. But wit wel þat bitwene vryn *rubea* & *vrina*
subrubicunda is no difference, or vnneþes eny.
   Vrina rubicunda or *subrubicunda*, spis and droubly and swartisshe
abouen, somdel towarde blohede, and also wiþ a stynk or elles a wickede
odoure or an euel eyre by þe nose, it seiþ a febre þat is callede *synochus*,   15
a synoch. *Sinochus* is a febre continuel causede þorogh corrupcioun of
blode in þe veyns in þis wise: when it is so þat blode is so wickedly disposede & so hugely distemprede þat kind is noȝt of myght for to ouercome
it, ne for to maistri it, ne reule it, þat blode turneþ into filþe and corrupcioun in þe vesseiles. And þerof comeþ vile corupt vapoures enflawmyng   20
þe hert continuely. *Synochus* is saide of þis worde *sin*, i. wiþouten, and
of þis worde *choos*, i. trauail, as who say a febre wiþout rest. For among
al roten febres, *synocus* is so trauaylouse þat he hath leste reste. *Febris*
[f. 74rb] *putrida*, a roten febre, is þat þat is causede of roten humoures in
þe body. & also it is callede *synochus*, i. *choabens* (*anglice*: hauond togedre,   25

---

1   more] M7CgHGSc, more more R
2   brennyng] *catchword*: and more scaldyng
3   CgH *cease being alpha texts at this point. Cg is grafted smoothly into the next sentence*
     in the beta version here, but retains the alpha chapter numbering; H begins the Rubi-
     cund chapter again, from the beginning of chapter 70 in the beta version and continuing
     with beta chapter numbering. They are omitted from the apparatus henceforth.

or elles hauand diuerse poyntz, diuerse condicions), for *synochus* haþ alle
þe poyntz & condicions þat longen to a febre continuel. Poyntz longand
to a febre continuel ar þise: continuel bullying & rolying of ouerdone hete
and of wickede humores in þe body, continuel walmyng of fumosites in
þe body vp to þe hert, and also huge plente of corrupte blode. *Et* alle þise   30
3 causes ar in no maner febre so, namely os *in synocho*. *Et* by þat skil it
is callede *synochus*. *Et* os *synochus* hath 3 causes, riȝt so it haþ 3 spices,[4]
and euery of þo 3 spices hath his propur name, s. *homothena, augmas-*
tica, and *epamastica*. In *homothena*, þe vryn is bloyshe, i. swart and dym,
fro þe myddes of þe vryn vpwarde, & þat bot menely & menely tinct, &   35
oueral aliche rede be cause of menly corrupcioun and menely consumpcioun of þe blode. But *in febre augmastica*, in a febre augmastik, þe vryn is
mykel more Blo þan *in febre homotetica*, in a febre homoton, or þan in a
febre epamastik eiþer, and but little tinct, be cause **[f. 74va]** þat þer is lesse
corrupcion & lesse consumpcioun of blode þan is in febre homotoun. In   40
epamastica, þe vryn is but litle Blo or elles vnneþes, and also it is mykil
tinct, s. high rede, & wonder bright be cause þat þer is more consumpcioun of substancial humidite of þe blode þan in eny of þe toþer tweyne.
But comunly in an homoten, þe malady[5] is stondand til it passeþ, or to lif
or to deþ, & þe coloure of þe vryn halt him in one þerafter. In *epamastica*,   45
comunly þe malice of þe malady encrecit & waxeþ wode more & more, &
þe vryn hyer & heyer after hym; but *in augmastica* it is *e contrario*.

   Et þerfor tak gode hede for a general reule þat whateuer vryn it be, & it
be spisse, if it clere hymself abouen, i. if þat ilk þikhede, þat droublihede,
draw to residens in þe botume and wax thennyssh and clerish abouen, it   50
seiþ warshing & scaping of þat malady. For þat þe vryn pureþ & clereþ
himself abouen, it seiþ þat þe bolying and þe roryng & þe hurlyng of þe
humores in þe body cessen. Whiche humores werne afornhand so squalprede & rolyede and distemprede, & so destourbled in þe body, þat þe
vryn **[f. 74vb]** myght noght schew him equal for þe tyme. And if þe con-   55
trarie befalle, s. if þe vryn dwel stille þik abouen and clere himself beneþe,
it seiþ deþ. For it is tokne of stying vp of mater into þe heuede and into
þe brayns, and þan it is for to drede of þe frenesy or of þe *manya* or elles
of þe litargy. Wherfor often tyme it befalliþ þat vnwise leches – þat in þise
dayes ar callede dogg-leches,[6] os þise entremetoures & þise bolde braggers   60
þat stonde in chateryng & in clatering & noght in connyng, and þat onely
for mony wynnyng – oþerwhile þai se þe vryn ferst þik and afterward

---

4   3 spices] *marg.*: 3 spices of synoc
5   malady] m *with four minims* R
6   dogg-leches] *marg.*: dog leches

þenne & cler donward, þai wene þat it were tokne of warshing and is *e contrario*, for it is verrey tokne of malice of þe sekenes, & but þe grace of God, of deþ.   65

Frenesis in c. *de albo colore*, lef {39}. *Mania*,[7] þe manye, is a turnyng vp-so-doune of þe brayn, wiþ rauyng and wodehede. *Litargia*,[8] þe litargi, is a stonying of þe brayn, wiþ forȝetilhede & wiþ grete exces in slepyng. *Maniachus* & *litargicus* ar þai þat haue þo malidies, os *freneticus* is he þat hath þe frenesie.   70

Þat þe vryn is Subrubicund *in synocho* is by cause of huge hete [f. 75ra] & bullying & hurlyng of þe[9] blode. The þikehede is be cause of humidite of þe blode, for os Y often haue saide, humidite þickeþ þe vryn. *Et* þat þe vryn is þikisshe in a hote febre is noble tokne, for it seiþ þat þere is sufficient moysture of þe blod in þe body. Þat it is droubli is os Y haue   75 often seide in oþer c.; þe blohede, os Y said, is causede of myxtion of roten blode. Þe euyl sauour of þe vryn is of corrupcioun of blode.

Et tak hede þat *synochus* is causede euermore noȝt principaly of quantite of blode, i. noȝt of ouerdon litlehede of blode, ne of ouerdone mykelhede of blode, but onely of wickede qualite of blode, os when the blode is went   80 and chaungede out of his owen kynde and turnede into filþe & corrupcioun. Þus seiþ Egidius. Noȝtforþan, som saie þat *synochus* cometh bothe of wicked qualite of blode, i. of wicked distemperure of blode, & eke of quantite of blode, s. of ouermykelhede þerof.

Item, þe same maner vryn, saue wiþouten blohede & wiþouten wickede   85 sauoure, seiþ a febre þat is callede *synoca*.[10] Take hede þat þer is differens bitwene *sinocha* & *sinochus*: for *sinoca* is a hote febre enflawmand þe hert, causede of plente of wickede blode in þe vesseiles, peynant & tur- [f. 75rb] mentand more by cause of quantite of wicked blode þan by cause of qualite of wickede blode, i. more be resoun of mykelhede of wickede blode þan   90 þorogh wickedhede of euel blode. And *synochus* is an hote febre, continuely enflawmand þe hert, causede of corrupt blode in þe vesseiles, peynand & turmentand more bi cause of wickedhede of wik blode þan by cause of plente of wickede blode. And also *in synocha* ar vapowres noȝt corrupt enflaumand þe hert; *in synocho*, vapoures corrupte. Also *in synocha*, þe vryn   95 is noȝt bloysshe ne it hath no wicked weif at nose, but *in synocho* is bothe. Also *in synocha*, þe vryn is lesse þik & lesse drubly þan *in synocho*, and also *in synocha* is som interpolacioun, but *in synocho* is none or elles vnneþes

---

7 Mania] *marg.*: Manya
8 Litargia] *marg.*: litargia
9 þe] *foll. at line end by* biu *canc.* R
10 synoca] *marg.*: synocha

eny. Constantinus seiþ þat comunly þise ar þe signes of *synocha*: ake and
anguisshe in þe hede, os it schulde tocleue and tobresten, rede chekes and   100
bolnyng in hem, & bolnyng and blouthede in þe veyns, and huge bolnyng
& beting, and stoppede at brest and o þe spirituales, and a maner of swetehede in þe mouthe. [f. 75va] And his body and alle hese lymes ar so heuy, so
greuouse, and so fortrauailed, þat vnneþes may he welde himself.

Þat þe vryn is swich colour & þicke and droubly is by þe same skil þat I   105
saide in þe nexte reule beforne. Þat it is noght Blo ne of euel sauoure is by
resoun þat þe blode is noʒt corrupt, os it is *in synocho*, for of corrupcioun
of blode is blohed and stynk of vryn causede. Also what seiþ stink in vryn,
se in c. *de nigro colore*, lef {*om.*}. Of blohede: in his propre c. & in þe 2 c.
next byforn.   110

Item, *vrina rubicunda* or *subrubicunda* menely spisse, but noʒtforþan
somdel more þenne þan þik, seiþ a febre þat is called *causonides*. Cau-
sonides is an hote febre continuel, causede of colre and of blode, but principaly of colre. And by cause þat *causonides*[11] is causede more of colre þan
elles, þe vryn is more thenne þan thik.   115

Item, *vrina rubicunda* or *subrubicunda*, saue somdel more þik þan
thenne, seiþ a febre þat is callede *synochides*.[12] *Sinochides* is a hote febre
continuel, causede of blode and colre, but principaly of blode, and be
resoun þerof, þe vryn is mo- [f. 75vb] re thick þan thenne, os it is *e contrario in causonide*. & noghtforþan, in boþe þise 2 febres, s. in *causonides*   120
and *synochides*, þe vryn is euermore wiþ a mene body. & as it is in *synocha*,
riʒt so it is in þise 2 febres, *causonides* & *sinochides*, saue þat, os Y saied, in
sinocha is interpolacioun, but in *causonides* & *synochides* is none interpolacioun. & in þise 2, s. *causonides* & *synochides*, þe mouthe is bittre, but in
synoca þe mouþ is swetesh.   125

Item, *vrina rubicunda* or *subrubicunda* & then & clere þroghout, and
schynand rede os fier, seiþ a febre þat is callede *causon*.[13] *Causon* is an
hote febre continuel, & most scharp & most brennand of alle febres. And
it is causede of huge plente of rede colre, which rede colre is corrup[te][14]
in þe smale veynes of þe mouthe of þe stomak, & of the lunges, and of   130
þe lyuer, and of þe mydrede, and of oþer membres þerabouten, and principaly of þe spirituales. *Causon* is seide of þise 2 wordes *cauma*, i. *calor*
(*anglice*: hete) & *insencio* (*anglice*: brennyng or setting on fier). And þise
be þe tokenes of a febre causon: hosehede & ake in þe hede, so scharp þat
him þenkeþ his forhede schulde tocleue, riʒt as who tocleue it [f. 76ra] wiþ   135

---

11   causonides] *marg.*: causonides
12   synochides] *marg.*: synochides
13   causon] *marg.*: Causoun
14   corrupte] M7GSc, corrup (*line end*) R

an hamer or elles thirle it wiþ a persoure. And þat is by cause of huge hete
& of violence of hote fumosites, smytand vp into þe heuede and distemperand þe veynes & þe synowes of þe cerebre, and huge þirst and no drynk
mai it quench. & it is bi cause of huge hete þat comeþ of þe brennand colre,
enflammand continuely the mouthe of þe stomac.   140

   And the tunge is somtyme blak and mykel filþe þervpon be cause of
brenand hete. *Et* also forberyng of slepe be cause of huge hete and peyn &
violence of þe malady, and when he slepeþ, him þenkeþ þat he is in diuerse
& strange place & þat he seeþ wonder þinges & rede þinges and brennand
þinges. & al is by cause of huge desiccacioun and feblisshing of þe cerebre, 145
and al is causede þorogh exces of hete. And þogh[15] al þis 5 maner febre
be callede and ar acuis, i. hote febres, noȝtforþan *synochus* and *causoun* ar
moste wik & moste perilouse, but *causon* is most brennand. And who so
hath eyþer of þise 2 febres, it is but grace if he scape.

   Þat þe vryn is swich colour is be cause of huge hete and brennyng and 150
bulying of þe mater in þe body, and principally in [f. 76rb] the places afor-
said. Þat it is thenne & clere and bright os fier, is for narowhede and st[r]eyt-
hede[16] of þe vesseiles of þe blode, bi cause of whiche streithede þer
comeþ noþing aweie þorgh hem, but þat þat is most suptil and þenne. And
when þat is myxt wiþ þe vryn, it makeþ hym suptil & thenne & ferrene. 155
Forþermore, vnderstonde þat os dyuerse auctoures teche, þogh it so be
þat *vryna rubicunda* or *subrubicunda* signifie þise forseide maladies more
propurly & more certeynly, noȝtforþan al þo poyntz þat *rubea* & *subru-*
bea seyne, al þo same poyntz may *rubicunda* & *subrubicunda* seyn. And
þerwiþ wel acordeþ experience fro wiþoutward. For often tyme we se att 160
eye þat in terciens, þe vryn sheweþ him riȝt os in *sinocha* or in *causonides*
or in *sinochides* & tokenes in þe pacient nerhand as in eny of alle þise 3
maneres, owtaken þat in terciens is interpollacioun.

[2.13]

De colore inopos, Swarte Rede colour: c. 13

Urina ynopos is most like wyne þat is þik & blakish, os wyne of Calabre
or wyn Grek, or elles like mody water þat is swart redish, os we se in
some contre [þer][1] þe soyl is rede clay. Ino- [f. 76va] pos (*anglice*: swart

---

15   þogh] þorogh *with* ro *underpuncted* R
16   streythede] Sc, steythede RM7, *om.* G

---

1   þer] GSc, *om.* RM7

rede). And it is componede of þis 2 coloures, s. Blak and Rede, and os Blak   5
colour haþ euermore a thik body, riȝt so euermore haþ Inopos, for þai ar
causede nerhande al of on þing.

Theophilus seiþ þat when þe blode is aduste, i. al toscorclede and brende
& corrupte, & colre also, þai ar myxt togedre and of hem comeþ *color yno-*
pos. And þerfor, riȝt as Blak colour þat I spak in þe j c. of þis boke, and in þe   10
2 c. also, is causede of mortificacioun, riȝt so colour Inopos in vryn is causede of adustioun. And þerfor his general significacioun is euermore of hete.

Kyanos is þe same colour in al poyntes, saue þat Kyanos is ȝit more
blak, for Kyanos is most like roten blode or elles purpre. Kyanos is no
more for to saie þan purpre. And þe same dome is of þe ton þat is of þe   15
todre, saue þat Kyanos is somdel worse. And þerfor al auctoures treten of
boþe vnder on. And Gilbertus seiþ, and diuerse auctours also, þat Kyanos
often tym haþ diuerse coloures, for in some party of þe vryn in Kyanos, þe
vryn is Rubicund os feir, in some party swart rede, & in som party bloysh
& [f. 76vb] in som partie wiþ a grenehede.   20

Item, Inopos & Kyanos ar sometyme causede þorowȝ congelacioun of
blode, os when eny veyn is bursten & blode passeþ oute. Which blode,
whan it is oute of his kynde vesseil, i. out of his veyn, he is out of his kynde
place. & þan þat blode congeleþ, i. waxeþ colde & cluddeþ and clompreþ
togeder, & swart and blak in coloure, and causeþ swiche coloure in þe   25
vryn. And somtyme by cause of adustion of blode, os when þe blode is
scalt & scorclid & brent þorogh exces of vnkynde hete, os it is in acuis.
For ofte in acuis, þe hete is so brennand & stronge and so violente þat he
wendiþ and chaungeþ þe vnctuosite of þe blode, i. þe kynd colour and
þe kynde brightnes of þe blode, into an exces of colre, be cause wherof   30
þe blode is mykel distemprede & distourblide and so is oute of his owen
kynde, boþe in qualite & in coloure ek. *Et* þerfor þe superfluyte of þe
blode, i. þe vryn, nedes cacheþ colour.

And somtyme also colour Inopos & Kyanos ar causede þorogh feblenesse o þe lyuer, os when *epar* is so feblisshede & so distemprede þat it is   35
noȝt of myght for to depart ne [f. 77ra] dyuyse pur fro vnpur, as it comuly
befalleþ in hem þat ar ydropik and in scabbid folk. And þerfor if an vryn
apere Inopos or Kyanos in an acue and bifore þat he hade a grete scabbe,
it is a noble tokne. And also þe same vryn in ydropisi is but gode tokne,
for it seiþ he is esie for to be holpen, & þat namely wiþ swich þinges os ar   40
comfortatif and helply to þe lyuer.

An vryn Inopos or Kyanos in an acue [seiþ deth],[2] and namely if þe vryn
beforn were *rubea* or *rubicunda*[3] (and þis reule is for t[o][4] vnderstonde bot

---

2   seiþ deth] GSc, *om.* RM7
3   rubea or rubicunda] M7, rubea or subrubicunda *with* sub *canc.* R, rubie or subruby GSc
4   for to] M7GSc, fort R

it so be þat þere went biforn a scabbe, os Y saide riȝt nowe, and þan it seiþ
warsching). For it seiþ so huge adustioun in þe body of þe humores þat þai   45
may no more be aduste, but kynde faile & þe body be destroiede. Bot wiþ
no febre, Inopos & Kyanos ar noght so wik.

Item, vryn Inopos or Kyanos, sumdel more þik in þe mydde region
þan elles, seiþ ydropisy. And þan it is gode tokne, for he is curable, &
namely wiþ swich þinges þat bene comfortatif & strenhen þe lyuer, os I   50
saide while ere. Þe regions of vryn & mannes body in c. *de karopos,* lef
{55}. *Ydropi-* [f. 77rb] *sis:* in c. *de albo colore,* lef {36}.

Item, vryn Inopos or Kyanos wiþ a maner of blohede seiþ a *leucofleuma. Leucofleuma:* in c. *de albo colore,* lef {36}.

Item, vryn Inopos or Kianos in on þat is calculouse, þogh it be so þat þe   55
malady haue longe tyme durede, & þo þe stone be ful growen, it seiþ þat
þe stone is dissoluede and brusten, or elles þat it is in bresting. *Calculosus,*
calculouse, is he þat haþ *calculum. Calculus:* in c. *de albo colore,* lef {38},
& in c. *de karopos,* lef {54}.

Item, *vrina inopos* or *kyanos* wiþ smale long resolucions, os I saide in þe   60
7 reule, in c. *de albo colore,* lef {om.}, seiþ þe *nefresis. Nefresis,* þe nefresy:
se in þe same places þer I saide riȝt nowe of *calculus.* & þat is but deþ.

Item, vryn Inopos or Kyanos, wiþ smale chesel or elles a maner of smal
so[n]de[5] in þe botume, seiþ dissoluyng of þe ston in þe vesie.

Item, vryn Inopos or Kyanos, more dresty & droubly in þe botume þan   65
elleswhere, seiþ brusting or brusshing or elles stonying of som veyne, or
þat kiles or som braunche of hem is astonyed [f. 77va] or mystrauailede.
Kiles in c. *de liuido colore,* lef {43}. If kiles be brosten, he dieþ wiþin 24
houres or elles be þe 3 day. If som braunche of kiles, he feleþ grete peyne
in þe bak, & namely in þe 7 ioyntoure of þe rigebone, telland fro benethe   70
vpward. If eny oþer veyn or braunche in þe body be broston or bresede or
astonyede, he feliþ grete peyne þeraboute.

Grete worship and honor is to him þat wel can deme þis poynt. Þis
forseide reule techeþ þe Comentour vpon Giles. Also dyuerse auctoures
teche þat often tymes vryn scheweþ him Inopos or Kyanos in hole folk, i.   75
in folk þat ar noȝt seke, by cause of mych destemperur of humores in þe
body, os somtyme be cause of brustyng or brisur, or myswriste or mystrauailyng of som veyn in þe reynes or in þe vesie, or elleswher. For often
it befalliþ þat þorogh rennyng or skippyng or liftyng or swiche oþer, and
somtyme þorogh exces in lecherie, þer bresteþ som small veyn or smal   80
synow in the reyns or in þe vesie or elleswher in þe body. And þogh þer
brest riȝt none, noȝtforþan [f. 77vb] ȝit be cause of exces and of violence
of mystrauailyng, þe veyns ar oþerwhile so rarefacte, i. so scheer and

---

5 sonde] M7GSc, somde R

so thenne, þat þe blode sweteþ & sweltiþ and seweþ þrouȝ hem, and so
causeþ swych coloure in þe vryn.   85

And namely exces of lecherie excitith and stereþ þe blode & al fortra-
uailes þe veyns and þe synowes of þe body and mathe the lendes and al þe
waies of þe sparme rawe & rede. And so comeþ colour in þe vryn. And
þan is he but dede but þe more happ be. *Et* when it is of lecherie, þise ar the
tokenes: þer appereþ in the vryn os it were ropand þingz, os it were parties   90
of white glett, and þat is of his sperme, and also long resolucions redish
and rawish, mych like wasshing of rawe fleish & þo ar of þe substance of
þe reynes. & þat is werst signe, for it seiþ þat his kynde is consumpt.

Item, *vrina inopos* or *kyanos* somtyme seiþ *epatica passio*, somtym
pleuresis, somtyme *peripulmonia*, and somtyme *yliaca passio*. *Epatica pas-*   95
sio: in c. *de liuido colore,* lef {33}, & in c. *de citrino colore,* lef {67}. But
take hede þogh *epatica passio* be taken largely in phisik for euery maner of
malady and sekenes of þe [f. 78ra] lyuer, noghforþan vnderstond it here
for aposteme of þe lyuer. *Pleuresis:* in c. *de liuido colore,* lef {33}; *peripul-*
monia: in þe same c., lef {32}; *iliaca passio:* in c. *de karopos,* lef {53}.   100

Item, vnderstond *yliaca*[6] here in þis c. noȝt os I saide in c. of Karapos,
but for aposteme of þe reynes. *Yliaca,* os it is taken here, is saide of þis
worde *yle. Yle* is the pith and þe mayn of a þing, what þing it be. & þerfor
yle is often tyme taken for þe reynes & þe lendes. For oute of þe reyns
& þe lendes comeþ principaly þe pith & þe myȝt in generacioun, bothe   105
of man & of best. Þan *iliaca passio,* os it is taken here and often tyme in
phisik, is aposteme of þe yles, i. þe reynes. And *ylycus* is he þat hath *ylica*
passio. But if þow wilt knowe wel and deme sikerly bitwene þis forsaide
maladies, s. when Ynopos & Kyanos seyn *epatica passio* or ellez pleuresy
or peripulmonie or elles *yliaca passio,* þou most be war, os techeþ þe   110
Comentour vpon Giles. And þou moste e[n]quyren[7] if he fele eny pricching in þe riȝt side or in þe left side, and if eny streythede of onde, or if he
fele eny greuance in þe reynes, and also by oþer tokenes [f. 78rb] as þou
schalt se anone.

If he be strete-onded & fele grete streythede and penaunce at breste   115
wiþ swich an vryn, he is *pulmonicus* and his spirituales ar ouercomen
wiþ wicked materis. *Pulmonicus* is he þat hath *pulmonia* or *peripulmo-*
nia: in c. *de liuido colore,* lef {32}, þer I saide while ere. If he haue grete
pricching & peyne in þe reyns, he is *yliacus,* os Y saide whil ere, and
þan comunly þe colour of þe vryn is mykel lik fine synopre, & þan is   120
but deþ, & namely in aged folk. And þo þat han þis passioun, comunly

---

6 yliaca] *marg.*: yle
7 enquyren] enquere G, inquire Sc, equyren RM7

when þai pisse, þai gronten and grone & make noyse as þai schulde tobrest or die for peyn. And þay wene, and meny folk eke, þat it were þe stone, and often tyme it is noȝt so. But sometyme it is þe stone in þe reynes, & somtym it is only *apostema* in þe reyns, & somtym it is boþe. 125 & when it is boþe, it is but deþ. And mykel more peyne is when it is an emposteme þan when it is onely þe stone. And when both, ȝit more, if it more may be.

Item, whene þe forsaide vryn seiþ *epatica passio* & when *pleuresis*, þou schalt know **[f. 78va]** in 4 wise, s. by 4 tokenes,[8] os auctores treten. On[9] is 130 by betyng of þe pouse, for euermore in aposte[m][10] of þe lyuer, þe pouse veyn smyt but skilfuly softe, and for þis skil: for *epar* is a membre þat is nesche and softe. Wherfor it causeþ but nesche & softe stroke, and so his beting of þe pouse is but esye. But in *pleuresis*, þe pouse beteþ wonder harde and, as techeþ þe *Tretee of Pouses*, þat tokeneþ grete perile. For if 135 it be wonderly and oute of course harde, it seiþ a perilouse pleuresie, & þat þe mater is hard & wickede for to dissoluen & to ouercome, & þat þe malady wil longe laste and ouercome þe myȝtes of kynde.

Item,[11] if it be of þe lyuer, þe body is of bettre colour þan if it be o þe ribbes. 140

Item,[12] if it be o þe lyuer, his kowyng is more dry þan in pleuresie, for þan is þe mater aboue þe mydrede. And in pleuresi þe mater is more vndre þe mydrede, and þerfor his kuoghing is more moyste þan of þe lyuer. Noghtforþan in boþ is þe kowh dry.

Item,[13] if it be of the lyuer, þer is noȝt so mykel peyn and priching as 145 if it be *pleuresis*. For whan it is o þe lyuer, it **[f. 78vb]** is[14] noght so nygh þe mydrede, and eke for þo places about the lyuer ar noght so neruose, i. noght so ful of synowes, os aboute þe ribbes.

Item, Galienus techeþ 5 dyfference or elles 5 reules[15] for to knowe aposteme of þe lyuer fro aposteme of þe ribbes. Þe j[16] is þat aposteme of þe 150 lyuer is in schap like a bent bowe or elle[s][17] like þe nowe mone, but in pluresie it is rounde.

---

8 4 tokenes] *marg.*: 4 difference atwene apostema of þe lyuer & of þe ribbes

9 On] *marg.*: j

10 apostem] Sc, aposte RG, a poste M7

11 Item] *marg.*: 2

12 Item] *marg.*: 3

13 Item] *marg.*: 4

14 is] M7GSc, is *foll. by* s *or partially erased* is R

15 5 reules] *marg.*: 5 maners of apostem of the lyuer

16 j] *marg.* j

17 elles] GSc, elleþ R, elles þe M7

Þe 2[18] poynt is þat if it be of þe lyuer, his egestioun is somtyme blodisshe
or elles redisshe. And þat is be cause of wasting of þe substance of þe lyuer,
or by cause of resudacioun, i. of sweltyng & meltyng, and vanysshyng   155
awaie of þe aposteme, or elles by cause of bothe. But in pleuresi noght so.

Þe 3[19] poynt is þat if it be o þe lyuer, þe body is wonder lene & wan and
bleik. But in pleuresi nor nygh so mykel.

Þe 4[20] condicioun is that if it be o þe lyuer, it is euermore onely in þe riȝt
side, for *epar* liþ on þe riȝt side. But if it be of þe ribbes, it is sometyme on   160
þe riȝt syde and somtyme on þe lifte side & somtyme in bothe.

Þe 5[21] poynt is þat if it be o þe lyuer, he maie [**f. 79ra**] neyþer reste ne
lien on þat side þat it is, s. on þe right side, and þat is be cause of schouyng
and pressing of þe stomak & þe entrailes and of oþer membres þeraboute.
But if it be o þe ribbes, he may bettre reste him and lie on þat side þer it is   165
þan on þat side þere it is noght. And þat is by cause þat it is noght schouen
ne crodede of eny oþer membre þeraboute. Þus seiþ he.

Os techen auctoures of phisik, aposteme of þe lyuer is causede in 2 wise:
or fro wiþouteward or elles fro wythinward. Fro wiþoutward, as þrough
some smyting wherof is causede colleccion of blode and so gendreþ into   170
aposteme; fro wiþinward, of wikede humores in þe lyuer gedrand togedre and turnand into corrupcioun, and so causeþ aposteme. And þan þo
wicked humores in þe lyuer, if þai be of sanguine complexion, þai cause
apostema þat is callede *flegmon* or elles *apostema sanguineum* (*anglice:*
apostema of humour blode). *Flegmon* also is anoþer þing, as I saide, j bok,   175
4 c., lef {*om.*}. If þai be colrik, þan þai brede aposteme þat is callede *her-*
isipula. If fleumatik, apostemes þat ar squob and nesche. If melancolik,
apostemes hard þat turneþ oþerwhile into cancres.

Sumtyme þe aposteme hongeþ & cleueþ wiþ- [**f. 79rb**] oute on the bak
of the lyuer as a pokete, and somtyme it hongeþ and cleueþ wiþin þe lip-   180
petes of þe lyuer. And somtyme þai ar causede of gros ventosites þat ar
closede and sperede þer, and wolde oute, & þai mai noȝt. *Et* cause of þat
is mykel etyng & drynkyng and litle defying. If it so be þat þe aposteme
of þe lyuer be wiþoute on þe lyuer, os I saide riȝt now, he may fele it
wiþ toching of honde on þe ribbes. When it is o þe wombe of þe lyuer   185
or bitwene þe lappates of þe lyuer, noȝt so. But be it on þe bagge of þe
lyuer or be it bitwene þe lappatz of þe lyuer, alwaie he feleþ huge peyne
& greuance in þe riȝt side bitwene þe lyuer & þe ribbes when he draweþ

---

18 2] *marg.*: 2
19 3] *marg.*: 3
20 4] *marg.*: 4
21 5] *marg.*: 5

his onde, & namely when he sikeþ, and when he ete, & when he goþ ȝerne
or hasteþ him oute, & swiche þinges wil sle him. & he is a party streite-   190
ondede and kowhing wiþout spatlyng, or elles wiþ litle spatle, & þe face
wan ȝelowishe. Þise ar þe tokenes of aposteme of the lyuer, be it wiþin or
wiþoute. But if it be wiþin hym, wlateþ his mete hugely, and whan he hath
eten, it greueþ and chargeþ **[f. 79va]** him gretly, and litle he defieþ, and þat
he defieþ is dry and hard.   195

If þe aposteme be causede of hote mater, it hath wiþ him an hote febre
and huge þirste, and first his tung is redisshe and afterward blakissh. It
it be a colde aposteme, he feliþ but little hete & but litle þriste. If it [be]
causede of ventosite,[22] he feleþ grete peyn in þe riȝght ypocondre, and
his coloure in face is citrinyssh or bloysshe. And euery maner aposteme,   200
in what place & in what membre so it be, it is but colleccion of wickede
humores and principaly of blode.

Of aposteme of þe rybbes þat is callede *pleuresis*, in þis wise spekeþ
Ysaac in þe 4 boke *Of Febres: pleuresis* is an hote aposteme, bredand on
þe mydrede, caused of wickede humores comand fro þe cerebre, somtyme   205
to þe longes, and somtyme to þe mydrede, and somtyme to þe fleishe o þe
ribbes. When þai come to þe lunges, þan is it callede propurly *pulmonia* or
peripulmonia, <u>os Y seide in þe c. of Blo coloure, lef</u> {*om.*}. *Et* þan he feleth
but litel peyn os to reward, for *pulmo* is a membre þat may soffre mykel
sekenesse on, and longe **[f. 79vb]** tyme or he wete it or parceyueþ it oght   210
mykel, and þat is be cause þat it is noȝt neruouse. And so mykel is sekenes
o þe lunges more perilouse, for it is more thinnysh.

And þogh sekenes of þe lunges be but litle felde, noghtforþan þe *spiri-*
tus ar þe more streit and þe onde þe more schort, for *pulmo* is þe instrument of þe *spiritus*. And þai þat ben gretly sekenessede on þis maner   215
malady, here face is rede and lippis ar blo, & hete in the extremytes,
litle egestioun, slowe in pyssing & mykel in quantite. & often tyme þai
loue for to liggen noselyng, & hard þai slepe, and open mouth, and þe
pouse is feble & feynt. And somtyme þai ar as it wer oute of hemself &
astonyede of here witt, and þat is be cause of siccite of humidite of hem.   220
And ageyn here deþ, þai swete, and her extremitees wax cold, and here
powse litle & þik.

And þan if his spatle[23] be sty[n]kand[24] and euel colourede and sanyouse, i.
glettissh & attrishe and ropand, & þerwiþ feblehede of kynde, it is tokne

---

22   be causede of ventosite] G, be causede of a ventosite M7, be caused of grett ventosite
     Sc, causede of ventosite R
23   spatle] *marg.*: Of tokenes of spatle
24   stynkand] M7, stynkyng GSc, stykand R

þat deþ is²⁵ nere. And if it be *e contrario*, god tokne. Wherfor vnderstond 225
þat þat spotel is gode þat is litle & white and liȝt & hongand **[f. 80ra]** togedre & liȝtly comand oute at the first or þe 2 reysing, and namely if him
þink or fele eny liȝtsomhede þerafter, and principaly if þe spotel schew
him wiþ swich tokenes in þe 3 dai or in þe 4 dai, for þo ar þe daies nunciatyues. <u>Of whiche þou hast as [I]saac²⁶ techeþ in þe c. of Blac colour, lef</u> 230
{22}. And in hem comuly kynde fulfilleþ his wirkyng of digestion. And it
is more siker demyng to þe spatel after þat it is digestede þan biforn. For if
it come owte or it be digestede, it seiþ þat kynde is yrke þerof, and kynde
is noȝt of myght for to wiþhold it to þe tyme of digestioun. If it passe þe
4 day and aper in þe 7 dai, it seiþ warshing schal comen, but longe ferst. 235

Þat it is wel coct and digest, it is tokne of warsching; þat it passeþ þe
4 day, it seiþ þat þe mater of þe sekenes is compact and inobedient to þe
wirkyng of kynde, and þat kynd is noght of power for to fulfil digestioun
in þe 4 daye. For þe more nere þat tokne of digestioun be þe bigynnyng
of þe malady, þe more nere is warsching; and þe ferþer fro þe bygynnyng, 240
the mo late warshing. For kynd most nede haue alse mykel tym **[f. 80rb]**
fro þe nunciatif day to þe dai of creticacioun as was fro þe bigynnyng of
þe maladi to þe nunciatif dai. *Crisis* & *dies creticus* & *dies nunciati[u]us:*²⁷
in c. *de nigro colore*, lef {om.}.

Wickede colour in spotle a[r]²⁸ þise: grene, blo, & blak & bitwe[ne]²⁹ 245
grene & blak. Somtym þe spotel apereþ first grenysshe and afterward
chaungeþ into colour bytwene grenysshe and blakishe, like water of þe
see, and þan turneþ into more blakishede. And þat seiþ euermore adustioun of a rede colre and of blode. If it be first bloisshe and þan turne
to grenysshe, like water of þe see, & þan to blak, it seiþ extinccioun, i. 250
fordoyng of kynde hete. And þerfor þe coloures in spotel³⁰ ar tokenes
of deþ.

Mene tokenes in spotel ar citrin & whit wattri or elles þik & viscouse
& rede colour. Þise colours in spotle seiþ stronge malady & þat þe mater
is herde for to maistri. But noȝtforþan, rede colour is leste wik of hem & 255
citrin werst. Re[de]³¹ colour seiþ þat þe malady is causede of blod, & blode
is worþiest of al humores & eþiest for to tak digestioun. For the kynde

---

25 is] *foll. by* ne *canc.* R
26 Isaac] M7G, asaac R, *om.* Sc
27 nunciatiuus] GSc, nunciatius RM7
28 ar] Sc, ben G, a RM7
29 bitwene] M7Sc, atwene G, bitwe R
30 in spotel] M7GSc, in spotel in spotel R
31 Rede] GSc, re. M7, re R

complexioun is hote & moyst & wiþ hote & moyst wirkeþ myȝt & kynd
of digestioun. For lif stant principaly in hote & moist.

Citrin colour in spotle seiþ a rede colre & þat [is]³² werst of al humores   260
for to defie, saue blak colour, [f. 80va] for it is moste dry, & dry is most
vnable to digestioun, for it is most harde to diuisen or to departe or entren,
and þerfor when it is indurat, i. harded & clabbed, i. is more inobedient.
And þerfor rede spotle in þe bigynnyng of þe malady is gode, and namely
if he haue tempre slepe, eny appetit, & in swich tyme os when he was hole.   265
If þe spotel schew him rede in þe 7 dai or in þe 14 dai & no gode tokenes
þerwiþ, it seiþ groshede & hardhede and compaccioun of þe mater, and þat
it wil be longe or he warshe, and þat it wil be first aboute þe 40 daies or 60
daies. But what tyme, seiþ Ysaac, ar we noȝt siker, for often tym the seke
mysreuleþ him or he is myskept, tymes changeyng þe eir chaungeþ, and   270
meny oþer poyntz befalle, wherfor þe malady changeþ also. But if wikkede tokenes come þerwiþ, it is grete drede.

Item, þogh þe spotel schewe him citrin in þe bygynnyng & at þe 4 dai
chaunge into rede, and gode tokenes þerwiþ, it seiþ warshing, saue longe
tyme ferst. For citrin colour in spotle seiþ a scharp malady causede of a   275
rede colre, wherfor kynde nediþ [f. 80vb] longe tyme to chaunge it out of
citrin into rede & out of red into white. If it dwel stil citrin to þe 7 dai, it is
wik tokne, and namely wiþ oþer wickede tokenes, os wiþ strong febre and
feblenesse of kynde, grete þirst, and streithede of onde, and Whit vryn.
For þan deþ is more ner, s. in þe 14 day or þeraboute, and somtyme or þe   280
14 day & somtyme after þe 14, vpon þe strengh & malice of wiked signez.

Spotel white & þenne is bettre þan thik and viscouse, for it seiþ þat þe
mater is obedient to accion of kynde. And grose and thik seiþ compaccion. If it so be þat þo ilk wiked humores þat falle don fro þe hede, os Y
saide, holde hem at þe mydrede and þer gader into a gobat, a bage, it gen-   285
dreþ into aposteme þat is called *pleuresis*. And sometyme þat hote mater
falleþ doun to þe fleish of þe ribbis, & þan it is called *pleuresis* vnpropurly,
for þe veray *pleuresis* is no³³ þing but an hote aposteme brennande on þe
mydrede, os Ysaac seiþ. And comunly, þai þat ar of hote complexioun
raþest haue þis malady. And comunly it is gendred in yeme & in vere,   290
i. in þe last ende of [f. 81ra] þe ȝer and in þe first ende of þe ȝer (se in j
bok, þe 4 c., lef {*om.*}), and namely when yemps is moiste & wete and ver
gros & rokish and ouerhote or oue[r]³⁴ moist. And þerof is causede exces

---

32 is] GSc, *om.* RM7
33 no] nogh *with* gh *canc. and underpuncted* R
34 ouer] M7GSc, oue R

of wikede blode[35] and of wiked humores in mannes body, and gader in
swyche place of þe body þer kynd hete is lest myghty. *Et* þerof ar causede 295
wickede humores and fumosites styand vp to þe heuede. And somtym
when þai fynde þe pores open þer, þai holde hem and gedren apostemes
in þe heuede. And if þai fynde þe pores closed and spered, þai descende
doune to þe body, right as we see in þe rofe of a couertoure of a bath, for
when þe fumositees of þe bath stieþ vp to þe rof, be cause þat þai mowe 300
noȝt go þorogh [n]e perisch,[36] it ne hath here issue out abouen, þai turne
donward agayn. Which mater or materes somtyme drawe to þe lunges and
somtym to þe mydred & somtym to þe ribbes, os Y said whil ere.

And þan if it be a verai *pleuresis*, os I saide, it hath þise 4 tokenes wiþout
eny faile: a strong febre, and þat continuely be cause þat þe mater of þe 305
aposteme is nygh þe hert; [f. 81rb] streithede of onde, by cause of passioun of þe instrument of þe spirites, i. of þe lunges; prykyng and peyn
in þe side, so mykel þat he may noght meve himself byneþe fro þe [on]
side[37] to þe toþer, be cause þat þe aposteme bredeþ in þo membres þat
ar mykel neruouse or elles in þat membre or place þat is nervouse, s. þe 310
mydred, which mydred hath certeyn synowes comand fro þe cerebre &
fro þe mydred com synowes and veyns to þe he[r]t[38] and to þe lunges;
and also a continuel cowh, by cause þat þe mater is in þe instrumentes of
þe *spiritus*, i. in þo membres þat draw and hale þe wynd and þe *spiritus*, of
which þe mydrede is on.   315

And take gode hede þat if þe forsaid priching and peyn in side come to
þe self poynt of þe ribbes, i. if þe priching be felt at þe extremytes of þe
ribbes, it seiþ þat þe aposteme is aboue the mydrede; and if it be about þe
ypocondres, þe aposteme is vnder þe mydrede. And þis malady, s. *pleuresis*, bredeþ rather [f. 81va] and more comunly in the lifte half þan in the 320
riȝt halfe, by cause þat þe lift is noght so hote kyndly os is þe riȝt, as þou
hast in the c. of Karopos.[39] And but selden in the lift halfe for þe same
skil: for in þe left half, kynde hete þat comeþ fro þe hert & fro þe lyuer
disquasseþ it and wasteþ it awaie. And in þe bygynning of þis malady, or
þe mater is digestede, þer comeþ vpon him a drye cowh, and in þat drye 325
cowh he spotleþ somtyme. And þat is gode tokne, for it seiþ þat þe mater
is eþi for to breke and wast awaie and wil noght longe tym dwel. For kynd
fondeþ for to helpe and comfort himself, for to delyuer awaie þat wikede
mater in the body and for to kache it and dryue it out wiþ þe cowh and

---

35 blode] M7GSc, bloded R
36 go þorogh ne perisch] perysshe G, perse Sc, go þorogh þe perisch RM7
37 fro þe on side] fro the oo syde GSc, fro þe side RM7
38 hert] M7GSc, hent R
39 Karopos] *foll. by* lef *canc.* R

wiþ þe spatlyng fro þe places þer it gadereth. Somtym it is long tym and 330
meny day or spatle come oute, and somtyme it comeþ noght, and al is by
cause of grosehede and gleymousehede & hardehede of þe mater, þat it wil
noght oute.

And þerfor him most haue longe tyme in medycynes for to ripe
[f. 81vb] it and dissolue it. And þerfor if þe pasient delyuer him of spotel in 335
þe bygynnyng of þe bredyng of apostem, as in þe 3 or 4 daie, it is noble signe
and principaly if it be skilful, litil, and liȝt, and cleuand togeder and white and
esie for to delyueren oute at þe j or at þe 2 cowhynges. For þat saiþ euermore
þat þe mater is noght ouerdone grose ne ouerdone viscouse, but þat kynd is
myȝty for to diuise him and breke him vp and dylyuer hym owte benethe.   340

Wheþer þe mater in pleuresi be causede of[40] on humoure or elles of
menye, or of what mater, þus schalt þou know: if it come principaly of
blode, his face is redishe and rodyish, his spotle redish, moyst kowh,
rounde body, litle þirst, pouse grete and large, i. gret betyng of þe pouse
veyn, and vryn like vermylon or Ynopos or Kyanos and a party grose; 345
if it be of colre, þe face is citrinyssh, spotle citrin, drye kowh, lene face,
scharpe hete, grete þirst, powse swifte and smert, vryn Rede and bright; if
it be of *fleuma*, the face white, þe spotle whit, moyste kuowh, body fat and
feble of coloure & wiþ a feynt febre, litle þirst,[41] [f. 82ra] pouse large and
slow, vryn vitellyn, i. like þe ȝolk of an eye, and þerwiþ gros and somtyme 350
thenne and White; if it be causede of melancolie, þe face blak or leden, þe
spotle also, cowh drye, body lene and drye, mykel thirst, pouse litle and
slowe, and vryn ȝelowh or ȝelowh a partie greny[s]h.[42]

If it be of diuerse humoures or elles of alle humores, þerafter hathe him
the face and þe spotle and oþer condicions in þe pacient. If so be þat in the 3 355
or in þe 4 dai þe spotle appere whit and holdand togedre, it seiþ þat he schal
be parfitly heil and hoole by þe 7 dai. For it seiþ þat kynde hath wroght and
digested þe mater in þo 3 daies or in þo 4 daies, and oþer 3 dayes or elles
oþer 4 daies ar sufficient to him for to cache oute þe mater, and þat namely
if it so be þat in þe 3 or in þat 4 dai, with þe spotle apperede eny gode 360
tokenes, os swagyng of þe febre, or amendyng of oonde, amendyng of
appetit, slakyng of thirst, amendyng of rest, or eny gode tokne in þe vryn.

If þe spotle appere rede in þe bygynning of þe sekenes, i. in þe 3 or in the
4, and þerwiþ eny gode signes, it [f. 82rb] seiþ þat kynde wil fulfil digestioun
of þe mater in þe 7 day and turne it into whit, & ende his wirkyng & make 365
parfite warshing in þe 11 or elles in þe 14 dai. If it appere citrin and in þe

---

40 of] M7GSc, of (*line end*) of R
41 þirst] *catchword*: pouse large &
42 grenysh] M7GSc, grenyh R

bigynnyng, s. in þe 3 or in þe 4 dai, of þe malady and eny gode tokenes þerwiþ, it seiþ warsching att þe 40 or at þe 60 day after.

Item, if þe spotle schewe hym in þe bigynnyng gros and sone afterward
thene, or elles thenne in þe begynnyng and sone after þat turne into þik,   370
it is gode tokne for his smerte changeyng or it seiþ þat þe mater is obedient, i. liȝt & ese for to be ouercomen, or elles þat kynd is strong & myȝty
in himself. For myȝty wirkyng of kynd oþerwhile engroseþ mater þat is
suptil of himselfe & theneþ mater þat is gros, and namely in þe 3 or in þe
4 day. And þat is tokne þat þe mater is obedient & þe kynde myȝty, and   375
principaly, os Y saide, if it be whit and holland & hongand wel togedre, &
comand oute, os Y saide, at on plechching or at 2. And when it is so, it is a
verrai tokne þat kynde is myȝty and þe mater obedient.

Þat þe spotle is litle is tokne þat þe mater is litle & esie [f. 82va] for to
ouercome. Þat it comeþ esely, s. at þe j or at the 2 kowhyng, þat þe kynde   380
is of power for to make delyuerance. *Et* if þe spotle schew him so in þe 3
or in the 4 daie, by þe 7 daye deme hym hole; if in þe 7, helþ in þe 14. If it
schew him so in the j dai, helthe in the 4 day.

If it schewe him in þe j or in þe 4 day wattrish and rawishe and thennysh & in þe 4 daie turne into redishede, and at þe 7 daie come oute skilly   385
digeste & whit, it seiþ warshing by þe 14 dai. If it be so þat he schewe him,
os Y saie, rawe and thenne in þe j or in þe 2 dai & dwel so stil to þe 4 dai,
& chang noȝt at þe 4 day, it seiþ þat the malady wil longe laste. If it schewe
him in the 4 noght chaunged, os Y saie, but þat it haue some tokne of
digestioun: vppon þat þe tokne of digestioun is, vppon þat wil the malady   390
laste. And if it dwelle stil crud and indigest til þe 7 daies ende, and þan it
com oute wiþ grete streytnesse and wo & peyn, it seiþ failing of kyn[de][43]
and it is no sikerhede of his lif. Alle þise forsaide thinges seiþ Ysaac in the
4 *Bok of Febres*, nerhand worde for worde.

Of þis forsaide maladyes and of al [f. 82vb] oþer maladyes þat ar toched   395
in þise 3 bokes, if God gif me lif and myn ordre me suffre, I shal teche by
themself.

Item, vryn Inopos or Kyanos, wiþ a bloyshede abouen, and þerwiþ he
be *sansugiosus* or *octomicus* (*anglice:* sansugiouse or octomyk), it seiþ þat
he wil fal[44] in *omothoiam* (*anglice:* in þe omothoye). *Emothoia:* se in c. *de*   400
karapos, lef {54}. *Sansugiosus* is he þat hath *sansugium; octomicus* is he þat
haþ *octomiam*.

Item, vryn Inopos or Kyanos, wiþ Froþ somdel ȝelowisshe, seiþ gret
chaufyng of þe lyuer. Of whiche chaufyng wil brede a sekenesse þat is

---

43   kynde] M7GSc, kyng R
44   fal] *foll. by* it seiþ þat he wil falle *canc.* R

callede *ictericia glauca*. Þer are 3 spices of þe jawnys,[45] as þou shalt se in the   405
folwend c. Which jawnys or which of alle þe 3 spices it be, if it come vpon
him wiþin þe 7 daye of an acue, it is a wik tokne, for it seiþ þat þe mater
of the sekenesse hath taken al þe body, and þe malyce þerof is smyten and
spred and disperplide be alle þe parties of þe body. And þerfor it enfectis[46]
þe hide of þe body and so scheweþ him outward. But if it so be þat kynde   410
be myȝty and waste and dry[u]e[47] oute **[f. 83ra]** þe mater and þe malice
of þe febre after his 7, and after þat come a ȝelowh jawnys, it is tokne of warshing. How & wherof þe ȝelowe jawnys comeþ, se in[48] þe c. folewand.

Item, vryn Inopos or Kyanos in women somtyme seiþ an hote febre
and somtyme sekenesse of here floures. And þis is þe difference atwene: 415
in þe floures, þe vryn is more þik and more droubly donward þan if sche
haue þe febre. *Et* vnderstond and take gode hede þat vryn Ynopos or Kyanos is euermore suspecte more in men þan in women, but if it be so þat
wommanes vryn be swiche be cause of febre and noȝt be cause of floures.
For if woman haue swych vryn by cause of malady on here floures, it is   420
wicked tokne and werse þan if it schewe him swiche in a man, riȝt in as
mykel os mannes kynd and wommanes kynde ar different. þus seiþ Giles.
Gilbert þus: os seiþ Ypocras in his *Pronostikes*, an vryn Inopos or Kyanos
in a febre causon seiþ warshing by bledyng at nose. Causon in þe next c.
aforne. Theophilus seiþ þat þis warshing comeþ wiþ hu- **[f. 83rb]** ge ake   425
in the heuede & peyn þat is caused in þis wise: be cause of þe huge hete
walmand and bulyand and hurlond in þe body, þe humores in the body ar
forscalt and scorclid and brende, whiche scaldyng & brennyng of humores
cause meny vapoures wonder subtil and thenne, drawand þe mater þat is
aduste vp to þe hede, which mater draweþ wiþ him also colre and blode   430
by myȝt of his owen kynde. Of which vapoures and of which mater þe
heuede is replete, and namely þe forme partie, for þer ar meny veynes
and arteries and also þere regneþ blode more principaly þan in eny oþer
partie of þe heuede. And by cause þerof, þe forme partie of þe heuede
is hote and moyst. & þerfor, by reson of similitude, i. likness in kynde,   435
when the forsaide mater is liftede vp and hent vp into þe heuede, kyndly
[it][49] drawiþ him most to þat party of þe heued þat is moste answerond to
him in kynde. And þan comunly he is *scothomicus*, s. he þat hath *scotho-
miam*, in c. *de albo colore*, lef {41}. And þorgh huge strengh & violence
of þe grete hete **[f. 83va]** and of the mater, and by cause of exces of hem,   440

---

45   3 spices of þe jawnys] *marg.*: 3 spices o<f> þe jawny<s>
46   enfectis] s *poss. written over* þ R
47   dryue] GSc, drye RM7
48   in] M7GSc, in in R
49   it] G, he Sc, *om.* RM7

þe mouþes of þe veyns and of þe arteries openen and tobresten, and so gussheþ oute the blode at þe nose.

Item, if a mannes vryn schewe him Inopos or Kyanos, wiþ mykel residence in þe botme, it seiþ warshing to com and þorogh brestyng out of þe emoraides.   445

Item, þe same maner vryn in woman seiþ sekenesse of her flours to comen of warshing.

Item, if a wommanes vryn be Inopos or Kyanos, wiþ mykel residence in þe botme in an acue, and sche haue noght here floures þerwiþ, it seiþ þat sche schal warsh by brysting out of here floures. If þer be vnneþes eny   450 residence in the gronde of þe vryn, or elles right none, if sche be, os Y saie, in an acue and þerwiþ noȝt here floures, it is tokne of deþ. O þe same wise, in a man þat hath the emoraides, if it so be þat his emoraides be stoppede, i. if þai renne noght, it is for to demen.

And þerfor schortly for to speke, vnderstonde þat vryn Inopos and   455 Kyanos þat haþ no residence in þe grounde, be it of man, be it of woman, he scapeþ noght, for it seiþ þat dyuerse materes, i. humo- [f. 83vb] res, in the body ar so wik and so corupt and so fordon þat it is impossible kynde hem to ouercome or for to maistri. And þerfor in swich cas þe seke is noȝt for to take on honde. Þus seiþ Gilbert.   460

[2.14]

De viridi colore, of Grene colore: c. 14

Yn as mykel as auctoures bigynne at Blak colour and ende in Blak colour, þai make os it wer a cercle. When on goþ aboute a cercle, he comeþ ageyn there he bigan.

Now if þou wilt witterly knowe Grene colour in vryn and also Blak   5 colour in vryn – as þis chapitle trethe of Blak colour, for Blak colour here & Blak of which it is sei[d][1] in þe 2 c. of þis boke ar noght on, ne of o þing causede, os it is saide in þe c. of Blak colour; but Blak colour here & Grene colour ar nyh al on, as þou schalt se by þis c. – vnderstonde þat Grene colour in vryn seiþ euermore adustioun of colre. What is adus-   10 tioun & how meny maneres adustioun þere is, se in þe furst c. of this boke, lef {18}.

---

1   seid] GSc, seiþ RM7

Item, take hede þat þere bene 3 maners of grenehede in vryn.[2] For when
colre is adust, it receyueþ 3 maners of grenehede, which alle 3 maners
of grenehede is vnkyndly and contrariouse to him. For as [**f. 84ra**] oure   15
leches and Grece and alle leches, outtak leches of Araby, seie þat þe kynd
coloure of colre is citryn, leches of Sarasyns teche þat *rubeus color* is þe
kynde coloure of colre. But if þou wilt vnderstond þis 2 bok os it is seid
byforn, and if þou take gode hede to here site and to oure site, and to here
complexioun and to oure complexion, þou schal se þat þer is no contradic-   20
cion in owre opynyoun and in here opynyon.

In this wise is Grene colour: first when the colre bigynneþ for to brenne
thorogh vnkynde hete in the lyuer and in the veyns of þe lyuer, þan first it
takeþ a maner of thikhede, wiþ a coloure bytwene Rede and Kyanos, and
wiþ a maner of dymhede abouen, somdel toward grenehede. And þan is it   25
callede *vryna subuiridis*, os som wilen (*anglice*: grenysh vryn).

When the colre is mykel brent, þan it tath a more fyne grenyshede, and
þan is þe vryn called propurly *vryna viridis* (*anglice*: Grene vryn). But
when it is so þat the colre is al fullik aduste, þan the colre turneþ into
sward blakishcde, like a grene cole lef or elles most like an herbe þat is   30
callede *pras*- [**f. 84rb**] *sus* or *prassius* or elles *marubium* (*anglice*: prassyn
or harhoune). And þan is þe vryn propurly callede *vryna prassina* or *vrina
eruginosa* (*anglice*: þe prassyn or þe rousty vryn). Also it is callede *vrina
nigra*, Blak vryn, for it is swart grene, mykel toward blak, os is ruste of
bras or horhoune, riȝt as we se in a thing þat is swart blak grene.   35

Þan *v[r]ina viridis*,[3] a Grene vryn, seiþ *ictericiam* (*anglice*: þe jawnys).
But vnderstond þat riȝ os þe colre hath 3 maner of adustioun, os Y saide
riȝt now, & vpon þat 3 maner of adustion, þe vryn scheweþ him Grene
in 3 wise, os Y seid riȝt now. Eke riȝt on the same wise, þer ar 3 spices of
the jawnys. Þe j spice[4] is *ictericia glauca*, þe ȝelow jaunys. And þis spice is   40
lest maliciouse and most esy for to hele. And þe more party of þe peple
calleþ it þe jawnys onelik, for þai wene þat þer wer non oþer jawnys but
þat. And þat is for þai knowe no ferþer. But it shuld be callede þe ȝolwe
jawnys.

Þe 2 spice[5] of þe jawnys, Grekes calle it *pegaseleon*, i. *mustela agrestis*   45
(*anglice*: a wesel of þe felde or elles a wilde wesel or elles a feld mouse, for
euery wessele is mouse but noȝt *e contrario*). Þe Grekes haue swich maner

---

2 3 maners ... vryn] *marg.*: 3 maner of grenehede in vryn
3 vrina viridis] M7, vryn viridis GSc, vina viridis R
4 j spice] *marg.*: j spice of þe jawnys
5 2 spice] *marg.*: 2

bestes **[f. 84va]** amonges hem þat ar of swich coloure an like weseles and
mees. We and our auctoures calle it *agriacam* or *ictericia viridis* (*anglice*: þe
grene jawnys). *Agriaca* is seide of þis Latyn word *ager* (*anglice*: þe felde)   50
and of þis word in Gru *achos* (*anglice*: grene), as who saie grene os þe felde.
For when on hath þis 2 spice of þe jawnys, þe colour in him is os Y saide,
and his vryn is Grene as þe felde when it is grene os grene gresse. And þat
is strong peril.

Þe 3 spice⁶ of þe jawnys is called in Gru *melanchimon*, in Latyn *mel-*   55
anchima (*anglice*: þe melanchyme or elles þe blak jawnys). *Malanchima* is
said of þis word in Gru *melan* i.⁷ *nigrum*, blak, and of þis worde in Latyn
chimus, i. humor, os who saie a blak humoure, for riȝt os in þe first spice
of þe jawnys, þe vryn is grenyssh, and in þe 2 spice more grene, riȝt so in
þe 3 spice þe vryn is alþermost grene, i. alþer-depest grene, riȝt os we seyn   60
swart grene. Which swart grenehede in vryn is callede *prassium color* of
prassyn, or os Y saide while ere.

Vnderstond þat þe blak jawnys is euermore causede principaly of 2
humores þat **[f. 84vb]** ar blak be waie of kynde, [s. of blak colre & of
blak melancolie. Melancolie is blak of his owen kynde,]⁸ os Y haue often   65
seide. And colre is citrin or elles redissh of his owen kynd, but when it
is so þat þe colre is al fully aduste, i. al forschalt and brent and scolcrid,
throgh exces of vnkynde hete, þan it takeþ a vile swart derk dymhede wiþ
a maner of grenehed, os I saide beforne. And þerof takeþ þe vryn þe same
colour.   70

And in euery of þe 3 spices of þe jawnys, þou maist haue knowyng by
þe face⁹ what maner jawnys it is. For in þe j spice, his eyȝen ar ȝelowish,
but in þe 2 spice his eyȝen ar ȝelowish and grenyshe. *Et* in þe 3 mane[r]¹⁰ of
jawnys, the eyȝen ar wonder ȝelow, nerhand os a puttok fote, and wonder
grene, nerhond os gres, and al þe face ȝelowissh and grenyssh and puble   75
and bloute and more þan wone.

In þis wise is þe jawnys causede & þus enfecteþ þe eyȝen and þe skyn.
In acues and in bodies þat ar vnhele and mykel disposede to dyuerse maladyes, often it bifalleþ þat þe vnctuosite of the blode somtyme þorogh
strengh of kynd, and somtyme be cause of violense & of malice of þe mala-   80
die, changeþ and turneth into a colre. & **[f. 85ra]** þat is noght but throgh
exces of grete hete, throgh which huge hete þe humidite of þe blode is fordon, os I saide. And þan by cause þat þe colre is wonder liȝt of kynde – for

---

6   3 spice] *marg.*: 3
7   i.] GSc, in RM7 (*spelled out in* R, *abbrev. as* i *with suspension in* M7)
8   s. of blak ... his owen kynde] GSc, *om.* RM7
9   by þe face] *marg.*: token in þe face what jawnys it be
10   maner] M7GSc, mane R

euery maner of colre (in as mykel os colre) is liȝt be waie of kynde – throgh
mygh and malice of þe malady it [is] liftede vp[11] and borne forth aboute to   85
þe ouerest partyes of þe body, and principaly to þe face and to þe eyen and
enfecteþ hem. And vppon þat þe colre is more and lesse adust, os I haue
saide, vpon þat it enfectiþ þe eyen and þe hyde.

Of þe j spice of þe jawnys, folk scape al dai, but of þe toþer twyn vnneþes
on, & namely of the 3.   90

For Y spake of vnctuosite of blod, vnderstond þat os Gilbert seiþ, *vnc-*
tuositas sanguinis, splendor sanguinis, color sanguinis, and *flos sanguinis*
(*anglice:* vnctuosite of þe blode, bryghtnes of þe blode, colour of þe blod,
and flour or elles hewh of þe blode) ar al on. Som sai and Thade also þat
þe 2 laste spices of þe jawnys ar noȝt gendred in the lyuer ne in the veyns,   95
but only þe j spice, s. þe ȝelowe jawnys, and for þis skil: for þan the lyuer
and the veyns shulde [f. 85rb] tobresten thorogh exces & violence of hete,
and also be cause of venymoushed and malice of þe malady. But the more
dele seyn (and wiþ hem accordeþ Gilbert) þat euery maner jawnys is gendrede principaly in the lyuer, for þer is none humor gendred principaly   100
but in the lyuer. But the forsaide skil of hem þat teche þat þe 2 spices of þe
jawnys ar nogh gendrede in the lyuer ne in the veyns, it concludeþ noght
i[f][12] þou take gode hede.

Item, vryn Grene in an acue seiþ a malady þat is callede *spasmus. Spas-*
mus as som seiþ is þe cramp and *tetanus* þe schote. *Et* some seie *e con-*   105
trario. But whiche is which þou mayst se by here descripcions, þat [ȝeueþ]
nygh alle auctoures of phisik and Ysodre eke in þe 4 bok of *Ethimologyis,*
þe 6 c.:[13] *Spasmus est minor contraccio subita parcium corporis aut ner-*
vorum cum dolore vehementi ex replecione vel ex inanicione neruorum
causata (*anglice:* spasmus is þe lesse contraccioun of parties in þe body   110
comand sodeynly in þe synowes wiþ huge peyn, causede of replecioun of
wicked humores in the synowes and somtyme of anyntishing of kynde
hete in þe synowes). [f. 85va] *Tetanus est maior spasmus siue maior con-*
traccio neruorum a ceruice & vsque ad dorsum ex eadem causata (Tetanus
is þe more spasme or elles the more contraccioun in the synowes, fro the   115
hatrel byhynde doune to þe bak, causede of the same maner þing os *spas-*
mus is). Contraccioun (*anglice:* clyngyng and schronklyng togeder of þe
synowes), and it is euermore caused of consumpcioun of þe kynde substancial humidite in the body. Constantyn in his first *Boke of Medycyns,*

---

11 it is liftede vp] it ys lyft vp GSc, it liftede vp RM7
12 if] GSc, it RM7
13 þat ȝeueþ …Ysodre eke … þe 6 c.] þat nygh alle auctoures of phisik and Ysodre eke in
    þe 4 bok of Ethimologyis þe 6 c. RM7, that Isoder ȝeueth in the 4 book of Ethimologies
    the 6 c. and nygh alle auctours of phisyk GSc

þe last c. saue on, seiþ þat if *spasmus* or *tetanus* come sodeynly in on þat   120
is hole, as it ofte tym doþ, witt wel þat it comeþ of replecioun, if it come
after a febre of inanicioun, i. of consumpcioun of substancial humidite. If
on haue þe schote or þe cromp and þere come no febre, it is curable anogh.
If on haue þe schote or the cramp and þer come a febre, it is curable, for
hete of þe febre dissolueþ and discatereþ and vanisheþ awaie þe humores   125
þat cause þe schote and þe crampe. If it com in a febre, it is doute, but it be
so þat it come wiþ þe febre or elles sone after þe bygynnyng of þe febre.
Whi a febre comand in the schote or in the crampe is tokne of warshing, se
in [f. 85vb] c. de pallido colore, lef {om.}. If it come after an acue, it is tokne
of deth or elles nyghhand, for my3t of kynde is wastede & fordone, and   130
þe synowes moste haue longe tyme to recoueryng and þe kynd is noght of
my3t for to abide so longe tyme.

Item, vryn Grene and somdel toward Kyanos seiþ þe more emitrice,
and þat by cause of adustioun.

Of 3 maner emitrices: in þe c. of Blo colour, lef {28}. What difference is   135
bitwyx adustioun and adustioun complete: in þe j c. of þis bok, lef {18}.
Et take hede þat if þe vryn schewe hym Grene in the more emitrice, it is
wonder dredful. For it is verrai tokne of extinccioun & consumpcioun of
kynd hete causede of adustioun complet, os Y saide ri3t now. Wherfor
kynde faileþ & perisheþ but grace be.   140

Item, vryn Grene and litle seiþ no3t but deth, and namely if it stynke. Or
if þou tak a drop þerof & put it on þi nayle or on þi fyngre or on þi honde,
it blecheþ and barkeþ þe place. And þis reule is also for to be vnderstond
bothe in Blak coloure and in Blo coloure as wel as Grene coloure. If þe
vryn be Grene and mykel in quantite, and it stynk noght ne bark noght,   145
[f. 86ra] and þerwiþ his age be gode, 3it þer is hope. What fetor of vryn
signifieþ, I said in c. of Blak coloure, lef {21}.

Item, vryn Grene and mykel in quantite and mody and wiþ an euel sauoure seiþ parbrakyng and blemysshing of som noble membre in the body.
Be cause of whiche blemysshing, þe substancial humidite of þat membre   150
squaterith awai and passeþ forth wiþ þe vryn. And þerfor it seiþ deth and
þat sone. *Nobilia membra,* noble membres: in c. of Blak colour, lef {19}. Of
þis mater þou haste in þe c. of Blak coloure, lef {19}. *Nigredo quot modis
causatur* and eke in the next c. aforn, lef {om.}.

Explicit liber secundus.   155

Book 3

[3.1]

Incipit liber tercius

In the first boke is saide principaly how and what wise is vryn genderede in man and in the 2 boke of coloures in vryn and of here significacions. Now in þis 3 boke we þenken for to speke þorogh gift of him þat mannes ende haþ in hande of þo þinges þat ar callede in Latyn *contenta* [f. 86rb] 5 *vrine* (*anglice*: thinges conteyned in þe vryn).

It is for to vnderstond þat, os auctoures in this faculte seyne and techen, þat it is wel more verray and certeyn demyng by þe bodyes, i. by þo þinges þat schewen ham and apere in the vryn, þan by þe colour of þe vryn, and þat for diuerse skilis. For colour is a þing þat now is and now noght is, for 10 it is a thing þat is but schadewand and superficial. For it fadiþ & vanyssheþ and passeþ awaie at euery alteracion of the body, i. at euery chaungyng.

Item, the colour of þe vryn often tyme makeþ the leche for to fallen in his crafte. For often tyme neyþer þe colour ne þe body of the vryn wissen ne certefien the leche what humor is in[1] cause of þe sekenes. 15

Item, often tyme boþen þe colour and þe body of þe vryn varien and dyuersen, now by enchesoun of streythede of þe pores of þe veyns, now by resoun of largehed of poris of þe veyns, now by cause of streythede of þe waies of þe vryn.

Item, somtym the colour & the substance of þe vryn varien som tyme 20 be cause of digestioun & somtyme by cause of indigestioun. Be cause of alle þise [f. 86va] poyntes, often it falleþ þat whan[2] þe vryn shulde be þik it is thenne, & *e contrario*. And also often tyme it shuld be wel colourede whan it is discolourede, *et e contrario*.

First Y saie the vryn is often tym thik when it schuld be thene and þat 25 is in 2 wise: somtyme be cause of myxtioun of dyuerse humores, os when humores colde in kynd and humores hote in kynd (but noghtforþan þai crud and indigest) ar myxt togedre. Somtyme also by reson of feblenes of kynde, os when kynd is noght of myght ne of power for to reteynen, i. wiþholden, þe vryn but passeþ forth all or elles half indigest. *E contrario* 30 it i[s][3] in childern, for in childerne þe vryn is thik by cause of plente of humidite þat is in hem, by cause þat childern ar *calidi* and *humidi* <u>as þou</u>

---

1 is in] M7GSc, is *foll. by partially erased or rubbed in* or is R
2 þat whan] M7, thenne whenn GSc, *foll. by* þat whan *partially erased* R
3 it is] M7GSc, it it R

hast in þe first bok, þe 4 c., lef {9}. And noghtforþan, be cause þat her vryn
waies ar wondir streit and narowe, her vryn is thene.

Item, þe vryn is discoloured whan it shulde be wel colourrede, as it   35
befalleþ often tymes in hote maladies þe<re>⁴ þe vryn shulde, be waie of
kynde, be high in colour, no3tforþan it is *e contrario*. And þat in 4 wise:
somtyme by cause þat þo materies of sekenes **[f. 86vb]** is hent vp to the
hede, os it is in þe frenesi; somtyme by cause of adustioun and of consumpcion of þe mater in þe reynes; somtym be cause of chaungyng and of   40
turnyng of humores in þe body; and somtyme also be cause of consumpcioun of kynde hete in the body. Which kynde hete is ofte tyme consumpt
þorogh vnkynd hete, os it is in the etik. For in þe etik *calor accidentalis*, i.
vnkynd hete, is so habit, i. so rotede and so mykel broght in vse & in vsage,
þat it bicomeþ as it were *calor naturalis*, i. os kynde hete. And þat is þe skil   45
whi þat kynde hete of him þat haþ þe etik is consumpt and fordone, as
þou haste in þe 2 bok, in þe c. of Blo colour, þer Y spake of *etica*, lef {32}.

And *e contrario*, it is wel coloured whan it schulde be discoloured, os in
maladies þat comen of colde, and þat in 4 wise eke: somtyme by cause of
strong ake & peyn, os in *colica passione*, of whiche it is saide⁵ in þe 2 bok, c.   50
of White colour, lef {*om.*}; somtyme be cause of feblenes of þe lyuer, for as
mykel os þe lyuer is vnmy3ty for to purgen & clensyn himself or for to son-
dren or twynen þe pur fro þe vnpur; somtyme be cause of oppilacioun of
[f. 87ra] humores, os whan an or elles dyuerse humores be gadrid in a place
& ar stopped þere þat þai mai noght awaie; and somtyme be cause of swich   55
thynges os causeþ god colour in vryn, os doþ vse of cafuist and of spices &
oþer þinges þat þorogh hete coloryn the vryn. *Cassia fistila* (cafuist) is fruit
of a tre þat groweþ in the londe of Ynde, hote and colde but tempre; *cassia lignea* (cassia ligne) is þe bark of þat tre and it is hote & moyst in þe 3 gre.

But þo þinges – þe bodies þat schewen hem & apperen in the vryn –   60
which þinges ar called *contenta vryne* (*anglice*: þinges conteyned in þe
vryn), os techeþ Ypocras and al auctours, or þai ar parties of þe membres
and of parties in the body or elles þai ar þinges & parties þat holden ham
in þe membris of þe body. Wherfor þai tellen and techen more sekirly þe
disposicioun of membres & of parties in þe body þan doþ coloure of vryn.   65

Contenta vrine bene 18 in nombre, as þou may sen in þise 4 verse in
Latyn, & afterward Y þenke for to vndo hem by and by:

Circulus ampulla granum quoque nebula spuma
Pus pinguedo chimis sanguis arena pilus

---

4 þere] M7GSc, þe(*2–3 illeg. chars.*) R
5 saide] *foll. by* of which it *canc.* R

Furfura [f. 87rb] *crinnoydes squame necnon attomique*   70
Sperma cinis sedimen ypostasis octo decem.

[3.2]

De circulis vrine, of Cercles of vryn: c. 2

Circulus vrine, þe Cercle of þe vryn, <u>os Y said in þe ende of þe c. of Karopos, lef</u> {60}, is þe ouerest region[1] of þe vryn, i. þe ouerest place of þe vryn.
Þe regions of þe vryn, what þai be and how þai answere to þe regions
of mannes body, <u>I said in þe c. of Karopos, lef</u> {59}. Þe Cercle of þe vryn   5
seruit euermore to þe membres of lif: it telleþ and scheweþ disposicioun
and principaly of þe hed and of þe cerebre, for þe cerebre is principal of al
membres of þe lif; <u>membres of life in c. *de karopos, lef*</u> {56}.

  Þan take þis for a reule: þat if it so be þat þe Cercle of a vryn be spisse
wiþ a feynt wan whitish coloure, it seiþ sekenes in þe heued & namely   10
in þe hender party. Which sekenesse is causede þorogh wicked materes
of fleume and of exces of fleume, for principaly in þe hender party of þe
heuede regneþ *fleuma*, <u>os I saide in þe 2 bok, c. *de albo colore*, in þe laste
ende</u> {44}. Þat þe Cercle is spis is bi cause of ouerdone humidite of fleume
ouergoand & ouerswymmand þe cerebre. Þat þe Cercle is remys in colour,   15
i. bleik and wan and mykel to- [f. 87va] ward water is by cause of frigidite
þat letteth & febleþ þe kynde hete þat schulde be in the cerebre, so þat by
þe cause þerof, kynde hete is noght of myȝt for to purgen ne clensen the
cerebre ne for to cache oute þo superfluites fro him.

  Item, if þe Cercle be spisse and mykel like purpur colour, it seiþ seke-   20
nesse and greuance in þe prore of þe hede. *Prora capitis*, þe prore of þe hed,
is the former partie of þe heuede and þat malady is þrogh exces of blode.
For as mykel os blode hath his principal se & place in the former party of
þe hede, kyndly þat parti of the hede is moste hote. And whan þat party of
þe heuede is distemperede and ouergone wiþ vnkynd hete,[2] it is more hote   25
and distemprede and causeþ purpre Cercle. And by encheson þat blode
hath þere his principal se and place in þat party and by resoun þerof more
plente of hete is in þat party þan in eny oþer partie of þe heuede. And þat
is þe cause whi me[n][3] wax ballede raþer þer þan byhynden. Wemen ar

---

1 os Y said ... is þe ouerest region] as I sayde ... is Supprema regio GSc, is os Y said ... is
   þe ouerest region RM7
2 vnkynde hete] *marg. contains two chars. in red, poss.* 70, *but without the usual points used
   around numbers and unparalleled in other witnesses; poss. an errant scribble by rubricator*
3 men] M7GSc, meni *or* mem R

more colde in the hede kyndly þan men and also þai ar more hote in þe   30
he[n]der⁴ parti of þe hede þan in þe prore. Also, os Gilbert seiþ, be cause
þat kynde hete is mykel lesse and more feble in women þan [**f. 87vb**] in⁵
man be waie of kynde, þe vapoures mow noght sperplyn ne spreden ham
as in men. And þat is þe skil whie wemen berden noght as men and eke þe
kynde hete in hem gadriþ þo vapoures into the hede, and namely into the   35
former party. And þat [is] þe cause þat⁶ þer groweþ more plente of heer
þere þan bihynde and þat is þe cause whie wemen ar noght balled os men.

Þat þe Cercle is purpre is bi cause of superfluyte and of exces of blode
destourband þe hede, but namely þe prore. Þat it is sp[i]sse⁷ is by cause
of humidite of þe blode and þat bitokeneþ huge turbacion in þe cerebre.   40
For þe kynde fode and norisshing of þe cerebre schulde be blode col[d]e⁸
and moyst, but whan þe Cercle of þe vryn scheweþ him purpre, it seiþ þat
cerebrum is fede wiþ and fodede with blode bolyand and brennand. *Et* if
it so be þat þe Cercle be no3t fully purpre, but somdele more toward red,
it seiþ grete peyn also in þe prore and gret priching in þe noseþirles. And   45
him thenkeþ as his ey3en bolne and his veyns ar wonder stepe and bolne
and blout and oþerwhile him þenkeþ as he sei rede þingez aforn him. And
al þise þinges bitokne bledyng at the nose.
[**f. 88ra**]

De rubeo circulo

Item, vryn wiþ a rede Cercle and thenne seiþ ake and peyn in the hede but   50
principaly in the ri3t half. And colre is in cause, for he regneþ principaly
in that partie of þe hede, os melancolie in the lefte half, blode in the prore,
and fleume in the hatrel.

Þat þe Cercle is rede is by cause of calidite of rede colre. Colre is hote
of kynde and when þat partie of the hed is ouertrauailede and ouercharged   55
wiþ exces of colre, þer is more hete and more distemperur & þerfor it is
causede a rede Cercle. That it is thenne and clere and bright is by cause of
siccite of colre, for *colra* is *calida* & *sicca*.

De palido circulo

Item, vryn wiþ a Cercle pale and thenne seiþ distemperur and peyn in þe   60
hed, and principaly in þe left half. And exces of melancolie is in the cause,

---

4 hender] hindre GSc, heder RM7
5 in] M7GSc, *in* in R
6 And þat is þe cause þat] And þat þe cause þat RM7, wherefore GSc
7 spisse] M7GSc, spsse R
8 colde] GSc, colre M7, cole R

for in þe left half of þe hede regneþ melancolie and when he is in exces, he
causeþ sekenesse principaly in þat side. Þat it is pale and wan coloure is be
cause of coldehede of þat humour; þat it is thene is bi cause of siccite of
þat humor. For *melancolia* is *frigida & sicca*. And if it be so þat þe Cercle   65
last longe tyme swiche, þis poyntes wil sewen: drede & dasthede, suspeciousehede, feynthede of hert, mykil waking, [f. 88rb] and grete aueryce.

De plumbeo siue de liuido circulo

Item, if þe Cercle of þe vryn be bloysh, it seiþ *epilencia*, i. þe epilence. *Epilencia* & þe names þerof, se in þe 2 bok, c. *de liuido colore, in þe last ende*   70
lef {37}. *Epilencia* is noþing but mortificacioun of þe cerebre. Þe cerebre
is rote and ground of alle synowes in the body and of alle þe myghtes of
þe soule. And þerfor afte temperur and distemperur of him is temperur
and distemperur of alle þe oþere, riȝt as if a wel faile, al þe grounde and
þe ryueres þat comen of him most nedes failen and deyn. *Cerebrum* and   75
his propurtes: þe 2 boke, *de colore karopos,* lef {17}. mortificacion:[9] þe 2
bok, lef {56}.

   If þe Cercle of þe vryn apere first blo and 2 daies or 3 daies after or
more it scheweþ him rede, þogh it be in *apoplexia*, it is a blisful tokne; for
it seiþ þat myȝt and vertu of þe cerebre riseþ and comeþ agayn and þat   80
kynde hete & þe *spiritus* coueryng & tak agayn here myȝtes and ouercomen and maistrien the malady. *Apoplexia* is a sodeyn fallyng out of blod
wiþ a strangelyng and chekyng wiþ his owen blode, and it is saide of þis
worde in Gru, *apoplexim*, i. *percussio*, [f. 88va] a smytyng. For when it
comeþ vpon, comenly he is smyten wiþ deþ and þat sone or ellez wiþin 3   85
or 5 at þe ferrest.

   Item, if þe Cercle seme blo and afterward pale & after þat citrin and at
þe last rede, it bitokeneþ þe same þing.

De viridi circulo

Item, if a Cercle schew him grene in a tercien or in a continuel or in a   90
causon or elles in eny hote febre,[10] it seiþ greuance and peyn in þe hede
causede by exces of hete of colre hent vp to þe cerebre. And by cause þerof
he schal fallen into a frenesie. Som seyn þat it is tokne þat þe mater is hent
vp into þe hede and to þe cerebre and þer wil gadren and gendren into
aposteme. And biforne or it gadre into aposteme, þere comeþ vpon him a   95
frenesy. *Febris terciana & febris continua:* þe 2 bok, c. *de liuido colore, lef*

---

   9 mortificacion] M7GSc, mo *underpuncted and canc.* R
  10 febre] *foll. by* for *canc.* R

{29}; febre causon & of hote febre, c. *de rubicundo colore*, lef {74}. Colre & *frenesis* in c. *de albo colore* {39}.

De nigro circulo

Item, if þe Cercle schewe him blak & afornhand grene, it seiþ adustion 100 complete. If it schewe him blak & biforhand schewe him blo, mortificacioun. What is adustioun and mortificacion *et*[11] difference atwene adustioun and mortificacioun complet, I said in þe 2 boke, j c., lef {18}. Þe grenehede cometh alwaie of adustioun, [**f. 88vb**] for adustioun causeth first a maner of grenhede and after þat a maner of blohede or elles a coloure þat 105 is mene atwene boþin, riȝt as þou seest at þe eye in liȝtnyng of a candel.

De circulo tremulo

Item, *circulus tremulus* (*anglice*: a quauand Cercle or elles a quakend Cercle, þat al on is for to saie), os if þou schagge menely mewand þe vrynal & al þat is þerin quaue & quake and tremble, it seiþ sekenes and peyn in þe bak 110 as fer os *nuca* lasteþ. *Nuca* (*anglice*: þe nuk): se in c. *de liuido colore*, lef {27}. Þis malady in þe bake is causede of wickede humores and of fumosites of wicked humores þat hurlyn & rennen in þe rigebone and in þe ioyntoures of þe bak, vp and doune fro þe hatrel, i. fro þe hender party of þe hede and agayn. And fonden al þat in hem is for to parbraken and for to 115 bresten þe ioyntoures of þe bak and bryngen hem oute of lith, so fayn þai wolden haue her issu oute in the hatrel, i. in the hendre partie of the hed. And þere abouten þe nek is þe principal place and ground and foundy[n]g[12] of myȝt and vertu in mevyng and stering of al þe body. And þerfor if þo parties be at male ese, nedes al þe parties of þe hede and of þe body[13] 120 [**f. 89ra**] ar the worse. & þat is the skyl þat þe Cercle tremeþ & tremblith and quauyþ. In þe formere partie of þe heuede is apprehencioun, i. takyng and vnderstondyng of wit and wisdom and skil and resoun. And if þat partie of þe heuede be aggreuede and stuffede & stymede wiþ wik humores and fumasites, it is hard for þan he falliþ liȝtly into frenesie and rauyng or 125 to wodnes. And if so be þat swich wikede mater of þe wicked humores and fumositees passen and fleten forth into þe hynder partie of þe hede, þan is it worse and more perilouse, for þan it hath no issue wher it may passen out of þe body, but holde him in þe nuk, os Y saide. But if swich wicked mater

11 et] & GSc, a M7, *poorly formed* et, *similar to 2-compartment* a R
12 foundyng] M7GSc, foundyg R
13 body] *foll. by* ar þe *canc.* R

of humores in the hender party of þe hed flete hem into þe former party of 130
þe hede, it is noble tokne. For þe former partie of þe hede haþ dyuerse waies
and issues, as þe eyen, þe eeres, þe mouþ, and þe nose, by which þe mater
haþ his issue and þerfor when eny smyte out of a litarge into a frenesie, it
is a gode tokne; *e contrario*, wicked. <u>*Litargia* in þe 2 boke, c. *de rubicundo*</u>
<u>*colore*, lef</u> {73}. *Litargia* is gendrede in þe hendre partie of þe hed, os *fre*- 135
[**f. 89rb**] *nesis* in the former partie of þe hede. *Litargia* is causede of ouerdone
frigidite and humidite of humores fleumatik, os seiþ Constantyn in þe j *Bok*
of Medecynes. *Frenesis*, os seiþ the same auctour in þe same bok, comeþ of
incensioun, i. brennyng, of a rede colre styand vp to þe cerebre or elles of
brynnyng and bulying of blod in þe hert steyand vp and persand þe cerebre. 140

[3.3]

De ampullis, s. of Burbles in vryn: c. 3

Ampulla or elles *bulla* is þe Burble in þe vryn. It schuld be said *ambulla*
(which .b.) and noȝt *ampulla* (which .p.). For it is seide of þis worde *am*,
[i.][1] *circum* (*anglice*: abouten), and of þis word *bulla*, þat haþ meny significacions but here it is for a Burble. For it is rounde abouten, riȝt as þou 5
seist of þe water when it reyneþ. And take god hede þat þer is 2 maner of
Burbles in vryn, one þat is called *bulla residens* or *bulla permanens* and
anoder þat is called *bulla non residence* and *bulla non permanens* (*residens*
& *permanens* as on in þis purpos); *anglice*: a Burble dwelland, a Burble
noȝt dwelland. 10

Bulla residens is when þe Burble hold himself stille hoole til þe vryn
haue his kynde residence, [**f. 89va**] i. resting, <u>os I saide in þe 2 bok, c. *de*</u>
<u>*nigro colore*, lef</u> {18}. And swych maner of Burble is euermore causede of
myxtioun of humores and of ventosite inclosede in the body. *Bulla non*
residens is þat dwelleþ noght til þe vryn haue his kynde residence, but van- 15
isheþ awaie sone after þe vryn is made, for it is caused but only of course
and of fallyng in the water-makyng. And þerfor of þis last maner of Burble
phisik tretiþ noght.

Item, vnderstond þat *bulla residens* is somtym callede *bulla tumens* or
bulla tumida. *Tumens* & *tumida* al on for to seyne (*anglice*: bollen). & som 20
tyme it [is][2] callede *bulla non tumens* or *bulla non tumida*. *Bulla tumens*

---

1 i.] GSc, & (*shaped like i with stroke above and bar across*) RM7
2 it is] GSc, it R, is M7

or *tum[i]da*[3] is when the Burbles ar grete and bolen and bloute; *bulla non tumens* or *non tumida* when þai ar but litle & smale, riȝt as þou seest in water podelles when it reyneth. But be it *tumens* or not *tumens*, if it be *bulla residence*, os Y said, it is euermore caused and gendred of interclu-   25
sioun, i. enclosyng of eire and wynde & humores crud and indigest & viscouse and gleymouse, i. clamysh. Ventosite & viscosite ar 2 þinges of whiche principaly Burbles ben causede.

Þan tak this for a reule: þat if the Burble be *residens*, os I saide, [**f. 89vb**] and it be water-wan in coloure and grete & bolne and þerwiþ it cleueþ hard to þe   30
Cercle of þe vryn or to þe side of þe vrinal, in so mykel þat wiþ a stik wapped in herdes or in a clout, it wil vnneþes awai or vnneþes breken, it is wicked tokne, for it seiþ huge crudite of materes and þat þe sekenesse wil longe last-yn and a nefresie, i. þe passioun of þe reyns or elles disposicioun toward.

Þat þe Burbles stond longe and noght wil awaie, it is tokne þat þe mal-   35
ady haþ taken dwellying and i[s]4 roted in þe body. Þat þe Burbles bene watrish, i. bleke and watre, wan & gret and bolne, it seiþ þat þer is mykel grete ventosite in the body; þat it is cleuand and hard to atwynnen is bi cause of mykel ventosite of þe materes, i. of þe wicked humores.

Item, þe same maner of vryn seiþ disposicioun toward[5] ake and seke-   40
nesse in þe hed, for it seiþ mykel ventosite enclosede in þe body and meny fumositees þerwiþ. Which fumosites, in as mykel as þai be liȝt, þai wil stien vp into þe hede and distempren the cerebre and so cause huge peyn in the hede. But when it seiþ malady in the hede for to com, as I saide, þe vryn is a party more high in colour þan when it seiþ[6] [**f. 90ra**] crudite of humores   45
and somtyme more froþi þan burbli.

But propurly and principaly Burbles euermore signifien the nefresi, þat euermore is causede of humours crude & indigest. Whiche crude humores haue answeryng in kynde to þe reynes, syn þat þai ar cold in kynde and þe reyns also ar cold & drye in kynd, <u>os Y saide in þe 2 bok, c. *de karopos*,</u>   50
<u>lef {59}</u>. And also þe reynes ar fer fro the wel of hete, i. fro þe hert, and by þat cause þo crude humorez þat causen þat malady, s. the nefresie, ar colde be way of kynd. For as Gilbert seiþ in his Coment, þai ar humores flu-matik, gros, and viscouse; þai drawen hem kyndly to the reynes. Whiche humores, sen þai mowe noght be ouercomen ne be ouermaistried be kynd,   55
be resoun þat he is noght sufficient and þai ar mykel in quantite & in mal-ice eke, þai beleuen ther still in the reyns and so causen þe *nefresim*.

---

3 tumida] M7GSc, tumda R
4 and is roted] G, & his rote Sc, and it roted RM7
5 toward] GSc, toward of RM7
6 seiþ] *catchword*: crudite of humours

Item, if þou schagge menely þe vrinal and þe Burblis hurlyn & rennen abouten hastely and swiftly, it seiþ but litil crudite and viscosite of
humores. *Et* at þe lesse mewyng of the vrinal þat þai done so, þe bettre   60
tokne it is euermore & þe lesse viscosite it betokeneþ.

[3.4]

[f. 90rb]

De granis, of Greyns in þe vryn: c. 4

Grana vrine (*anglice*: kirnelles in the vryn, *gallice* greyns) ar noþing elles
but smale parties of Froth diuised in diuerse parties in the vryn. And swich
maner Greyns in the vryn euermore bitokne course of wicked humores
flowand fro the hed to þe oþer parties in þe body. And in þis wise þai ar   5
gendrede: the cerebre, os Gilbert seiþ, is kyndly *frigidum & humidum*, for
it acordeþ mykel toward in kynd grece and marie, and by cause þerof, his
fode & norisshing is cold & moyst. Now cold & moyst causyn[1] fleume
and flux and watrishede. & whan it falleþ þat plente & exces of humores
flumatik, s. cold & moist, be in þe hed, þan is þe hede ful of wickede dis-   10
posicioun, ake, & peyne. But when it is so þat kynd wil helpen and is of
myght and fondeþ for to wirken into that wicked mater of þo wickede
humores, for to maistrien and fordone[2] hem in as mykel os in him is, he
diuiseþ and minusheþ litle & litle and twycheþ awaie þe mater by smale
litle partes. And þan þo partis fallen doune to þe oþer parties of þe body,   15
and namely to þe parties þat þai fynde most feble: to þe nose, to þe eyen
or abouen the ey3en in the forhede, to þe eres, to þe mouthe, to þe throte
golle or to þe þrote, or [f. 90va] elles to þe chikes and to þe jowis, and so
of the rema[na]nt.[3]

Þan if þat ilk mater passe to the nosethirle, it causeþ a malady þat [hat]   20
corexa.[4] *Corexa* is a reume in the hede, passand out by þe noseþirle and
þerwiþ nesyng amonge; if it [passe][5] to þe ey3en, a malady þat hight *optalmia*.[6] *Opitalmia* is when on thenkeþ þat his ey3en schuld tobresten oute

---

1 causyn] causen M7, causeth GSc, causyng (*with* g *canc.*) R
2 fordone] M7, for (*to canc.*) done R, for to doo G, & to do Sc
3 remanant] M7GSc, remaunt R
4 þat hat corexa] M7, callid corexa Sc, þat corexa R, Corexa G; *marg.*: Corexa
5 passe] GSc, *om.* RM7
6 optalmia] opitalmia *with first* i *underpuncted* R; *marg.*: optalmia

of his hede. If þat mater hold him abouen þe eyȝen, ake & peyn in þe eye-
bryen and þerabouten. If it go to þe eres, tynnyng[7] & hurling and wynd   25
and queynt swoyng in eres and lettyng in heryng. If it come often & longe
last, it causeth defhed. If into the mouth and to þe tunge, rawhede and
flawand in the mouthe & in þe tunge and þeraboute. If to þe þrote golle or
to þe þrote, streythede and hoshede, grete disese.

Item, o þe same wise, swich maner mater falleþ into þe þrote and þan   30
a sekenes þat is called *ismonia*,[8] þe ismonie; and somtyme a sekenes þat is
called *squynancia*,[9] þe squynancy; & somtyme a sekenes þat is callede þe
cinancya,[10] þe cynancie; and somtyme a malady þat is called *vuula*[11] or
vua, þe vuel or elles þe rotel. *Vuula:* se in c. *de karopos,* lef {*om.*}; *ysmonia
squynancia* & *sinancia* in þe same c., lef {57}.   35

If [f. 90vb] it passe to þe chekes, ake & peyn and bolnehed in the chekes
and in þe iowis and þe gomes and about the tethe. And somtyme it passeþ
to the trachearteries and into the lunge pipis, and þan it causeþ cogh wiþ
streitnes of onde and disese at the brest. *Trachearteria:* in þe 2 bok, c. *de
karopos,* lef {57}; *fistule pulmonis* & *canales pulmo:* þe lunge pipes in þe 2   40
boke, c. *de liuido colore,* lef {32}.

If it go to þe lunges, it causeþ *asma* and *disma*. Se *asma* & *disma:* in þe
2 bok c., *de liuido colore,* lef {28}. If it passe to þe *yliones,* i. to þe guttes,
lienteria & *dissenteria* and þan his egestioun is fro[þ]i.[12] Ypocras geueþ his
reule in his *Afforismis* þat whensoeuer þe egestioun is froþi, it is a verraie   45
tokne of flux and wicked humours fleumatike, comand fro þe hede into
the guttes. *Lienteria* is þe reye, s. when it schet fro on as a bolt. *Dissenteria
in þe 2 bok, c. de liuido colore,* lef {31}. If it passe to þe stomak, it causeþ
ake and peyn and inflacioun of þe stomak.

And in al þis causes, þe Cercle of þe vryn is granelouse & ful of smale   50
Greyns, for os Y said, þai betokne euermore distillacioun, i. course of
droppyng and fallyng, of mater [f. 91ra] reumatik fro þe hede to þe oder
parties in the body, and namely to þo membres or parties þat ar most feble
in kynd for þat tyme & most able for to vnderfongen þat reumatik mater
and ar noght of myght at þat tym for to cachen it oute ne to dryuen it forth   55
awaie. Þai ar moste like Burbles but þai ar wonder[13] litle & smale. For os
Y saide, þai ar riȝt noȝt but smale desicions, i. litle chippynges, of spume

---

7 tynnyng] GSc, twynnyng RM7
8 ismonia] *marg.*: ysmonia
9 squynancia] *marg.*: squinancia
10 cinancya] *marg.*: sinancia
11 vuula] *marg.*: vuula
12 froþi] M7G, frothe Sc, frori R
13 wonder] M7GSc, swonder R

and þai holden hem comunly abouen in the vryn. And þe philosophie is by cause þat þai ar first and principaly gendred abouen in the cerebre, for when it is so þat kynde and myght of þe cerebre cacheþ out fro him þat ilk   60
reumatike mater by þe veyns of þe rigebone to þe places þat comen fro þe hatrel dounward.

Otherwhile in bak feble and colde causeþ sekenesse grete; if þe bak be god and hote, it is cached forthe to the nose or to þe ey3en or elles to þe oþer parties, os Y haue saide. And þan ar the Greynes formed & gendred   65
in the membres & places þer þe course of þe mater is, and ri3t vpon þat þo membres or places to which þat mater draweþ to ar more high or more lowe, [f. 91rb] holden hem þe Greynes in the vryn.

Þan tak þis for a reule certeyn: þat if þe Greyns be in the Cercle of þe vryn or elles a litil beneþen (for in the botume be þai neuer), at a schagg-   70
yng of þe vrinal þai go doun to þe botume or nerhand to þe botume and sithen vp a3eyne to þe Cercle þere þai were bifore, it seiþ malady in the hed caused of wicked reumatike maters, os Y haue saide. If þai be wiþin the Cercle & at a schaggyng of the vrynal beneþen þe Cercle and þai come ageyn þer þai were beforne þe schaggyng, it is a tokne of flux of humores   75
colde & reumatik comand fro þe hed to þe parties of þe body, vppon þat þe Greynes holden hem hier or lower in the vryn, os Y said.

[3.5]

De nebula, **of Cloude in vryn: c. 5**

Nvbes vrine, the Sky in the vryn, is a fumows (a vaporouse) superfluyte dymmysh and swartishe and fatish, houand abouen on þe vryn, mykel like an arayne web or elles a poudre wer strewed þeron. And it is but super-fluite of þe 3 digestioun, caused & gendred þorogh wirkyng of vnkynd   5
hete, which vnkynd hete is gendred only in 2 places in the body: in the brest and þe lyuer. What is þe j digestioun & what 2 & 3 digestion [f. 91va] þou hast in the j bok, þe 3 c.

Auctoures callen it *corpus aereum* (*anglice*: þe eyrisshe body) or elles *nubecula spiritualis*, a spiritual Sky. And þerfor it seiþ euermore exces and   10
distemperur of vnkynd hete of þe spirituales & of the lyuer. And þus it is caused & gendred, os Tadeus seiþ: when it is so þat whan þe vapoures passen out of þe body wiþ the vryn, frigidite of þe eir gadereþ him togeder and so sweyth abouen on þe face of þe vryn, mykel like a cop-web or elles a poudre or dust strewed þeron, os Y saide. & whi it halt him abouen on   15
the vryn is by cause þat it hath mykel of kynde of the eire.

And þus þou schalt knowe when it signifieþ of þe spirituales and when of the lyuer: if þe vryn haue a maner of dymhed abouen & þerwiþ þe Skye be bloysh like powdre of askes or poudre of pomys or of blank plum, it is o þe spirituales. And þat maner of Sky is þe j tokne of disposicioun toward   20 the etik. Þat þe vryn is more dymmysshe abouen is by cause of more feble-nesse of the spirituales; þat þe Ski is os Y said is be cause of vnkynd hete in the brest, i. in the spirituales. Of the etik and of the pthisik is said suf-ficiently in þe 2 bok, c. of Blo coloure, lef {32}.

If þat Sky apper [f. 91vb] somdel wiþ a maner of fathed, it seiþ þat þat   25 ilk vnkynd hete haþ [pershede &][1] entred þe spirituales, i. þat he is soken in hem & þat he wasteþ and fordoþ þe kynd substancial humid[ite][2] of hem or elles it is in poynt.

If the Sky seiþ sekenesse of the lyuer, þan is þe Sky ȝelowish & redish, mykel toward saffran chies or elles swart redissh, mykel toward blak pur-   30 pre or saundres and þerwiþ Froth ȝelowish or grenysh; and þan it is called *nubes rubea*, a rede Sky. And þerfor wete wel þat euermore when it is o þe spirituales, it is more bloish in colour and more thenne in substaunce and the vryn more dymyssh abouen þan beneþen. And when it is o þe lyuer, it is more redish and swart in colour & more þik in substance & more fattish,   35 in so mykil þat þou maist taken it wiþ þi fyngre, mykil toward as þou seest on fat potage after þat it hath stonden a while vncouered & abouen gadred as it wer a fate ryme. And os Isaac seiþ, when þe Sky appereþ rede in the vryn, it is tokne of malady ha[r]d & scharp.[3]

[3.6]

De spuma vrine, of Froth in vryn: c. 6

Spuma is Froth þat houeþ abouen on the vryn. But tak god hede þat þer ben 3 maners of Froth in vryn:[1] on[2] þat is called spuma [f. 92ra] ven-tosa or spuma ambulosa (anglice: spume or elles Froth ful of wynde and ful of Burbles), of which maner Froth it is said in c. de [b]ullis.[3] And   5

---

1 pershede &] GSc, & is RM7
2 humidite] GSc, humid RM7
3 hard & scharp] M7, ?hasd & scharp R, scharp & strong GSc

---

1 Froth in vryn] *marg.*: 3 maner of froth
2 on] *marg.*: 1
3 bullis] ambullis GSc, pullis M7, pullis *with* p *written over canc.* b R (*but see Daniel's stricture on spelling at beginning of chap. 3.3 above*)

swich maner of spume seiþ euermor[4] more ventosite and more viscosite of humores in the body þan eny oþer maner Froth.

Anoþer[5] maner of [Froth][6] þer is, þat is as who seie no Froth, but it is as it were litil smale desicions, i. smale chippinges, smale particlez of Froth, as it were wonder smale Greynes holdand hem in diuerse places in the vryn, so smale þat a man þat can noȝt þeron[7] vnneþes may perceyue hem. And swiche maner of Froth is callede *spuma granulosa*, spume granelouse or *spume de greyne* or *greyn de spume* (*anglice*: Greynes of Froth). And of þis maner of Froth <u>it is said in c. *de granis.*</u>

Þe 3[8] maner of spume is neiþer of þise 2: neiþer Greynes os Y saide riȝt now ne burblisshe, os Y said while ere, but Froth wiþouten eny Burblis, mykel lik þe foom of a bor. And þis maner of spume in vryn is called *spuma continuata* (*anglice*: Froth holdyng himself togeder), for it halt and cleueþ togedre & goþ noȝt in diuerse partes. And of þis maner of spume, vnderstond by this chapi- **[f. 92rb]** [t]le,[9] s. of þe Froth that hath no Burbles. And þerfor, in alse mykel as þis word *continuus* or *continua* is alse mykel for to saie os lastand or alwaie holdand on or elles holdand togedre, som seyn þat *spuma continuata* schulde be þat spume þat haldeþ himself so hard togedre þat oneþes brekeþ, þogh on stere it wiþ a stik wappede in herdes or in a cloute, <u>os I said in c. *de bullis.*</u>[10]

But vnderstond þat swich maner of Froth þat cleueþ so hard to þe Cercle of þe vryn or to þe sides of þe vessel is noght propurly callede *spuma continua* but it is propurly called *spuma viscosa* or *spuma glutinosa*, <u>os Y said in c. *de bullis,* lef</u> {88}. *Viscus* is birdlym and þerof comeþ *viscosus* (*anglice*: ropand and cleuand togedre) and *gluten* is glue & þerfor it is saide glutinowse, byndand. And os Gilbert aleggeþ þat Galien seiþ, þat spume is euermore caused of ebulicioun of vnkynd hete, i. þorogh bulyng & walmyng & hurlyng of exces of vnkynd hete in þe body, and namely aboute the lyuer, riȝt os we seen in a buliand pot or elles bi cause of agitacioun of humores, i. þorogh rulyyng and hurlyng and distemperur of humores in the body, as we seen in the see, or elles **[f. 92va]** be cause of boþen, s. of bulicioun of vnkynd hete and by cause of agitacioun of humores.

---

4   seiþ euermor] *foll. by* seiþ euer *canc.* R
5   Anoþer] *marg.:* 2
6   Froth] M7GSc, *om.* R
7   þat can noȝt þeron] G, cannot þerron Sc, þat is can noȝt þeron RM7
8   3] *marg.:* 3
9   chapitle] M7, c. GSc, chapi (*page break*) le R
10   bullis] *foll. by* lef *canc.* R

Eke Gilbert seiþ þat when spume i[s]¹¹ causede of litle hete, it is gros
in substance and remys in colour, i. mykel & thik in body and feynt in   40
colour. If it be caused of mykel hete, i. of grete bulicioun of hete, it is
more thenne and more high in colour. Wherfore ȝet tak hede þat spume is
in dyuerse wise, for somtyme it is thik and somtyme thenne. If it be thik,
it seiþ ventosite, & þe more thik þe more ventosite. If it be thenne and
smale, it seiþ incensioun, i. brennyng, of vnkynd hete, for hete thenneþ it   45
euermore and ventosite thikkeþ it.

If it be ȝelowish, it seiþ *ictericiam glaucam*, þe ȝelwe iawnys, causede of
an vnkynd hete of þe lyuer. If it be grenyssh, *agriacam, i. ictericia viridis*,
þe grene iawnys, causede þorogh¹² grete hete of þe lyuer.

If it be blakish, *melanchima, i. ictericia nigra*, the blak iawnys, caused   50
þrogh huge hete and brennyng o the lyuer. *Ictericia glauca* and *ictericia
viridis* & *ictericia nigra*: in the 2 boke, þe last ende lef. *Melanchima* is nothing elles but combustioun o þe lyuer, vppon her opinioun þat seine and
techen þat euery of þe 3 spices **[f. 92vb]** of the iawnys is gendrede in the
lyuer.   55

Item, vryn subtil and wonder thynne & wiþ *spuma continua* seiþ exces
of hete.

Item, vryn high in colour os Citrin and vpward wiþ *spuma continua* seiþ
exces of hete.

Item, vryn discoloured wiþ *spuma continua* seiþ mykel ventosite and   60
feble digestioun.

Item, vryn wiþ a maner of ȝelowishede and wiþ *spuma continua* seiþ
vnkynd hete o þe lyuer.

Item, spume wonder thik and mykel in quantite seiþ mykel ventosite in
the body and euel disposicioun, bot it wil esely passen, for þe mor white   65
þe bettre tokne.

Item, þe same maner of spume wiþ smale Greynes in the vryn and wiþ
resolucions somdel lik Heres seiþ feyntesse and feblenesse in body and
wicked disposicioun, & namely of the spirituales.

And if the vryn schew him so longe tym togeder or elles often tym, it is   70
tokne of mykel disposicioun toward the etik – & principaly in hem þat ar
lene and haue narwe & streite brestes.

Item, vryn wiþ spume lik snowe seyth sekenesse of the reyns. And þan
if þe vryn be þicke donward & more then vpward, is tokenyng of warsching; if *e contrario*, stronge perile.   75

---

11   is] GSc, it RM7
12   þorogh] M7GSc, þorogh þrogh R

[3.7]

De sanie vrine, **of Quyttur in vryn: c. 7**

Pvs & sanies in vrina ar al on (*anglice*: Attre & Quyttre). It is comunly lik
attir and quytter, thik and ropand and gleymouse and hongand togeder,
mykel like an hame or the white of a rawe ey or elles glet, and in þis wise
speke auctoures þerof. Giles in þe Coment seiþ þus: when *sanies* apereþ in   5
the vryn it seyth vlceracioun, i. blemysshing and sorehede, o þe vesie or o
þe reyns or elles o þe lyuere, of which 3 membres vlceracioun is causede
þorogh superfluite of vile mater þat gadereþ in the places & þerabouten.

But when it is o þe vesie and when o þe reyns and when o þe lyuer, þus
techen þai: if it be o þe vesie or elles o þe reyns, it haþ a grete sauour and   10
þe pacient feleþ grete peyn abouten þe vesie if it be o þe vesie,[1] or abouten
the reyns if it be o þe reyns. If it be o þe lyuer, it haþ no sauour, but in the
riȝt ypocondre is gret holding of peyn and betyng and grete heuynes, and
þe lyuer hath lost mykel of his kynd digestioun and no wonder [f. 93rb]
þogh þe stomak eke. Ypocras in the ende of þe 4 particule of *Afforismys*   15
seiþ þat whosoeuer make *sanies* or *pus* and scales in his water and it gif a
grete sauour, it tokeneth vlceracion o þe vesie.

Gilbert seiþ þus: *sanies* somtym is o þe lyuer, somtyme o þe reyns, and
somtyme o þe vesie. When it is o þe lyuer, it is noght elles but corrupcioun o þe lyuer, os when his kynd hete faileþ and þe substance of þe lyuer   20
wasteþ and vanysheþ & musseleþ and falleth awaie. And þan it is in the
botume of the vryn, moste like drestes of oyle, and drublish and drestish
and modissh. And somtyme *sanies* is gadred and gendred in the webbes
þat þe lyuer liþ in, wiþouten eny wastyng or weryng awaie or blemyshing
o þe lyuer. And som tyme þat corosioun and corupcioun þat brediþ so in   25
þe webbes of þe lyuer cometh to þe veyne þat is on þe body of the lyuer,
þat þe substance of þe lyuer swelteþ and melteþ and wastiþ and droppeþ
awaie, and so passeth forth wiþ þe vryn.

Item, *sanies* is somtyme o þe lyuer and eke somtyme in the webbes of
the lyuer, os when þer brediþ aposteme o þe lyuer and also when þer is   30
oppilacioun [f. 93va] o þe lyuer, i. when the lyuer is stoppede and stuffede
wiþ mater of wicked humors. & in þus many wise is *sanies* of the lyuer.

---

1 vesie] *foll. by* or elles of þe reyns, it hath a grete sauour and þe pacient feliþ grete peyne
abowte the vesie If it be o þe vesie *canc.* R

Also fele wise it comeþ o þe reyns: if *sanies* be o þe lyuer, it smelleþ but ful litil, and if it do it is onely by cause of corrupcioun & corosioun of the² lyuer. If it be o þe reyns, it smelleþ more þan if it be o þe lyuer. And þat is   35 be cause þat þe reyns ar more colde in kynde þan is *epar*, þogh it so be þat þe reyns ben *calidi & sicci* and *epar* is *calidum & humidum*. And also for *renes* ar ferþer fro þe wel of kynd hete, i. fro þe hert. If it be o þe vesie, it is more stynkand þan if it be o þe reyns, by cause þat the vesie is ȝit ferþer fro þe wel of hete, i. fro þe see of blod, þan ar þe reynes. And euermore   40 *sanies* is blodish, i. redishe, saue when it is o þe reynes.

Also euermore of whiche of alle 3 forsaide membres it be, þerabouten feliþ þe pacient huge wo and peyn. Which peyne forbarreþ him his myȝtes & his poweres and vanyssheþ his digestioun & appetit, and somtyme distroiþ him al fully. Þus techeþ he.   45

Tadeus & eke dyuerse auctors thus: Thre thinges schewe hem in vryn þat ar somdel like to sight: *ypostasis, humor, & sa-* [f. 93vb] *nies*. Whiche 3 þus shalt þou knowe a-sondry: when þou sest swich þik mater in þe grond of þe vryn, schagge þe vrynal, and if þat thik mater in þe grounde sty vp into þe vryn and diuise him in meny smale partes and sone after go doune   50 ageyne into þe same forme as it was biforne, it is *ypostasis*, for *ypostasis* is liȝt of kynd and þerfor he stieþ liȝtly vpward when þe vryn is shagged. Of ypostasis in þe j bok;³ & in þe 2 bok, þe 2 c. de nigro, lef {24}; and in þe last c. in þis 3 bok, lef⁴ {110}.

And if it diuise him in meny smale partes and noght turne ageyne as   55 it was biforne, wit wil þat it is *humor*, of which *humor* se inward in his propre c.

If it be so þat it wil noght breken nor gladly asundren it if þe vrinal be schagged wonder sore – and perauentur it wil be no waie sundre but it qwobbeth & quauiþ in the botme of the vryn, like mater gleymouse and   60 slippish os a hame or os the white of a rawe eye or as it were gleyme or glett, os it bifalleþ often in olde folk vryn – wete wel þat it is *sanies*. And þan comunly it hath a sauour.

And take hede þat *sanies* cometh of 3 places of þe body,⁵ s. of þe vesie, of þe reyns, or of the lyuer. And [f. 94ra] in 5 wise thow may wyten &   65 knowen for a certeyn of which of al it be: by his residence; by his incorporacioun wiþ þe vryn, i. by þe medlyng of him wiþ the vryn; be þe sauour; by þe peyne felyng; and by wirkyng of þe 2 digestioun.

---

2 of the] *foll. by* of the *canc.* R
3 j bok] *foll. by* lef *canc.* R
4 lef] *poss. canc., though leaf reference is correct (Ypostasis begins on the verso of old leaf 110).*
5 body] *marg.:* þat quytter comeþ of 3 places & is knowen in 5 wise

By þe residence: for when *sanies* comeþ of the vesie, þan anon as þe vryn
is made, he halt him beneþe in the grounde. And þat is be resoun þat þat   70
ilk mater, s. *sanies*, comeþ of a membre, s. of the vesie, which is fer fro the
wel of hete, i. fro the see of blode, s. fro þe hert and fro þe lyuer. If it com
of the reyns, it draweþ noght so sone doune to þe botme os when it is of
the vesie, and þat is by resoune þat it cometh of a place and of a membre
þat is more nere þe wel of hete and þe see of blode þan is þe vesie. Item, if it   75
be o the lyuer, it draweþ noght doune, but nerþeles it is more þik donward
in þe vryn þan vpward, by cause þat þat comeþ of a membre and of a place
þat is see of blode and eke is ner þe wel of hete. But bi cause þat þat ilk
membre þat is þe see of blode is refte of his kynde hete & is distemprede
& ouergone wiþ colde or elles wiþ wickede mater of colde humours, of   80
which *sanies* is causede & gendrede, þat ilk vile mater, i. *sanies*, is[6] more
heuy þan liȝt; and also by [f. 94rb] cause þat *sanies* goth more space wiþ þe
vryn when it is of þe lyuer þan when it is o þe reynes, and more when it is
o þe reynes þan when it is o the vesie.

Item, by his encorperacioun wiþ þe vryn, for if it come of þe vesie, it is   85
as who say nothing menkt wiþ vryn, but it is also in the botme of þe vryn,
os Y saide while ere. And for the same skyl os Y saide, if it be o þe reyns,
it is more incorporate wiþ þe vryn for the same skiles þat I seide. If it be o
þe lyuer, it is mykel incorperat wiþ þe vryn be cause os I seide.

Item, by his odour: for if it be o þe vesie, it hath grete odoure by cause   90
þat þe vesie is a membre colde in kynde and fer fro the wel of hete, i.
fro þe se of blode, and also oþerwhile colde ouergoth þe kynd hete. For
þise ar þe causes of þe stynkyng odour in vryn. And tak gode hede þat
often tyme it semeþ os þe vryn hade a fetoure, and þogh it haue no fetour
proprely, as it is comunly whan *sanies* appereþ in the vryn, and namely   95
o the vesie. Þus þou myght prouen it sone: for somtyme when *sanies* is o
þe vesie or of þe reyns (but namely of the vesie), tak and poure sliȝly þe
vryn fro *sanies* and put the þin in a [f. 94va] vessel and þe thik in another
and smel at þe tone and at þe toþer. If it come of þe reyns, it smelleþ but
litil & somtyme noȝt, by cause os I saide. If it be o þe lyuer, it hath no   100
fetour but if it be so þat þe substance of the self lyuer vanysh & dwyne
and dropp awaie. For þe lyuer is principal after the hert, grounde & wel
of kynd hete.

Item, by felyng of sore and peyne: for if it be o þe vesie, þer is grete peyn
aboute the schore and about þo parties. If it be o þe reynes, þerabouten is   105
the peyn. If it be o þe lyuer, þe peyn is abouten the riȝt ypocondre. *Ypocondria*: in þe 2 bok, c. *de liuido colore*, lef {29}.

---

6 is] *foll. after line break by* is *canc.* R

Item, by wirkyng of þe 2 digestioun. For if it be o þe vesie or elles of the reynes, þe 2 digestion is noght lettede þerby; but if it be o the lyuer, þe 2 digestioun is fordon or elles ful ner.   110

And vnderstonde þat it is of þe lyuer or elles of þe reyns, þan is þe malady propurly callede "vlceracioun" (*anglice*: sorehede); when it is of þe vesie it is callede propurly "scabbyng": þus sai þai. & os I haue saide beforn, Gilbert seiþ þat only *sanies* of þe reyns is wiþouten eny blode.

[3.8]

De pinguedine vrine, of Fatnes in vryn: c. 8

Pinguedo in vrina, os seiþ þe Comentour vppon Giles, is a maner of Fathede, a maner of greci- [f. 94vb] hede abouen on the face of the vryn, resoluede of membres in the body and swymmand out forth wiþ þe vryn. And it is nogh elles but consumpcioun of þe grees in the reines and in the   5
body of man. And þerfor it seiþ euermore consumcioun of kynde, <u>os Y saide in the 2 bok, c. of Blak colour, lef {21}</u>.[1]

Nowe tak hede þat þer ben 2 maners of fat vryn: on þat is called *vrina pinguis* (*anglice*: fat vryn) and anoþer [þat is][2] callede *vrina oleagena* (*anglice*: oylish vryn). & þus schalt thou knowen when it is on and when   10
it is anoþer: when þe vryn hath a maner of Fathed or grecyhede abouen, as þou seest on lene browes, when þou maist noght sene þe grece for litilhede of greece, but if þou loke aȝeyne the liȝt, þan it is callede *vrina pinguis*. But if þe vryn haue wiþ þe Fathed a maner of swarthed, mykel toward colour of oyle, þan is it callede *vrina oleagina*, os it is comunly in lent febres in   15
hem þat haue lene and drye bodyes. And þe more vnkynd hete þat regneþ in the body, oute-taken hote febre, þe more Fathede is o þe vryn.

We sene at eye þat hete resolueþ grees & talow, but cold clammeth & clatteþ [M7, f. 62r][3] & clumpreþ it togeder. & þerfor euermore fat vryn betokeneth feblisshing & wastyng of kynde & þe etik, or elles þe disposi-   20
cioun toward, & namely in lene bodyes & streit breste. Vnderstond þat Fathede in vryn somtym is only of þe reyns [& of the lendes and sumtyme of alle the body. But whenne it cometh of þe reynes & of the lendes],[4] it is

---

1   of blak colour lef 21] 21 *somewhat smudged* R, of blak colour lef 22 M7; of blak
coloure leef G, de nigro co. (*blank space*) Sc
2   þat is] M7GSc, þer it R
3   R *wants one leaf here* (lef 94 *in the old foliation*). *Missing text supplied from* M7.
4   & of þe lendes ... of þe lendes] G, and of þe lendes and sumtyme of alle thoo But when
it comith of þe reynys and of þe lendis Sc, *om.* M7 (*eyeskip*), *wanting* R

mikel; & wan of al þe body, it is but litle. & þis is þe philosophie: in þe reyns
& þerabouten is plente of grees or of talow, os þou seest in bestes bo-   25
dies þat ar opynd, þe which grees þorgh mislikyng melteth awaie & passeþ
forth wiþ þe vryn. & also by cause þat þe grece of the reyns is fast by þe
waies of the vryn, & þerfor by cause of more plente of grece is in the reyns
þan elleswhare, & also by cause þat it is more nere þe vryn waies, for in þe
reyns is no hete consumptif, i. no hete wastand þe grees, s. no hote febre.   30
For þe febre is noзt in þe reyns ne in the lendes, þogh it so be þat þere be
distemperure of vnkynd hete resoluand & meltand & wastand þe grees &
þe substance of þe reyns, it passeth the more largely & [in]⁵ þe more plente.

But when [it]⁶ comeþ of al þe body, it is but litle, bi cause þat it is ferre
fro þe vryn waies, & also by cause þat þer is hete of febre in þe body þat   35
lou[s]e[þ]⁷ him & wasteþ him. For euermore when Fathede comeþ of al þe
body, þe body is noзt wiþouten febre, al be it so þat often tyme he feleþ
no febre, or elles non but os it were disposicioun toward, but he is mykel
lenysh & wannysh & dedisch & feynt & euel disposed, for he hath appetite negh loste & swich maner tokenes.   40

And when *pinguedo* is of al þe body, it is called *pinguedo generalis*
(*anglice*: þe general Fathede or elles Fathede of al þe body). When o þe
reyns alone, it is called *pinguedo particularis*, particuler Fathede or elles
only o þe reyns. & þerfor vnderstond þat fat vryn euermore, or it is **[M7,**
f. 62v] wiþ a febre or elles wiþowten febre. If an vryn appere fat in a febre,   45
euermore it seiþ wasting & dwynyng. If it schew him fat & no febre, it seiþ
wastyng & vanishing only of þe reyns.

Item, in þe 3 wise þou schalt weten when it is o þe reyns & when of al
þe body. If it be onely of the reyns, þe Fathed is mykel, os I saide. If it be
of al the body, it is but riзt litle, os I saide eke, but it so be þat it be in the 3   50
spice of þe etik. Of þe etik & his spices it is saide sufficiently in þe 2 bok,
c. *de liuido colore*, lef {*om.*}.

Item, if it be o þe reynes, it sheweth him on þe face of þe vryn anone as
it is made; if it be of al þe body, noзt til þe vryn haue his restyng.

Item, when⁸ it is o þe reyns, þe vryn is noзt intens in coloure, but it so   55
be þat þe lyuer be achaffid & distempred of vnkynd hete. But if it be of al
the body, þe vryn is wele coloured & thenne.

Item, to knowen when *pinguedo* betoknes⁹ þe etik & wh[at]¹⁰ spice of
þe etik, vnderstond þat if *pinguedo* be disp[erp]lede¹¹ in meny smale

---

5 in] GSc, *om.* M7, *wanting* R
6 it] GSc, *om.* M7, *wanting* R
7 louseþ] lesseth GSc, louþes M7, *wanting* R (*see note*).
8 Item when] GSc, Item when (*line end*) when M7, *wanting* R
9 betoknes] *final s poss. written over, or overwritten by,* M7's *y-shaped* þ
10 what] GSc, when M7, *wanting* R
11 disperplede] disperpled G, disperled Sc, dispoilede M7, *wanting* R

sundry parties, in meny smale droppes in þe face of þe vryn, os we se in   60
iouse or in broth of fleish or in lene broth, it is tokne of þe j spice of etik.
If *pinguedo* occupie þe face of the vryn like an areyn web, it seiþ þe 2 spice
of þe etik. If *pinguedo* be disperpled oueral in þe body of þe vryn, it seiþ þe
3 spice of þe etik. & a verray tokne herof, þis is: þat if þou poure þe vryn
vpon a flat stone, it maketh a criceland noyse, like oyle if it be poured oute.   65
Þus seiþ þe Coment of Gilis & diuerse oþer.

Gilbert seiþ þus: Fathede in vryn somtyme is whitish, somtyme is
ȝelowish or elles citrin, somtyme grenish. When it is white, it is caused
\of/ feble & feynt hete; ȝelowish or citrin, of more myȝty hete; grene, &
of ouerdone hete. Os if þou tak grees al hote, os it cometh out of a bestes   70
body, & hange it or laie it in þe sone or in þe hote eyre, þe hete wasteþ
awaie þe wattrihed & þe moysthede þerof & maketh it ȝelowish or elles
citrinysh. I[f] þe hete o[r þe] eyre be riȝt st[r]ong & durable,[12] it caused
a grenishede. First, when þe spiritualis bygyn to take sekenes & disposicioun toward þe etik, *pinguedo* i[s][13] whitish. For euermore when it is   75
inward, it is subcitrin or citrin. & when it is at þe fulle, it is more citrin or
subrufa or elles rufa. & þus by colour of Fathede maist þou sene which
spice it seiþ of þe etik. Þus seiþ he.

Sum [seyn][14] þus: Fathede þat appereþ in vryn, somtyme it is in smale
gobates, in smale parties, os it were in smale Greynes, smale croteles, \&/   80
þan it houyþ noȝt abouen on the face of þe vryn, but it halt him beneþen
in þe vryn, s. in the body of þe vryn. & i[n] \þis/ wise,[15] it may be knowen
if it be *pinguedo* or not: tak it & multre it bytwys þi fyngres, & if it be
pinguedo, **[R, f. 95ra]** it multrith and melteþ awaie as it were lard of a
swyne. Anoþer maner of Fathede in vryn þer is, þat houeth on the face of   85
þe vryn os grees on broth. & swiche maner *pinguedo in vrina* somtyme
cometh of al þe body, and somtyme but of on part of þe body, as of þe
lendes. But when one, when oþer, þer is 5 maner of knowing: s. by his
residence; by his incorporacion; be colour of þe vryn; by a febre; & by a
quantite of þe Fathede, i. vppon þat it is mykel or litle.   90

By his residence þus: if þe Fathede draw to residence anone after þe
vryn is made, þe Fathede is of þe reyns. Þat it draweþ so sone doune is bi
cause þat it is but litle incorporat wiþ þe body of þe vryn. If it be of al þe
body, it is longe or it drawe to residence, and þat is by cause þat it is mykel
incorporat wiþ þe vryn.   95

---

12   If … durable] GSc, it þe hete of eyre be riȝt stong & durable M7, *wanting* R
13   pinguedo is] GSc, pinguedo it M7, *wanting* R
14   Sum seyn] GSc, Sum tyme M7, *wanting* R
15   & in þis wise] and þus GSc, & it þis wise M7, *wanting* R

Item, by his incorporacioun wiþ þe vryn: for if it be o þe reyns, it is incorporat but litil wiþ þe body of þe vryn. And þat is by cause þat he and the vryn comen but litle waie togedre. For *renes* ar noȝt fer fro þe vesie, ner fro þe ȝerd. If it be of al þe body, it is mykel incorporate wiþ þe vryn, by cause of longe course wiþ the vryn.   100

Item, be a febre: for if **[f. 95rb]** it come of þe reynes, þan cometh it noght by cause of febre, but by cause of sekenesse of vnkynde hete and con-sumpcioun of þe reyns. If it be of alle þe body, it is causede þorogh hete of an vnkynd febre wastand þe kynde.

Item, by þe colour in the vryn: for if *pinguedo* be of þe reyns, þan is   105 þe vryn wel coloured, s. Citrin or higher. And þat is by cause þat þe 2 digestioun is gode and is noght lettede. If it be of al þe body, þe vryn is discoloured, s. Subcitrin or Whitissh or Palishe, be enchesoun of lettyng of þe 2 digestioun.

Item, be quantite of Fathede: for if *pinguedo* be o þe reyns, *pinguedo* it   110 [is] in gode quantite,[16] by cause þat it ȝede noght fer waie wiþ þe vryn, and also for þan is þere no febre mynusshand the Fathede. But when it is of al þe body, *pinguedo* is but litle in quantite, by cause þat it passeth longe weie. For euermore when *pinguedo* cometh of al þe body, it passet more space and lenger waie in the body er it cometh oute at þe ȝerde or at þe   115 membre þan whan it cometh of þe reyns. For the ferthe[r][17] it passeth, þe more it is mynusshede. And euermore when it is of al þe body,[18] it is noȝt wiþouten a febre, which febre lesseþ & wasteþ þe Fathed.

[3.9]

[f. 95va]

De humore crudo, **of Rawe Humour: c. 9**

Understonde þat, os techeþ þe Comentour vppon Giles, 3 þinges appere in vryn lik *sedimen*: *ypostasis*, *putredo*, & *humor crudus* (*anglice*: Ypostasy, Corrumpcioun or elles Rotenhede, & Rawe Humor). <u>*Sedimen:* se in þe 19</u> <u>c.</u> Þan for to knowen veraily when it is *ypostasis*, when *putredo*, and when   5

---

16   pinguedo it is in gode quantite] M7, pinguedo it in gode quantite R, ther is myche
      fathede GSc
17   ferther] GSc, ferthe RM7
18   þe body] *foll. by* the body RM7

crudus humor, shagge softly þe vrinal, and if þe mater in the botume stye vpward and diuise him in meny partys and in meny porcions, it is *yposta-sis*. Ypostasis and sedimen: se in þe 19 c.

If it diuise him into parties thik and drestish or elle noȝt diuise him [but is] clammysh and squobbish like attri mater,[1] and þerwiþ it hath a   10
wicked odour, it is *putredo* or *humor putridus* or *humor corruptus* (*anglice*: Rotenhede or Roten Humor or Corumpt Humor), þat al is on. And þan is Humor Corupt in cause of þat sekenes. *Humor coruptus* & *putredo* and *sanies* al on. Of sanies: biforn in the 7 c.

If it dyuyse him in meny parties wonder smale, as motes in the sone, it   15
is *humor crudus* (*anglice*: a Rawe Humor) and of swich maner of humor vnderstonde by al þis c. Þanne when swiche maner of Humor apereþ in þe vryn, or it scheweþ him in the ouer party of the vryn or in þe myddes or in the neþer [**f. 95vb**] partie.

If Humor occupie þe ouer partie of þe vryn, it seiþ *artetica* passion (i.   20
sekenesse of the spirituales, os *asma* & *disma* and compressioun of the mydred, i. pressing & stuffing). Artetica passio: in þe 2 bok, þe 4 c. de albo colore, lef {39}; asma & disma in þe 2 bok, þe 3 c. de liuido colore, lef {28}.

If it holde him abouten þe myddes of þe vryn, it seiþ sekenesse of the stomak causede of replecioun of superfluytes, and wiþ disposicioun   25
toward brakyng and inflacioun in þe body and in the wombe and roulyng and crowlyng in the guttes.

If it ocupie þe neþer party of the vryn, sekenes of the reyns & abowt-ten þe lendes, & ake & feblenesse in the thies and in the knees and in the legges, & *nefresim* and *stranguiriam* and *tenasmon*. Þus seiþ Giles and þe   30
Comentour eke. Nefresis: in þe 2 bok, 4 c. de albo colore, lef {38}. Stran-guiria: in the j bok, þe 4 c., lef {7}. *Thenasmon* is when on may noȝt – or elles vnneþes wiþ croudyng and strong peyne – delyuer himself beneþen. Gilbert seiþ þus: if Humor apper in þe ouer partie of þe vryn and wiþ no febre, it betokeneth os I saide while er in the j reule beforn. If it hold him   35
in the mydward of the vryn, os Y saide in þe 2 rewle [**f. 96ra**] aforne. If it holde him in the botume bineþen, it seiþ sekenesse os Y saide in þe 3 reule aforn. Whiche sekenesse is causede of wicked raw humors fleumatik gadrid in the body, of which wickede humores kynde wolde delyuer him & cacheþ him þider.   40

If Humor apere in þe vryn and þerwiþ no febre, it seiþ grossehede & hardhede and viscosite of humores in the body and scharp malady. Noght-forþan if age or elles myght in kynde be gode, gode hope of saf, but longe

---

1   but is clammysh and squobbish like attri mater] clammysh and squobbish like attri
    mater RM7, but it (clammyth & Sc) quabbeth lyk attryssh matere GSc

first. If it so be þat in the bigynnyng of the malady þe Humor hold him
abouen in the vryn, it seiþ þat suptile & ese for to be ouercomen & defiede.   45
If it holde him in the botume, gros & viscouse, hard for to ouercome; if in
the myddes, menely.

If Humor schewe him in the botume of þe vryn in the stondyng of the
sekenes, þogh it so be þat kynde be myȝty, it is dredeful. <u>What is stondyng
of þe malady þou haste in þe 2 boke, þe 2 c.</u> *de nigro colore,* <u>lef {23}, þer I</u>   50
<u>saide what ar</u> *quattuor tempora morbi* (*anglice:* 4 tymes of sekenes). And
forthermore, Gilbert seiþ þus. But difference, seiþ he, is atwene *ypostasis*
and *sanies* & *crudus humor.* For if it be *ypostasis,* wiþ a softe mevyng it
s[tye]th[2] vp li- **[f. 96rb]** til and litil, and sone after þat it dessendiþ doune
ageyne into þe same forme os he was biforn. And if þou meve it hard, it   55
vanysseth awaie, anone as it were into noght, but wel afterward he gadreþ
him ageyne into his place. But noghtforþan so parfit ne so hole os he was
ere was broken wil he noght be al fullik. But if it be *humor crudus,* þogh
þow schagge it softly, it s[tye]þ[3] noȝt vp ne it stereþ noght. Ne þogh þou
meve it harde, it vanyssheþ noght os it wer into noght, os it doþ if it be   60
ypostasis, but it brekeþ into meny smale bodies, nygh as it were poudre.

And in þe 5 wise is Humor knowen fro *ypostasis:* be his figure, be his
substance, by his mevyng, be his breking, and by colour of þe vryn. By his
figure, i. by his forme and schap: for euermore a kynd *ypostasis* is schap
like a pere or a pynote, but *humor crudus* is neuermore of swiche forme,   65
but it is pleyne and brode[4] and thikkish.

By his substaunce, i. by þe body þerof: for *ypostasis* is continuel, i. hole
and holdand togedre, and oueral alike thik & thynne, and a body þat is a
mykel cloude or a sky, but Humor is grosse & gruttish and derkish & in
som place more thikkish þan sum.   70

Item, be mevyng: for if it be *y-* **[f. 96va]** *postasis,* anone at a litle schaggyng he stieþ vp and goth doune agayne; and at a hard schagyng, it vanyssheþ awaie to noght. But if it be Humor, it stieþ noght vp but wiþ a sad
schaggyng, and þan it goth vp os Y saide, like smale bodyes of powdre &
cometh ageyn as it was biforne.   75

Item, be brekyng: for if it be *ypostasis,* anone at a litle schaggyng, os Y
saide, it brekeþ os it were into noght. But Humor brekeþ os it were into
mode or into grutte and into bodies litle & smale, as it were poudre.

Item, by colour in the vryn: for *ypostasis* hath euermore vryn gode and
bright in coloure, for euermore *ypostasis* seiþ litle crudite of humors or   80

---

2 styeth] GSc, seyth RM7
3 styeþ] GSc, seiþ RM7
4 pleyne and brode] a pleyne and a brode RM7, pleyne aboven & brood GSc

none. But *humor crudus* hath alwaie vryn crude & indigest and ful selden
appereþ it wiþ Subcitrin or Citrin; & þogh it do, ȝit is vryn derke and
dym. But if it be wiþ an vryn Subcitrin or Citrin it is a noble tokne, for þe
malady dwelleþ noght longe. If elles, it is hard.

And for *sanies* is callede and is *humor in vrina* (of whiche it is saide in þe   85
7 c.) and Humor of which þis c. principaly treteþ of is called & is Humor in
vryn eke, Gilbert techeþ þat þus þou schalt know hem in sondry: euermore
when it is *sanies*, it stynketh; when **[f. 96vb]** it is Humor, noȝt so. For *sanies* is
os saide *humor putridus* and *coruptus*, *humor* corupt & roten; and Humor þat
propurly is callede *humor in vrina* is *humor crudus*, Rawe Humor. Þus seiþ he.   90

Sum saie þus: þis terme, þis word *humor* somtyme is taken in general
& somtyme in special. In general for euery of þe 4 humores, but noght so
here in this c. In special for one onely of þe 4 humours, os for humour of
fleume or elles of melancolie, crude & indigest, & in þis wise it is taken
here. (Of humor of blode, se inward in his propre c.) If it so be þat humor   95
of colre passe somtyme out wiþ the vryn, noȝtforþan be cause þat it is liȝt
and suptil in kynde, he is so litle incorporat wiþ þe vryn þat he may noȝt
be aperceyuede. And þerfor þis c. techeþ onely of humor fleumatik or
melancolic, crude and indigest, & of his significacions.

Þis Humor appereth somtym abouen in the vryn, and þan it comeþ of   100
þe membres of life. *Membra animata, þe membres of life: in þe 2 boke,
7 c. de karopos, lef* {55}. & somtyme in the myddes of þe vryn, & þan it
cometh of nutrityues. *Membra nutritiua*, þe membres nutritiues: in þe 2
bok, þe 7 c. de karopos, lef {58}. And somtym in the grownde of þe vryn,
&[5] **[f. 97ra]** þan it cometh of þe generatiues. *Menbr[a][6] generatiua*: in þe 2   105
bok, þe 7 c. de karopos, lef {59}.

And þerfor þe Humor halt him in þe vryn þer is þe sekenesse in the
þe body. And þis is þe principal significacioun of Humor. *Secundarie*,
þou schalt demen by Humores in the botume þe stranguirie, for when
wicked humores gaderen aboute þe nek of þe vesie, þai causen the stran-   110
guirie. *Stranguiria: in þe j boke, 4 c., lef* {7}. For somwhat of swich wicked
humour or humores mengen hem wiþ þe vryn and passeþ forth þerwiþ,
and bi cause þat it is rawe & indigest, it is kyndely heuy and so draweþ
donward & so scheweþ him in the botme.

Item, Humor in the botume seiþ *tenasmon*, for þe vesie lith euen on   115
longaoun, & oþerwhile humor gros and viscouse stoppen and stuffen so
longaoun þat þat mater þat schuld passe þorogh him is wiþstent & letted,
and so is *tenasmoun* caused. *Thenasmon I saide beforne longaoun, in þe j
bok, 3 c., lef* {3}. Þus techen þai.

---

5 vryn &] *catchword*: þan it cometh
6 Menbra] M7GSc, Menbr R

[3.10]

De sanguine vrine, of Blode in the vryn: c. 10

De sanguine vrine, of Blode in vryn, þus auctoures speken, þe Coment
vpon Giles þus: when Blode cometh oute of þe body wiþ þe vryn, or it is
of þe vesie or of þe reyns or elles of þe [f. 97rb] lyuer or elles of the kil.
What is *kilis* I saide in þe 2 bok, 3 c. *de liuido colore, lef* {28}. When it is of   5
the vesie, it is trumbouse, i. coldissh and clumish, in þe vryn and saggand
doun in the botme alse lowe as it may and wiþ an euel odour and wiþ grete
prichyng & peyn aboute þe schore and þe tail end and þe ȝerdes ende and
þe vesie.

   Þat it is trumbowse is by cause þat þe vesie is a membre þat is ful colde in   10
kynde, and þerfor it is noght of myght for to purgen ne to clenesyn himself
fro superfluytes of wicked humores þat gadren þerabouten. And þerfor
also it halt him in the botume and is noght (or elles ful litil) incorperat wiþ
the vryn. And also þat is þe skil whi it halt wicked odour, also for þe skil
os I said in c. *de sanie*. And for þe same skil, somtyme þe blode roteþ in   15
the vesie. And by cause þat þe blode is so trumbid, i. coldid and clomprid,
in the vesie and þe vesie is cold in kynde (and perauentur þe complexioun
of the man or of þe woman is also colde and feble), it gadereth into filþe
& corrupcioun.

   And often tyme mykel folk deyn þerof and mykel folk wenen þat it were   20
þe stone, but noþing so. And os Galien seiþ, swich [f. 97va] blode cometh
somtyme fro one mykel like a water leche. Ypocras techeþ þat whoso pisse
blod clomprish & coldish or poudrish or shalish or elles boþen blodish &
shalish and wiþ euel odour, it seiþ vlceracion and blemyshing of þe vesie. If
it come of þe reynes, it is noght so trumbouse os when it is of the vesie, &   25
þe priching and þe peyne is in the reynes & þereabouten and noght in the
schore ne þerabouten and þe Blode is more clere þan when it was of the vesie.

   If it be o þe lyuer, þe Blode is pur & clere and priching & peyn in the
right ypocondre. If it come of the kil or elles some of his veynes is brosten
or blemest or myswrenkt or mystrauailede, it is clere and pur as when it   30
cometh of the lyuer, but þan þe prickyng & þe pein is in the rig, [i.]¹ in the
bak, and principaly in þe 7 ioynte of þe rigebon fro þe neþer end vpward,
os Y said in þe 2 bok, 13 c. *de inopos & kianos, lef* {76}. Þus seiþ Gilbert
and þe Comentour.

   Gilbert þus: Blode aperand in þe vryn somtyme cometh of þe lyuer   35
and þat in meny wise: somtyme be cause of brusyng or brestyng of som
veyn of the lyuer, os when on is parbraked & ouer- [f. 97vb] trauailed and

---

1   i.] GSc, and R, & M7

longe tyme or in exces. And afte[r]² þat cometh to reste, þe blode þat was
chafed & mystraualid turneþ agayn to þe lyuer & scheweþ awaie by þe
veyn perauentur brosten. Or elles when blode hath holde his course by þe   40
nose or by þe course of womannes flours or by þe emoraides þat men haue
oþerwhile, perauenture þe blode is constreyned and wiþstand and letted.
& þan it fondiþ for to turnen ageyn to his wel þer he cam fro, s. to *jecur*.
Jecur and *epar*: al on to seyn, for *iecur* is wel of blode.

Item, somtyme þe lyuer is feblisshed & fadid and vanysch awaie, and   45
so his kynd mygh faileþ. And by cause þerof passeþ Blode wiþ þe vryn.³

Item, somtyme when a membre or a lym in þe body be hurt or ble-
mysshede, if it come of þe reyns, it is be cause of brestyng or brusyng of
som veyne or of som stryng of hem. When of þe vesie, also is be cause
of brusshyng o[r] brestyng⁴ of som veyn þerof. When of þe kil, þrogh   50
brestyng or bresur of him or of some of his **[f. 98ra]** veyns. *Et* tak gode
hede þat when Blode is of þe vesie, it is wonder litle. *Et* when Blode cometh
of þe vesie, it is wonder perilouse. And if it be mykel Blode and come of⁵
þe vesie it is incurable, but if he be cut.

Þe vesie is a membre þat hath bot litil of blode, by reson þat it is colde   55
& drye & skynnysh. But when it is of þe reyns, it is somdel more clerysh
& briȝtish þan when it is of þe vesie, & of þe kil more pur þan of þe reyns,
and of þe lyuer more pur þan of þe kyl, be cause þat þe ouer parties &
places haue more of kynd hete þan þe neþer. & be þe same skil, when it
is of þe vesie it is lompish & clompish & coldish & crudish & spottish &   60
more lowe in þe botme þan if it be of þe reyns or of þe kil or of þe lyuer.
Þus seiþ he. Som þus: Blod in vryn is somtyme of the vesie, somtyme of
the reyns, somtyme of þe kil, somtym of þe lyuer.

And be 5 maner⁶ it is knowen asundri: by þe body of þe Blode; by þe
colour of þe Blode; by þe odour; by his hasty or slake residen[ce];⁷ and by   65
felyng of peyne. First, Y saide, by his substance: for if it be trumbouse, os
it were gobates & clumpris, it is of the vesie, but if it be of þe reyns or of þe
kyl or of þe lyuer, it is noȝt trumbuse. And þat is by cause þat þo membres
ar more hote in kynd þan the vesie and more nygh to þe wel of hete þan is
þe vesie, and by **[f. 98rb]** cause þat þe vesie is more cold and more fro the   70

---

2 after] afterward GSc, afteþ RM7
3 vryn] *foll. by* Item somtym þe vryn is feblesshed as fadede and vanisseþ a waie and so
   his kynd myght faileþ and by cause þerof passeth blode wiþ þe vryn *canc.* R
4 brusshyng or brestyng] brusyng & brestyng G, brusshyng of brestyng RM7, *sentence
   om.* Sc
5 and come of] M7GSc, *foll. (after line end) by* and com of R
6 maner] *marg.:* 5 maner of knowyng of blode
7 residence] M7, residen (*at line end*) R, grounde GSc

welle of hete þan þai, and the Blod is more trumbouse þan when it is of
hem, os Y saide in the c. of *sanies.*

Item, by his coloure: for if it be blak, it cometh of þe vesie or elles of þe
reyns, be cause þat þe vesie and þe reyns ar ferre fro the wel of hete. And
þerfor here nurisshing and her fode, s. blode, is þe more colde and þe more   75
blak kyndely. But if Blode in the vryn be of the vesie, it is more blake þan
if it be of þe reyns, by þe same skil þat I said riȝt now; but if it be of þe kil
or of the lyuer, it is pure and clere.

Item, by his odour: for if it stynk, wiþouten faile it is of þe vesie, for þe
vesie haþ but litle hete of his owen kynde, and eke he is fere fro þe wel of   80
hete. And þerfor vnkinde hete fordoth his kynd hete, litil þat he hath, and
oþerwhile colde wasteþ & fordoþ his kynd hete and so causeth *fetor.* If it
be of the reyns or of þe kil or of þe lyuer, it stynkeþ neuermore, but if it so
be þat þe substance of hem rote and dwyne awaie.

Item, by his hastely or slakely goying doune into þe botume: for when it   85
is of þe vesie, it is doune in the botume anone as it is[8] **[f. 98va]** made, as who
seie, and skile whie is it þou myȝt wel seyn be poyntes þat ar saide both in
þis c. & in þe c. of *sanies* & in meny places moo. But if it be of þe reyns, it is
longer er it satle. If it be of þe kil, ȝit longer. If it be of þe lyuer, alþer-longest.

Item, by felyng of the peyne: for if it be of the vesie, þe peyn is in þe   90
schore and þerabouten; if of þe reyns, þerabouten. If of the kil, in þe 7 ioynt
in þe rigebone os Y saide biforne in þe 2 boke, 13 c. *de inopos,* lef {76}. If
of the lyuer, in the riȝt ypocondre and þerabouten. What ar þe ypocondres
often haue I said, as þou hast in þe 2 bok, þe 3 c. *de liuido colore,* lef {25}.

Þat Blode scheweþ fro þe lyuer is by meny causes: somtym be cause þat   95
he is so wastede and wanysshid in his substance þat he may noght conteynen
his kynde myȝt of wirkyng; somtyme be cause þat he is noȝt of myȝt for to
deceueren ne departyn þe blode fro þe oþer humores, os it is oþerwhile in ydropisi and also in scabbede folk; also be cause of feblenesse of myght in kynde;
also be cause of wicked materes of humores drawand & gaderand þerabouten. 100

[3.11]

De arenis vrine, of Grauel: c. 11

Arena vrine, Grauel in vryn, euermore bitokeneþ [oþer][1] **[f. 98vb]** *lytiasis*
or *nefresis. Lit[i]asis*[2] in þe j bok, þe 5 condicion, lef {*om.*}. *Nefresis* and

---

8 is] M7GSc, *foll. (after page break) by* is R

---

1 oþer] M7, orþer R, *om.* GSc
2 Litiasis] lythyasis GSc, Litasis RM7

nefresia in þe 2 bok, 4 c., lef {38}. And euermor it is like grauel or sonde
or chesel in þe botume of the vryn. But somtym it is whitish and somtym   5
redisshe and somtyme blakish.

If it be white, it is of the vesie and i[t][3] seiþ *calculus*. *Calculus* in þe 2
bok, þe 4 c. *de albo colore*, lef {39}. Þe vesie is kyndely white. Euery maner
þing þat is causede, it takeþ kynd & propirte of þat place & of þat þing
wherof þat þing is caused & gendrede, as apostemes mosten be of swich   10
kynde os ar þe places & þe materes wher & of which þai ar brede: if colde
place or colde membre, colde aposte[me];[4] if hote membre or hote place,
aposteme eke; and if aposteme brede in a place þat is bony, þat is most perilouse. And so of euery malady and sekenes. And þerfor when Grauel is of
þe vesie and þe vesie is white kyndely, þe Grauel is white kyndly.   15

If þe Grauel be redish and soft & nesch, as it were of fleish, it comeþ of
þe reyns. *Renes* ar kyndely redish and softe and nesche, and þerfor when
arena cometh þerof, he takeþ mykel of þe same kynd & forme.

If *arena* be blakish, it is causede of wick humores melancolik, viscouse,
and compacte, þat noght wil be dissol- **[f. 99ra]** uede but wiþ stronge   20
helpe and longe first. And þerfor blak Grauel is werst of al Grauelles and
werst tokne in the stone. And þerfor he is incurable but if he be cutte, and
namely if the stone be grete & ful waxen. But if the Grauel be whit, i[t][5]
is causede of humores fleumatik, raw and compacte, and eþiest for to dissoluen. When it is rede, it is werse þan whan it is white. But drede þe noght   25
þogh þou se rede Grauel in an vryn, ne gif noȝt anone dome of the stone,
for often tym rede Grauel in vryn apereþ in a double tercien, and somtyme
in a simple tercien,[6] be cause of discracioun of þe febre, and namely in hem
þat haue drie wombes, and þer lith gode helpe.

And vnderstond þat 3 causes þer be, or elles 4 att þe most, þat Grauel   30
appereþ in vryn: or by cause of þe stone, or elles in *artetica passione*, or
be cause of þe quarteyn long tym lastand. Þe febre quarteyn longe tyme
lastand is caused þorogh exces of melancolie, dryand and endurand, i. hard-
and, þe humores, as Alexandre telleþ of one þat had þe pthisik and þat
spited out þe stone at his mouthe. Which stone was gendred in þe pipes of   35
the lunges by **[f. 99rb]** cause of induracioun of humores.

And tak hede þat often tyme childerne haue þe *litiasi* or *litasi*, and þat
is be cause of viscosite of plente of humores in hem. Ȝonge folk often
tym haue *nefresi*, be cause of siccite of þe reyns and be cause of whiche

---

3 it] M7GSc, is R
4 aposteme] M7GSc, aposte (*line end*) R
5 it] M7GSc, is R
6 tercien] *foll. by* but *canc.* R

siccite, blode in the reyns is desiccat and mynushede in hem, more þan in   40
childerne. And be cause þerof, þe suptile parties ar consumpt, and þan þe
parties þat ar terrestre beleuen stille, and so ar indurate & so turnen and
breden into þe stone.

And 5 causes[7] þer be of gendryng of þe stoun: ouerdone plente of superfluytes of humores; viscosites of humores and streithed of the waies of þe   45
vryn; feblenesse of þe kynd; no my3t for to purgen ne to cachen ne for
to delyueren himself; and exces of vnkynd hete ouergoand þe moist and
wastand þe suptil. Þis causes are comunly most in childerne, al saue þe
last cause, þat is to seyn of hete. And þerfor comunly childern haue moste
þat passioun, s. *calculus*. Difference atwene *calculus* & *nefresis* or *nefresia*   50
& *lapis*: in þe 2 bok, þe 4 c., *de albo colore*, lef {38}. And how *calculus* &
nefresia ar causede and gendred: in þe same [**f. 99va**] bok, þe 7 c. *de karo-*
pos, lef {54}.

Item, take hede þat *arena* somtym seiþ þat þe stone is in breding; somtyme þat it is bredde; & somtyme þat it wil breken and lesne and vanis-   55
she awai. If it so be þat þe Grauel apperand in the vryn schewe him in
diuerse wise, s. alwai smaller & smaller or elles somtyme gretter & somtym smaller,[8] so þat þai be lesse & lesse, it seith þat þe stone is bredand. If
þe Grauel apere in þe vryn in diuerse wise, s. alwai g[r]etter[9] & greter or
elles somtym smaler and somtyme greter, so þat þai be more grete and mor   60
grete, it saithe[10] þat þe stone is vanishand. If it apere clene & smethe, as it
were purged & polisshed, it seiþ þat it is ful waxen. Þus seiþ þe Coment
vpon Giles; Gilbert þe same.

And if it so be þat þou my3t noght wel or redely knowe by þe colour
of þe Grauel, os I haue said, wheþer it be of the vesie or of þe reyns, tak   65
þis for a certeyn and verraie experiment þat Gilbert techeþ in his Coment:
make þe vryn for to be clensid þorogh a clene lynen clowte into a basyn
clene & bright & drye, & if þe stone be in the reyns, þou shalt se in the
grond of þe basyn Grauel as smale [**f. 99vb**] as eny poudre or dustc &
somdel toward redish. If it be of þe vesie, þe Grauel is more grete, mykel   70
toward smal grauel or sond, in colour somdel toward whitishede. Þus
seiþ he.

Som seyne in 5 wise Grauel appereþ in vryn, þogh on haue no3t þe ston:
somtyme in a simple tercien; somtyme in a double tercien; and somtym
in the febre quarteyn; somtyme in hard-wombed folk; and somtyme in   75

---

7 5 causes] *marg.*: 5 causes of gen<dryng> of the stone
8 smaller] *foll. by* and somtyme gretter *canc.* R
9 gretter] M7GSc, getter R
10 it saithe] *foll. by* it seiþ *canc.* R

artetica passione. Þe skil whie þou my3t se beforn. *Et* þogh þer be 5 causes
of gendryng of þe stone, os I saide beforn, noghtforþan som seyn þat þer
ar but 3, s. viscosites, groshede, & ouerdone exces of vnkynd hete. And þat
is false, for ouerdone streithede of þe waies of þe vryn is often tyme grete
cause of þe ston, as þe more party of auctours seyne, and ek os kynde skil   80
gifeþ it. And þerfor vnderstond þat, os techeþ Constantyn in þe 5 *Boke of*
Medicynes, þe 16 c., in wemen selden brediþ þe stone, be cause þat þe nek
of þe vesie in woman is more large þan in men, and her membres ar more
wide þan is þe 3erd of man, and here water waies ar no3t so wronge as in
men. & also **[f. 100ra]** wemen drynken no3t water os childerne, for no-   85
thing causeth so mykel þe stone os mykel water drynkyng, for it moste cause
humores gros and viscouse. <u>Of þe stone: þer I saide beforne; & which bene</u>
<u>disposede to þe stone: in c. *de karopos*, lef</u> {54}.

[3.12]

De pilis vrine, of Heres in vryn: c. 12

Pili vrine, Heres in vryn, ar smale and longe resolucions like hede heres,
and by cause þerof, þai ar callede *pili*. *Pilus* is an hede here. Þai comen
comunely of the reyns and þe lendes or elles of desiccacioun of humores.
And þis is þe difference and þe knowyng atwene: take & rubbe hem by-   5
twene þi fyngres softly, & if þou fele os it were a maner of saddehede, os
it were of fleish, it is of þe substance of þe reyns and þai signifien sekenesse & ake & pein abouten the reyns & þe lendes. Whiche sekenesse is
causede þorogh scharphede and exces of vnkynde hete in the lendes and
þerabouten, dissoluand & wastand þe substance of hem, & clippend and   10
chippand awaie þe smale partis of hem. & so passeþ forth wiþ the vryn &
apper in þe vryn moste like hede heres.

& comuly whan *pili* **[f. 100rb]** schewen hem in the vryn, þe vryn hath
a Fathede abouen. Þerof spekeþ Ypocras in *Afforismis*: whosoeuer make in
his vryn smale resolucions of fleishe, in schap and forme mykel like hede   15
heres, & þerwiþ þe vryn be fatt, þe Heres ar consumpcioun of þe reyns.
And somtyme swich maner *pili* apperen in *diabeta*, <u>of which I spake in þe</u>
<u>2 bok, þe 4 *de albo colore*, lef</u> {39}.

If it so be þat þou fele no maner of sadhede, no maner of fleishede,
betwene þi fyngres in þe felyng, but þai melten and vanysh into noght bi-   20
twene þi fyngres, wete wel þat þai come of humores, dried & baked & hard-
id þorogh exces of vnkynd hete. And þan if þai be longe, os half an vnche
& more, and of gode quantite, os wel more þan an here, it seith opylacioun

of þe reyns and of þe lendes, & þat somtym of þe riȝt half & somtyme
of þe lifte halfe and somtyme in boþen. Be cause o swich opilacioun, þe   25
synowes in þe body ar stopped & stuffed and letted, and be cause þerof,
þe spirites of lif ar astonyede and wiþstent & lettede eke. Which *spiritus*
schulden by here kynde course abouten by þe synowes of þe body giffen
myght and vertue & mevyng of soule to oþer [**f. 100va**] partis of the body,
and may noȝt, be resoun þai haue noght her fre course. Wherfor cometh   30
slepyng in the feet and steryng of lecherie in the lendes. If of þe riȝt half,
þan he feleþ steryng to lecherie & slepyng in þe riȝt fote; if in þe lifte halue,
on þe same wise in þat half; if in bothen, also in bothen.

And vnderstond þat, whan *pili* apperen in the vryn, or it is wiþ a febre or
elles wiþouten febre. If wiþ a febre, *pili* comen of al the body; if wiþouten   35
febre, onely of þe reynes. Þus seiþ þe Coment vpon Giles. Gilbert seiþ
þat *pili* come noght of þe reyns, but onely of membres þat ar synowy
and skynny, os is faxwax and os synowes ar and the reyns and þe arteries
and swich maner membres in the body. And þai ar caused by encheson of
wickede[1] humores, grosse & viscouse, beand in þe grete veynes of swich   40
maner of membrez. Þus seiþ he.

Som saie þer ar 3 causes of Heres in vryn: 2 þat þai comen of & ar of[2]
& þe 3 þat wirketh hem. Þe 2 þinges wherof þai be[3] ar þe membres or
elles þe place where and wherof þai comen, i. þe reyns & wicked humor
or humors of which þai comen. Þe 3 cause þat makeþ hem and wirketh   45
hem [**f. 100vb**] is longe dryhed. Isaac seiþ þat þe wirkyng of huge drihed
and þe wirkyng of hete ar alike. Þerof þou maist wel seen and knowen þat
euermore *pili in vrina* ar causede principaly of exces of vnkynd hete. And
when þai ar of þe reyns and when but of humores, os Y saide beforne, wiþ
felyng of þi fyngres.   50

[3.13]

De furfuribus, of Scuddes or Brenne in vryn: c. 13

Fvrfura vrine, Scuddes in þe vryn, ar white resolucions apperand in þe
vryn, most lik whete brenne or scuddes of a mannes hede. *Furfur* is brenne
& *furfur* is þe scuddez of an hede. Also þat þai ar white is be resoun þat þe

---

1 of wickede] *foll. by* of wicked *canc.* R
2 of] *foll. by* of *canc.* R
3 be] *foll. by* and *canc.* R

membre þat þai comen of, s. þe vesie, is white. And þai ar causede þorogh   5
exces of vnkynd hete, os when þe vesie is ouercharged wiþ onkynd hete,
þat ilk hete wasteþ þe humidite of the vesie. And þan risen scuddes and
royns of the body and of þe vesie, and violence of the hete chippeþ hem of,
and þai fallen awaie and so passen forth wiþ þe vryn.

Than when *furfura* apperen in vryn, or þai seyn consumpcioun of al the   10
body or elles but of þe vesie alone. But be a febre or wiþouten febre þou
schalte weten it. When *furfura* schewen in the vryn **[f. 101ra]** wiþ a febre
and[1] indigestioun, þai seyn consumpcioun of al þe body; wiþouten febre
and wiþouten indigestioun, scabbe & consumpcioun of þe vesie alone.
And take hede þat when *furfura* seyn consumpcioun of al þe body, it is no   15
more for to menen but euen þe 2 spice of þe etik. Of þe etike and of his
spices: in þe 2 bok, *de liuido colore*, lef {32}.

Item, fatt vryn and wiþ *furfura* seiþ a scabbede vesie & a consumpt
body. *Furfura* ar alwai causede of vnkynd humor of þe vesie or elles of al
þe body wiþinne, and þat somtym þorogh exces of vnkynd hete wastand   20
þe humidite, os Y saide while er, & somtyme þorogh exces of colde, crumblend and schrankeland togeder þe vesie. And so risen scuddes & roynes of
þe vesie. Þus seiþ þe Coment vppon Giles. Se more in þe 2 next c. folwend.

[3.14]

De crinoidibus in vrina: c. 14

Crinoydes & *furfura* ar mykel lik, saue þat *crinoydes* ar more þan *furfura*,
bothe in lenthe and in brede and in thikhede. *Crinnoides* ar saide of þis
word *crinium* (*crinium* is þe thrid part of a whete corn onely gronde),
and of þis worde *ydos*, i. *forma*, a schap or a forme. For *crinoydes* ar my-   5
[f. 101rb] kel of swyche schap. Also *crinoydes* haue another name in phisik,
cripine or *cripina* (*anglice*: cripyns), so þat þise 3 ar al on for to seyn: *crinoydes*, *crinium*, & *cripinum*.

Crinoydes ar causede os *furfura*, saue þat *furfura* comen somtym (and
þat for the mor del) of þe vesie, os I saide in the next c. beforn, but *cri-*   10
noydes onely of þe membres þat ar more thik or elles more depe þan is þe
vesie, os of þe brest and þe spirituales. & also þat *crinoydes* ar by more
violence of vnkynde het þan ar *furfura*, and by cause þerof, *crinoydes* euermore seyn more consumpcioun & destruccioun of þe body þan *furfura*.

---

1 and] *foll. by* di (*erased*) gestioun or *canc.* R

And þerfor when *crinoydes* aperen in the vryn, þai betokne þe 3 spice   15
of þe etik. Of þe etik and of his spices: þer I saide in þe next c. aforne. An
vryn wiþ *crinoydes* in a febre seiþ þe longe malady, i. þe etik, os Ypocras
seiþ. *Crynnoydes* ar comunely white in colour, but somtyme it is redishe
or blakkish, os in acuis. & þat is be² cause of incencioun of blod and þan
is it grete perile. And when *crinoydes* ar massif, i. grete & wel thikke, þai   20
comen noght of the vesie but onely of þe spirituales. And þerfor þe gretter
þat *crinoydes* be, þe more perile, for it seith the more was- [**f. 101va**] tynge
of the spirituales, be cause þat þe body³ is ful smyte and taken wiþ þe 3
spice of the etik.

[3.15]

De squamis in vrina, of Scales in vryn: c. 15

Squame & petala & petaloydes al on (*anglice*: scales or shalis), for þai ar
most like þe scalis of a fish þat we calle goiown. Wherfor tak hede þat
squame & *furfura* & *crynnoydes* ar mykel like, saue þat *squame* ar lesse &
thenner þan *furfura*, & *furfura* lesse & thenner þan *crinnoydes*. Of þe same   5
wise þat *furfura* ar caused ar *squame* causede, but *furfura* of more exces
of hete than *squame* and *crinoydes* of more hete þan *furfur*. And of þe
same membre or membres þat *furfura*, s. of the vesie or of þe spirituales,
saue þat *furfura* comunly come of þe vesie, but *squame* and *crinnoydes*
comunly of þe spirituales.   10

But when *furfura* ar of the vesie or noght, þus schalt þou knowe: if *fur-*
fura holde him lowe in the vryn, i. fro þe myddes dounward, and þerwiþ
sekenesse beneþen aboute þe schore, it ar of þe vesie. If þai be high in þe
vryn, i. in þe myddes or vpward, of þe spirituales. If þai ocupien al þe vryn,
bothe abouen and bineþen & in the myddes ek, it ar of bothen. [**f. 101vb**]   15

When the kynd humidite of þe vesie or of þe spirituales is consump[t]¹
and fordon by vnkynde hete, Shales & Scuddes,² Crypyns, fallen awaie
þerfro, ri3t os we se in scabbede folk.

And þerfor þou schalt demen of *squame* & of *furfura* and of *crynoy-*
des nerhand al like, saue þat *furfura* seyn more vnkynde hete & more   20

---

2   is be] M7, be is be R, by GSc
3   be cause þat þe body] *foll. by* by cause þat þe body *canc.* R

---

1   consumpt] M7GSc, consump R
2   scuddes] *foll. by* folk *canc.* R

consumpcioun þan *squame*, & *crynoydes* more þan *furfura*. And þerfor
squame seyn þe j spice of þe etik, *furfura* þe 2, & *crinoydes* þe 3. And
whosoeuer haue þe etik or be mykel disposede þerto, his vryn hath Scalis or Scuddes or *crinoydes* or elles alle. If he make Skales, he is curable
anogh. If he made Scuddes, it is hard. But if he make *crinoydes*, it is   25
incurable. & by cause of lykenesse of Scales and Scuddes & of Crypynes,
and by cause þat al 3 betokne þe etik, þe more del of auctours treten of
squame and *furfura* al vnder on, & somtym of al 3 vnder on. And vnderstond þat when *squame* or *furfura* or *crynnoydes* betokne þe etik, þai ar
n[e]uermore³ caused þorogh cold, but only þorogh vnkynd hete, os Y   30
haue saide.

   Theophilus (os Gilbert reherceth) seiþ **[f. 102ra]** þat *squame* & *furfura*
& *crinoydes* al 3 comen somtyme of one membre, os of þe vesie, of þe
spirituales, os it is seid. Bot Ypocras and Galienus þat were more knowyng
in anatomyes, i. of þe inder partis of man, þai seyn þat *crinoydes* comen of   35
me[m]bres⁴ þat ar carnouse, i. fleshy, and longe & brode & massif, os ar
þe spirituales, & *squame* of membres þat ar webby and skynny, os veyns
& arteries and synowes and swiche oþer. But *furfura* comen of membres
þat ar of kynd mene atwene boþen. Þus seiþ he & accorden wiþ þe þing
aforsaide.   40

[3.16]

De attomis in vrina, of Motes in vryn: c. 16

Attome or *attomye* ar smale & white & rounde bodies in the vryn, and
þai ar smale & litle os motes in the sone, and þerfor þai ar callede *attome*
or *attomie*. *Attomus* is a mote in the sone. Þan vnderstond þat swich smal
white Motes, when þai apperen in þe vryn, oþer of man or of woman, þai   5
seine comunly þe goute: in man alwaie but nogh in woman. Wherfor take
hede þat when þai apperen in þe vryn, oþer þai apperen in the botume or
in þe myddes or abouen or elles ouer al þe vryn.

   If þai schewen hem in þe neþer regioun **[f. 102rb]** of þe vryn þai seyn
the goute in þe neþer regioun of þe body. Of þe 4 regions in body of man   10
and of þe 4 regions of vryn answerand to hem, Y saide in þe 2 boke, þe 7
c. *de karopos*, lef {55}. If in þe myd regioun of þe vryn, þe goute is in þe

---

3   ar neuermore] ar nermore M7, arn (e *eras.*)uermore R, *om.* GSc (*chapter ends after
    preceding sentence in* GSc)
4   membres] M7, mebres R, *om.* GSc

myddes of þe body, s. fro þe lendes to þe myddred. If in þe ouer regioun
of the vryn, riȝt so in the body. If *attome* ocupie al þe body of þe vryn, þan
al þe body is taken wiþ þe goute.   15

Attome ar causede & gendred þrogh continuel distillacioun, i. þrogh
euery fote fallyng & course & rennyng of humores vpon sad membres, as
vpon þe bones & on oþer membres þat ar hard & sadde, os paxwax, synowes, & swich oþer. Þat *attome* ar white is be resoun þat þai comen of swich
membris þat ar white of kynd, for kyndely þai sewen þe colour of þo mem-   20
bres fro which & of whiche þai ar desicede fro. Smale & litle, for whan kynd
hete wirketh and doth his myȝt for to dissoluen & to defien and fordon þe
malady, s. þe goute or elles disposicioun þertoward, alse mykel os in him is,
& þat membre or elles þo membres into which he wirkeþ ar sadde and hard,
and eke þerwiþ þe wirkyng of kynd hete is but **[f. 102va]** litle and feble, þat   25
þat is resoluede and desicyd of þe wicked colde humores þorogh kynde
hete is but litle, s. þo smale white resolucions. & þat is þe skil whie þai ar so
smale. Herof it folweþ wel þat þe grettre þai be, þe bettre tokne. For it seiþ
þat kynde is redy and þe more of myght for to delyueren the mater.

Þe more rownde, be cause þat hete wirketh into þat mater in virown, i.   30
in rownde abouten, and also be cause of he[re] fa[l]lyng,[1] as we seen in fallyng of reyne droppes. For when þe smale resolucions or elles decysions
(þat al one ar for to seyne) ar resolued & desicyd fro þo membres & parties in þe body þat þai comen of, þai stonde noȝt ne stynt but continuely,
i. euery fote, þai rollen and trendelen, falland doune til þai comen to þe   35
vesie. And in þat ilk trendelyng and rollyng downe, be cause þat þai ar
bodies vaporows, is þe roundehede causede.

But take hede þat þogh it so be, þat euermore wemenes vryn is more
wick or more wrowe for to gif dome of þan mannes vryn. For swich maner
of vryns, s. in woman, begyle[n][2] most man of þis craft, of alle vryns þat   40
ar, <an>d most hard is for to gif dome of, boþ for þe skil þat I haue sayde
in þe j bok, þe 4 c., lef {*om*.}, **[f. 102vb]** and also for *attomye* in vryn of
woman seyn meny þinges, as þou schalt seen.

Et þerfor womenes vryn – and namely wiþ Attomys – ar called of auctoures ful cursed & froward vryns, but mennes vryn wiþ Attomys ar euer-   45
more esy and redy anogh. For wiþouten faile, it signifien euermore in men
os it is saide.

And þerfor vnderstond þat in vryn of women, *attome* seyn 3 þinges:[3]
oþer *gutta* (*anglice*: þe gowte), or conseyuyng of childe, or elles sekenesse
of þe matrice. Þan take this for a reule, þat if *attome* apere in vryn of   50

---

1   here fallyng] GSc, heyȝ failyng RM7
2   begylen] gyleth G, begildith Sc, begylem RM7
3   3 þinges] *marg.*: Attome seyn 3 þinges in wome<nes> vryn

woman so þat þai be þike, and namely donward, lik water þat amydown
were wasshen inne, and wiþin a litil while afterward, þai gadren and cletten
hem togedre, it is tokne þat sche haþ conceyued. And os Auicen[4] seiþ, þan
þer apereþ in the vryn a suptil body, whitishe, mykel toward rawe silke, i.
vnwroght silk.   55

And þan if þo Attomies ben redisse or rodyish, it is verai tokne þat sche
is wiþ a knaue childe. Þat þai ar redish or rodish, it is tokne of myght &
vertue of kynd hete. If *attomye* seme as þai wer wanne bloysh, she is wiþ
a femel. Þat ilk colour in Attomys seiþ feynthede & feble- **[f. 103ra]** hede
of kynde hete. If sche haue noȝt conceyued and her vryn appere swiche, it   60
seiþ þe gowt. If þer appere in her vryn a þing whitish, flakend or ropand,
haue þe vryn Motes or no Motes, it seiþ þat she hath late be seruede of man
or elles þat here sperme passed late fro here. And of þe same wyse it is of
vryn of man, saue þat comuly white þing halt him more high in mannes
þan in womannes.   65

Item, þe same maner of vryn, saue more þikk & mor swart & droublish,
seith humorosite of þe matrice, i. appetit & wodnesse to man. But os Gi[l]-
bert[5] seiþ, when Motes betokne concepcioun, þai ar caused oþerwise þan
when þai seyn þe gowte. When þai seyn *gutta*, þai ar causede os I said, and
þai ar white be 3 skiles: or be cause þat þai ar desisede þorogh wirkyng   70
of hete, be it kynde hete or vnkynde hete, fro membres þat ar white of
kynde; or elles be cause þat here mater, i. þe humor or þe humores þat
attomie comen of, ar white and fleumatik. For in euery maner of reume
& course & flowyng of humores reumatik (and namely in the goute, þat
alwaie cometh **[f. 103rb]** þrogh course and gaderyng of wikkede humores, 75
colde & fleumatik, to þe synowes and to þe ioyntes), fleume medlith him
and is principal maystre. And be cause of his coldehede & moysthede and
neshed, he floweth & swymmeth and makeþ oþer humores also, if kynd
hete be noȝt of myght for to wasten him & fordon him. Or elles þai be
white be cause of proprete and of vertue of þe hete of þat membre þat þai   80
comen of, be it kynd hete, be it vnkynd hete. For hete wirkand into þat
crude mater, i. into þat humor or humores, comprehendith him & becloseþ
in virown abowten, and giffeþ to þat ilk mater into whome he wirkeþ his
fourme and his coloure. And also þat is one skil whie þai ar rownde, whie
þai ar white & smale & rownde, os Y seide.   85

Gutta,[6] os speken diuerse auctoures of phisik and of sirurgie, bredeth
in diuerse places of þe body, but moste in þe ioyntoures, os in the albowe,

---

4 Auicen] Auiceñ R (*susp. over* -n *taken as otiose, to match* R's *usual spelling* Auicen)
5 Gilbert] M7GSc, Gibert R
6 Gutta] *marg*: þe goute þe podag\<ra\>

in the wristes, and in þe fyngres, somtyme in þe þombe, somtyme in the litle fyngre, and somtyme in þe kne, somtyme in þe hele, & somtyme in the toos. & it is callede *gutta*, for also mykel os it is causede of wickede   90
humores guttand, i. [f. 103va] seweand and faileand, litil & litle into þo places and þo parties in þe body. Somtyme it cometh of humores colde, fleumatik, & viscouse, & þan it is called þe colde goute. And þan it is strong gnawyng and anguishand bolnyng, and þe place is pale or palish and þe vryn is discolourede & wiþ Attomis. And somtyme it is causede   95
of hote humor, os of humores of blode or of red colre menk togedre, os Constantyn seyth in his *Antitodarie*, in þe 6 bok, þe 18 c. And þan it is called þe hote gowte & þan is more peyne þan in þe colde gowte and þe place is redishe.

Boþ in colde gowte and in hote goute, þe vryn is euermore bloysh   100
abouen, i. dymmysh & derkish, and soumetyme in þe riȝt half and somtym in þe lefte half and somtym in boþe. In þe lifte half, it is euermore more perilouse þan in þe riȝt half. Constantyn, in þe forsaide bok, þe 19 c., seiþ þat þe gowt & þe podagre brediþ comuny in hem þat leuen softly & in mykel reste and haue no trauaile, and in hem þat wil noght vsen pur-   105
gacions ne medycynes agayn wicked humores, and in hem þat eten mykel & drynken, for swich thinges causen wicked humores and fordon gode; & [f. 103vb] in hem alse þat ar of moyst & fleumatik conplexion, & namely in hem þat vsen mykel lecherie and meny dyuerse metes and drynkes when none nedith.   110

Þe synowes and þe ioyntes ar chaufed þorogh ouerdon trauailyng, & þat chaufyng is noght helpyng to þe kynd but wastyng & fordoing of kynde. For þe synowes ar trauailede, slakked, & dryed and dwynede, & þan wicked humores, colde & fleumatik, drawen & gaderen to þe places þat ar destitute & refte fro here kynde hete. And þan if þo places be moste   115
feble and kynde hete encreseth noght, þei beleuen þere stille and causen sekenesse or elles þe gowt. If hete encrece & cache hem þens, þai passe to þe feblest places of þe body, and namely to þe hondes or to þe fete if þai be moste feble, as it is comunly boþe be cause þat þai ar neruouse & by cause þat þai ar moste ferre fro þe wel of hete. And þerfor as Constantyn seiþ,   120
þai þat leuen chaste, þai ar noȝt guttowse ne podagre but wil onneþes; and if þai be, it is noght but be cause of wicked diete and of wickede humores.

Childerne ar noȝt guttouse ne podagre but it be þorogh wicked [f. 104ra] humoures causede of wicked diete. And ȝitt be cause of ȝouthe, myȝt in kynde cacheþ hem & scatereþ and disperpleþ hem awaie. Wemen   125
ar noght guttouse ne podagre by cause of lecherie as men ben, for þai tra-uaile noȝt þerin os men done; and also for þai haue purgacioun of sperme by here floures euery monyth ones. And on þe same wise is often tyme *ciatica passio* causede.

Now vnderstond þat *gutta* haþ meny namen:[7] *gutta* and *artetica* & 130
gutta artetica & *artetica passio.* It is callede *gutta* for þe same skil os Y
saide. It is callede *artetica* of þis word *artus.* *Artus* is a litil lym of man, os
þe fyngre or þe too and þe ioyntes of hem, so þat be it wiþin the body, os
abouten þe spirituales or þe nutritiues or þe reyns & þe lendes, or elle in þe
vttre parties of þe body, os in þe hondes or in þe feet or in eny whirlebone, 135
it is callede *gutta* & *gutta artetica* & *artetica* & *artetica passio.* But when
it is of þe spirituales, os Y saide, it is propurly callede *malum spirituale.*[8]
Malum spirituale is euery maner of sekenes of the spiritual membres, os it
is saide in þe 2 boke, þe 3 c. *de liuido colore,* lef 31. When it is of þe nutrityues, os I saide, it is called *malum* [f. 104rb] *nutritiuorum* and *malum* 140
yliale & *yliaca passio.* When it is *yliaca passio* & how & wherof it is causede, I saide in þe 2 boke, þe 7 c. *de karopos,* lef {53} and in þe 13 c. *de
inopos & kyanos,* lef {77}. If it be of þe reyns and abowten the lendes, os Y
saide, it is callede *malum renum* and *malum lumborum* or elles yle or *iliale*
or *iliaca passio.* Yle: os I saide in þe 2 bok, þe 13 c., *de inopos* and *kyanos,* 145
lef {77}. Yle is often tyme taken in phisik for þe reyns and þe lendes, and
so may euery malady of þe reyns & þe lendes be callede yle or *yliale* or
yliaca passio. And so is *iliaca passio* taken in meny diuerse significacions,
os often haue I saide.

If it be on þe hande or on þe handes, it is propurly callede *ciraga.* If in þe 150
fote, *podagra.* If it be in *cia,* it is called *sciatica* or elles *sciatica passio. Scia*
is propurly þe whirlebon in þe hepe, þat we callen þe hepe-bone, and it is
taken comunly for euery maner of knokel bone. And so *scia* and *vertebrum*
& *condilus* ar al on (*anglice:* þe knokel bone, þe whirlebone), and þerof is
saide *sciatica* and *sciatica passio* (*anglice:* sekenesse of þe whirlebone). And 155
al þise ar spices of þe goute and ar causede os I saide.

Also *sciatica passio* [f. 104va] is causede somtyme þorogh a drop of
blode falland into a ioynt or into a whirlebone, os if one take a colde after
a grete hete or a chaufyng. And somtyme þe colde [f]leumatik[9] humores
þat passen so to þe whirlebone, þai holden hem þere so longe þat þai roten 160
awaie þe synowe þat halt þe whirlebone togedre; and þan þe vryn is wan
and dede and blo and þer is not bote deþ. Galien & Constantyn seyn þat
podagre, if it bigynne *in vere* or *in estate,* it is helede in 40 daies or lesse. If
it com in autumpne and laste to wynter, it is harde for to helen. *Ver* & *estas*
& *autumpnus* & *yems:* se in þe j bok, þe 9 condicion, lef {11}. 165

7 namen] *marg.*: names of goutes
8 spirituale] *foll. by* is *canc.* R
9 fleumatik] GSc, sleumatik RM7

And be cause þat þe gowte somtyme is causede of blode, somtyme of colre, somtym of *fleuma* or of melancolie, and also meny knowen noȝt whan it is one ne when it is oþer, þus techen auctours for to knowen: if it be of blode, by bolnehede & redhede of þe place þer it is and also by stirt- ing þerof, by swetishede in þe mouþe, and by fulhede and blowthed of þe 170 veynes, & by apperingz of rede bodyes and rede þinges in slepyng, and by tokne þat hote þinges harmen him and cole þinges helpen him. And in þe houres & tymes of blode, it noyeþ & greueth moste. [**f. 104vb**] <u>Which</u> <u>ar þe houres of þe 4 humoures, I saide in þe 2 boke, c. *de lacteo colore*,</u> <u>lef {45}. Which ar þe 4 tymes of þe 4 humores, þou mayst knowen by þe</u> 175 <u>proces þat I saide in þe j boke, þe 9 condicioun, lef {10}. And by þe figure</u> <u>& þe proces in þe 13 condicioun, lef {13}.</u>

And take hede þat in no spice of þe artik is grete hete. For neyþer by hete ne by kolde schalt þou haue knowyng what gowte it is; and if it be, it is ful selden.   180

If it be of colre, litle bolnyng or non, peyne none like, by cause of which peyn he falleþ in febre and somtym feleth priching and prynging in þe synowes and in the ioyntes, þorgh violence of þe bitand colre. And þe hide is citrinysh owtward, and þe mouthe bittre, hote þinges noyen, colde helpen. In þe hours & tymes of colre, him is werste. In slepe, cytrinyshe 185 & redish þinges appere.

If it be causede of *fleuma*, grete bolnyng, more þan of blode or of colre, & peyne, but lesse þan of colre. And þe place is wan, white, & pale and squobbe, nesshe, euel sauour in the mouthe; in slepe, appering of white & pale þinges. Colde þinges disconfort him & hote þinges confort. In hours 190 & tyme of *fleuma*, he is most traualede. And tak hede þat in colde cause, be reson of mykel wakyng causede of peyn, þe vryn often tym is skilfully wel colourede. & þerfor by[10] [**f. 105ra**] colour of þe vryn may þou noȝt certeynly demen ne knowen when it is in colde cause or when in hote.

If it come of melancolie, huge bolnyng, more þan in eny oþer cause; 195 þe place is wonder drye and bloish or blakish, and grete greuance & scharphede & sowrehede in þe mouth, appering of swart and blak þinges in slepe, & somtyme noyse in slepe. Colde noyeth & hote helpeþ. In hours & tymes of melancolie, it is most hard wiþ him.

Anoþer spice of þe goute þer is þat is called *gutta rubea* or *gutta rosata* 200 or *gutta rosacea* (*anglice*: þe rede gowt or þe redegownd). Þe more partie of folk, when þai seen a childe haue it, þai callen it þe radigownd; when þai sene a man haue it, þai calle it þe salse *fleuma*; when a woman, þe lepre. In man & woman, it appereþ in þe nase & þerabouten. In childern, hit

---

10 þerfor by] *catchword*: colour of þe vryn

seyen fro wiþout- **[f. 106rb]** ward; in women of age & in hem þat often
haue conceyuede and mykel ar wont to swich seruise, it is but litle seen or
aperceyuede fro wiþoutward. But noȝtforþan, þai felen it wel in hemselfe.
Hereby þou maiste se whie som women haue gretter pappes þan som, s.
by cause þat þai ar more spongiouse.   285

Item, os techeþ Ypocras in his boke of *Afforismis*, in þe 5 particule,
aboute þe mydward: if þou wilt weten witterly if a woman haue conceyuede, when she schal slepen, ȝif here to drynk a drynk þat is callede in
phisik *mellicratum*, in oþer facultes *meldo* or *medo* (*anglice:* mede). And if
sche fele grete crowlyng and rolying and peyne in her wombe, sche hath   290
conceyuede; and if she fele no peyn, sche haþ noght conceyuede. But tak
gode hede þat þis experiment is euermore sothe in the negatif, but noȝt
euermore in þe affirmatif. For it folwe[s]¹⁵ noȝt: "Þis woman feleþ distemperure in her wombe of þis drynke, *ergo* sche hathe conceyuede." For perauenture sche hath sekenesse in here wombe of som oþer cause. But in þe   295
negatif, it is euermore sothe. For þis is a gode skil and euermore sothe: "Þis
woman feles no fretyng ne no distemperure in her wombe of þis maner of
drynk, *ergo* **[f. 106va]** sche hath noght conceyuede."

And also take hede þat þis worde *mellicratum* is often tyme taken for
euery maner of pocioun þat is made onely of water and hony, and so is   300
mede euermore made. But os *mellicratum* is taken her, is 4 {oz.} of rawe
hony wiþ 8 {oz.} of rawe water. And þis drink shulde be geuen her when
sche goþ to reste. And also it schulde noght be geuen bot to swych a
woman þat is noȝt wonte for to drink mede ne swich maner drynkes os
ar maade of hony. For þan it wirketh noght so in here wombe. And also   305
sche oweþ noȝt to weten whie it is giffen her. Þat it causeth swyche distemperure in here wombe, þis is þe skil, os techeþ Gilbe[r]t:¹⁶ for it causeth
grete ventosite in here stomac, and þat only when she hathe conceyuede
and elles noȝt, and namely if it be wel waxen. And þan þe guttes shronklyn
and draw togeder. And by cause þerof, þat ilk ventosite may noȝt awaie,   310
and so it causeth distourbling in here body.

Þis ar general signes of concepcion. Special tokenes¹⁷ of concepcion in
women, s. wheþer sche be wiþ male or wiþ femal, ar þise. If her face seem
more rody and more bright after sche haþ conceyued **[f. 106vb]** than it
was biforn, or elles if she kepe stil her colour as she was beforn, certeyn   315
she is wiþ a knaue child. For þe male is euermore conceyuede & gendrede
of blode more hote and of þe bettre partie of þe seede of þe man and of

---

15 folwes] foleweth GSc, folwel RM7
16 Gilbert] M7GSc, Gilbet R
17 Special tokenes] *marg.*: Special tokenes of concepcioun

þe woman, and also he lieþ in the more warme place of þe matrice þan þe
femal. And be cause þerof, kynde hete more stereth and spredith abowte
in þe womannes body and þe bettre digestion is. And also, os Gilbert seiþ, 320
þat by cause of gode hote mater, s. of gode hote humores and principaly of
gode blode, wirkand in þe matrice, hote vapores stien vp about to þe lyuer
and to þe hert and to oþer membres, and namely to þe spirituales & warme
hem. And when þo membres and places ar so chaufede & warmede, hote
vapores stien vp to þe hede and to þe face. And so is caused rodihede and 325
brightnesse in the face.

Item, if she be wiþ a male, sche is more liȝt in body, be cause of gode
hote blode & gode digestioun. For gode blod & gode digestion causen
gode norishing in kynd and gode temperure of þe spiritz, and þerof
cometh lyghthede in body. Item, if sche be wiþ a male, her mylk is þikk, 330
for it is more and bettre excocte and digestede, be cause þat kynde hete
mynusheþ and wasteþ awaie þe [f. 107ra] aquosite, i. the wattrihede, of
þe melk. For if þou take a drop of here mylk and pour it on þi nayle
or elles on a pleyn thing, if it breke noȝt but holde him stille togedre in
rounde and sche be wiþ childe, it is a certeyn tokne and a verray tokne 335
þat sche is wiþ a mal.

Item, if sche be wiþ a male, sche feleth in maner of a bolnyng, a rysyng
in þe riȝt side. & þat is os it were in rounde & in þe ryght half, for þe knaue
childe euermore lith more in þe riȝt side. Þat it is in rounde is bi cause þat
þe masculyn bodies ar more hote in kynde & more stronge & myȝty and 340
holde hem þe more togedreward and ar noght scaterede ne disperplede
aboute in the matrice þrogh frigidite. And be cause þerof, þer is in þe riȝt
half a risyng in round, riȝt as we se in fleishe when it is soden or rostede,
it is more stiffe and more sad & rounde þan when it was rawe, be cause
þat hete maistrieþ and ouercometh þe moysthede and draweþ it oute and 345
saddeth him & al math hete. And þat is þe skil whie men ar more hard and
sad in fleishe þan ar wemen; and also whie þai ar more liȝt & clene & noble
in kynde þan women.

And [f. 107rb] vnderstonde þat kynde hete when he is aggregate, i.
gadred togedre, and halt him in on, he is more stronge and more myȝty 350
þan when he is discatered and disperplede in brode. For os Aristotil seiþ,
Omnis virtus vnita forcior est se dispersa (*anglice*: euery þing is of more
myght & virtue when it is togedre þan when it is atwynnede). If she be wiþ
a femal, þe forseid signes befal *e contrario*.

Item, if sche be wiþ a male & sche be sodeynly callede, sche stepeth 355
forth firste þe riȝt fote. For in the riȝt half is more kynde myght &
strengh & vertue of kynde hote blode þan in þe lifte half. If wiþ a femal,
e contrario. Item, if wiþ a male, sche feleth mevyng & steryng more
toward þe riȝt side, for þe forsaide skiles. If wiþ a femal, more toward þe

left. Meny oþer experimentes auctoures giffen and techen, which I passe   360
be cause of prolixite.

If þai may noght gendren and þou wilt wete whiche of hem is bareyn,
þis experiment techeþ Maistre Bartholome in his *Boke of Genecyes*: tak 2
pottes & put bren in bothe pottes and put þe mannes water in þe tone &
þe womannes watre in þe toþere pott, & lat stonde 7 daies or 15 daies. And   365
if it be þe mannes defaute, [**f. 107va**] þou schalt fynde wormes þerin wiþ a
foule stynk & sauour. If she, in þe same wise. If in bothe þe vryn, both. If
neþer vryn be so, neyþer he ne sche is bareyn, but þai mowe be holpen as
þou schalt se in our *Medycynarie*.

Bareynhede is comuly rather in woman þan in man: som woman mow   370
noght conceyue be cause of ouerdon lenehede & dwynyng and shronkelyng togedre of þe matrice; *et* som be cause of ouerdon fathede and gres
þat is so clattede aboute þe mouþ of þe matrice þat þe sede may noght
entren. And þogh it somtyme entre, þat gres stuffeþ & strangeleþ it, so þat
it mai noght cleue. And som tyme þe mouth of þe matrice is so narowe   375
& so strite þat it may noght vnderfonge þe ȝerdes ende, and namely if þe
ȝerde be riȝt schort & right grete, wherfore it sokeþ noȝt þe ȝerd ne receyueþ noght þe seede. And somtyme þe matrice is so gleymouse and so
slyper wiþin þat it may noght kepe ne holde þe seede, but slit awaie. Item,
þe seed of þe man is somtyme so thenne þat when it is in þe matrice, it glit   380
awaie os water; and som mennes ballok stones ar colde & drie in complexioun, and swiche men ar neuermore or elles vnneþes gendryng. [**f. 107vb**]
For þe seede of swiche complexionede folk is noght able to generacion.

[3.17]

De spermate in vrina, of **Sperme in vryn**: c. 17

Sperma, <u>os I saide in þe 2 bok, in þe c. of Blo coloure, lef</u> {36}, is white
blode. Þe seed of beste is decysede of þe pur substance of al þe membres
& lymes of him. It is white bothe be cause þat al þe membres & lymes of
whiche it cometh of ar kyndely white (for fleish is noght rede but only   5
because of blode) and also by cause of grete agitacioun, i. of trauailing
& chaufyng in mevyng and stering, and also by reson þat þat membre of
which he cometh principaly of is white.

For, os auctoures speken & techen, *sperma* hath his first grounde and
bygynnyng at þe principal membre of lif, s. in þe cerebre, <u>of whiche Y</u>   10
<u>saide in þe 2 bok, c. *de karopos*, lef</u> {55}, and so passeth forth to þe genera-
tiues, s. to þe reyns and to the ballokkes, berand wiþ him mater & kynde

of euery membre þat is bitwene þe cerebre and þe generatiues, redy for to
make generacioun. And þan in þo generatyues, but principaly in þe ballok
stones of him & of here (<u>of which I saide in þe 2 boke, c.</u> *de liuido co-*   15
[f. 108ra] <u>*lore,*</u> lef {13}), it is swongen and trauailede and wroght and
knoden os dowh or paste, þorogh trauayling and mevyng of bodies and
þorogh myght and wirkyng & lykyng in kynde. Þan oþerwhile some of
þis Sperme passeþ oute wiþ þe vryn. For when þe Sperme passeþ fro on,
som þerof cleueth & hongeþ aboute by þe sides of þe ȝerd and of þe value,   20
wiþin þe eye of þe ȝerde and wiþin þe lippes of þe value. Riȝt os þou
seest when foule licour is poured out of a vessel or os filth passeth oute
of a goter, & after þat water washeþ it awaie, riȝt so after pissing oute
of Sperme: when one makeþ vryn, þe vryn bereth forth wiþ him þat þat
hongeþ on þe sides of þe membre in his waie. And þan it scheweþ him in   25
þe vryn.

And somtyme it appereth in þe vryn somdel [l]ike[1] a part of spotle or
like on part of filth of a nase when one hath þe pose, somtyme long & large
& somtyme schort[2] and smal. Þan when resolucions of Sperme appere in
þe vryn, it seiþ þat he or she was late at þe seruise, or elles þat in som wise   30
þe Sperme passede, oþer þrogh wirkyng [f. 108rb] wiþ woman or of passing in slepe thorogh þoght and liking and desire had biforn in wakyng,
or in dremyng in slepe, or þrogh plente and kraskehede in kynde, or elles
þrogh *gomorre*. *Gomorria* and *sodomia* al on: *gomorrea* is a pouryng oute
of sede of man or of woman wilfully ageyne kynde. Of þis forwaried   35
doyng, meny ar schameful & wil noght shryue ne amende hem þerof.
Wherfor þai perish but þai hem amende.

And somtyme *sperma* passeþ fro one, sewond & droppand out by
þe ȝerde or by þe value, and þat al wakand when þai þink on none such
þingez. And þat is be cause of grete plente of blode. For grete plente of   40
blode, & namely in rank blode, os it is in ȝonge folk, causeth grete plente
of sperme. And when spcrme is so plentuouse in þe body, it seweth oute
& sweteþ oute at þe priue membres, somtyme wiþouten eny þinkyng or
stering to synne. Item, *sperma* passeth somtyme bothe in wakyng and in
slepyng because of feblenes in kynde, os it ofte tyme falleþ in seke folk.   45
For oftym in sekenesse, þe vesseles of þe sede, os in þe reyns & þe womanes bollok stones, & when þe <ballok stones>[3] ar dedish & feble & kynd
is noȝt [f. 108va] of myght for to wiþholden it. And so it glitt awaie or he
wote. And þis passioun haue þai comunly þat ar in þe falland euel, and þai

---

1 like] M7GSc, kike R
2 somtyme schort] M7GSc, *foll. by* & (somtyme *canc.*) schort R
3 ballok stones] M7Sc, stonys G, *illeg.* R

þat haue *apoplexia*, and also þai þat haue þe palsie, and namely þai þat haue   50
þe palsie in here cod.

Also often tyme folke haue it be cause of feblenes and feyntnesse &
dedenesse of here synowes, os in hem þat ar sekish and þai þat gif hem
mykel to penance and to fastyng, for kynde is noght of myght for to
receyuen þe seede. But in hem þat mesurabli sustene þe body, kynd haþ   55
wheron to wirke and is besy aboute digestioun and giffeþ myght to al þe
body, and so is þe body of my3t for to wiþholde & kepe þe seede. *Epilencia, þe falland euel: in þe 2 bok, c. de liuido colore, lef* {37}. *Apoplexia:
in þe 3 bok, þe 2 c. de circulis, lef* {87}. *Paralisis, þe palsie: in þe 2 bok, c.
de pallido colore, lef* {61}. *Paralisis virge vel testiculorum: in þe j bok, þe*   60
15 condicioun, lef {15}. *Paralisis* is noþing elles but destruccioun and fordoyng of þe synowes.

Than take hede þat *sperma* appereth in þe vryn in dyuerse <u>wise</u>: somtyme in meny smale litle parties, noght incorporate wiþ þe vryn but hold-
and hem in þe grounde of þe vryn; & [f. 108vb] þat seiþ þat she or he   65
was late at þe seruise. If it appere in gode grete parties, mykel like flakes,
hangond & ropand & but fewe and somdel incorporate wiþ þe vryn, i.
noght fullik in the grounde but drawand more dounward þe gro[wn]d,⁴ it
seiþ þe *gomorre*, of which I said while er.

[3.18]

De cineribus in vrina, of Asshen in vryn: c. 18

Cineres vryne, Askes in vryn, ar smale resolucions, smale bodyes, litle partis gaderand and holdand hem in þe botum of þe vryn, like a plot of askes
or elles of poudre. And euermore when Askes appere in þe vryn, þe vryn
is remys in coloure, i. feynt & wan and dedishe.   5

Than when an vryn scheweth him wiþ a maner of Askes or poudre in þe
botume, b[l]akkish¹ or bloysh, it seiþ *emoraidas* or *attrices* or *condilomata*
or elles *ficus* (*anglice*: þe emorays or þe attrikes or þe condilones or elles
þe fikis). Þat þe vryn is remys in coloure is be cause of exces in melancolie.
For *sanguis melancolicus* is so habundant in þe body þat þe kynde hete is   10
strangeled & stuffede, and be cause þerof is dygestioun fordon; & by cause
of fordoyng of diges- [f. 109ra] tioun is þe vryn remys and discoloured. Þo

---

4   grownd] grounde M7GSc, gronwd R

---

1   blakkish] blakish M7GSc, bakkish R

poudrishe resoluciouns in the botume ar þe remanauntz and þe bleuynges
and þe dregges of melancolik blode terrestre; and blak be waie of kynd, os
I haue said in diuerse places of þe 2 bok, and ar diriuyede to þe vesie and 15
so passen wiþ þe vryn. And by resoun þat þai ar terrestre and powdrowse,
for þai ar causede of melancolie, and melancolie is kyndly erþish and heuy
and drawand donward, þai holde hem beneþen. Þat þai ar blakish & bloish
is by þe same skil, s. for þai ar causede of melancolie.

   Emoraide ar taken in 2 wise: som for certeyn veyns þat comen fro *kilis* 20
to þe ers and ende in the ers hole; and somtym for a sekenesse of þe same
veyns. & alle is called emorayes in the speche._Kilis:_ in þe 2 bok, c. *de
liuido colore,* lef {27}. *Emorayde* ar saide of þis worde *emath*, i. blode,
&² of þis worde *roys*, i. a flux, a course of rennyng, os who saie "a flux of
blode." For þo ilk veynes þat I saide riȝt nowe, þat ar callede *emoraide*, ar 25
somtyme gretly charged and ouerdon, replete wiþ plente of blode melancolik. Which blode melancolik is wonder habundant in þe kil of þe rigebon. Þe rigebone, for alse mychel os it is þe hen- [**f. 109rb**] drest part of
mannes body, it is colde in complexioun; and þerfor be cause of frigidite
þerof and of his parties, þat ilk *sanguis melancolicus* gadereþ and congeleþ 30
in þe veynes. And when þo veyns ar in þis wise ouerchargede and ouerdon, replete and distemprede, þai also swellyn and bolnen, in so mykel þat
þe heuedes of þo veyns ar knoddishe and knarlish and somtyme þai bud
oute like sowes bigges. And þan is huge peyn þeraboute and heuynesse of
al þe body and colour in þe face dede and wan. And somtyme þe veynes 35
bresten by cause of huge plente of swich maner of humor, be cause þat
kynd is vnmyghty for to wiþhold it, or be cause of huge hete, or be cause
of gnawyng & peyn, or be cause of frigidite fro wiþoutward; or by³ cause
of compressioun⁴ blode cometh out in grete quantite. *Et* þai comunly haue
þis passioun þat somtyme were wonte for to sit hard & lie hard and colde; 40
and somtyme be cause of exces and plente of melancolik blode, and þai
ar comuly holpen and helede þerof, for þai ar purgede þerby of wikked
humores of melancolie, riȝt os wemen be by here floures. But þai þat haue
it bi cause of harde sittynge & hard lying and colde takyng [**f. 109va**] þai
ar incurable or elles nerhand. 45

   Atrices is 2 spice of þe emoraies. *Atrices* ar colleccioun of melancolik
blode þat is collecte and gadred in þe tail ende, causand knoddes and
knarles in þo parties. *Condilomata* is þe 3 spice of þe emoraies & þai ar
also collecciouns in the bottokes, sad and harde and round, lik akcornys.

---

2 &] M7GSc, & (*line end*) and R
3 by] M7GSc, be by R
4 compressioun] M7, compressioun of R, compressioun & thenne GSc

And þai ar callede *co[n]dilomata*[5] of þis worde *condiloun*, i. round, and of   50
þis worde is saide *condilus*. *Condilus*: in þe c. *de attomis*, lef {104}. *Ficus* is
þe 4 spice of þe emorais. Þai ar colecciouns of the buttokes, nesshe, here
& ʒonde ful, þe fleish lik greyns in a fike. *Et* take gode hede þat in the
atricis & in þe condilonis and in þe fikes, þe vryn sheweþ him riʒt os in
þe emorays, and is disposed in þe same wise, bothe anentes colour & þe   55
resolucions of poudre, and for the same cause os I saide.

Item, þe same maner of vryn seiþ feblenesse and sekenesse of þe splene,
saue þan ar þe resolucions askish and poudrish, more toward purpre þan
when it seiþ þe emorays. Item, vryn remys in colour, wiþ poudre like Askes
in the botume blakish, if it be a womannes water & it haue schewede swich   60
long tyme togedre, it seiþ stopping **[f. 109vb]** of her floures. For be cause
of drihede and of stoppyng of her floures, *sanguis melancolicus* haþ nogh
his kynde course ne purgacioun os he schulde haue, & by cause þerof, parties of þat ilke *sanguis melancolicus* swelt awaie wiþ þe vryn and appereþ
in þe grounde of þe vryn like poudre blakish or bloysh. Wiþ þise forsaide   65
signes accordeþ Gilbert, & for the more he seiþ þus: swich maner of resolucions in vryn ar wonder suptil & smale, os dust of grauel, somdel like
Grauel & noʒtforþan it ar noght Grauel, for þai ar neiþer stony ne erþi, but
moste like dust or poudre of grauel.

Þat þai holde hem lowe in þe botume is by cause þat þe mater, þe humor   70
þat þai comen of, is gros & indigest. And vnderstonde þat *attricis*[6] ar colleccions or elles oppilacions of melancolie & þai ar mykel like wrottes.
Condilonys ar more like sores þat we calle smale kiles or pusshes or elles
harde buddes and warres in the fleishe, causede of blode melancolik congelede and clomprede and knoddede in þe heuedes of þe veyns, i. in þe   75
endes. *Et* it may be in euery membre of mannes body. And somtyme þai
waxen os a mannes hede, and þe membre moste be cut þat it **[f. 110ra]**
draw noght ouermykel blod and þe stomp moste be brent. For in þis wise
bene many warshed þerof.

And when þe pores þat ar bitwene *epar* and þe splene ar stuffede &   80
stoppede wiþ blode melancolik, þan is þis sekenesse, s. þe condilons. Þus
seiþ he. Som speken þus: asky resolucions in vryn ar mykel like Grauel,
þogh it so be þat þai be no Grauel; and it ar noþing elles but humores
aduste. And somtyme þai ar whitisshe, and þat is tokne of fleume aduste;
and som tyme blakish, and þat is tokne of blode adust or elles of melan-   85
colie adust. But for alse mykel os þai ar comunly blak, by cause þerof þai
seien principaly þe *attrices* and þe condilones and þe fikes, which sekenes

---

5 condilomata] M7GSc, comdilomata R
6 attricis] attrices GSc, atri *(line end)* tricis R, atritricis *(on one line)* M7

ar causede comunly þrugh adustioun of blode, os it comunly befalleþ after
long chaufyng of þe lyuer and also after continuel febre. For in swiche
maner of maladies, comunly þe blode is wont for to be scorclide and adust   90
by þe sides & in þe extremites of þe veynes.

Attrices ar colleccions of melancolie in þe hed of *longaoun*, i. in þe ende
of *longaoun*. For þerabouten is *humor melancolicus* wonte for to gadre into
hard buddis & [f. 110rb] knottes. And often tyme men haue þis maladi.

Emoraydes ar 5 veyns þat ende in þe selfe cercle of *longaoun*, i. in þe   95
sides of þe ers-hole. Þe cercle of *longaoun* & þe ende of *longaoun* and þe
sides of þe ers-hole ar al on. And þise 5 veyns ar somtyme so replete wiþ
plente of melancolie comand doune oute of þe body to þo parties þerabouten, þat þai bene bolne & bloute and step and breste oute, and blode
þerwiþ. Anoþer spice of þis sekenes þer is þat is callede *ficus*, þe fikes, be   100
cause þat when one hath this euel, his tail end is ful of smale knarles like
kirnelles of a fike. *Condilomata* or *condilomate* ar hard colleccions, harde
buddes & knarles in þe fleishe lik acornes. And al þis maladies ar causede
of exces of melancolie or of blak humor, and of swiche humor ar askish
resolucions þat appere in þe vryn resoluede.   105

Som sai þat *attrices* ar saide of þise 2 wordes: *ad* & *trica*. *Ad* is toward
gretely; *trica* is a tresse of here & a lettyng, a tarying. Þan it is saide &
callede *attrica* of *ad*, i. toward, & of *trica*, a tresse, by cause þat when one
hath þis spice of þe emoraies, his tail end is buddy & knotty, in liknesse
mykel toward a tresse. [f. 110va] Or *attrices* ar saide of *ad*, i. wel or   110
gretly, and of þis worde *tero, teris, triui*, for to bere doune and for to do
sorwe. For who so haue *attrices*, he is wel gretly and wel hugely borne
doune wiþ sorwe and peyne & wo. Or *attrices* ar saide of *trica*, for a
tresse, by resoun þat os a tres is of thre, riȝt so he þat hath þe *attrices*, he
felith 3 buddes, 3 knottes, or 3 knarres in his fleishe beneþe. Herewiþ[7]   115
accordeþ som auctoures.

Þe Coment vpon Giles seiþ þus: *attrices sunt 3 collecciones* (*anglice*:
attrices ar 3 hard buddes or knottes in þe tail end). Herwiþ accorden also
þai þat seyne þat *attrices* ar said of þis word *tris*, i. *tres* (*anglice*: 3). Herwiþ accorden also þai þat saien þat *attrices* ar saide of þis worde *a*, i. *sine*   120
(*anglice*: wiþouten) and of *trica* by þe contrarie, os who saie noȝt wiþouten
tresse, i. noght wiþouten buddes ne knoppes ne knoddes in þe tail ende.
Item, *atrices* ar saide of *trica* for letting and tariing. For who so haue þe
attricis, he is so lettede and tarried þat he may riȝt noght done, but lien and
tholen. And þerfor wet wel þat *attrices* ar alse mykel for to seyne os *atroces*   125
(*anglice*: schrewede & greuouse & gryme).

---

7 Herewiþ] *foll. by* he *canc.* R

Emoraide os it is saide, fikis also Y saide. *Condilomate* ar saide of þis worde *condilon* or elles [f. 110vb] of þis worde *condilus* and of þis worde *meta*, i. a merke or elles a likenesse. For þai ar knoddes and knorles in the fleshe, like þe hedes of whirlebones. *Condilon* & *condilus*, I saide beforne. 130

[3.19]

De ypostasi in vrina: c. 19

Ypostasis, <u>os I saide in þe first boke, þe 3 c., lef</u> {2}, is but superfluyte of þe 3 digestioun. How fele digestions and which þai ben <u>þou hast in þe j bok, þe 3 c., lef</u> {2}. And euery of þe 3 digestions hath his propre superfluyte and purgacioun and clensing and his delyuerance, <u>os I saide in þe same c.</u>   5

And for to know parfitely *ypostasis* in vryn, þise ar þe 5 propretes[1] þerof: colour, substance, place, tyme, & figure. Os anentes þe j poynt, vnderstonde þat þe kynde colour of *ypostasis* oweþ euermore for to be white. Þe philosophie is þis: alle þe membres in man ar white be waie of kynde. For þogh it so be þat it be rede to þe sight, noghtforþan þat is noȝt þe kynde   10
colour þerof, but it is coloure of blode þat is disperplede by þe pores of þe fleishe. For when þe blode is wrongen oute, as the Yrish men serue here fleishe þat þai eten, or elles if it be soden or rostede os we Englismen done, þe fleishe blecheþ & torneth toward his propre colour.

[f. 111ra] Now þe fode in mannes body turneþ noght into þe kynd of þe   15
membres and lymes of þe body til it be so þat it haue firste taken swiche colour os is kyndly answerand to þo membres and lymes, wiþ þe whiche membres & lyms þat fode schal be incorporat wiþ. For þe fode is noþing elles but an assimulacioun, i. a kyndely liknesse, a kyndely turnyng of þat þing þat nursheþ into þat thing þat is nurshede. *Ergo*, syn þe membr[e]s[2]   20
and þe lymes of þe body ar kyndely white, þe fode also moste be kyndely white.

Þan ferþermore, euery *ypostasis* is desisede & dyryuyed fro þe fode and fro þo membres, s. of alle þe membres of þe 3 digestioun. *Ergo*, syn þo ar white kyndely, þat oweþ for to be white kyndely. For *ypostasis* is noȝt elles   25
but superfluyte of þe 3 digestioun. And euery superfluyte spekand to þis purpose oweþ for to be like and answerand in kynde to þat þing or to þo þinges of which he is desisede and diriuiede, i. þat he cometh of. And þis

---

1 5 propretes] *marg.*: 5 propretes of ypostasy
2 membres] GSc, menbres M7, membrs R

is þe cause whi þat none *ypostasis* in vryn is gode ne kynde *ypostasis*, but whit alone. For onely swich *ypostasis* seiþ euermore parfit assimulacioun,   30
i. accordyng of þe fode wiþ þe **[f. 111rb]** membres vpon the mater and the kynde of bothe. And also it is verray tokne þat kynde hete is of myght and power for to make gode digestioun and maistre þe malady.

But one may saie aʒeyne me, "*Contra!* Alle auctoures in þis faculte seyen and techen þat *extremi colores* (*anglice*: þe vttereste coloures),[3] s.   35
White colour and B[l]ake[4] colour, þat ar callede so for alse mykel os al oþer coloures ar but mene atwene hem and componede of hem 2. And þo 2 ar þe werste colours þat ar or may be in vryn or in Ypostasy, for White colour in vryn or in Ypostasy seiþ frigidite and indigestioun, & Blak colour, mor-tificacioun, as þou haste in þe 2 boke, þe j c., lef {17}, and in c. *de nigro*   40
colore in diuerse places, and in c. *de albo colore*, in þe j ende."

I answer þat þer is 2 maner of whitehed[5] in vryn and in Ypostasi: one þat is watrish and wannysh and þis is noght propurly Whit colour, in Ypo-stasy no more þan in vryn, but it is propurly watrish colour or wan white colour, be it in vryn, be it in Ypostasi. Of which maner White colour spek-   45
eþ al þe 4 c. of þe 2 bok. And som saie þat wan whit colour in Ypostasi or in vryn, wheþer it be, it seiþ bigynnyng of digestioun.

Anoþer maner of whitehede þere is in **[f. 111va]** Ypostasy and in vryn: þat is brigh mylk white. And þis maner of whitehede, be it in vryn or be it in *ypostasis*, auctoures callen it *candor* (*anglice*: bright white or elles   50
schynand white). And þis colour in Ypostasi alle auctours comenden. For it seiþ euermor þat wirkyng of kynde hete is as parfit & as redy toward as possible is, for þe wirkyng of kynde hete is kyndly to þat ende for to make & wirke. White and whithede is of þe kynde of lyʒt and of brighnesse.

Þe secunde condicioun, þe 2 proprete, of *ypostasis* is his substance, i.   55
þe body þerof, þat þe body of him be continual & equal, i. þat it be hold-and togedre, and oueral alike hole and noʒt tobroken, here a clod & ʒond anoþer. For when it is wiþouten interrupcioun, i. wiþouten eny brekyng, it seiþ þe 3 digestion is gode and parfit and þer is no ventosite for þe tyme, for to breken ne for to letten him. For if he be interrupt, þat is noght but   60
by cause of ventosite in þe 3 digestioun.

The propre and þe kynd place of *ypostasis* is þe botume. *Et* vnderstand þat *ypostasis* somtym halt him beneþe in þe botume of þe vryn, & somtym in myddes of þe vryn & somtym it houeþ abouen in þe vryn. & vpon þise 3 maner of **[f. 111vb]** places, Ypostasy hath 3 maner of names. Whan it is in   65

---

3   coloures] *foll. by* ar *canc.* R
4   blake] blak GSc, brake RM7
5   2 maner of whitehed] *marg.*: double whitnes

þe botume, it is propurly callede *ypostasis* or *sedimen*. *Ypostasis* is saide of þis word of Gru *ypos*, i. *sub* (*anglice*: beneþen or vnder) and of þis worde *stasis*, i. *stacio* (*anglice*: stondyng). For *ypostasis* propurly stant beneþe in þe botume. *Sedimen* is saide of þis worde in Latyn *sedere* (*anglice*: sitten), for it halt him in þe grounde of þe vryn.   70

When it is in the myddes of þe vryn it is called *eneorima* and *ypostasis dependens*. *Eneorima* is as mykel for to sai as *dependens* (*anglice*: hong-and), for when it is in þe myddes of þe vryn, it is os it were hongand. & so *ypostasis dependens* & *eneorima* ar al on for to saie. But when it houeþ abouen in þe ouer parti of þe vryn, þan is it callede *nephilis*, i. *nubes*   75
(*anglice*: a sky). For wete wel euermore þat be it *sedimen* or be it *eneorima* or be it *nephilis*, os Y haue said ryȝt nowe, euermore it is moste like a roke or a cloude or a sky. And euermore when it is lowe in þe botume, it is tokne þat digestion is noght desturblid ne letted wiþ ventosite. For þe hier þat *ypostasis* be in þe vryn, þe more tokne it is of ventosite.   80

Tyme of *ypostasis* is longe [f. 112ra] lastyng, s. be dyuerse daies togedre, os 2 or 3 or mo. Os if one make an vryn þis dai wiþ gode *ypostasis*, & þe vryn þat he maketh tomorwe appere þe same maner of *ypostasis*. And þe mo daies togedre, þe bettre. For if it do so, it is tokne þat kynde is strong and myghty in himselfe and of power for to cont[i]nuen[6] his wirkyng   85
in defiying. For if it so be þat *ypostasis* apere one dai wiþ gode tokenes and anoþer daie wiþ wickede tokenes, it kepeþ noght his tyme, but he is vnstable & vnstedefaste. And þat ilk vnstedfasthede is tokne of feblenesse of kynde, and þat kynde is vnstedefaste & vnmyghty for to fulfille his wirkyng. Þe gode tokenes of *ypostasis* ar þise 5 propretes þat I spak of,   90
wicked tokenes *e contrario*. And wete wel þat if *ypostasis* laste longe and gode, it is þe beste tokne þat mai ben in vryn; longe and wicked þe werst þat may ben. Item, litil while gode is wik and litil tyme wik is gode.

Þe 5 condicioun or elles þe 5 propurte of a kynde *ypostasis* is his forme, his schap. For if it be a kynde *ypostasis*, it begynneth brode be- [f. 112rb]   95
neþen and euen alike round al abouten, euer þe longer þe scharper and scharper vpward, lik a pere or a pynote. And þat seiþ parfite digestioun.

And os Y saide in þe j boke, 3. c., lef {4}, in hele folkes vryn is none *ypostasis* or elles oneþes eny. For in hole folke is þe superfluyte of þe 3 digestioun disquasht and consumpt þrogh mygh of kynd hete and also be   100
cause þat þe membres in hole folke ar of gode fode. Wherfore þer beleuyth no superfluytes and by skil þerof litle *ypostasis* or elles non. And þerfor if *ypostasis* faile eny one of þise forsaide 5 condiciouns, þogh it haue alle þe toþer 4 condiciouns, it is noȝt kynde *ypostasis*, but it is callede *ypostasis*

---

6   continuen] contynue GSc, contnuen R, coninuen M7

innaturalis (*anglice*: an vnkynd *ypostasis*), for if it haue noȝt þe schap, os Y 105
saide, it is tokne þat þe 3 digestioun is noght gode. If it kepe him no while,
os but one daie or 2 att þe most, it is os Y saide. If it kepe him noght in his
kynde place, as I saide also. If it be interrupt, os I saide. If he haue noȝt his
kynde coloure, os I saide.

And also riȝt os[7] auctours techen, nerhand al coloures mowe ben in 110
ypostasis. Of white Ypostasi is sufficiently saide. Þe beste colour in *ypo-*
stasis after white colour is rede coloure, [**f. 112va**] for it is leste wicked.
Noȝtforþan *rubea ypostasis*[8] euermore seiþ longe sekenes, and þat be cause
of plente of mater, noȝt be cause of crudite, for *sanguis fleumaticus* is in
cause. But þogh it saie longe sekenesse, os comunly a febre, noȝtforþan it 115
is but *febris eucrita, febris eutrica*, or *egritudo eutrica*, i. a febre or a sekenesse þat wil wel enden & scapen. *Eutricus morbus est bene terminabilis.*
Eutricus is saide of þis worde *eu*, i. *bonum* (*anglice*: gode) and of þis word
crisis (*anglice*: warshing of sekenes or elles a demyng, <u>as þou hast in þe 2</u>
<u>bok, c. *de nigro colore*, lef</u> {23}). 120

And þerfor *ypostasis rubea* seiþ discrasioun of body, i. sekenesse in
body, but noȝt to deþ. For þe mater þat causeþ þat sekenes, s. *sanguis*
fleumaticus, is light and resolubile and tempre. Liȝt in himselfe be resoun
þat it is *calidus & humidus*, by þe kynde of blode; resoluble, i. eþi for to
be resoluede and defiede and for to be ouercomen, be cause of þe qualitees 125
of blode, s. calidite & humidite. For þo 2 qualites principaly causen and
make gode digestioun.

If þe mater, s. þe humor, were crude and compacte and harde for to
resoluen and to defien, þe vryn shulde be wattrishe. If þe mater wer adust,
þe vryn schulde be grose and þik,[9] and so schulde þer none *ypostasis* 130
appere. For *ypostasis* neuermore appereth but in vryn cler [**f. 112vb**] or
elles menely cler. But be cause þat þe matere is resoluble, os Y saide, þe
vryn is mene and *ypostasis* rede. Item, the mater is tempre, for it stant be
þo qualities þat ar moste wirkyng and moste tempre in kyn[d],[10] s. calidite
& humidite, for in hote and moyst stant lif of euery beste. 135

This is temperure and þe proporcioun of þe 4 qualitees in man, s. þat
mannes body haue double of blode to *fleuma*, and double of *fleuma* to
colre, and double of colre to melancolie.

Now perauentur one wil saien þat it is agayn resoun þat eny *ypostasis*
shulde be rede or of eny colour saue white alone. For *ypostasis* is euermore 140

---

7 os] *foll. by* as *canc.* R
8 rubea ypostasis] *marg.*: rede ypostasis
9 þik] thikke GSc, þrik RM7
10 kynd] kynde M7GSc, kyng R

superfluyte of þe 3 digestioun and is desi[s]ed[11] fro þe membres, and þe
membres ar white be waie of kynde and þe fode is white, and þat þat is
desisede fro hem schulde be swich colour os þai ben. Wherfor it semeth
wel by skil and os I saide beforn, þat *ypostasis* schulde euermore be onely
white. I answere þat þer is som *ypostasis* þat is digested & parfit & som þat   145
is indigested and vnparfite. For to speke of þe j maner *ypostasis*, so is none
ypostasis but white; for to speke on þe 2 wise, so is none *ypostasis* white.
Herewiþ accordiþ Gilbert in his Coment vppon Giles, and he folweþ þe
sentence of Ysaac, þat putteþ 2 maner of colours[12] [f. 113ra] in Ypostasy
or it come to white colour, s. rede and ȝelowe. For when *sanguis* is but a   150
partie digestede, firste he takeþ a rede colour or elles a rody colour somdel
toward white; and whan þat colour is more digestede, it is ȝelow; and att
laste it is white. *Et* þerfor, when on seiþ þat *ypostasis* is euermore superfluyte of þe 3 digestioun or elles þat euery Ypostasi is superfluyte of þe 3
digestioun, þat is soth. But os it semeth wel by Ysaac and by Gilbert, os   155
Y saide riȝt now, þe conclusioun of the argument suyth noght. For þer is
dyuerse maner of digestioun, s. gode and feble & more feble, and vppon
þat is þe colour in Ypostasy.

　Subrubea ypostasis[13] hath but litle or elles vnneþes of redhede, but it is
moste wan watrish & it is werse þan *ypostasis rubea*. For it seiþ distem-   160
perure and sekenesse of sausfleume, wattri and rawe, and also indigestioun. And þerfor it bitokeneþ longe sekenesse and stronge, be cause of
crudite of þe mater, but noghtforþan stronge perrile is þere none, in alse
mykel os it is of mater sanguine, þat moste is tempre of alle materes.

　But wonder þing it semeth þat *subrubea ypostasis* schulde be werse and   165
more perilouse þan *rubea ypostasis*. For syn [f. 113rb] *ypostasis alba*, os it
is saide, is þe beste *ypostasis* þat may be, & *rubea ypostasis* is ferther fro
alba Ypostasy þan is *subrubea ypostasis* (for *subrubea ypostasis* is a mene
coloure bitwene *alba & rubea*, for he may noght passe ne change oute of
rede colour into whit colour but by þe mene atwene boþe), *ergo*, *subru-*   170
beus ypostasis is more nere and more answerand kyndely to white *ypostasis*
þan *rubea* Ypostasy. For þat þat is more answerand and more ner to best
is bettre of þe 2. *Ergo*, syn *subrubea ypostasis* is more nere to whit þan is
rede *ypostasis*, it is lesse wicked þan is *rubea ypostasis*.

　Þus answeren auctours and seyn þat *subrubea ypostasis* is ferþer fro *alba*   175
Ypostasy þan is *rubea ypostasis*. For *subrubea ypostasis* is noȝt of mene
digestioun os *rubea ypostasis* is, but it is of a sang aquouse and crude,
whiche sang aquouse & crude, be cause of his crudite, may noght be
decocte ne defiede ne couenablie vnderfongen þe kynde colour of rede.

11　desised] decysed GSc, desided RM7
12　colours] *catchword*: in ypostasy or
13　Subrubea ypostasis] *marg.*: redishe ypostasi

And þerfor os be waie of digestioun, *rubeus ypostasis* is more ner white   180
ypostasis þan *subrubea ypostasis.*

Noghtforþan vnderstonde þat þer is 2 maner of subrube: one þat goth
aforn rube, vppon þat it takeþ rede colour litle & litle, as we sen at eye in
meny þinges; and þis maner [**f. 113va**] of *subrubea* is fer fro decoccioun.
For it is but toward redehede os redehede is toward whitehed, and þerfor   185
subrubea ypostasis on þis wise, os be waie of decoccioun, is more fer fro
alba ypostasis þan is *rubea ypostasis*, and in so myke is *subrubea ypostasis*
werse þan *rubea ypostasis.*

Anoþer maner þer is of subrube þat cometh after rede in decoccioun.
For in decoccioun and digestioun, rube passeth by subrube or he come to   190
white. And o þis maner for to take subrube, is *subrubea ypostasis* bettre
þan *rubeus*, os þou seest. But vnderstonde þat subrube, os it is taken in þe
j wise, it is wan wattry and dedish in colour, and in þe 2 wise it is more
quyk [bryȝttisch].¹⁴

*Liuida ypostasis*¹⁵ is wel werse þan *subrubea*, for it seiþ mortificacion.   195
<u>Mortificacio: in þe 2 bok, þe j c., lef</u> {18}.

Ypostasis viridis or elles *ypostasis nigra*,¹⁶ wheþer it be, is moste perilouse. For it seiþ mortificacion in so mykel þat kynde hete is so consumpt and quenchede þat þer is no recouerer. And take gode hede þat
somtyme þer appereþ in the vryn *sedimen nigrum* and somtyme *eneorima*   200
nigrum. Sedimen and *eneorima* I saide before. *Sedimen nigrum* is werse
þan *eneorima nigrum* and noghtforþan *eneorima nigrum* hath [**f. 113vb**]
mo wicked tokenes þan *sedimen nigrum*. For *eneorima nigrum* is wik in
2 poyntes: for his colour is wik & his place is wik. But *sedimen nigrum*,
his colour is wik & his place is gode. But þat one defaute þat *sedimen*   205
nigrum hath is werse þan bothe defautes þat *eneorima nigrum* hath. For
his one passeth þe toþer two in malice. Þat *sedimen nigrum* halt him so in
þe botme is bi cause of plente of malice & of terrestrihede & of vnablete of
decoccioun & digestion. For it is tokne þat kynd is so mykel consumpt þat
þer is noȝt so mykel kynde hete in the body that may maken or sufficiently   210
helpen for to make eny resolucion of þe wickede humores. And for alse
mykel os þer is no resolucioun ne no helpe toward, þrogh kynde hete þer
is no ventosite in the body ne no maner cause þat may helpe for to dryuen
ne for to cache vp ne for to put vp þat ilke *sedimen* vpward into þe vryn.
And þerfor it is bot tokne of deth.   215

But *eneorima nigrum*, þogh it so be þat it be tokne of consumpcioun
of kynde hete, os doþ *sedimen nigrum* also, noȝtforþan be cause þat þer is
impulsioun, i. caching vp, which vp-caching is caused of som ventosite (for

---

14 bryȝttisch] G, bright Sc, byttriche R, bittrische M7
15 Liuida ypostasis] *marg.*: blo ypostasy
16 ypostasis nigra] *marg.*: Grene & blak ypostasy

alwaie when it is on **[f. 114ra]** lofte in the vryn, þat is tokne of somme ventosite), þat is tokne of som myght of kynd & of kynde hete, þogh it be litle.   220

Et þerfor, os Gilbert seiþ, *sedimen nigrum* is worse in himself þan *eneorima nigrum* or þan *nephilis nigra*. For þer is no helpe of kynde hete
for to resoluen ne to suptilen ne for to maistreen þe humores. But if it be
eneori[m]a[17] *nigrum* or *nephilis nigra*, in som wise ʒit it may, for myʒt of
kynde hete somdel helpeþ vp þe *ypostasis* in þe vryn, os we seen in ʒonge   225
folk þat gone vpriʒt be cause of myʒt & plente of kynde hete. But olde
folk, be cause of failyng of kynd hete, gone stoupand.

But when *ypostasis nigra* holt him low in þe botume, it seiþ þat þe mater
is wel heuy & wol mykel, and þat kynde is wel feble and impotent for to
wirken and wiþouten help & þat kynde faileþ and þerfor þer is noght but   230
deþ. How & wherof is ventosite causede & gendred in þe body þou hast in
the 2 bok, c. *de albo colore,* lef {40}. And þerfor auctours techen þat *nigra*
ypostasis, þe hier þat it be in þe vryn, þe lesse peril it is.

Item, tak þis for a reule, os al auctoures teche, þat riʒt os noght euery
whitehede in *ypostasis* is for to preise **[f. 114rb]** (as þou maist se by þe proces   235
aforn, þer I spake of 2 maner of whithede in *ypostasis*), riʒt so noʒt euery
blakhede in Ypostasi is for to blame ne for to doute of. For sumtym *ypo-*
stasis appereþ blak by cause of melancolie, & þat comunly in dissoluyng
þerof, os in curyng of þe febre quarteyne, & also in drying of þe floures
agayn bristing oute of hem towarde helth, or elles in þe bresting oute of þe   240
floures after dryng of hem. *Et* somtyme *ypostasis* is blak by cause of adustioun & somtym by cause of mortificacioun, as þou haste in þe 2 bok, c. of
Blak colour. In þe 2 first wises, it is tokne of warshing; in þe 2 laste wise, it
is tokne of dying. For if *ypostasis* be blak by cause of adustioun, kynde hete
is consumpt to þe ful; if it be blak by cause of mortificacioun, kynde hete is   245
quenchede & consumpt þrouʒ plente & malice of mater of þe malady.

[3.20, "The Rules of Isaac"]

[Prologue]

I haue spoken al þe hole doctrine of alle þe doctours þat I myʒt haue in
handes of þis faculte. Now shal Y saie the reules þat Isaac ʒeueþ in þe laste
ende of his *Bok of Vryn*, so þat whoso may noʒt conyn þe substance &
þe wel of þo þinges þat ar saide beforne or ellez perauenture he may noʒt

---

17 eneorima] M7G, eneorma Sc, eneorina R

reporten hem by hert, lat him holde him paiede wiþ comune reules shortly   5
ʒifen. As whoso may noʒt tochen þe gode myʒty marow wiþin þe bone, lat
him be paiede wiþ þat þat is wiþouten. And whoso may noʒt haue of þe
gauelles, let him glene after þe bynderes.

**Of general reules which Isaac putteþ in þe 10 bok of his *Vryns*, and
first of vryn citryne**   10

Urina citrina & suptil & thenne and clere in a febre seiþ þat þat malady
   wil longe laste. In a febre acue we ar noght certeyn wheþer þe
   [**f. 114va**] pacient may scape or noght.
Item, vryn citrin or subcitrin and suptil wiþ a white *ypostasis* in on þat is
   trauailede wiþ a febre is wickede tokne.   15
Item, þe same maner of vryn in þe bigynnyng of þe febre it betokeneþ
   spasmus. *Spasmus & tetanus* in þe last c. of þe 2 bok, lef {84}.[1]
Item, citrin and suptil in an acue is euermore wik.
Item, citrin and suptil with a[2] white ypostasy & þe body of þe vryn
   diuerse, i. somtyme more and somtym lasse, & wiþ *furfura* it is drede-   20
   ful. *Furfura* in þe 13 c., lef {101}.
Item, colrik vryn, i. citrin, in a febre trauailouse: wik & in þe bygynnyng
   of þe malady, forþan it seiþ þat he shal falle into a spasme.
Þe same vryn in paralitik folk hauand none appetit and also stiptik is
   noble tokne.   25
Item, *vrina colerica* & spumouse, i. froþi, abouen & beforn þat vryn went
   a white vryn and if he berst oute of blode at þe nose, it is wik.
Item, *vrina colerica* in dai of creticacioun, and namely in þe 4 daie for
   to telle by ordre, and þerwiþ þer appere a rede skie on þe vryn: gode
   tokne. Of creticacioun and of cretik daies os techeþ Isaac in þe   30
   [**f. 114vb**] 2 bok, c. *de nigro colore*, lef {22}. *De nebulis* (*anglice:* of
   skyes in þe vryn): in þe c. *de nebulis*, lef {90}.
Item, *vrina colerica* in an acue wiþ a white *ypostasis* is ful wik, for it seiþ
   þat þe mater is compacte and crude.

De alba vrina   35

Alba vrina in an acue wiþ ake in þe hed and wiþ litle slepe and wiþ
   rauyng & wilhede is tokne of sone deth.

---

1 *Most of the leaf cross-references in the "Rules of Isaac" are written on the line in the
   text, rather than in the margins.*
2 with a] *foll. by* wiþ a *canc.* R

Vryn whit & suptil in þe jawnys wik, for it [be]tokneþ³ a wik ydropisi
folwend.

Vryn white and subtil in an acue euermore wik.   40

Vryn white & suptil wiþ ake and peyne aboute þe reynes and þe lendes
seiþ oppilacioun [in]⁴ the waies of þe vryn be cause of gros fleume; in
a febre, oppilacioun of gros colre.

Vryn white & gros apperande in cretik dai, and namely in þe 4 day, seiþ
warshing of *passio artetica* and delyuerance of gadring of wicked mater   45
in þe hede and in þe eeris.

Þe same maner of vryn, if it appere after a warshing, it seiþ þat þe malady
wil come agayne.

Vryn white and gros, wiþ icche aboute þe neþer parties of þe wombe, it
seiþ þat grauel is for to brede in þe vesie.   50

Vryn white and grose in a **[f. 115ra]** lent febre is anguyssh & dredeful.

Vryn white and gros wiþ non *ypostasis*: peyne & drede of dethe.

Vryn white and gros and derk and dym lyke oyle: deþ.

Vryn white, grosse, & nebulouse or spumouse: wol wik.

Vryn white with a sky like an oynyoun: sekenes in þe reynes and longe   55
lastyng.

Vryn white and with an euel sauoure: wik, for it seiþ þat þe humores in
þe body ar wicked & dede & roten.

Vryn white & gros and os it wer spumouse: lesyng & failyng of kynde.
And comunly when an vryn scheweþ him so, ther is sekenes & peyn   60
[in]⁵ þe riȝt ypocundre.

Vryn whit & groos in an acue & in a frenesy & peyne in þe ypocondre,
and namely if it be in bothe þe ypocondres, it is drede.

Wryn white os attre and quyttre in an hote febre: wik, and namely in a frenesi.

Vryn white & gros & none *ypostasis* seiþ humors gros & viscouse.   65

Vryn white & gros and longe tyme lastend so and noght chaungeyng seiþ
þat þe stone is for to brede in þe reynes.

De alba & aquosa vrina

Vryna cruda & aquosa, i. vryn wan and wattri, and subtil, i. thenne &
bright, if **[f. 115rb]** it kep[e]⁶ him so eny while, it is tokne of super- 70
fluyte of moyst humores.

---

3 betokneþ] GSc, is tokneþ RM7
4 in] GSc, *om.* RM7
5 in] GSc, and RM7
6 kepe] M7GSc, kept R

If in a lente febre, collecioun of ewe citrin in þe body.

Vryn aquouse wiþ peyn in þe ypocondre seiþ ouerdone humidite of
humores in þe veyns.

Vryn aquouse and afor þat went rede vryn and þat in a febre: scapying of   75
þe febre.

Vryn aquouse if it come out litle & litle & longe and it so be in the jawnys, it seiþ þat he schal falle into an ydropisi.

Vryn aquouse continuely: ravyng and woodhede. But if kynde rise and
encresce & maistrie þe wicked humores, it seiþ warshing of þe febre   80
and mendyng of mynde.

If þe vryn haue no sky in þe bygynnyng of þe acue, it schal be wik.

Vryns aquose & hauand in him like a water leche or elles like a wilde
fecche in an acue: wik.

Vryn crude in þe bigynning of a febre and oþer tokenes be gode, he schal   85
be travailede wiþ þe febre.

Vryn crude in þe bigynnyng of a febre is gode. Inwarde in þe febre &
negh creticacioun: ful wik.

Vryn crude & dym in colour and none *ypostasis*: ful wik.

Vryn crude in the begynning of an acue and wiþ *ypostasis* mykel [f. 115va]   90
like thik mele: þat he schal smyte into a ravyng & into a spasme.

De rubea vrina

Rubea vrina in an acue: gode.

Rubea vrina & mykel and wiþ a white *ypostasis* and þe more white þe
bettre: warshing of þe febre.   95

If þe vryn turne & change into litle & suptil, þe febre wil be more stronge
and haraiouse and after þat slaken.

Rubea vrina & pure & bright and suptil is ful perilouse.

Rubea & suptil & liȝt: *artetica passio* and rauyng & woodnesse. <u>*Artetica
passio* and his spices in c. *de attomis,* lef</u> {104}.   100

Rubeu and stynkand & wiþ a blak *ypostasis* & drubly and wiþ bodycs
like heres or elles lik thynges muselynges of paxwax: ful wik tokne &
deth.

Rubea vrina in yleoun: ful wik. Yleon & <u>*yliaca passio* al on: se in þe c. *de
inopos & kyanos,* lef</u> {77}.   105

Rubea wiþ none *ypostasis*: wik.

Vrina rubea & gros, not clarifiand himself, and þerwiþ ake aboute þe eres
and þe þonewynges & defhede & peyne in þe hede & peyn in þe epi-
condre seiþ þat a wik & perilouse jawenys is for to comen [f. 115vb]
wiþin þe 7 day.   110

If he change & turne into more suptil and wiþ a kynd *ypostasis*, dym in
   colour & wiþ oþer gode tokenes, it seiþ þat þe sekenesse wil aslaken &
   þat rauyng wil him taken.
Vrina rubea & gros in an acue seyþ ake in þe hede and peyne in the
   ypocond[r]e⁷ and heuynesse & greuance aboute þe nek.   115
Vrina rubea & litle & pur in ydropisy: deþ.
Vryn rede as blode or elles os wyn & none ake in the hede seiþ þat þe
   febre wil be trauailouse, i. it wil him trauailen & al toschaken.
If þe vryn kepe him so stil longe tyme: þat þe stone wil brede in þe vesie.
Vryn rede like colour of blode & litil & suptil: wik & namely in hem   120
   þat ar sciatik and in women þat delyuerne hem of childe longe or here
   tyme: ful wik.
Vryn rede os blode in an acue: sodeyn deth.
Vryn rede & in þe 3 region aboue white: sekenesse & peyne in þe hed &
   ravyng & wodenesse.   125
Vryn rede wiþ braking, rede, rousty, & wiþ ruhhed [**f. 116ra**] &
   scharphede in the tonge: deth.
[Vryn rede like colour of blode in an acue & with quakyng at þe hert &
   peyn in þe riȝt ypocondre: tokne of deþ.]⁸
Whoso make blode & þat sodeynly, it seiþ þat som veyn in the reyns or   130
   in þe lyuer or elles som veyn by which the blode of womannes floures
   passen by is bur[s]ten⁹ or quayste & brusede.

De rufa vrina

Rufa vrina seiþ maistre of colre.
Vryn ruf and subtil with an acue & none Ypostasi seiþ þat day shal be   135
   stronge & haragiouse to him. And if his vryn laste longe tyme swich
   vertu and kynde shal faile.
Vryn ruf & litle in a jawnys seiþ warshing.
Vryn wiþ a febre & wiþ a frenesi: ful wik; with ake in the hede: ful
   perilouse.   140
Vryn ruf & spumouse, in coloure mykel like spume of wyn: raveyng &
   wodenesse.
Vryn ruf wiþ a blak *ypostasis*: wik & namely in a frenesie.

---

7 ypocondre] M7GSc, ypoconde R
8 Vrin rede … deþ] GSc, *om.* RM7
9 bursten] M7, berst Sc, brostyn G, burten R

De viridi vrina

Grene vryn in þe cretik dai & with hede ake seiþ swageing & reles of   145
    peyne.
Grene vryn in a brennand febre: rauyng & wodenesse.
If it be a lent febre & þerwiþ he drynk mykel water, it seith consump-
    cioun of al the body.
Grene vryn or elles like sulphur in a brenand febre, if þe pacient be   150
    mykel ouergone therwith and wonder lene & feble & he swete on his
    body and [f. 116rb] fele colde in the extremytees, it seiþ þat he schal
    smyte into a wickede & perilouse spasme.
Grene vryn and os þoȝ it wer rousty, seith þat he schal smyte into a
    spasme.   155

De nigra vrina

Blak vryn in mykel folk is tokne of deth.
Blak vryn in an acue with a blak *ypostasis* noght in the botme but vpward
    in the vryn & þerwiþ mykel wakyng, i. litle slepe, and wiþ defhede, it
    is tokne þat þe malady wil longe laste and solucioun, i. warshing, and   160
    cesyng of the malady with a bledyng att the nose.
Blak vryn in a brennand febre and greuance in the hede, anguysshe
    and rauyng and failyng of mynde and of wit in tyme of creticacioun:
    warshing wiþ a bledyng, and þat principaly in women þat haue for-
    gone her floures.   165
Vryn blak and grose in an acue: þe spasme. And if he suffre rauyng, it
    seiþ wlatyng of mete & after þat, deth.
Vryn blak as blode that is swart & dym in a pleuresie: deth.
Vryn blak in an acue and wiþ an ypostasi diuerse, i. noȝt hoole but in
    dyuerse plottes and parties, & [f. 116va] if swich ypostasi chaunge   170
    often tyme his coloure: deþ.
Vryn blak in an acue & wiþ an euel sauour & swetynge in þe neþer par-
    ties: deþ.
Vryn blake & stynkand & no sekenes of þe vesie: deth.

De oleagina vrina   175

Vrina oleagina (anglice: oilish vryn) & wiþ an ypostasi hool & noȝt
    brekyng ne diuersede in diuerse parties and it so be þat þe pacient
    befor colde: gode.

Vrina oleagina with as it were an areyns web abouen: consumpcioun of
   substancial humidite in þe body.   180
Vryn viscouse os oyle, i. towȝ & byndand as oyle: also consumpcioun of
   substancial humydite.
Vryn euery dai chaungeand his [colour]¹⁰: consumpcioun of body and
   wastyng of kynde.
Vryn euer[y]¹¹ day chaungeable: ful wik, & namely in aposteme of the   185
   myddrede.
Vryn dym in an acue: a ful wik crise is for to come.
Vryn lik rust of [yren]¹² in an acue: þe spasme for to comen.
Vryn swart & dym & like roust of yren in a lent febre: þe stranguyrie.

De lucida et clara vrina   190

Vryn briȝt & clere in an acue seiþ ake & peyne in the hede.
Vryn briȝt & clere & white shiere in an acue: a perilouse **[f. 116vb]** alienacioun. Þan is þe pacient alienat when he is oute of witte & hath lorn
   mynde.
Vryn brigh & wel cocte: gode splene.   195
Vryn bright in masing & stonyng of mynde: alienacioun wiþ a febre.
Vryn bright with *ypostasis* viscouse, & þe vryn be lik briȝt metal or swich
   a þing & þerwiþ ake & sekenesse in þe wombe or aboute the splene
   or the schore or the ȝerde or þe value or elles wiþ peyne aboute al þo
   places, seyth consumpcioun of þe reynes or elles scabbe or sekenesse   200
   of the vesie. If it so be þat þer be no peyn in the forsaide places, it seiþ
   consumpcion of oþer membres & places in the body.
Vryn subtil & bright & clere: peyne & sekenes of membres in the body,
   and namely in the spirituales.
Vryn subtil, liȝt, & wattri & more in quantite þan þe water þat he drank: 205
   stronge perile.
Vryn subtil in an acue wiþ ake in þe hede & aboute þe nek & þe bak: wik.
Vryn subtil in the ende of a febre seiþ þat him shal brede aposteme of the
   lyuer.
Vryn subtil in an acue wiþ *ypostasis natant*, i. swymmand or houand, in   210
   þe vryn: alienacioun.
Vryn subtil with alienacioun: wick.

---

10   colour] GSc, *om.* RM7
11   euery] M7GSc, euer R
12   yren] Sc, irn *or* iru*n* G, vrey (*with* v *underpuncted*; y *written over* n?) R, vrey M7

Vryn subtil wiþ alienacioun & it haue an *ypostasis* grosse **[f. 117ra]** and
crude: drede.

Vryn subtil & mykel in a pleuresie and þerwiþ a drie coghe: alienacioun   215
of mynde. If þer come a bledyng at þe nose or elles a gode swete, þe
malady passeþ [awey].[13]

Vryn subtil turnede into a rede coloure & wiþ *ypostasis* whit and grosse:
warshing is nere & þat with a swete.

Vryn subtil saue os it were blak in colour & wiþ greuance in the hede and   220
in þe bak: grete gusshing of blode for to come at þe nose.

Vryn subtil saue as it were blakish & wiþ ypostasy *natant* & þat in an
acue: grete gusshing of blode at þe nose & swetyng and warshing.

Vryn subtil somde[le][14] blakish or toward colour of blode & wiþ a blak
ypostasis & wiþ a wik sour odour: grete drede.   225

Vryn subtil wiþ a brennand febre & blakish & mykel oylish: deth. In
olde folk seke: the falland euyl.

De turbida vrina

Vryn alwaie grosse & droublie and wiþ greuance in the hede seiþ þat a
febre is for to comen.   230

Vryn grosse & droublie & noʒt changeand himself & þe tokenes ben
gode: gode.

Vryn grose & noʒt clerand himself & wiþ a maner of *ypostasis* abouen
seiþ ventosite in þe body grete & inflatif, i. swelland, and bolnand the
body. Þat ilk *ypostasis* that **[f. 117rb]** wolde schewe him in the vryn is   235
so lifte alofte in the vryn þrogh ventosite & is so myxt wiþ grosehede
& trublishede in þe vryn þat it may noʒt descende ne appere kyndely[15]
as he schulde in the vryn. And þerfor swich vryn seiþ, os Y saide, ake
in the hede or þat now i[s][16] or þat is for to comen.

But so is it noʒt in þe vryn of hole folk, for þogh þe vryn be þik & drou-   240
bly when it is hote & newe made, it clereþ when it coleth and þat is by
reson þat hete lifteþ vp and meueþ vpward & colde downward, riʒt os
we sene þat water, be it salt or be it freish, comunly when it is warme,
it is more þik; when it is colde, thenne & clere.

[Vryn gros wiþ greuance in the hede: gode.][17]   245

---

13   passeþ awey] Sc, passeth G, passeþ .v. (v *poss. underpuncted*) R, passeþ .v. M7

14   somdele] M7GSc, somde R

15   kyndely] M7GSc, kyndely (*line end*) kyndely R

16   now is] is now GSc, now it RM7

17   Vryn gros wiþ greuance ... gode] GSaSc, *om.* RM7, *conflated with next sign* T (*this and
      the four following signs from the* Regule Isaac *are preserved fully in beta texts* AG6EW,
      but with varying omissions in alpha witnesses GSaSc T)

[Vryn gros and mykel wiþ ake in the hede or wiþ sekenesse of the lyuer: warshing.]¹⁸

[Vryn gros & droubly & none *ypostasis*: wik.

Vryn gros & mykel in an acue: wik.

Vryn gros & wiþ *ypostasis* & wiþ as it were sheuedys or bren seiþ whelk-   250
es & smale sores on þe vesie.]¹⁹

Vryn whiei white in the bigynnyng of an acue: deþ.

Vryn gros and wheie white & wiþ brakyng, mykel lik roust in colour & wiþ grete drihede in the tunge: deth.

Vryn grosse & mykel & wheie whit wiþ hede ake or sekenes of the lyuer: 255
wik.

Vryn viscouse wiþ peyn of þe reyns: wik.

Vryn mykel in quantite more þan wont or elles litil vryn in the febre: wik.

Vryn more than the water dr[u]nk[e]:²⁰ consumpcioun of body.   260

More than wonte: mundificacioun and clensyng of body in hem þat faste mykel or in [f. 117va] hem that swete mykel, anyntisshyng of substancial humidite, and consumpcioun of body.

Vryn mykil and spisse and none consumpcion seiþ grete multitude and plente of moystehede in þe body.   265

Vryn mykel and spisse wiþ heuyhede and sorehede in the nek and in the body and þe vryn be gode in body and com oute wiþouten peyne, it seiþ warshing, and namely if it haue a white *ypostasis* or grosse or viscouse.

Vryn mykel and viscouse and fattish *in colica passione*: gode.   270

Vryn mykel and viscouse and wiþ ypostasy viscouse in *artetica passione*: gode.

Vryn mykel & grosse in yleon [gode]:²¹ and namely with a white ypostasy.

Vryn [mykel]²² and spisse and aquose or elles a litil redisshe: plente of   275
blode.

Vryn mykel in tyme of cretyng of the febre and wiþ a grete *ypostasis* seith hete and failyng of kynde.

---

18 Vryn gros and mykel … lyuer warshing] A, *om.* RM7GSaSc

19 Vryn gros & droubly … þe vesie] TGSaSc, *om.* RM7

20 the water drunke] þe watir þat he dronke GSc, the water ?drynker *with poorly formed final* r *or* þ R, þe water drynkeþ M7

21 gode] GSc, *om.* RM7

22 mykel] M7GSc, *om.* R

Vryn longe tym apperand wiþ a grete ypostasy in a long lastand febre:
    warshing of the febre.   280
Vryn white and mykel [f. 117vb] and saniouse: þe epilence.
Vryn mykel and comand hastely or elles sodeynly and as blode: brestyng
    and brusshing and blemysshin[g]²³ of som veyne in the reyns or
    þereabouten.
Vryn in hem that haue þe jawnys, if þe vryn be more þan nede and   285
    comune course, is ful wik and namely if it be citrin or toward, for it
    seiþ þat he shal smyte into an ydropesie. And when that cometh, it is
    nedeful þat the vryn be mykel. Wherfor it behoueth for to make and
    for to done þat the vryn may be mykel, os by swich þinges þat cause
    mykel vryn.   290
Vryn somtyme mykel & somtym litle in an acue: ful wik; in a lent febre:
    longe lasting of þe febre.
Vryn litle in an acue: ful wik; if þe ypostasy diuerse him in colour: þat þe
    febre wil be stronge & noyouse and namely in reumatik folk.
Vryn comand litle & litle and droppande: ful wik.   295
Vryn litle in þe bigynnyng & afterward mykel wiþ a rede ypostasy in an
    acue: drede.
Vryn litle & rubicunde: longe lastand malady.
Vryn litil & subtil & as blode in colour: wik.
[f. 118ra] Vryn litle & grosse in an acue: ful wik, & namely in a wombe flux.   300
Vryn stynkand seiþ he is roten wiþin & mortificacioun of kynd.
Vryn if he streyn himself in hem þat haue ake in þe hed, it seiþ þe spasme.
Vryn goyng out agayns his [wil]²⁴ & þerwiþ he haue no sekenes of þe
    reyns ne of þe vesie, it is ful wik & deþ nere.
Vryn sandarik, i. rede os mader: sekenesse & peyne in þe stomac & in þe   305
    hede & in þe brawne & in þe paxwax and in þe schuldres.
Vryn white bothe in men & in women seiþ peyn in þe sydes & somtyme
    in the reyns, but when on þe reynes, it is more drubli in þe botume.
Vryn if it be clere abouen and cloudishe donward & bloish: sekenesse
    aboute þe reyns & þe lendes & þe þies and the knes wiþ defaute of þe   310
    stomak.
Vryn blakish abouen & clerish beneþen: sekenes of þe reyns and ake &
    greuance in þe hede & stopping in þe nose & in þe²⁵ eeris. Fumosite of
    þe stomac makeþ al þat.

---

23   and blemysshing] GSc, and blemysshin RM7
24   his wil] M7GSc, his (line end) R
25   Sc ends here, with the catchword nose & þe

Wryn white and bloish euermore seiþ colde & feblehede.   315
Vryn white & fatish or elles like a horses vryn: sekenesse of þe vesie & of
    þe reyns and somtyme in þe hede.
[f. 118rb] Vryn signifiand sekenes of þe lunges is euermore white &
    pingwse (*anglice*: fatt) & froþi. & þerfor swich maner of vryn seiþ
    peripulmonie.   320
Vryn spoumose abouen seiþ ventosite in þe stomac and sumtyme desire
    to lecherie & somtym colde & coghe.
Whoso be seke of þe lyuer, his vryn is rede & dymysh.
Vryn rede os fire: a tercien.
Vryn rede os blode: *synoca* & causoun.   325
Vryn rede os rose & dym in a febre: þe frenesi. Whoso haue *sinochum*,
    comunly he falleþ into þe frenesi.
In euery maner of acue, if þe vryn be bloysh in colour, it seiþ a frenesie
    for to comen, for *frenesis* is long tyme in comyng.
Vryn in þe pleuresy is kyndely dreggy & dresty in ȝonge folke but   330
    selden die þeron. Elde folk but selden scape. But þai þat scapen of þe
    quarteyn & þerwiþ a pleuresi, þai scapen it noght.
Vryn in ydropisi, if it be ful litil & ruf: noght but deth.
Vryn rusty and with peyne aboute þe hert and aboute þe riȝt ypocondre:
    sodeyne deth.   335
Vryn of ham þat ar cardiac or in a dissenterie or in a yleoun or in ydro-
    pisi, if it be ruf: deth.
Vryn þat stynketh & longe tyme [f. 118va] lasteþ wiþouten chaungeyng,
    it seiþ þat him schal com on sodeyne colde; and by þat colde, brekyng
    of þat malady, but noght to gode.   340
Vryn mykel & white in þe bigynnyng of sekenesse in ȝonge folke: gode
    tokne. & if þer come swich an vryn in þe cretik day or after þat, þe
    malady wil passen. If it be blakish or bloysh, þer shal be perile.
Vryn spumouse after warshing, and it chaunge noght, þat febre wil
    comen aȝein.   345
In alle þise sekenes, s. in þe pthisik, ydropisi, apoplexie, epilence, *peri-*
    pulmonia, palsi, *colica passio*, & in þe dissenterie, if þe vryn be *rubea*, it
    betokeneþ deþ.
In frenesi, in pleuresi, in *cynoca*, & in a tercien, if þe vryn be white &
    bright: deþ.   350

De ypostatibus

Ypostasis os it were þik mele in a longe lastand febre wiþ gode toknes:
    warshing of þe febre. If þe pacient haue aposteme and þe apostem

breke & *ypostasis* in þe vryn kepe him stille, s. os gros mele, þat aposteme shal be his deth, & namely if wik tokenes appere þerwiþ.   355

Ypostasis mykel wiþ a continuel febre, if þe febre abate noght ne slake
noght: consumpcioun of body.

Ypostasis þikke os blode or as [**f. 118vb**] attre or quyttre: longe lastand
malady.

Ypostasis os bren & colour os attri & quytter & þerwiþ helþe in þe reyns   360
& in þe vesie: harde hacches and stronge peyn and trauaile with þe
febre.

Ypostasis mykel & rede, and þe vryn be god & clene in qualite & quantite, i. in colour & in substance, i. in body, seiþ warshing of a febre
after 7 daies.   365

Ypostasis natant, i. noght goand doune to þe botme, wiþ swetyng &
akyng and brennyng & peyne aboute þe ypocondres is dredeful.

De nebulis

A sky apperand o þe vryn after a warisshing scith comyng ageyn of þe
malady.   370

Sky ruf: scharphede of þe sekenes.

Sky lik þik mele: longe lastyng malady.

Sky blak: alienacioun of meende.

Sky blak in a febre interpolate, and þe febre kepe noȝt his interpolacioun,
it seiþ changeing & turnyng into a febre quarteyn.   375

De vrinis mulierum

If a woman make an vryn like an horse or like a nete, it seiþ a febre wiþ
sekenesse of þe value and the matrice.

Vryn of a woman late seruede is a party drubli but litle, wiþ sperme of
the man [**M7, f. 78v**]²⁶ & of here in þe botme, of heir kyndely in þe   380
grounde & of þe man a partie hier.

If þe vryn be mykel droubly & thik, sche had som oþer sekenes when
sche was seruede.

Vryn of a woman when sche hath her floures is os it were blody & dym
& swart & al droubly in þe botume.   385

Vryn of a woman with childe in þe j monyth & in þe 2 & in þe 3 is with
meny smale skyes & cloudys & wiþ a white & clere ypostasi.

---

26 R *ends here, due to the loss of the final leaf of the text.*

In þe 4 monyth hire vryn is bright & clere & gode of colour, & with a
white ypostasi & beneþe gros & dymmyssh.
Vryn of a woman clere & goldene coloure, þoght it be a partie dym   390
toward þe botume: frikehede & likyng for to be seruede.
Vryn of a therue clene mayden is cler & sheir & bright & þat wonderly.

Þus fonde I in Ysaac, nerhand worde for worde in þe laste boke of his
Vryns.

[Epilogue]

Si quid transiui tradidi tramiteve decliui,   395
Si quid reliqui, si quid scribendo deliqui,
Emendent hij qui non sunt sermonis iniqui,
Sed tantum hij qui sensu litteraque periti.
Nec scriptura docet sed nec natura docebit
Si fetus pregnantis presbiteri vel militantis   400
Aut si sacerdos vel quis maculauerit illam;
Quod pluries tu scire potes sed quociens nunquam,
Aut si niger erit vitulus rubeus masculusve.
Quisquis oppositum facit pomposus erit.
M. tricenteno . septem . x . atque noueno,   405
Regis recardi anno secundo secundi,
Anno primali constanti papa duali
Aut papa francorum sed non anti romanorum.
Laus tibi in gente quoniam labor explicit iste;
Tu qui eterne manes hunc conseruare digneris.   410

Explicit *Liber Vricrisiarum* **a fratre Henrico Daniel, ordinis Fratrum**
Predicatorum, ex Latino in wlgare translatus. Deo gratias.

Appendix 1

Liber Uricrisiarum Prologue (Latin Original)

The Prologue to the *Liber Uricrisiarum* survives in three Latin versions and an English translation of the second Latin version. Witnesses to Prologue 1 are M6G3 GTSaSc; witnesses to Prologue 2 are HCgCfB RM7; Prologue 3 has only two witnesses, AG6. The Latin version of the *Liber Uricrisiarum* in Glasgow University Library, Hunterian MS 362, contains an extremely abbreviated form of the Prologue, retaining only the dedication to Walter of Ketton and the final paragraph on the general contents of the work.

On stylistic grounds, including the absence of doublets and triplets in translating Latin words and of Daniel's typical alliterative synonym-strings, we believe that the English translation in RM7 was made by a different translator than Daniel himself. The Latin text below is taken from H, with emendations as needed from other witnesses to Latin Prologue 2. Paragraphing, punctuation, and capitalization follow modern usage; the Middle English Prologue provides a generally accurate gloss on the original (occasionally difficult) Latin, and on how one of Daniel's contemporaries understood it. For information on biblical allusions and other authorities cited in the Latin Prologue, see the Explanatory Notes to the Middle English Prologue (pp. 309–11 below).

[f. 1r]

Hic incipit prologus in librum vricrisiarum Ricardi Dodd[1]

Dilecto socio in Christo magistro Waltero de Ketene, Frater Henricus Daniell Ordinis Fratrum Predicatorum seruulus Jhesu Christi & Virginis matris eius:

Amantissime socie, pluries & instanter rogasti me vt de iudicijs vrinarum saltem manipulum vnum florum tibi carpam atque vel breuiter tibi

---

1 The reference to Dodd in the rubricated heading is an attribution of ownership or commissioning of the manuscript. Dodd is probably Richard Dodd (or Dod), the mid-fifteenth-century London barber-surgeon who also owned BL, Sloane MS 5 and Longleat House, Longleat MS 174.

scribam & hoc ydiomate in uulgari. Quod vtique faciendo ad opus certe difficile et obtrectatorum latratibus immo & derisionibus patule ipse me inpulisti, tum quia quicquid scripto traditur in doctrinam nisi sit mulcens aures hominum aut multorum transcendens ingenium reputatur totaliter in derisum, tum quia hanc scienciam nec in Anglico traditam memini me legisse sed neque audisse; tum quia huius lingue neque gnarus neque sum disertus, tum quia secundum Aueroys (& habetur a Gilberto in suo commento super Egidium) quod hec facultas non potest lingua explicari. Nam vt scientificis satis est manifestum, nulla sciencia hac lingua sufficienter valet explicari. Et hoc vt reor ratio est: aut quia ydioma in se insufficiens est aut quia eam perfecte nescimus, tum et quia neque ab homine accepi eam ego neque didici, solo sed [v]t^2 in ceteris scientificis interpretacionis dono Spiritus Dei, qui singulis ad salutem diuidit prout velit.

Sed certe, magister amantissime, amor et caritas simplices vincunt, huius autem seculi filios nisi que lucri temporalis laudis aut fauoris existunt; immo quisquis quid appetit et ipse idipsum erit. Legimus in scripturis plures et sanctos propter eorum dicta et scripta grauissime fuisse perpessos multa mala sed a malis. Ipsos etiam Christi apostolos sine litteris et idiotas comemorat scriptura sacra inproperanter fuisse reputatos. Si ergo tanti et tam sancti, immo Spiritu Sancto pleni, ob dicta eorum atque scripta malorum contumelias superborum derisiones presumptuosorum et inuidorum atque mente coruptorum uilipensiones ac linguarum serpentinarum sibilos atque detracciones nequaquam euadere valuerunt, ego quidem qui tantillus utputa minimus seruorum Christi, articulus primus (vt estimo) hanc facultatem in Anglica lingua docens – obloquia & inproperia [eua]-dere^3 quomodo quiuero? Nequam & gratia lucri ac etiam ut alijs,^{4} sapi[en]-tes^5 uideantur solum linguacitate languencium^6 hominum modernorum. Sed certe dum mala a malis illata bonis ipsis i[n] meritum^7 cumulantur, ne prauorum propter mores opera bona a discretis retrahenda iudicantur.

Igitur, karissime, ego considerans multos & diuersos in vrinarum iudicijs expertos esse cupientes, eo quod sciencia pulcra sit & mirabilis – immo

---

2   **vt:** HCgCfB all read *et/&*, but the English version's *as* (= Latin *ut*) makes better sense.

3   **euadere:** (suade *canc.*) evadere Cf, suadere CgB, suaue pro neque dere H

4   **Nequam ... ut alijs:** A vexed passage in all four witnesses, as well as the other versions; the Middle English translator appears to have had a better text or to have imposed a reasonable meaning on the passage: "Certeynly in no waiez, for I do it noʒt for cause of lucre of fauour as oþer men doþ."

5   **sapientes:** CfB, sapi^{tes} Cg, sapites H

6   **languencium:** Although this word, on which all witnesses agree, appears to be a form of *langueo* "grow weak, languish," the Middle English translator clearly understood his source to mean "speaking," as if from a verb *linguere* (cf. *DMLBS*, s.v. *linguare*).

7   **in meritum:** CgCfB; imeritum H

[quasi prophetabilis hominibus quia multum proficua. Videns esse eam quamplurimos – ymmo]⁸ quasi omnes – eius filios circa eius veritatem cecutienter,⁹ & quod quam apertius quid docetur, tam facilius & a pluribus capietur,¹⁰ idcirco ne lucerna accensa sub modio abscondita [f]iam,¹¹ [tuis precibus condescendam. & non solum tue tuique similium]¹² sed et omnium in hac facultate proficere cupiencium noticie in Deo adaugeam.

Presens opus multorum auctorum libris eorumque comentatorum [f. 1v] dictis multo labore prout potui excolegi per tres annos non solum obedie[ncie]¹³ ordinis mei laboribus verum diuersis infirmitatibus quandoque & fere ad mortem frequenter interceptus quibus ex causis magis quam ex penuria ydiomatis multa dimittens uel de meo addens quod auctores no[n]¹⁴ affirmant. In quo quidem opere patent regule & doctrine de iudicijs vrinarum secundum tradiciones auctorum istius sciencie cum diffinicionibus & exposicionibus terminorum morborum seu infirmitatum atque membrorum humani corporis interiorum & cum alijs multis in hac arte notabilibus. Quod opus *Librum Vricrisiarum* censui appellari.

Istum enim librum lingua uulgari Anglica scilicet scriptum qui bene perspexerit & perfecte perfectus iudex in hac arte erit, honoremque apud homines, opes et diuicias, animeque salutem proculdubio consequetur. Si tamen vita pomposa, verbosa, fallosa, & mendosa (vt medici moderni solent) fuerit non abusus.

Sapiens enim Aristotiles, sicut ex fine primi et principio 2ⁱ *Methaphisice*, patet manifeste regraciatur hijs qui ante ipsum non solum sapienter sed & qui non sapienter scriptis tradiderunt quoniam ex hijs que alij scripserunt materia data suptiliora adinuenit. Quoniam secundum eundem etiam in fine 2 libri *Elenchorum*: Que inueniuntur ab alijs prius elaborata particulariter augentur ab eis qui accipiunt postea. Et sequitur: Que autem primo in[u]enivntur¹⁵ paruum in primis augmentum sumere solent, vtilius autem ille quod postea ab hijs fit augmentum. Hec ille.

---

8 **quasi prophetabilis ... ymmo:** CgB, -que prophetabilis ... imo Cf; *om.* H.
9 **cecutienter:** blindly, in a groping fashion (from *caecutire*). The sentence remains ungrammatical in Latin Prologue 2, but Prologue 3 omits *esse eam* and adds *illanguentes insuper* after *cecucienter*, which more closely approximates the English translation: "I seand ful meny men ȝe, as it were alle men – languishand doutously aboute þe sothfastnesse or trewþe of it," and may suggest a better reading for Latin Prologue 2.
10 **& quod quam ... capietur:** only in H and the RM7 translation.
11 **fiam:** Cf; siam HCgB
12 **tuis precibus ... similium:** CgCfB; *om.* H
13 **obediencie:** obedieᵉ CgCfB; obedie H
14 **non:** CgCfB; not (!) H
15 **inuenivntur:** CgB, ineniuntur H, ineiuntur Cf

Nam de meipso hoc non dico quod noua, sed quod nouiter sum scripturus. Collegi nuper & pro hijs qui capere sciunt in Latino tractatum breuem huius facultatis medullam plenius continentem & scripsi in lingua vtique mihi kara. Nec miretur quis si morbis & egritudinibus in hoc libro tactis medicinas non subsequor pertinentes yperapistem imploro.[16] Quapropter, iuuante Deo & obedientia ordinis mei non obstante, vnum opus per se ad hoc me facturum promitto.

In hoc ergo opere veracem lectorem semper expostulo, humilem auditorem desidero, & benignum correctorem semper adopto, quoniam plus caritas quam audacitas ad hoc me induxit. Rogo insuper omnem huius transcriptorem siue copiatorem quatinus (nisi alterius patrie ydiomatis sit) seruet graphiam meam. Namque pro omni ydiomate Anglice lingue apud discretum & donum linguarum habentem vera atque perfecta ars arthographie docetur in libro isto. Qui non intelligit, oret vt interpretetur, inquit tuba Christi.

Presens ergo tractatus [in] 3 libros siue [in][17] 3 particulas diuiditur. In j libro docetur de vrina, vnde dicatur & quid sit, vnde & quomodo generatur, que et quot sunt a medico consideranda, et quomodo [f. 2r] se debet habere in judicando. Et habet 4 capitula. In 2 libro de iudicijs & significacionibus colorum & corporum vrinarum. Et habet 14 capitula. In 3 vero libro de iudicijs & significacionibus contentorum vrinarum & habet 20 capitula. In quorum 20 capitulorum vltimum est de regul[i]s[18] Ysaac, quas ipsemet dat in decima particula libri sui *De vrinis*.

Explicit prologus in librum vricrisiarum.

---

16 **yperapistem imploro:** This phrase ("I beg for an interpreter/expounder"), which occurs here in all witnesses to Latin Prologue 2 but is omitted in the English translation, presumably belongs in the later sentence seeking good readers, hearers, and correctors, which is its position in Latin Prologue 3.

17 **in ... in:** Cf, a ... a H, a^i ... a^i Cg, a^i ... a B. RM7 agree with Cf, translating *in* as *into*.

18 **regulis:** CgCfB, regulas H

Appendix 2

Regule Isaac (Latin Original)
(Isaac Israeli, *Liber urinarum, particula* 10)

The Latin text of Isaac's *Regule* below is taken from the 1515 edition of the *Liber urinarum* (U) in the *Omnia opera Ysaac* (Lyons), 1: 201rb–202va,[1] selectively supplemented and occasionally corrected from Bodleian Library, MS Laud lat. 106 (O), ff. 207vb–209va; BL, Harley MS 3140, ff. 65v–67v (H); Vatican City, Vat. Pal. lat. MS 1260, ff. 300vb–302vb (V); Pavia, Fondo Aldini MS 449 (P, ed. Fontana 1966, 229–39); and Leipzig, Universitätsbibliothek MS 1154 (L, partially transcribed in Peine, ed. 1919, 74–5). Emendations are made and reported variants are selected primarily for the purpose of shedding light on Daniel's English text of the *Regule Isaac*, and secondarily to suggest some of the variability of the Latin text. Minor reorderings of signs in different versions, though not uncommon, are not reported here.

[f. 201rb] Decima particula de vnaquaque vrina & hypostasi quid significent.

Coloribus & liquoribus & vrine hypostasibus monstratis: & que temperamentum monstrant complexionis non regiminis: corruptione quoque & sanitate: vel infirmitate vniuersaliter dictis: oportet librum compleri coloris hypostasis & liquoris: & incipiendum de citrino colore morbum significante.

Urina citrina & subtilis in febre diuturnitatem portendit. In febre acuta non sumus certi vt [O: utrum, V: si] ad statum perueniat.

---

1 Peine's 1919 edition of the *Liber urinarum* is also based on the 1515 *Omnia opera*, but because Peine occasionally misreads his source, we have gone directly to the early print for our copy text, collated against selected manuscript copies and Peine's limited transcription of L.

Citrina & subtilis cum alba hypostasi malum significat in febribus
laboriosis.

Si in initio sit spasmum significat.

Citrina & subtilis in febre acuta est mala.

Citrina & subtilis cum alba hypostasi in liquore diuersa & furfurea
timenda est.

Urina cholerica in febribus laboriosis: maxime initio morbi spasmum
ostendit.

In paralyticis appetitum non habentibus: & stipticis est laudabilis.

Urina cholerica [V: *foll. by* intensa] si in die cretica: maxime quarta in
ordine: nebula rubea apparuerit: laudabilis erit.

Urina citrina [OHPV: colerica] in superficie spumosa: & antea alba: si
sanguis e naribus effluat mala.

Cholerica in [f. 201va] febre acuta cum hypostasi alba pessima est: quia
crudum esse morbum nunciat.

De alba

Alba vrina non cholere significatiua: cum ardore febris: dolore capitis:
vigilia: & cum alienatione mentis: mala est & vicina morti.

Subtilis & alba in yctericia mala: cum hydropisim pessimam demonstrat
esse futuram.

Alba & subtilis cum febre mala.

Alba & subtilis in hancharum dolore oppilationem significat in via vrine
de grosso phlegmate. In febre oppilationem de cholera grossa.

Alba & grossa apparens in die cretica: maxime quarta: a dolore artetici
liberat: & ab apostemate post auriculas.

Post crisim reuocationem significat morbi.

Urina alba [HV: *foll. by* & grossa] si cum prurigine [O: pinguedine] sit
corporis: & in inferioribus ventris: arena in vesica futura erit.

Urina alba & grossa in febribus lenibus angustiam & timorem
demonstrat.

Urina alba et grossa sine hypostasi dolorem & timorem demonstrat.

Urina alba & grossa quasi oleagina mortalis est.

Urina alba & grossa nebulosa sicut spuma pessima est.

Urina habens nebulam quasi niueam [PH: uveam; O: unam/uuam uel
?crassam; V: ?vneam *corr. to* ?uueam]: dolorem in renibus significat &
morbi diuturnitatem.

Urina alba & putrida mala est: quia humores sunt marcidi.

[V: Urina alba & grossa & sicut spuma perdicionem ostendit & plurimum
?hec urina apparens cum dolore in dextro ypocondrio; UHOP: *om. sign*;

V: Urina alba & grossa in acutis febribus in frenesi & dolorem ypocon-
drie timorem nunciat; UHOP: *om. sign*]

Urina alba & putrida cum febribus alienationem mentis demonstrat. [*not
in English text*]

Urina alba sicut sanies in incendio febris mala est: maxime in freneticis.

Urina alba & grossa sine hypostasi humores grossos & viscosos
significat.

Urina alba & grossa non mutans se longo tempore: lapidem in renibus
futurum portendit.

Urina aquosa & subtilis: si in vna qualitate permanserit: superflua est in
humoribus humidis.

Si cum febre leni: adunatur aqua citrina in corpore.

Urina aquosa cum dolore hypocundrie: nimij humores sunt humidi [P:
huiusmodi] in venis. [V: humores humidos esse in uenis.]

Urina aquosa si tamen [OPV: ante; H: *om. sign*] fuerit rubea & in febribus: febres auferentur.

Urina aquosa in continua alienationem mentis significat: sed tamen
confortari debet natura in subtiliandis humoribus [V: ?humoralibus, O:
foll. by vrina alba & grossa in febribus lenibus timorem & angustiam
ostendit]: & deponi nebulam in inferioribus: nuncians liberationem
febris & reuocationem mentis.

Si non habeat nebulam in initio [V: medio] acute febris: mala erit.

Urina aquosa si paulatim [OHPV: *foll. by* & diu] exeat in ycteritia in
hydropisim infirmus incidet.

Urina in febribus acutis aquosa: si quasi sanguisugam vel orobum habeat
mala est.

Urina in initio febris cruda: si bona sunt signa alia: laborem demonstrat.

Urina cruda in initio febris non [UVP; O: *om.* non; H: non *subpuncted*]
laudabilis est: in statu & in vicinitate crisis pessima erit.

Urina cruda colore obscura: neque hypostasim habens: pessima est.

Urina cruda in initio acute febris: si hypostasis sit quasi farina grossa:
futura est alienatio mentis & timor spasmi.

De vrina rubea

Rubea vrina cum febre acuta bona est.

Rubea vrina cum hypostasi multa: nimium alba febris dissolutionem
significat.

Si mutata paruam & subtilem se fecerit: febris habet confortari & post
alleuiari.

Rubea vrina pura si subtilis sit: pessima est.

Urina rubea & subtilis & lenis. i. vnctuosa dolorem arteticum significat: & alienationem mentis.

Urina rubea & fetida cum hypostasi nigra: & turbida quasi pili: vel in vnctuositate [V: muscilagines, P: vel mutationes, O: uel ?inuictiones uel *blank space*, H: uel muccaciones \uel muscilagines/] pessima est & mortalis.

Urina rubea cum hyleon pessima est.

Urina rubea & si- [f. 201vb] ne hypostasi mala.

Urina rubea & grossa neque clarificans in dolore auricularum [HV: aurium, O: ?articularum] & surditate: dolorem capitis ostendit: & tenuatione [H: ?retinnacione, V: ?rethinatione, O: in dextro latere ?retinatione] hypocundrie pessimam yctericiam ante diem septimum significat.

Mutata & subtiliata cum natatili [OVP: naturali] hypostasi: in colore obscura cum alijs signis similibus morbum [V: *foll. by* potest] reuocari: & mentem significat alienari.

Urina grossa & rubea in febre acuta dolorem capitis & hypocundrie colli grauitatem significat.

Urina pura rubea [OHVP: *foll. by* parua] in hydropisi mortem significat.

Urina rubea sicut sanguis siue sicut vinum sine dolore capitis [OHP: corporis] laboriosa, si in qualitate illa permaneat: futurus est lapis in vesica.

Urina rubea quasi color sanguinis parua & subtilis mala est: maxime in sciaticis.

Urina rubea sicut sanguis in febribus acutis mortem subitaneam denunciat.

Urina rubea in tertia [V: inferiori] parte superiori alba: dolorem capitis & mentis alienationem significat.

Urina rubea cum vomitu quasi eruginosa: lingue asperitatem & mortem significat.

Urina rubea quasi color sanguinis in acuta febre & tremore corporis [OHPV: cordis] & dolore in dextra hypocundria mortalis.

Si quis sanguinem mingat multum & subito: venam in renibus habet incisam vel in epate vel in menstruis [H: uiis].

De rufa vrina

Rufe vrine cholera rubea dominatur.

Urina rufa & subtilis cum acuta febre sine hypostasi molestatio die illa erit: si diu permaneat virtus deficiet.

Rubea [OHPV: rufa] vrina parua cum yctericia dissolutionem morbi significat.

Rufa vrina cum febre & frenesi est pessima. Cum dolore capitis periculo-
sissima erit.

Rufa vrina & quasi vini spuma: alienationem mentis significat.

Urina rufa cum hypostasi nigra in spleneticis est mala.

De vrina viridi

Vrina viridis in die apparens cretica: si infirmus in capite doleat: solutionem doloris denunciat.

Urina viridis in incensione febris alienationem.

Si febris sit lenis: et infirmus multam aquam bibat: consumptionem corporis significat.

Urina viridis vel sulphurea in incensione febris: & si infirmus subtiliatus
fuerit: & in superioribus sudauerit: & in extremis friguerit: pessimum
spasmum et inanitione [OHP: pessimum futurum] significat.

Urina viridis & eruginosa spasmum futurum nunciat.

De vrina nigra

Vrina nigra in pluribus est pessima & mortalis.

Urina nigra in acutis febribus hypostasique nigra & natante: cum vigilijs
& surditate: longitudinem morbi significat: & solutionem sui cum
fluxu sanguinis.

Urina nigra in febre incensa & cum capitis grauitate: angustia mentis:
alienatio erit in crisis tempore cum sanguinis fluxu: maxime in mulieribus quibus menstrua sunt ablata.

Urina nigra et grossa in acutis febribus spasmum: & si alienatio adfuerit
desiderium auferendi cibi & mortem significat.

Urina nigra sicut sanguis obscurus in pleuresi mortale.

Vrina nigra cum febre acuta & hypostasi diuersa sepe mutans colorem est
mortalis.

Urina nigra et fetida [O: in febre; P: in febribus; V: in omni febre &
fetida] in anhelitu et sudore in membris superioribus mortalis. [H: *om.
sign*]

Urina nigra & fetida sine [V: cum] dolore vesice mortalis.

[f. 202ra] De vrina oleagina

Vrina oleagina cum hypostasi iuncta: si infirmus rigeat [*so also in* OHVP]
bonum.

Urina oleagina in superficie quasi aranee tela consumptionem pinguedinis significat.

Uiscosa quasi oleum apparens pinguedinis [V: corporis, H: *om.*] consumptionem significat.

Si vrina alternatim mutet colorem: consumptionem corporis & dissolutionem significat virtutis.

Urina quaque die mutabilis pessima est: maxime in apostemate dyaphragmatis.

Urina obscura in febre acuta pessimam crisim futuram nunciat.
  [H: *om. sign*]

Urina clara et lucida in febre acuta dolorem in capite significat; cruda et indigesta alienationem pessimam significat.

Urina turbida colore obscura in febre mala. [*not in English text*]

Urina sicut rubigo ferri in febre acuta spasmum futuram significat.

Urina obscura & quasi rubigo ferri: in febre leni stranguriam significat venturam.

Urina lucida & bene cocta in magnitudine splenis [P: lenis] bona.

Urina lucida in mentis stupore: alienationem mentis cum febribus significat.

Urina lucida cum hypostasi viscosa [O: muscosa, HP: muccosa, V: unctuosa]: vel sicut eris scintilla in ventris [O: *foll. by* uel ?exteris] & pectinis [OP: splenis] dolore atque virge consumptionem renum vel scabiem vesice significat. Si autem in his locis non sit dolor: membra alia consumuntur.

Urina subtilis & cholerica: dolorem membrorum significat.

Urina subtilis & [O: lenis subtilis &, P: subtilis et lenis et, HV: subtilis lenis &] aquosa maior aqua bibita pessima est.

Urina subtilis in acuta febre cum dolore capitis & colli atque dorsi mala.

Urina subtilis in fine febrium: apostema epati significat futurum.

Urina subtilis cum hypostasi in febribus acutis alienationem portendit.

Urina subtilis cum alienatione mala.

Si grossa & cruda hypostasis fuerit: timenda est.

Urina subtilis multa in pleuresi & sicca tussi: alienacionem significat mentis. Si sanguis ex naribus superuenerit & sudor nimius: morbus dissoluetur.

Urina subtilis in ruborem versa cum hypostasi grossa & alba vicinitatem crisis: & dissolutionem morbi cum sudore significat.

Urina subtilis quasi nigra in grauitate capitis & dolore dorsi: plurimum fluxum e naribus ostendit.

Urina subtilis cum acuta febre quasi nigra cum natante hypostasi conturbationem corporis & plurimum sanguinem e naribus & crisim cum sudore significat.

Urina subtilis pertinens nigredini: vel colori sanguinis: acuta in odore: acida in sapore & pungitiua cum hypostasi nigra timorem significat.

Urina subtilis cum incensione febris & quasi nigra & multum oleagina: mortem demonstrat: in infirmo sene [OHPV: seniore] epileptiam significat.

De vrina semper grossa

Vrina semper grossa cum grauitate capitis febrem superuenturam ostendit.

Urina grossa & turbida que nunquam fit clara & alia signa habet bona: laudabilis est.

Urina grossa & non clarificanda ventositatem grossam et inflatiuam & hypostasi mixtam significat: quam sursum leuat ut non deorsum descendere permittat. Vnde dolorem capitis ostendit presentem vel futurum.

Commixtio huius ventositatis sanorum hypostasi: prohibet ne clarificetur dum egreditur: sed cum exeat turbida: & clara fit cum refrigescat, quia calor semper eleuat & mouet: frigitudo facit quietam: vnde aqua dulcis siue salsa cum calefiat est turbida: cum frigescat clara.

Urina grossa cum grauitate **[f. 202rb]** capitis bona.

Urina grossa multa cum dolore epatis dissolutionem monstrat doloris.

Urina grossa & turbida sine hypostasi, mala.

Urina grossa cum hypostasi furfurea [O: sulfurea] pustulas in vesica significat.

Urina quasi lactea in principio febris mortalis.

Urina grossa & multa in febre acuta mala.

Urina grossa & lactea & in vomitu eruginosa siccitate lingue superueniente mortalis.

[Daniel's rule for gross, copious, whey-white urine signifying headache or liver sickness: No obvious equivalent in UOHVP.*]*

Urina viscosa cum dolore renum mala.

Vrina multa plusquam [O: postquam uel plusquam] sit consueta vel parua in febribus mala.

Vrina maior aqua bibita consumptionem [O: mundificationem] corporis significat.

Plusquam soleat mundificationem corporis in ieiunantibus [P: vicinantibus] vel sedentibus [UO; P: descendentibus; HV: sudantibus] inanitionem [HV: minoracionem] humiditatis substantialis [O: subtilis]: & consumptionem membrorum.

Vrina multa & spissa sine [UHP, O: in, V: cum] consumptione: multitudinem humiditatis [HPV: humidam, O: habundare] significat.

Vrina multa cum grauitate corporis & colico [OV: colerico] dolore: bona. In liquore & colore exiens sine dolore: dissolui dolorem significat maxime cum hypostasi alba & grossa & viscosa vel mucosa [HV: unctuosa].

Vrina multa & grossa in passione colica laudabilis. [O: *om. sign*]

Vrina multa & viscosam habens hypostasim vel mucosam: laudabilis in dolore artetico. [OV: *om. sign*]

Vrina multa & grossa in yleo laudabilis: maxime si albam hypostasim habeat.

Vrina multa & spissa grossa vel [O: multa spissa aquosa &, HV: multa & spissa aquosa uel] parum rubea abundantiam sanguinis demonstrat.

Vrina multa in tempore augmentate [O: augmentante] febris: & cum multa hypostasi: calorem & defectionem significat.

Vrina diu exiens cum hypostasi multa in febre diuturna: dissolutionem febris significat.

Vrina multa & alba & saniosa [O: *foll. by* uel squamosa] epileptiam significat.

Vrina multa & subita & quasi sanguis incisionem [O: incensionem] venarum in renibus significat.

Vrina in yctericis plusquam oporteat etsi citrinitati attineat: pessima: quia hydropisim significat: que cum venerit: multitudo vrine laudabilis est: quam aliquando oportet artificialiter fieri multam.

Vrina aliquando multa aliquando parua: in febre acuta pessima est: & in leni diuturnitatem morbi significat.

Vrina parua in acutis febribus est pessima: si hypostasis alternetur in diuerso colore molesta erit: maxime in reumaticis.

Vrina parua paulatim exiens & guttatim pessima.

[OHV: Urina parua cum (O: in) ypostasi rubea cum acuta febre timenda est; UP: *om. sign*]

Vrina parua & rubicunda longitudinem morbi significat.

Vrina parua & subtilis & quasi sanguis mala.

Vrina parua & grossa in febre acuta: pessima est: maxime in fluxu ventris.

Vrina fetida putredinem [V: corruptionem humorum] & nature mortificationem significat.

Vrina si se tinxerit [OPV: strinxerit; H: *om. sign*] dolorem habentibus capitis: spasmum denunciat.

Vrina sine voluntate exiens cum renum sanitate & vesice pessima est: & morti vicina.

[V: *adds* Urina ?in ?unicam plumbea cum febre acuta pessima est & timenda.]

[L:[2] Urina alba et in masculis et in feminabus sine febre laterum dolorem et renum aliquando significat.

---

2 In L, the next thirteen signs follow the urines of women at the end of the text (Peine, ed. 1919, 74, lines 2674–96); most of them occur in the *LU*, but appear directly before the section on hypostasis, where we have inserted them here.

L: Urina si superius citrinitatem habuerit et inferius nebulosa et sublivida fuerit inferius dolorem hancae et geniculorum et stomachi defectionem significat.

L: Urina si superius fuerit subnigra et plana inferius claritatem habuerit inferius [*sic*], dolorem renum et capitis gravitatem, aurium obscuritatem et narium similiter significat, quia fumus stomachi hoc facit.

L: Urina alba et cruda in omnibus debilitationem et frigiditatem in toto corpore.

L: Urina alba et pinguis ut iumenti dolorem renum et vesicae et capitis aliquando significat, quoniam saepius ad urit [*for* uritandum?] vadit hoc habet ex frigiditate vesicae, qui patitur vitium epatis, habet urinam obscuram et rubeam.

L: Urina pulmonis pinguis et alba peripleumoniam significat.

L: Urina si spuma superius fuerit, ventositatem stomachi significat et aliquando desiderium veneris et frigiditatem et tussim.

L: Urina quasi ignea tertianam significat.

L: Urina sanguinea turbata sanguinem, lucida vero causon significat.

L: Urina pleuresis quasi fex est et iuvenes citius senes vero tarde moriuntur, sed de pleuresi, qui quarta decima die solutione[m] non habuerit, non evadet.

L: Urina rosea et obscura in acuta febre frenesim significat.

L: In omnibus his aegritudinibus ptisica, ydropica, apoplexia, epilempsia, colica, dissinteria si urina rubea fuerit, mortem significat.

L: In pleuretica, frenetica, synocha, causonide, tertiana si urina alba fuerit aut sublucida mortem significat.]

De hypostasi grossa

Hypostasis quasi farina grossa in febre diuturna cum signis alijs bonis: dissolutionem febris significat et apostematis: si in illa qualitate permanserit post eruptionem [UHV; OP: apparitionem] apostematis: mortale & pessimum [OH: mortale apostema] erit [V: *foll. by* apostema]: maxime si cum vrina alia appareant signa pessima.

Hypostasis multa cum febre continua: si febris non mutetur vel minuatur: consumptionem corporis significat.

Hypostasis quasi sanguis & sanies longitudinem morbi significat.

Hypostasis furfurea: & vt sanies [O: & non sani] colorata cum sanitate renum & vesice: rigorem febris significat.

Hypostasis multa & rubea cum laudabili liquore & naturali post septem dies dissolutionem febris significat.

Hypostasis natans [**f. 202va**] & non in fundum descendens: cum sudore & accensione [O: ascesione &] hypocundrie & dolore timenda est.

Nebula preter [OHPV: post] crisim apparens morbi demonstrat
reuocationem.

Nebula rufa acumen morbi significat.

Nebula quasi farina grossa morbi diuturnitatem.

Nebula nigra alienationem mentis.

Nebula nigra in febre peryodica [O: modica] & sue interpolationis cus-
todia [OV: custoditam, H: custodita(m *subpuncted*), P: custoditiva]:
febris mutationem [O: mundificationem] in quartanam significat. [P
ends here]

Latin signs not in the English text:

Urina in superficie spumosa in febre acuta dolorem capitis nunciat.

Urina spumosa si sit viscosa & sine mala significatione alia bona [H: sine
alia significatione mala] erit.

Urina spumosa in superficie sicut vuea dolorem renum significat. [U *ends
here*; V: *adds* & cetera deo laus. Expliciunt vrine Ysaac finita & completa anno domini M° cccc° 6° in crastino sancte [*sic*] remigij. (= 12 Jan.
1406/7); H: *adds* Vrina si per se fluxerit dolorem habentibus capitis
spasmum denunciat. Explicit.]

[LO *add several gynecological rules at this point*:

L: Urina puellae virginis lucida est et nimio serena.

O: Virgines faciunt vrinas lucidas & nimis serenas.

L: Urina mulieris co[n]cubitae turbulenta est et in fundo vasis viri semen
apparet.

O: *om. sign*

L: Urina mulieris menstruatae est quasi sanguinea.

O: Menstruate quasi sanguineas.

L: Urina pregnantis in secundo vel quarto mense et nebulam habens et
minutam hypostasim et albam erit minus [*lege* nimis] clara.

O: Pregnantes in primo mense uel secundo uel tercio nebulas minutas
habent & ypostasim albam & ipsa urina est nimis clara.

L: Urina pregnantis post quartum mensem serena est et vini similitudinem habet et hypostasim albam, sed septem menses habuerit, intrinse-
cus grossa et lucida est.

O: Que uero quartum mensem habent serenas & uini colores habentes
& ypostasim albam inferius & grossam & liuidam. Expliciunt vrine
Ysaac.]

Appendix 3

Liber Uricrisiarum Epilogue (English Translation)

The translation in this appendix renders the Latin epilogue in the edition above, taken from M7 because of the lost folio at the end of the text in R. Other witnesses contain additional lines or omit some of the lines in the M7 epilogue or both, though most of them run to similar lengths of twenty-one to twenty-nine lines, aside from the simple couplet in the beta texts EW and the sixteen lines in M7.[1]

The translation is heavily indebted to a literal English version provided by Professor A.G. Rigg to Harvey in the early 2000s. Professor Rigg notes that the verse is sometimes ungrammatical or unmetrical, perhaps with a deliberately jocular purpose not untypical in poems of this type and period.

If[2] I have omitted anything or transmitted it on a slanted path,
If I have left out anything, if I have erred in the writing,
Let those who are not of wicked speech emend it,
But only those who are skilled in wit and letters.
Writing does not teach, nor will nature teach
If the fetus of a pregnant woman is a priest's or a knight's,
Or if a priest or someone else debauched her;
You can know that she has often had sex, but never how many times,
Nor if a calf will be black or red or male.[3]
Whoever proposes the opposite will be an arrogant fool.

---

1 The Epilogue appears in M7 GTSa (alpha texts); AG6 (beta); the final couplet only in EW (beta); and M6G3 HBCg (beta*). Some omissions are caused by loss of leaves (e.g., R, Sc, and possibly Sb), while others appear to be deliberate exclusions (e.g., Cf, J).

2 All other copies of the Epilogue except EW begin with four or five lines, omitted in M7, expressing Daniel's purpose of passing along everything he has learned about urines to those who cannot understand it in Latin.

3 M7's reading *masculusve* "or male" is probably an error for *maculusve* "or spotted," found in other witnesses. See the explanatory note on 1.4.502–7.

One thousand, three hundred, and seventy-nine,
In the second year of King Richard the Second,
The first year that constantly had two popes,[4]
The Frenchmen's pope an "anti,"[5] but the Romans' pope not an "anti."[6]
Praise to You among the people[7] because this work is over.
May You who remain eternally deign to protect this.

---

4 The Great Western Schism, which led to the election of competing popes by cardinals
   of different nationalities, began in the fall of 1378, but the first full year of two popes
   would have been 1379.
5 M7's reading "Aut" is nonsensical and clearly an error for "Anti." Later versions of the
   epilogue alter this line to refer to popes of the *Franci* and the *Angligeni*, the French and
   English people (England supported the pope who resided in Rome, not the Avignonese
   pope).
6 Later versions of the epilogue add up to four lines here referring to events in 1380 (a
   brawl of some kind among preachers), 1381 (the Peasants' Revolt or Great Uprising),
   and 1382 (the earthquake in May of that year), suggesting that Daniel added dating
   lines as he continued to revise his text or that scribes may have inserted the updated
   lines.
7 "Among the people," translating M7's *in gente*, makes a certain amount of sense, but
   most witnesses read *ingenite*, the vocative form of "unbegotten one," or God the
   Father.

Appendix 4

Astronomical Measurements in *Liber Uricrisiarum* 2.6 and Other Astronomical Authorities

The following tables show the variations between Daniel and several Latin astronomical authorities: Ptolemy, *Planetary Hypotheses* (ed. Goldstein 1967, 11); al-Farghānī, *Differentie scientie astrorum* (ed. Carmody 1943, 38–9); Roger Bacon, *Opus maius*, part 4 (trans. Burke 1962, 250, 255–7; ed. Jebb 1733, 143, 146–8); and Robertus Anglicus, Commentary on Sacrobosco *De sphera*, lectio 14 (ed. Thorndike 1949, 193–5, 242–3). Although all columns differ somewhat from each other, Daniel's figures appear to be closest to those of al-Farghānī and Bacon.

Table 4. Volumes of the Planets (as a ratio to the volume of Earth)

	Ptolemy, *Plan. Hypo.*	al-Farghānī, *Differentie*	Bacon, *Opus Maius*	Rob. Angl., comm. on *De sphera*	Daniel, *Liber Uricrisiarum*, f. 50ra
DATE:	2nd cent. CE	(trans. c. 1135)	1267	1271	1378
Planet:					
Moon	1/40	1/39	1/39.25	no volumes given	1/39
Mercury	1/19,683	1/22,000	1/22,000*	–	1/22,000
Venus	1/44	1/37	1/39	–	1/37
Sun	166.33	166.	166.375**	–	166.
Mars	1.5	1.625	1.5625	–	1.625
Jupiter	82.3	95.	94.	–	95.
Saturn	79.5	90.	91.	–	91.

*Burke gives this proportion as 1/22, but Jebb's edition (Burke's source) reads 1/22,000, in line with the rest of the tradition.
**Bacon acknowledges that other authors give this number as 166 or 170.

Table 5. Nearer Distances of the Planetary Spheres from Earth (and Daniel's alleged inter-sphere distances)

Planet	Ptolemy, *Plan. Hypo.**	al-Farghānī, *Differentie*	Bacon, O*pus Maius*	Rob. Angl., comm. on *De sphera*	Daniel, *Liber Uricrisiarum,* f. 50ra
DATE:	2nd cent. CE	(trans. c. 1135)	1267	1271	1378
Planet:					
Moon	156,000	109,037.50	109,037.50	107,936	109,036
Mercury	373,750	208,541.67	208,541.67	209,198	742,000
Venus	2,023,125	542,750	542,750	57,930**	528,750
Sun	3,932,500	3,640,000	3,640,000	3,892,866	3,000,740
Mars	16,380,000	3,965,000	3,965,000	4,248,629	1,865,000
Jupiter	37,388,000	28,847,000	28,847,000	32,352,079	28,847,000
Saturn	55,334,500	46,816,250	46,816,250	52,529,881	46,816,250
Stars	65,000,000	65,357,500	65,357,500	73,387,747	65,357,500

* Distance in miles calculated by multiplying Ptolemy's mean distance in Earth radii by 3250.
**Robertus or a later scribe may have erred in assigning the rank of the first digit in this number, mistaking hundred-thousands as ten-thousands.

Appendix 5

The Language of the Royal 17 D.i Scribe

The scribe of R is a well-disciplined writer with a highly consistent ortho-graphic practice. Many of the items in the *LALME* Questionnaire are given by this scribe in spellings found widely across the country, or at least widely across counties south of the Wash.[1] For example, the scribe consistently uses the following non-northerly spellings and forms:[2]

---

1 Examples of widely occurring spellings used by the R scribe, for *LALME* items 1–56 (up to Forms): *þe, þise, þo, sche/she, it, þai, man, ar, wer(e), is, art, was, schal/shal, schalt/shalt, schuld(e)/shuld(e), wil, wilt, wold(e)* sg., *wolde/wolden* pl., *to, fro, after, þan* "then," *þan* "than," *þogh, if, whil(e), noȝt/noght, world(e), þenk-* "think," *werk* sb., *wirk- pres. stem, þer(e), wher(e), myȝt, þor(o)gh, when* (and less common *whan*). The familiarity of these and other spellings suggests a certain degree of standardization, or at least avoidance of narrowly regional forms, by the scribe.

2 The localizations of different words discussed here are based both on *eLALME*'s general Dot Maps, many but not all of which are also found in the print version of the Atlas, and on the interactive, User-defined Maps available only in the web version, especially when the general Dot Maps conflate several spellings of a word. The tallying of forms has been made possible through the use of R.J.C. Watt's Concordance program (v3.2). In the following quantitative estimates, "extremely rare(ly)" means less than 2 per cent of all instance; "very rare(ly)" = 2 to 5 per cent, "rare(ly)" = 5 to 10 per cent, "less common(ly)" = 10 to 25 per cent. We use the term "East Anglia" to mean Norfolk and Suffolk; county names are based on the pre-1974 boundaries, as in *LALME*.

It should be noted that "localization" of a Middle English text according to *LALME* maps (more precisely, of its scribe's written language) refers to orthographic features that the text shares with "anchor" texts, whose place of production is known from internal evidence. Such shared features need not mean that the text under consideration was produced in the same place as similar anchor text(s): a scribe might learn how to spell in one location, and then move and work elsewhere while retaining some, most, or all of his early orthographic habits. As the General Introduction to *LALME* points out, "the *Atlas* tells us, in essence, *where the scribe of a manuscript learned to write*; the question of where he actually worked and produced the manuscript is a matter of extrapolation and assumption" (1:23, section 4.1.1; original emphasis).

o for OE/ON *ā* (*LALME* Questionnaire Item 48);

-*þ* and -*th* (with very rare -*t* and extremely rare -*þe*/-*the*) for the *pr.3sg.* ending (Item 61): over 2400 instances; -*es* occurs only about five times in the entire text outside the Prologue (and only once in the Prologue);[3]

hem (very rarely *ham*) for THEM (Item 8): a form that reaches into south Yorkshire and south Lincolnshire but is found mainly further south; the only non-*h* initial spelling outside the Prologue is *themself* in 2.13.397;

her and *here* for THEIR (Item 9), with distribution similar to that of *hem/ham*; no *þ*-/*th*- forms outside the Prologue;

here and *her* for HER (Item 5), with extremely rare (1x) *hir*: *her(e)* distribution similar to that of *hem/ham*;

swich(e) and *swych(e)* for SUCH (Item 10), alongside rare *such(e)* and extremely rare *sich(e)*/*swhich*/*swche*: *swich(e)*/*swych(e)* typically occur in East Anglia, Essex, Cambridgeshire, along the southern and southeastern edges of Lincolnshire, and south of a line that then runs through Bedfordshire, southern Northamptonshire, south Warwickshire, Worcestershire, and the northern part of Herefordshire;

which(e) and extremely rare *whyche* for WHICH (Item 11), with the -*ch(e)* ending in all but two cases (*whilk* and *whilke*, Northern/Northeastern spellings found only in the list of conditions in 1.4.6 and 13, perhaps reflecting an element of the scribe's exemplar that he felt was worth preserving);[4] some *which(e)*/*whyche* spellings do occur further north than most of the features listed here, but in a more scattered fashion, and mainly south of a line from the Wash to Morecambe Bay (in and south of Lancashire, southern Yorkshire, and southern Lincolnshire);

eny for ANY (Item 15), with *any* and *ony* each only once: *eny* is typically found south of a line that runs west from the Wash and then turns northwest through Lancashire;

---

3 The Prologue and the suppletions of R's gaps by M7 have slightly different spelling systems from R; they are discussed briefly below (pp. 307–8). We have also inventoried five-folio runs from the beginning, middle, and end of the manuscript; those samples do not reveal any significant differences in major and minor spellings and forms across R's work on the main text, though the scribe uses *os* (for AS) and -*th* (*pr.3sg.* ending) with some increasing frequency across the course of the text.

4 The spelling *whilk(e)*/*whylk(e)* in the Conditions list occurs not only in R but also in its descendant M7, the proto-alpha witness G3, and the alpha subgroup CfCgBH; the proto-alpha witness M6 and alpha subgroup GTSaSc have forms of *which*. Beta texts change the phrase "which(e)/whilk(e) it is" to "what hue it is," clarifying the sense.

meny for MANY (Item 13), with rare *many* and one instance of *menye*:
meny(e) is normally a more southerly form than *eny*, occurring mainly
south of a slightly wavy line running across Suffolk and west through
Buckinghamshire, Oxfordshire, and the northerly parts of Gloucestershire and Herefordshire; however, *LALME*'s Dot Map for the item
shows one Linguistic Profile (LP 73)[5] with *meny* as a minor form in
north Cambridgeshire (Isle of Ely);

cherche and *chirche* (one each) for CHURCH (Item 108), with no *k*-
forms (though only two instances, they agree with the general non-
Northern orthography).

Several *LALME* items help to limit the general southward and west-
ward extent of the language:

os and *as* for AS (Item 34), both frequent (664x and 475x respectively), as
well as very rare *alse* and a single instance of *also*: *os* is typically found
in Northern and Northeastern counties, including the more northerly part of Norfolk; parts of Cambridgeshire/Isle of Ely, Huntingdonshire, and Northamptonshire; and counties north and east of
Leicestershire, Derbyshire, and Yorkshire (inclusive). The spelling *as*
is widespread across *LALME*'s NOR survey points and presumably
continues on into the south.

-and(e), the somewhat less common *-end(e)*, and the less common
-ond(e) for the *pr.ppl.* ending (Item 58), together with less common
-ing/-yng and very rare and extremely rare *-ant* and *-ynd*: *-and(e)* is
usually found north or east of a curving line running to the northwest
of most of Gloucestershire, Oxfordshire, Northamptonshire, north of
most of Huntingdonshire, and then turning southward to run west of
most of Cambridgeshire/Isle of Ely, East Anglia, Essex, the Middlesex/
London area, Kent, and parts of Surrey and Sussex, thereby excluding
a large portion of the southern and central Midland shires;

-end(e) has a smaller, more easterly footprint, with a narrow "finger" of
instances reaching out to the northwest: broadly shared with *-and(e)*
are parts of Sussex and Surrey, Kent, the Middlesex/London area,
Essex, East Anglia, and Cambridgeshire/Isle of Ely; further north, the
form is limited to the northern areas of Northamptonshire, Rutland,

---

5   Linguistic Profiles (henceforth LPs) are given in *LALME* vol. 3 and explained in the
    Introduction to that volume; both the LPs and the Introduction to vol. 3 are also avail-
    able in *eLALME*.

south Lincolnshire, northeast Leicestershire, and southeast Nottinghamshire (-*and(e)* also occurs in these counties).

-*ond(e)* occurs in an even more restricted area, in four LPs from Lincolnshire and Leicestershire and another two from Lancashire.

CALL (Item 103) is represented almost entirely (more than 320
instances) by the root *call-*, with only four instances of *clep-* forms,
all in the first part of the text (1.3.31, 2.3.55, 2.3.59, 2.3.352): most
LALME records of *call-* forms occur in Surrey, London, Essex, East
Anglia, and north of a line running north of all or most of Hertford-
shire, Buckinghamshire, Oxfordshire, Gloucestershire, and Herefordshire, though very scattered instances can be found in Oxfordshire and
the southwest;

mykel(-) for MUCH (Item 16), along with rare *mykil*, very rare *mych(e)*,
and extremely rare *mikel*, *mykyl*, *myke*, and *mich*, *mychel*, *mychil*:
forms like *mykel/mykil/mykyl* and *mikel* are normally found north of
a line from the Thames estuary to the mouth of the Severn.

Based on these forms, especially *os* and -*end(e)/-and(e)* combined with
the broadly non-Northern spellings and forms noted above, R's language
is best explained as coming from an area that would include the northern
half of Norfolk, the borders between southern Lincolnshire and northern
Cambridgeshire (Isle of Ely), Northamptonshire, Rutland, and Leicestershire, and possibly a small part of southeast Nottinghamshire.[6] Two
individual items deserve special notice: *meny* for MANY and the -*ond(e)*
ending for *pr.ppl.* As mentioned above, the spelling *meny* (R's majority
form of the word) is usually found further south than the region suggested
here for R's language, but its occurrence as a minor form in LP 73 (Isle of
Ely) suggests that it could have been familiar to the R scribe. Perhaps he
found the visual analogy between *eny* and *meny* a persuasive argument for
writing the two words with the same vowel.

The -*ond(e)* ending occurs 36 times in the text, out of 285 total *pr.ppl.*
forms – a not insignificant minority form (13 per cent), though substan-
tially outweighed by -*and(e)* (151x) and -*end(e)* (54x). The very restricted
distribution of -*ond(e)* in the *LALME* Dot Maps overlaps slightly with the
dialect area described above, which could mean that the area should simply
be narrowed down to south Lincolnshire and northeast Leicestershire, but
it is also possible that the -*ond(e)* spellings are inherited from R's source and
were familiar enough to the scribe that he did not always translate them into

6 Our dialect analysis differs somewhat from that of Norri, for whom "The dialect has
   Norfolk features, and perhaps comes from the southern part of the county" (1992, 71).

his more common *-and(e)/-end(e)* spellings. The fact that Stamford and Ketton, places associated with Daniel and his dedicatee Walter Turner of Ketton, are in south Lincolnshire and Rutland (and only three miles apart) may lend possibility to the hypothesis that Daniel's text was originally written and initially copied in the Dominican convent at Stamford, but no documentary support has yet come to light as to where Daniel himself learned his letters or where he resided when writing the *Liber Uricrisiarum*.

One last observation concerning the scribe of R should be made, namely that he appears to avoid spellings that might be seen as strongly Northern, Northeastern, or East Anglian. If his writing system is based in Norfolk, for instance, he eschews the characteristic East Anglian spellings *xal-/xul-* for SHALL/SHOULD; nor do spellings for SUCH and WHICH with *-lk-* (aside from the Conditions list in bk. 1.4) or *qu-/qw-/qwh-* for WH- appear anywhere in his text, even though such forms are easily found in counties such as Lincolnshire, Norfolk, the Isle of Ely, and Leicestershire. In this behaviour, he seems to move in the direction of the kind of "colourless" regional writing that Samuels discusses in the context of later fifteenth-century examples (1981, 43–4).

Two sets of folios in our edition diverge from the dialect features of the main text described above: text transcribed from M7 and the text of the Prologue.

As indicated in the Introduction (p. 31), we have substituted text from M7 for ten missing or mutilated leaves in R. The M7 scribe is generally very faithful to the text of R, including most of the forms inventoried above,[7] but differs in one particularly striking feature: he uses the character <*y*> for both *y* and *þ* in R, which may well have been his immediate exemplar (based on the carryover of many marginal "lef" cross-references, even though they no longer apply to folios in M7). According to Michael Benskin, the scribal practice of conflating *y* and *þ* in a single letter-form "characterizes the writing of scribes from the northerly and some easterly parts of England, and from Scotland" (1982, 14). Based on Benskin's map showing the general distributions of the spellings <*þ*> and <*y*>, the "easterly parts of England" include large portions of Norfolk, a narrow band stretching across mid-Suffolk into Cambridgeshire, and two very small regions of southern Essex. Benskin's map may be further refined for our purposes with the User-defined Maps in *eLALME* for the *pr.3sg.* ending,

---

7 We have concorded and compiled a separate Inventory of Forms for the M7 material, but omit its details here, as they generally agree with R aside from the conflation of *y* and *þ*. As noted in the Introduction, our edition normalizes M7's *y* as *þ* as appropriate, for ease of reading.

limiting the forms to -ey/-iy/-yy.[8] These endings appear in only eleven
LPs, ten of them in Norfolk, Cambridgeshire, Isle of Ely, south Lincolnshire, north Huntingdonshire, south Nottinghamshire, and Staffordshire,
with one outlier (-yy as a minor form) in Herefordshire.[9] Such findings
may imply that the M7 scribe learned to write in an area similar to or
slightly west of the R scribe's language, an area where (or under a teacher
for whom) y and þ were not distinguished, but was otherwise comfortable
with the rest of R's spellings, reproducing them with little or no variation.

The Prologue also diverges in small but significant ways from the language in the main text of R, particularly in its use of þam (8x) and þaym
(1x) for THEM, and þair (2x) for THEIR, instead of R's usual hem/ham
and her(e).[10] Although þam and þaym can be found across the country,
they are somewhat more common in the Northern areas, consistent with
their origin in Old Norse þeim. The spelling þair, with both initial þ- and
medial -ai-, is also found primarily in the north. The Prologue is in the
hand of the R scribe, so these variations from his practice elsewhere in the
text suggest that his exemplar for the Prologue was written in a slightly
more northern dialect than that of the main text. A minor linguistic vari-
ance of this sort from the main text might be explained if the English version of Daniel's Latin Prologue was created by a translator other than
Daniel, slightly later than the *Liber Uricrisiarum* proper, and then grafted
on to a copy of the main text either by the R scribe or by a predecessor.

---

8 M7's *pr.3sg.* endings are -ey (136x), -th (24x) , -t (5x), -es (5x), -iy (2x), -ith (2x), -yth
   (2x), -yy (1x).

9 The infrequency of -y endings for *pr.3sg.* verbs, despite the common y/þ conflation
   in Northern Middle English, is explained by the even more common use of -es as the
   pr.3sg. ending in the north: most scribes who use the same character for y and þ would
   have used -es in the *pr.3sg.*, and it is not surprising that the -y endings for *pr.3sg.* occur
   in counties between the broadly Northern and Midland dialect areas.

10 The form *hem* for THEM occurs only once in the Prologue.

Explanatory Notes

The Explanatory Notes provide information on Daniel's named sources, glosses of difficult or unusual words and phrasing, occasional commentary on medical content, and some of the more interesting variations among the versions of the *Liber Uricrisiarum* (*LU*). Quotations from the Standard Commentary on Giles of Corbeil's *Carmen de urinis* and Gilbertus Anglicus's Comment on Giles are based on transcriptions made by E. Ruth Harvey from BL Sloane MS 282 and Wellcome Library MS 547. Unless indicated otherwise, translations are our own.

Prologue

Daniel's Latin prologue can be found in three versions, each expanding somewhat on the preceding one, and reporting different periods of time that Daniel had spent on his book. The earliest version appears in manuscripts M6G3 (with the proto-alpha text to bk. 2.6) and TGSaSc (alpha text); it gives two years as the time invested in the work. The second version occurs in CfCgHB (alpha text) and reports a three-year period of work; the English prologue in RM7 (alpha text) was translated from this second Latin prologue. Finally, two beta witnesses, AG6, begin with a third version of the Latin prologue, in which the number of years spent is given as a blank space (A) or five (G6). The text of the second Latin Prologue is provided in Appendix 1.

15–16 Aueroys ... Gilbert in his Coment vpon Giles ... schewede by tonge: The only analogue to this ineffability claim in Gilbert's Comment on Giles appears to be a passing remark near the end of the commentary, concerning a certain transparency in urine derived "a natura corporum supracelestium dancium elementis suam diaphanitatem, que est res sicut dicit Aueroys que nominari non potest" (from the nature of the heavenly bodies giving their diaphanousness to the elements, which is a thing that Averroës says cannot be named) (Wellcome 547, f. 144va). Galen makes a similar remark in the *De crisibus* 1.12: "Et non est possibile quidem vt in sermone fiat declaratio quantitatum harum permixtionum [of blood and choler in urine]: Vnum non est necesse tibi vt addiscas ab alio considerationem ad naturalem urinam: uerum experiaris tu eam per te ipsum tentando et experiendo in urinis sanorum" (And it is not possible to express in language the quantities of these mixtures: you do not need to learn from someone else how to judge natural urine: you will experience it yourself by testing and experiencing it in the urines of healthy people) (*Opera* 1490, vol. 1, sig. nn ij vb). It may be that noting the limitations of language alone in learning about urine was broadly traditional – or at least unsurprising – in medical discourse.

20–1   **sciences of interpretacions by þe gifte of the Holy Gost ... as he will:** 1 Cor. 12:10–11.

27–9   **Holy Writte makeþ mynde þat þe selfe aposteles ... wiþouten letres and ydiotes:** Acts 4:13.

28–9   **arectede reprouabli:** "mockingly accused."

48–9   **þat I be noȝt made a liȝtede lantern hide vnder a busshel:** Matt. 5:15.

52–3   **meny auctoures & þe sayingz of þe comentours of þam:** In the earliest version of the Prologue, extant only in Latin, in GTSaSc and the hybrid texts M6G3, Daniel names his sources as the texts of Galen, Isaac, and Giles with their glosses and commentaries, together with Constantinus (Africanus), Theophilus, Thaddeus (presumably Taddeo Alderotti), Gilbertus (Anglicus), and "as many other authors as I could find, as will be clear to the reader."

67   **neuerþeles if he mysvse noȝt ... lif or bostful:** "provided that he doesn't (wrongly) live an ostentatious or boastful life"; *mysvse noȝt* is a double negative used for emphasis, a common Middle English construction.

70–3   **Wise Aristotel ... *ex fine primi & principio secundi Methaphisice*, he þankeþ ... þat oþer wrote bifore:** Aristotle, *Metaphysics* 2.1, "It is just that we should be grateful, not only to those with whose views we may agree, but also to those who have expressed more superficial views; for these also contributed something, by developing before us the powers of thought" (trans. Ross, in Barnes, ed. 1984, 1570).

73–8   **þe same Aristotel *in fine 2ⁱ libri Elenchorum*, þo þinges ... more profitable, *hec ille*:** Aristotle, *Sophistical Refutations* 34, "For in the case of all discoveries the results of previous labours that have been handed down from others have been advanced bit by bit by those who have taken them on, whereas the original discoveries generally make advance that is small at first though much more useful than the development which later springs out of them" (trans. Pickard-Cambridge, in Barnes, ed. 1984, 313).

81–2   **þe tong þat forsothe is riȝt dere to me:** I.e., Latin, not English, referring to Daniel's "schorte tretice" containing the marrow or essence of his subject matter. The sole extant copy of this Latin version of the *LU* is Glasgow University

Library, Hunterian MS 362, ff. 1r–83v; it is significantly less expansive than the Middle English version of the text, presumably because of the greater expertise of its anticipated audience.

83   sewe: A variant spelling of *sheue/shewe* "show, tell of, describe" (*MED*, s.v. *sheuen* [v.(1)], sense 7).

85–6   I bihete me for to make a werk: Daniel will not "show" remedies for the maladies described in the *LU*, but plans to write another book – a promise he may have fulfilled in compiling his herbal, the *Aaron Danielis*, though he refers to his own collections of remedies with several different titles, including *Medycynarie* (see 3.16.369 below) and the beta readings *Pra(c)tyke* (= "Practica": G3HCfCgB, bk. 3.1) and *Praptyke* (Sb, bk. 3.1).

86–92   I aske euermore … ortographie is taugh in þis bok: Daniel's desire for careful readers, correctors, and scribes anticipates comments by Chaucer (*Troilus and Criseyde* 5.1793–9; "Adam Scriveyn"). Hanna suggests that Daniel and Chaucer are atypical among Middle English writers in their concern for accurate transmission of their texts (1996, 175).

92   taugh: Omitting the final *-t* after *-gh-/-ȝ-* appears to have been a regular option in the spelling system of the Royal scribe, though less common than his *-ght* and *-ȝt* spellings. See, for example, *lengh* (1.3.26), *noȝ* (1.3.216), *wrogh* (1.4.244), *brygh* (1.4.312), *riȝ* (1.4.678), etc.

92–4   he that vnderstondes it noȝt, praie … þe trompe of Criste, i. Seynt Poule: Adapting 1 Cor. 14:13: "And therefore he that speaketh by a tongue, let him pray that he may interpret."

102–3   þe reules of Ysaac, which himself giffeþ in þe 10 partie of his *Boke of Vryns*: Isaac Israeli, *Liber urinarum, particula* 10 (in *Omnia opera Ysaac* 1515, 1: 201rb–202va; ed. Peine 1919, 69–75, lines 2461–2696). See bk. 3.20 and Appendix 2.

1.1

30–2   as saiþ þe Comentoure vpon Gyles … and womennes membres: "Aut vrina dicitur ab urendo quia uritiuam et desiccatiuam habet naturam, unde urina valet contra inpetiginem et serpiginem et contra pustulas, si paciens membrum laverit. Et contra uirge ulceracionem. Cum felle autem aucipitris coliriata panum et maculam delet in oculo" (Or it is called "urine" from *urendo* "burning," because it has a burning and drying nature, which is why urine is good against impetigo, serpigo, and pustules, if the patient washes the body part with it. And it is good against ulceration of the penis. If it is made into an eye-salve with hawk's gall, it removes the membrane and the spot in the eye) (Sloane 282, f. 19v).

33–4   as Gilbert seyþ, it fordoþ also þe webbe … here chyldyng: We have not found a mention of *webbe in þe eye* (clouding or cataract) as a symptom of childbirth in Gilbert's commentary on Giles or in the Middle English or Latin versions of his *Compendium medicine* or *The Sickness of Women* (an excerpt from the Latin *Compendium*), although *webbe* appears several times in the *Compendium* as a generic eye-disease and Daniel mentions the ailment as a consequence of childbirth in his herbal (*Aaron Danielis*, BL Add. 27329, ff. 164vb, 207vb). For the *Compendium*, see Getz, ed. 1991, 34/8, 45/19, 47/1, etc. On Gilbert's biography and writings, see McVaugh 2010.

34–6   Also if *spleneticus* ... drynke his owen fastande water ... my3ttely: Cf. the Standard Commentary: "Potata spleneticis confert" (When drunk, urine is good for those with spleen disorders) (Sloane 282, f. 19v).

38–45   whit clay ... blake clay ... wollen clout ... Peyto salt: Mixing urine with clay or soaking a woollen cloth in urine are methods for preparing plasters that can be bandaged to a wound, sore, or aching joint and allowed to remain for a period of time. *Peyto salt* is an imported variety of sea-salt harvested from salt pans on the Atlantic coast of Poitou; the salt trade there dates back to at least the thirteenth century, especially at Ile de Ré. Both fine white salt (*fleur de sel*) and coarser grey salt (*sel gris*) are produced. Dissolving a half-quart of salt in a half-gallon (*potel*) of urine, and then boiling the solution down to a half or a third, would yield a very concentrated liquid.

39–40   and þat þe clay be clene piked: "and see that the clay is picked clean (of stones, grit, etc.)."

43   awasshyn: RM7's clearly written *clena wasshyn* may be an error for *clene wasshyn*, as the readings in other witnesses suggest, but we have taken it as a mis-division of the past participle of the verb *awashen*.

1.2

2   Giles in his texte and alle auctores and comentoures: Giles's definition: "Sanguinis est urina serum, subtile liquamen / Humorum, quos conficit ars regitiva secundi / Et princeps operis" (Urine is the watery part of blood, the subtle fluid of the humours, which the controlling and principal power of the second digestion creates) (*Carmen de urinis* 6–8; ed. Choulant 1826, 4; ed. Vieillard 1903, 272).

27–8   þis forsaide descripcioun of vryn þat Gilbert 3eueþ accordeþ wel: "Gilbert" (found only in RM7 J) is an error for "Giles" (attested by M6 GCfH AEWP, inserted in SaSc). B and Cg omit the name entirely, while T and G6 read "Gyl" with a barred *l*; G3 rephrases and refers to Egidius. Cf. the Standard Commentary's gloss on Giles's definition, "Hec est diffinicio que hic assignatur, et bene consonat diffinitionem Theophili et Ysaac que talis est, Vrina est colamentum sanguinis ... " (This is the definition that is assigned here, and it agrees with the definition of Theophilus and Isaac, which is as follows, "Urine is a filtrate of blood ... ") (Sloane 282, ff. 19v–20r).

28   þe diffinycioun þat Ysaac and Theophile 3euen: Theophilus, *Liber urinarum* (ed. Dase 1999, 3; *Articella* 1483, f. 5va): "Urina est colamentum sanguinis [*add* & *aliorum humorum* (*Articella*)]" (Urine is a filtrate of the blood and other humours); Isaac, *Liber urinarum, particula* 1, f. 157va (ed. Peine 1919, 10, lines 24–5): "Vrina est colamentum sanguinis ceterorumque humorum de nature quidem actionibus natum" (Urine is a filtrate of the blood and of other humours, produced by the actions of nature).

The definitions given in the Latin translations of Theophilus and Isaac continued to be used by later uroscopic writers, such as Johannes Platearius, Maurus of Salerno, Bernard de Gordon, the author of the brief treatise "Omnis urina est colamentum sanguinis," and its Middle English translation "All/Every Urine Is a Cleansing of Blood" (Tavormina 2014, 3n3 and item 3.3; ed. Tavormina 2019, 9–10, 50–1, 57), etc.

1.3

23–4   Galienus in *Libro anathomiarum suarum,* **in þe** *Boke of His Anathomy*: Most of Daniel's references to Galen's "Anatomies" are actually citations of the brief twelfth-century text known as the *Anatomia porci*, sometimes called the First Salernitan Anatomical Demonstration, which was erroneously attributed from the Renaissance on to Copho of Salerno. Medieval copies of the text typically assign it to Galen or leave it anonymous. For careful discussions of the text and its history, see Corner, ed. and trans. 1927, O'Neill 1970, and references given in both. Quotations from the ps.-Galenic *Anatomia porci* are drawn from Corner's revised edition and translation. (The text uses the pig as a structurally similar proxy for human anatomy.)

24   calleþ it *portonarium*: "Sub stomacho est intestinum quod dicitur portanarium, sub portanari est duodenum, sub duodeno est ieiunum, sub ieiuno est orbum, sub orbo saccus, sub sacco longaon" (After the stomach comes that part of the intestine called *portanarium*; next is the duodenum, after the duodenum the jejunum, after the jejunum the *orbum* [caecum], after the orbum the *saccus*, after the saccus, the *longaon* [rectum]) (*Anatomia porci*, ed. and trans. Corner 1927, 49, 52). Later medieval anatomy treatises began to approximate more closely the modern breakdown of the intestines into duodenum, jejunum, ileum, caecum, colon (ascending, transverse, descending), and rectum, but it is not uncommon to find terminological variations and confusions in pre-modern descriptions of the intestinal tract.

In other medieval anatomy treatises, the term *portanarium* is more often applied to the duodenum, though still in the sense of a passage from the stomach into the intestines. See for example the pseudo-Galenic *Anatomia vivorum*, §35 (ed. Töply 1902, but misattributed there to Ricardus Anglicus; also in Galen, *Omnia quae extant opera*, vol. 10, *Ascripti libri*, Venice 1565, ff. 43v–56v, at 50r); Guy de Chauliac, *Cyrurgie* (ed. Ogden 1971), 59. However, the *De iuuamentis membrorum* (the Latin translation of an abridged Arabic version of Galen's *De usu partium*) also uses the term *portanarius* to gloss the "via que est inter ipsum stomacum & intestinum" (Galen, *Opera* 1490, vol. 1, sig. ee 6vb; the glossing phrase does not appear in the copy of the text in Harley MS 3748, ff. 168rb–190rb, at f. 176rb).

42–3 Isaac and þe auctour of *Anathomys*: Isaac, *Liber urinarum, particula* 1, f. 158va–vb (ed. Peine 1919, 11, lines 54–5): "[intestinum] quod est tortum, rotundum et globosum a medicis vocatur ieiunum" ([a gut] that is twisted, round and globular, called the jejunum by doctors).

The *Anatomia porci* names the jejunum as the intestinal section between the duodenum and the caecum (*orbum*), but does not describe its physical form.

49 buddy fleissche: Lumpy or irregular flesh, tissue covered in small protuberances.

53 mylke ȝate: Daniel rather confusingly uses the term *mylke ȝate* for three distinct parts of the body: the jejunum (here); the portal vein, which he understood as bringing chyle from the stomach to the liver via the meseraic veins (2.3.56–60); and the rectum (2.3.60–6). He acknowledges the multiplicity of meanings both here (line 1.3.56) and after the last definition, saying "Also, *l[a]ctea porta* is anoþer þing, as Y saide, þe j boke, þe þrid c." (2.3.66–7).

81–2 þogh Isaac say þat *duodenum* is on & *ieiunum* anoþer: Although the majority of witnesses in all versions include the word "another" here, the reading in M7H (also seen in Cf) could have been understood by scribes to mean "the duodenum is one thing and the jejunum is one (separate) thing." The key point for Daniel is that Isaac treats the duodenum and the jejunum as separate sections of the intestines (*Liber urinarum, particula* 1, f. 158va–vb; ed. Peine 1919, 11, lines 45–55), in contrast to the *Bok of Anathomis*, as he understands that text (see next note).

82–3 þe *Bok of Anathomis* saiþ þat þai arne boþe on: If Daniel is still referring to the ps.-Galenic *Anatomia porci*, this assertion conflicts with Corner's edition of that work, whose description of intestinal anatomy is quoted above (1.3.24n). A corrupt copy of the text might have conflated duodenum and jejunum in some way, or Daniel may have had access to some other anatomical work (though his primary source for anatomy remains the *Anatomia porci*).

111 as Galien saiþ in his *Anatomis*: On the relative positions of the liver and the stomach, see *Anatomia porci*: "Ex dextra parte sub fundo stomachi est hepar positum" (At the right side under the pouch of the stomach the liver is placed) (ed. and trans. Corner 1927, 49, 52).

For the fire and cauldron simile, compare the twelfth-century *Anatomia Magistri Nicolai physici*: "[Stomachus] habet etiam epar sibi suppositum, quod est quasi ignis suppositus lebeti, unde quidam olla cibi stomachus, fel cocus, ignis epar" ([The stomach] has the liver below it like a fire underneath a cauldron; and thus the stomach is like a kettle of food, the gall-bladder is the cook, and the liver is the fire) (ed. Redeker 1917, 49; trans. Corner 1927, 79).

159–60   **pissing places:** This phrase for the ureters (vessels from the kidneys to the bladder) is probably an error for *passing places*, the phrase used in other witnesses and supported by the verb *passeþ* later in the sentence. See also 2.3.403.

181–2   **saiþ Galien þat vryn of hole folke ... lytil *ypostasis* or none:** We have not found this assertion in the *De crisibus* 1.12, though Galen does discuss *ypostasis* there. The point may be made elsewhere in Galen's works, such as his comments on the Hippocratic books or in the *Tegni*, which Daniel could have read in a commented *Articella*.

195–6   **haþe purgacioun ... & þe neþer hole:** "has the upper and lower hole as the purgation for its superfluities." Emending the text by inserting *by* before *þe ouer hole* would yield easier syntax, but no witnesses (alpha or beta) support such an emendation, and all but four manuscripts agree verbatim with M7's syntax.

262–3   **Nerehonde al ... Isaac techeþ nyȝ worde for worde:** Bk. 1.3 in Daniel corresponds more or less closely to *particula* 1 of Isaac's *Liber urinarum*, after its first paragraph on the definition of urine (ed. Peine 1919, 11–14, lines 37–176), although Daniel tends to expand on Isaac's physiological explanation of how digestion works and how urine is generated, especially in the first half of the chapter. As Hanna observes, the last half of the chapter is more closely rendered (ed. 1994, 216).

1.4

4   **þe moste knowe:** "it is necessary for you to know, you must know"; *þe* is the objective form of *þou* "thou, you (sg.)." For the impersonal construction using a grammatically past tense form with present sense, see *MED*, s.v. *moten* (v.[2]), sense 8.

5–6   **as techeþ Giles & Gilbert ... comentoures, i. expositoures:** For identical or similar lists of "conditions" to be considered by physicians in the judgment of urine, see Giles, *Carmen de urinis* 10–14; Standard Commentary, Sloane 282, f. 20r–v; Gilbert, Comment on Giles, Wellcome 547, ff. 106rb–108ra; Bernard de Gordon, *De urinis*, ch. 5, in *Lilium medicine* (1574, 728–824), at 746–50.

Other uroscopy treatises recommend shorter lists, such as the "four things" recommended by the widely disseminated *Dome of Uryne* (colour, contents, "substance" or density/opacity, and region in the flask), or the five or six primary and eight or seven secondary considerations recommended by Ricardus Anglicus or in *Barton's Urines* (the "four things" plus equality [Ricardus] or taste and pulse [Barton]; age, complexion, sex, habit, time, diet, region in the flask, and custom of the patient [Ricardus] or age, complexion, occupation, diet, sex, "cure" or emotional state, and medications [Barton]). See Tavormina 2014, items 2.0, 7.5.3, 20.0, 25.0; *Dome of Uryne*, ed. Tavormina 2019, 30.

8   **Kynde, s. wheþer it be man or woman:** In RM7 and the sixteenth-century witness J, the term *kynde* is used here to mean the patient's sex (*s. wheþer it*

be man or woman), and is preceded by *complexioun* (temperament). All other witnesses omit the term *complexioun* and use *kynde* for temperament, reserving the phrase *he or she* for the condition of sex.

10–11   If þou wilt wise-man ... wel and fyne: Possibly a couplet rhyming *vryn/fyne*, although Daniel has not followed his usual practice of labelling verse as such (as in 1.4.418 and 426, 1.4.687, 2.2.316, 2.6.293–5, 3.1.66–7). The sentence appears in most of the alpha witnesses (not in T or J) and one irregular beta witness (Sb), but not in the proto-alpha or other beta witnesses. It is a reasonable English rendering of lines 13–14 in Giles of Corbeil's *Carmen de urinis*, "Debent artifici certa ratione notari, / Si cupit urinae iudex consultus haberi" ([The conditions] should be noted by the master with sure knowledge / If he wants to be considered a skilful judge of urine).

55–6   þe quantite of þe colour ... the more it meneþ: RM7's readings *quantite* and "the more it meneþ" (= "the more significant it is") make general sense, but variants elsewhere in the tradition suggest that some corruption has entered the text here: aside from the late witness J, all other witnesses across all versions read "the more mater it menith [H AEW: mevith, *prob. in error*]" for the phrase (i.e., more intense colour means there is more material in the urine). A small group of alpha witnesses (GSaSc J) read "qualite" for "quantite" in line 55.

77   but þe more grace be: "unless (God's) grace is greater."

122–4   *Breuiarius medicine ... Breuiarie of Medycyn*: John of St Paul, *Breviarius medicine* (= *Breviarius Ypocratis*), "De paralisis": "Fit paralisis sepe ex flegmate. uel melancolia. senibus et ex precedente egritudine. raro ex sanguine et iuuenibus et nulla precedente egritudine diuerse lesiones sequentur secundum membrorum diuersitatem que ea occupantur egritudine. ut uocis et locule [*sic*] amputatio, urine et egestionis inuoluntarie emissio" (Paralysis often comes from phlegm or melancholy, and in old people also from a preceding illness, rarely from blood. Also in young people with no preceding illness, diverse sores follow according to the diversity of the members which are affected by that illness, such as the cutting away of the voice or testicles, the involuntary emission of urine and feces) (Montreal, McGill University Library, Osler MS 7627, f. 18v).

127–8   os techeþ Isaac: From here to line 1.4.180 ("Þus seiþ Isaac word for word"), on the procedures for collecting and inspecting urine, Daniel's text is roughly equivalent to *Liber urinarum*, *particula* 2, f. 163ra–rb (ed. Peine 1919, 15–16, lines 224–58).

146   Þe beste after þat is þat is made ... þenne: "The next best type of urine is that which is thick when produced and changes into thin."

168   But Ysaac in his texte techeþ: *Liber urinarum*, *particula* 2, f. 163ra–rb (ed. Peine 1919, 16, lines 252–8).

175   chaffede: Many witnesses (M6G3 GTSaSc J AG6EW PSb) add the phrase "at the fire or in hot (warme J) water" after *chaffede*.

235–6   Isaac techeþ … be day: *Liber urinarum, particula* 2, f. 163ra (ed. Peine 1919, 15, lines 239–41). The beta manuscripts AG6EW PSb and one proto-alpha witness (M6) add a summary paragraph here on external characteristics (age, complexion, speech, movements, eyes, diet, etc.) that should be considered or inquired about, whether at the bedside or at a distance from the patient. The physician is also advised to give comfort and spiritual counsel and to consult the Hippocratic *Prognostics* for more comprehensive instruction.

240–1   wel and parfitely digestede as kynde wil and may: The emendation "digestede" in the text is best supported by the late witness J ("welle & perfytely wroght & dygestyd as kynd askyth"; cf. line 244 in the following paragraph), with partial support from the proto-alpha witnesses and most beta witnesses ("wele digestyd"). The omission of "digestede" in RM7 CgH also occurs in CfB W6.

248–9   in þoght and dede vtwardes … to done: "in outwardly directed thought and deed that a person has to do."

256   it is said: "has (already) been discussed" (in conditions 7 and 5 above).

261   vppon þat þat kynde … in hem: "(based) on this: that natural heat is great or little in them."

303   of þise 3 4: "of these three groups of four."

324   of hem schal he … complexioun: I.e., a person's complexion is named for whichever humours or elements are strongest in his or her nature.

362–3   be be … be be: I.e., "be by" (twice).

366   This are þe condicions of complexions of man: The four couplets describing the complexions or temperaments are widely disseminated, both in Latin and in the vernacular. They were incorporated in the *Flos medicine* (Tavormina 2014, 69n48), but also often occur on their own or in other texts. For examples of their Latin distribution, see Thorndike 1955, 177–80. Besides their occurrence in the *LU*, they play an important role in *The Four Elements*, a substantial Middle English treatise on the elements and humours (Tavormina 2014, item 8.2), and show up in smaller texts and in margins of medical miscellanies.

385   gyle: Translating *non expers fraudis* "not without guile," possibly with omission of some phrase meaning *not without*.

388–94   4 ages of man … 7 ages of man … : The classic Anglocentric treatments of the various medieval classifications of the ages of man are Burrow 1986; Dove 1986; and with an art historical perspective, Sears 1986. As both Burrow and Dove note, one can readily find three-, four-, six-, and seven-age schemes for human life, each with one or more correspondences to natural and historical parallels. For a more recent treatment, with further bibliography and a focus on the theological aspects of the question, see Darby 2012, especially part I, "The World Ages Framework."

388   *decrepita*: "aged." This feminine adjective may be a scribal error for *decrepitas*, but it occurs in more than half of the witnesses; slightly less than half read *decrepitus*, presumably by analogy with *iuuentus* and *senectus*.

405–6, 421   4 ages of þe ȝere … 4 tymes … 4 quadres … : Here, as in the longer computistical passage in 2.6, Daniel probably draws from John of Sacrobosco's *Computus* (*Compotus*) *ecclesiasticus* (cited in these notes from BL, Harley MS 3647, and from the Wittenberg 1543 printed edition, both accessible online). In his section "De quatuor temporibus anni" (ff. 42vb–44vb; sigs. D 7r–E 3v), Sacrobosco describes all three of the seasonal schemes Daniel lists – liturgical, zodiacal, and monthly – but gives slightly different mnemonic verses.

The dates of the saints' days given by Daniel are as follows: Chair of St Peter: 22 February; St Urban: 25 May; St Bartholomew: 24 August; St Clement: 23 November.

436   be a þing neuer so hote: "no matter how hot something is" (it contains some degree of cold) and similarly throughout the paragraph.

442–4   ar callede *qualitates prime … quia primo & principaliter insunt omni elementato*: Although the Latin passage here has the flavour of a quotation, probably from some philosophical work, we have not yet traced its source.

502–7   And wite wel þat nouþer phisic … wheþer a blake or … a braynede: "Know well that neither medicine nor any medical writer gives either lore or rule to distinguish a man from a woman in urine, except as I said just now. For there is no medicine or author who gives a technique to tell, assuming a woman is with child, whether the child is choleric or melancholy or of any other temperament, nor, if a cow is with calf, whether it will be black or dun or a white bull or a brindled one." The participal adjective **braynede** is a form of the *MED* entry *brend* (ppl. as n.) and the *OED* entry *brinded* (adj.), but Daniel's use significantly antedates *MED*'s first recorded stand-alone instances, in Audelay and Lydgate (with dates of composition c. 1426 and c. 1430), aside from a mid-thirteenth-century surname, *Brendeskyn*.

It is worth noting Daniel's concern with what *cannot* be determined from the urine. In his verse epilogue (3.20.395–410), he warns readers that "Nec scriptura docet sed nec natura docebit / Si fetus pregnantis presbiteri vel militantis / Aut si sacerdos vel quis maculauerit illam; / Quod pluries tu scire potes sed quociens nunquam, / Aut si niger erit vitulus rubeus masculusve [*var.* maculusve]. / Quisquis oppositum facit pomposus erit" (Writing does not teach, nor will nature teach, if the fetus of a pregnant woman is a priest's or a knight's, or if a priest or someone else debauched her; you can know that she has often had sex, but never how many times, nor if a calf will be black or red or male [*var.* spotted]. Whoever proposes the opposite will be an arrogant fool).

The rationale behind patients' – or their relatives' – desire to know the paternity of a child in the womb is self-evident, and the temptation to seek or offer such diagnosis must have been strong. Responsible medical writers, however, emphasized that such specific knowledge could not be obtained uroscopically, even though pregnancy, menstrual status, and virginity *were* believed to be ascertainable.

The concern with the colour or sex of a calf may have had multiple origins. A common anxiety in uroscopic texts is that the physician not be fooled by patients who offer animal urine instead of their own, either to test him or simply to mock him. (For an excellent discussion of the complex dynamic underlying this concern, and the place of uroscopy within a broader investigation of patients' conditions, see McVaugh 1997.) Thus, short rules for distinguishing human from animal urine are not uncommon in medieval uroscopies or uroscopic sections of larger works; see following note. But in an agricultural society, it might have been just as useful – and less emotionally fraught – to try to find out in advance if one's cow would produce a bull-calf or not, or even what the appearance and perhaps the resulting value of that calf might be.

509–10   If þou wilt haue lore for to deme bestes water ... þus techeþ Aui-cen: Avicenna discusses differences between the urines of donkeys, cattle, sheep, goats, and humans in his *Canon of Medicine* (*Liber canonis medicine*, henceforth *Canon*) 1.2.3.2, c. 11, but does not mention how those urines appear when viewed close up or farther away from the eye. The more likely source for Daniel's criterion is the *Flos medicine*'s couplet, "De prope spissa magis hominis minctura videtur: / non liquor est alius cui talis regula detur" (Human urine appears more thick from close by: / There is no other urine to which such a rule is given) (ed. Frutos González 2010b, lines 1367–8; ed. De Renzi 1852–9, 1: 492, lines 1438–9, and 5: 65, lines 2273–4). Some short Middle English texts on the urines of men, women, and beasts also recommend versions of the density/distance test, at least once (in Sloane 2527) invoking Avicenna's authority; see Tavormina 2014, item 7.3.4 and n.

555   if he be myȝty and kene: Although the reading *clene* in RM7J makes grammatical sense, the more common *kene* "strong, fierce" (M6G3 CfCgHB G6EW PSb; *corr. from* clene A) fits better with *myȝty* in describing the ability of the liver to move excess moisture into the urine. Several witnesses (GSaSc W6) read *kynde* for *clene/kene*, taking Nature (or the liver and Nature together) as the force that drives the excess fluid to the kidneys.

583   4 principal wyndes: Daniel's list of principal and secondary winds corresponds to that given in a table and accompanying verses in Sacrobosco's *Computus ecclesiasticus* (Wittenberg 1543, sig. D 8r; for the circular diagram, see Harley 3647, f. 43ra, though that diagram omits the secondary winds, the east and west winds, and the verses found in the print edition and around the edge of Daniel's diagram). Sacrobosco's diagram is the most likely model for Daniel's, despite minor differences; both belong to a broader tradition of representing fourfold cosmic correspondences visually. For a stunning earlier analogue, with somewhat different information, see "Byrhtferth's Diagram" as preserved in BL Harley MS 3667, f. 8r (MS c. 1130; a copy of Byrhtferth's *Manual*, written c. 1011), viewable in the British Library's online gallery: http://www.bl.uk/onlinegallery.

594   pirnale wynde: "northeast wind." Although the *LU* does not provide sufficient evidence for the meaning of *pirnale*, its sense is clarified by three passages in Daniel's herbal (emphases added):

> [Rosemary] may with ["is strong against"] every time & weder, saue these some: þat is to sey, noth [*sic*] wynd, est, & *northest (þat is the pirnale wynd)*, these thre & blac frost arn deth to him . qwyt frost & snow arn refreschyng & norischyng to him. (*Aaron Danielis*, BL Add. MS 27329, f. 18rb)
>
> And euere [the almond tree] leueth, but þe gret cold esterne or norther or *northest wynd* in cold winter make it, & ȝet be 9 dayes after it leueth ageyn. (*Aaron Danielis*, BL Add. MS 27329, f. 150va)
>
> [The almond tree] is eueremore grene leuyd but if est wynd or north wynd *or pirnale wynd* in cold wynter tyme make it, and ȝut withyn þe 9 day after such weder it hath newe leuys agayne. (BL, MS Arundel 42, f. 24v)

(The Rosemary section of the herbal, which circulated independently and widely, has been edited by Mäkinen (2002), with the reading *priuale wynd* at lines 173–4. Further clarifications of sense and spelling may be possible by examining the other thirty-plus manuscripts of the treatise.)

Scribal forms for *pirnale* are somewhat ambiguous, due to the indistinguishability of *n* and *u* in most witnesses and the use of a barred *p* (abbreviating *pre-* or *per-*) in some of them. However, several witnesses, including R, spell out the first syllable as *pir-* or *pyr-*, which strongly supports the *per-* expansion, and the M7 scribe, whose *n* and *u* forms are well distinguished, transcribes the word as *pinale* (with an erroneous omission of *r*). The rest of the word varies slightly as well, from *-al(e)* (RM7GT CgHB) to *-ell* (SaSc) to *-hale* (G3M6). The scribe of the late alpha manuscript Wellcome 226 apparently did not recognize the word, and changes it to *pryncypall*.

The *MED* cites this passage (from G, which uses the barred *p* abbreviation) under the word *prevaile* (n.), and suggests the meaning "prevailing," but given the stronger support for *pirnale* or *pernale*, and the uses in the herbal, we would suggest that the entry requires correction. The etymology of the word remains uncertain, but compare Scots *birr, bir,* n. "a strong, sudden breeze," from ON *byrr* "a fair wind" and *pir(he* n., attested from the eighteenth and seventeenth centuries respectively (*Dictionary of the Scots Language*; https://dsl.ac.uk/entry/snd/birr_n1_v1, https://dsl.ac.uk/entry/dost/pirhe). See also *English Dialect Dictionary*, s.vv. *perry* sb.[1], *pirr* sb. and v.

617   vpon þat: "in so far as, based on the fact that, because." The phrase occurs with similar causal or etiological senses at 1.4.261, 1.4.322, 1.4.711, 2.2.104, 2.14.87, 3.4.76, etc. The phrase can also carry less causal senses, like "following that," "(up) on that," etc.

657   by þis word cure: The condition "cure" (Lat. *cura*) refers to worries and anxieties ("cares"), sometimes translated as "besynesse." This section is expanded in the beta versions to include the cares associated with *amor hereos*; on that expansion, see Walsh Morrissey 2014a.

667–8   Aristotil saiþ þat swonge wombe ... remytteþ þe vryn: Probably taken from Gilbert's Comment on Giles: "Inanicio et replecio [mutant corpus], quod patet per Aristotelem quia dicit, 'venter inanitus calefacit, repletus vero infrig[es]cat'" (Emptiness and fullness change the body, which is clear from Aristotle, because he says "an emptied stomach warms, a full one chills") (Wellcome 547, f. 107vb). Cooler urine was understood to be of duller or "remitted" colour.

The idea is also expressed and attributed to "the philosopher" (i.e., Aristotle) in the *Anatomia vivorum*: "et infrigidatio cordis per aerem atractum propinqua est infrigidationi stomachi [que] euenit ei in hora sue repletionis propter motum et descensum ciborum, vnde philosophus 'uenter uacuus calefit . repletus infrigidatur' propter motum ex partibus" (The cooling of the heart by the indrawn air is similar to the cooling of the stomach at the time it is being filled, by the movement and descent of the food [as the Philosopher says, "the empty stomach heats, the full stomach cools"], for the lung also has moving parts) (ps.-Ricardus Anglicus, ed. Töply 1902, 12, §25; trans. Corner 1927, 96).

687   *Lote cale sta paste vel i frigesce minute*: *Flos medicine* 1177 (ed. Frutos González 2010b, 292; also in De Renzi, ed. 1852–9, 1: 448, line 120, and 5: 6, line 209): "Lote, cale, sta, pasce (*var.* pranse) vel i, frigesce minute" (Bathe, heat, stand, eat or move, cool off, let blood). Daniel clearly takes this series of commands as indicating three separate pairs of sequential actions, of which only the first pair ("After bath, kepe þe hote") applies directly to the discussion here.

690   as Isaac techeþ: The *Liber urinarum*, *particula* 7, lists two causes for the failure of digestion in the stomach: *cibum humidum multumque inflatiuum* (moist and very gassy food) and *cibum inordinate acceptum* (food eaten immoderately), both characteristic of gluttons (*gulosi*) and people who stuff themselves with food (f. 184ra; ed. Peine 1919, 38, lines 1174–6).

709–10   in alse mykel as ... complexioun of þe body askeþ: I.e., the quality of the urine is based both on the nature of the food and the complexion of the body.

715   delyte: "a culinary delicacy, gourmet food." Only RM7 offer this reading; most other witnesses have the much easier *spices*.

739–52   Johannicius in his boke De ysagogis ... and garlik. Þus seiþ he: *Isagoge ad Techne Galieni*, §§35–6 (ed. Maurach 1978, 159; trans. Wallis 2010, 145–6). For a detailed analysis of the relations between the *Isagoge* and its Arabic source, see Jacquart 1986, suggesting that the text may have been an early translation by Constantine the African (233–6).

781–5   *Et stipticum* hote and moyste ... John de Sancto Paulo in his *Boke of Phisik Medycynal*: John of St Paul, *De simplicium medicinarum virtutibus*, s.vv. De laxativis, De constrictivis, De diureticis; ed. Kroemer 1920, 21–3, 36.

In these passages, John of St Paul indicates that diuretics are "sharp" (*aliquid acumen habere*) and that they thin the blood (possibly suggesting moisture rather than dryness) and heat the kidneys. Constrictives are cold, and consolidate or tighten bodily fluids and organs by virtue of their frigidity, sometimes strengthening the retentive power like styptic things (*ut similia stipticorum*) and by virtue of their *stipticitas*. John is thus in agreement with those who call "diuretik solutif and stiptik constrictif"; he also associates diuretics with heat and sharpness and possibly moisture, as Daniel indicates. On the other hand, he is explicit in linking constrictives with cold as well as with occasional styptic effects. He does not include a specific category of styptic simples.

John also describes a wide variety of mechanisms by which different types of laxatives work, including penetrating fumes, assistance to the expulsive power, the inability to tolerate an obstruction, viscosity, saltiness, sweetness, sharpness, compression, and so on, depending both on what laxative is used and what humours are being purged. This complex array of causation, if common in other treatises on simples, may help explain the uncertainty that Daniel feels about the terms "styptic" and "diuretic."

795–6 s. mykel toward: "namely, quite close to it (swartness)."

802–3 Gilbertus in his Coment vpon Giles … take in exces: Cf. Gilbert's comment that "[uinum] album aquosum facit vrinam albam tenuem quia subtilitatem sue \substantie/ euadit a digestione prima et secunda" (white, watery wine makes urine white and thin because the fineness of its substance escapes both the first and second digestion), followed by more detailed remarks about the specific effects of red, citrine, and sweet wines, and concluding with "et sic vina diuersificant vrinam, quia fere aliquam faciunt eam albam & tenuem, et maxime a[l]bum et aquosum, et maxime si multum sit bibitum" (and so wines diversify the urine, because they usually make it somewhat white and thin, and especially white and watery wine [does so], and especially if much is drunk) (Wellcome 547, ff. 107vb–108ra).

820 þe behoueþ to: "it behooves you to, you should."

2.1

77–9 Galienus in his *Boke of Anathomyes* … pipes of þe lunges: " … omnes aliae arteriae quae procedunt ad membra, in quibus fiunt pulsus, quibus mediantibus cor alligatum est pulmoni et aerem trahit a fistulis pulmonis" (… all the other arteries which proceed to the members; in these the pulse occurs. By means of these vessels the heart is connected to the lung and draws air from the cavities of the lung) (*Anatomi porci*, ed. and trans. Corner 1927, 49, 52).

2.2

34–8 Isaac in þe 4 boke *De febribus* seiþ þat noble membres … oþer places of þe body: The "noble members" are usually defined as the principal organs (heart, brain, liver, reproductive organs), but Isaac also describes arteries and veins as "noble" in *De febribus* 4.2: "Quia si natura illam nequit expellere materiam [morbi] extrinsecus propter suam grossiciem: mouet eam a nobilibus membris ad ignobilia … & vene & arterie sunt nobilia membra a quibus solet mouere natura materiam [morbi] ad alia loca" (For if nature cannot expel the matter of the disease outside the body on account of its grossness, it moves it from the noble members to the ignoble ones … And veins and arteries are noble members by which nature is accustomed to move morbid matter to other places) (*Omnia opera Ysaac* 1515, 1: 212va).

Isaac refers to the heart, lungs, and diaphragm as noble members in *De febribus* 4.1: "Ostendunt enim nobilia membra esse robusta de quibus vita procedit & monstratur .i. cor & pulmo & diaphragma & pectoris membra sunt cordis instrumenta. sano ergo fundamento sana eius sunt instrumenta: vnde flatus completur et pulsus confortatur & etiam cum fortitudine calor per totum corpus diuiditur" (For they [easy breath and strong pulse] show that the noble members, from which life proceeds and is proven, are strong, that is, the heart and the lungs and the diaphragm. And the organs of the breast are the instruments of the heart, and thus the instruments to a healthy foundation are themselves healthy, on account of which the breath is perfected and the pulse is strengthened and also heat is strongly dispersed throughout the whole body) (*Omnia opera Ysaac* 1515, 1: 210vb).

55   and boþe þo causen: Both the turbidity (*droublehede*) and the unnatural heat cause thickness in Black urine (RM7). Although this reading makes grammatical sense, the variant in CgHGSc, according to which the natural heat may be quenched either by great cold or by unnatural heat, is more likely on humoral terms: "… dymhede & drublyhede that is cawsid of disturblyng & distemperure of the humores as it is euermore in blak vryn. Item black colour in vryn or it is caused of grete colde sleyng the kende hete or els of vnkende hete skaldyng …" (Cg).

73–4   þere-awaie: "away from there, thence."

114–16   þe vryn þat he made nexte bifor … syth it bicom Blak: I.e., diagnosing mortification from Black urine is warranted if the urine that the patient was producing before he produced Black urine was Blo, even though the Black urine has been produced for many days.

146   de depressioun: Probably an error, shared only by RM7 and (as *depression*) the late witness J, for *de passione* (*of passiown* CgHGSc), though *depressioun* occasionally appears in medical contexts (see Norri 2016, s.v. *depressioun*, but with examples only in connection with prolapse of the uterus and depression of the cranium).

154–5   Of *fetor* and of Fathede … her propre chapitlez: Bk. 3, chaps. 7 and 8 (on Pus and Fat in urine).

156–7   What vryn it be þat stinkeþ from fer: "Whatever urine stinks at a distance."

191   os Ysaac techeþ in þe 4 boke *Of þe Febre*: From here to line 2.2.257 below ("seiþ Isaac nerhand worde for worde"), Daniel follows Isaac's *De febribus* 4.6, "De scientia cretice diei" (*Omnia opera Ysaac* 1515, 1: 213vb–214ra), relatively closely, with some selective omissions in the latter part of the chapter. Occasional divergences from the 1515 text, especially in numerals, may be due to variation in the manuscript tradition.

197   liʒten: Possibly an error for *fiʒten*, as found in GTSaSc, but all other alpha and beta witnesses agree with R. More likely an early form of the phrase *lightening before death*, referring to a revival of the spirits just before death (*OED*, s.v. *lightening* [n.2], sense b; first attested from 1597, in Shakespeare), but with death and the malady still ultimately victorious over nature. The Latin version of the *LU* (in Glasgow University Library, MS Hunter 362) speaks at this point in the text about *eis qui alleuiantur parum ante mortem* (those who are eased shortly before death), but whose illness will return in force (*potenter*) and conquer nature.

208   þe 13 and þe 19: Isaac's text here reads "tertia & decimaoctaua." All other witnesses of the *LU* agree with R's *þe 19*, but only RM7J have *(þe) 13*, in contrast to *þe 3* in other manuscripts.

224–8   Tak gode hede þat Isaac vseth þise termes al for on ... endyng of þe malady: A brief interruption to the material taken from Isaac's *De febribus* 4.6, defining terms used for some of the stages of disease. Medieval and classical medicine commonly distinguished four stages: the beginning (*initium*), increase (*augmentum*), peak or "standing" (*status*, which Daniel equates with *terminus, terminatio, crisis,* and *dies creticus*), and decline (*declinatio*). See below, 2.2.281–93.

238–9   Ypocras blameþ bledyng att þe nose in þe 2 dai of an acue: We have not located this statement in Hippocrates, but Daniel is taking it from Isaac, *De febribus* 4.6: "Ideoque vituperauit Hippocrates sanguinem de naribus in secundo die manantem in acutis febribus: dixit enim eum timoris fore nunciatiuum. Idcirco dies illaudabilis quanto fuerit longior a secunda die: tanto minoris erit timoris" (And therefore Hippocrates blames blood flowing from the nose on the second day in acute fevers: for he says that it is predictive of fear. Thus the further a bad day is from the second day, the less cause there will be for fear) (*Omnia opera Ysaac* 1515, 1: 214ra).

243–9   þus answereþ Isaac ... endeþ his wirkyng: *De febribus* 4.6: "Respondemus impares licet sint conuenientes naturaliter diei cretice: pares tamen sunt eis accidentaliter: quia si crisis incipiet in .xiij. die natura suam complebit actionem in xiiij. Unde crisis in .xiiij. die computatur: quia actionis nature complementum in eo ostenditur. Similitur in tertia natura incipit suam operationem: & in quarta finit eam" (We answer that although odd numbers correspond to the critical day naturally, nevertheless even numbers do so accidentally: because if the crisis were to begin on the thirteenth day, nature will fulfil its action on the fourteenth. And therefore the crisis is calculated as being on the fourteenth day, because the completion of nature's action appears on that day. Similarly, nature begins its operation on the third, and finishes it on the fourth) (*Omnia opera Ysaac* 1515, 1: 214ra).

Note that where R has "if it be so þat crisis begynne in þe 3 dai and fulfilleþ his wirkyng in þe 4 day" (lines 245–6), Isaac has the thirteenth and fourteenth day, which makes more sense of the next phrase, about attributing the crisis to the fourteenth day. Most other *LU* witnesses agree with Isaac.

254–5 Ypocras in his *Empidijs*: *Impares … forciores*: The Greek text of the *Epidemics* does not appear to contain any equivalent to this pithy phrase, but Isaac (or perhaps Constantine) attributes the notion to Hippocrates and the *Epidemics* in *De febribus* 4.6, following a passage that is clearly an insertion by Constantine: "causa diuersitatis diei cretice duobus modis est: aut propter debilitatem nature: aut propter diuersitatem figure lune inequali modo lumen a sole recipientis: quod vtrumque explanabimus in nostro libro pantegni. Quod si quis facillime intelligere desiderauerit: legat capitulum de yme[r]acriseos scriptum in eodem libro [*Pantegni*, Theorica 10.8]: ibi enim plene diximus & monstrauimus: quia impares sunt apertiores & certiores paribus: sicut Hippocrates in epydimia. 'Impares inquit sunt fortiores paribus'" (The reason for differences in the critical days is twofold: either from the weakness of nature or from differences in the shape of the moon, which receives the light of the sun unequally. Each of these we will explain in our book *Pantegni*. If anyone wants to understand it easily, let him read the chapter "De ymeracriseos" [Theorica 10.8] written in the same book: for we have said and showed it there fully, that odd numbers are clearer and more certain than even numbers, as Hippocrates says in *Epidimia*, "Odd numbers are stronger than even numbers") (*Omnia opera Ysaac* 1515, 1: 214ra).

The cited *Pantegni* chapter – chapter 10.8 in Constantine's translation of al-Majūsī's *Art of Medicine* – speaks at length about different ways in which the critical days can vary from each other, but the fuller discussion of odd and even numbers, with a citation of Hippocrates, occurs in 10.9: "Unde dixit Hippocra[tes]. Quecunque crisis in numero fit impari: securiores quam in pari nos reddit" (Whence Hippocrates said that when a crisis occurs in an odd numbered day, it makes us more assured than in an even number) (in *Omnia opera Ysaac* 1515, 2: 53va–54rb).

257 Alle þise poyntz seiþ Isaac nerhand worde for worde: I.e., from line 2.2.191 above to here.

259–62 And vnderstande … but for also mykel as *crisis* comunly comeþ in swich day, falleþ & eke in tokne of sauacioun: R's confusing syntax, with *comeþ* and the redundant (and presumably erroneous) *falleþ* in such close proximity, is paralleled only in M7 and H. All other witnesses have some version of *but for as myche as crisis comynly cometh (ther)in that (such T) day & that (eke CgCfB) in good tokene, i. (in)to sauacioun* (GTSaSc CgCfB) or (*but* AG6EWSb) *for os myche as crisis comynly comyth þerinne, and þat in gode tokun* (M6G3 AG6EWSb).

Daniel's Latin reads "Et nota quod non dicitur *dies creticus* quia tunc venit crisis solum, sed quia venit in bono signo" (And note that it is not only called *dies creticus* because the crisis comes then, but because it comes in a good sign) (Glasgow, University Library, Hunterian MS 362, f. 17r).

268   þus techeþ Isaac in þe same boke anone after: *De febribus* 4.7, "De cognoscenda crisi ventura." Daniel translates approximately the first fifth of the chapter, roughly twenty-three lines in the 1515 *Omnia opera Ysaac* (1: 214ra–rb), inserting a paragraph of his own giving a fuller explanation of the four stages of febrile disease (lines 281–93), and then returning to Isaac through line 307.

297–9   wiþin þe 2 houre afore ... by þe 2 hour byforne: The options appear to be within the two hours before crisis, within two hours (i.e., around crisis?), by the second hour (after crisis), or else before the second hour before crisis. All four options occur in RM7CfCgB, while other witnesses reduce the options to only one, two, or three alternatives.

306–7   Alle þise poyntz nerhand word for word techeþ Isaac in þe forsaide boke: I.e., *De febribus* 4.7.

316–17   *Qui bene digerit ingerit egerit est bene sanus*: Proverbial; see Walther 1963–86, no. 23836, citing source texts in manuscripts from the fourteenth to the sixteenth century.

320–1   But colde swete in þe heuede alone is perilouse, as Isaac seiþ, þe 4 bok *De febribus*: *De febribus* 4.4, "De signis nunciatiuis": "Vnde timorem nunciant sicut sudor non in die cretico apparens frigidus ... maxime si in solo fuerit capite" (For which reason they [other signs] lead to fear, such as a cold sweat not appearing on a critical day ... especially if it is in the head alone) (*Omnia opera Ysaac* 1515, 1: 213rb). This chapter includes most of the other signs that Daniel mentions here, including general strength or weakness, ability or inability to move the body, state of mind, breath, appetite, sleep, the appearance of the face, and various purgations from urine and feces to white, viscous sputum delivered in one or two coughings and vomit that alleviates the patient.

335–6   þise ar tokenes of deþ: The signs listed here are a version of the Hippocratic *facies*, the facial signs associated with impending death, classically described in *Prog.* 2, but disseminated widely in classical, medieval, and Renaissance medical texts and their vernacular offshoots.

338–9   more dere dere: Possibly a scribal error (dittography), or perhaps a play on words, "more costly harm" (see *MED*, s. vv. *dere* [adj. (1)], sense 3; *dere* [n.(1)]).

341–8   Galien seiþ *Vppon Empidijs* ... Item, Galienus ... 2 reules þat Galien techeþ by Blak colour: These citations of a Galenic (or pseudo-Galenic) commentary on the Hippocratic *Epidemics* are derived from the Standard Commentary on Giles: "Idem Galienus *Super epidimias* preponitis quod si aliquis infirmus in principio morbi faciat materiam nigram cum signis molestis et terribilibus, tamen sanatur si contingat uirtutem eius esse constantem, hanelitumque facilem, vel quando in inicio morbi venerit cum timore accidencium, & permanet vsque in diem vii. Sed materia superueniente cum alba ypostisi [*sic*] & virtute se expediente morbi decoccionem signat, & egri salutem" (Galen [says] the same as the foregoing points, in *Upon the Epidemics*: if a sick person at the beginning of the illness makes a black substance with harmful and terrible signs, nonetheless he will be healed if his natural force is constant and his breath easy, or when it comes in the beginning of the illness, with concern about the symptoms, and remains until the seventh day. But if other matter follows, with a white *ypostasis* and with the help of his natural force, it indicates digestion of the disease and the health of the patient) (Sloane 282, f. 22r).

Very little of the Hippocratic *Epidemics* (only book 6) was available to Western medieval audiences (Kibre 1985, 138–42). The commentary usually found with the Latin *Epidemics 6* was that of the Byzantine physician John of Alexandria (early seventh century); both works were translated into Latin from Arabic versions by Simon of Genoa.

357   propurlik onely when it is in þe ouer partie of þe vryn: Given what has just been said about *ypostasis* being the proper term only when it appears in the ground of the urine, this statement appears to be in error, but all alpha texts agree on the reading. The proto-alpha (M6G3) and beta (AG6EWSb) witnesses omit the entire phrase.

362–4   Theophilus in his *Boke of Vryns* … into a febre quarteyn: Theophilus, *Liber urinarum*: "Si uero in febribus causon nigras nubes habet, significat in quartanarium transmutari" (If it has black clouds in causon fevers, it signifies that it will change to a quartan) (ed. Dase 1999, 37; *Articella* 1483, f. 7ra).

374–5   Mo rewles … þis boke: Daniel may be thinking of the discussion of Black urine caused by heat in the chapter on Green urine, at the end of book 2 (2.14.5–12, 27–35), or of the "Rules of Isaac" translated at the end of the entire treatise (3.20). Several witnesses (CgCfHB W6) read "the laste chapitre of the 3 book" here, though CgCfHB do not actually end with the "Rules of Isaac" because of their switch to the beta* version of the *LU* in bk. 2.12, and W6 is atelous from bk. 2.8. The remaining full witnesses – proto-alpha G3M6, alpha GTSaSc, beta AG6EW, the possible hybrid Sb, and the Latin version of the text – replace the sentence about "mo rewles" with a series of approximately ten signs related to Black, turbid, oleaginous, and rusty urine, most of them drawn from the Urina Nigra and Urina Oleagina sections of Isaac's *Regule urinarum*, though with different translations from those in *LU* 3.20.

2.3

11–12   os be cause of turbacioun of humores: "such as on account of turbulence of the humours."

38   lef {1}: The cross-reference is an obvious error, as the Karopos chapter begins on f. 53r (old leaf 52). R's cross-references are usually accurate, but not always (as here).

98–100 os Galien seiþ, goþ inne ... vpward in þe body: "Et tunc videbis quandam venam quae concava dicitur, quae ab hepate venit per medium diaphrag-matis et subintrat inferiorem auriculam cordis et fit arteriam de qua fiunt omnes aliae arteriae quae procedunt ad membra" (Next you will observe a vein, called *vena concava*, which comes from the liver through the middle of the diaphragm and enters, from below, the inferior auricle of the heart. It then becomes an artery and from it arise all the other arteries which proceed to the members) (*Anatomia porci*, ed. and trans. Corner 1927, 48–9, 51–2).

108–9 þe pouce is more certeyn ... þan in þe riȝt wirste: All witnesses agree with R's text here, but only RM7 offer the conflicting marginal comment that the pulse is more certain on the right side; in other witnesses, the marginal note says that the left side has a more reliable pulse.

119 octomia: Daniel's form of MLat *orthomia* < *orthopnoea* "difficulty breath-ing except in an upright position." ME spellings of the root include *ortom-, ottom-, octom-,* and possibly *occom-* (as reported in Norri 2016 from R). Two or three of the instances of *octom-* words in R might use *-cc-,* but the majority are clearly spelled with a *-ct-* ligature.

141 kynirz: Cf. *DMLBS,* s.v. *kinelis, (vena ~is,* med.) "vena cava" (citing Gil-bertus Anglicus).

188 nuk: This word for the marrow of the spinal cord or the nape of the neck, from Latin *nucha/nuca* and ultimately derived from Arabic, often confused scribes unfamiliar with its medical meaning. The four minims of *nu-* were not infrequently decoded as *mi-,* leading to spellings such as the clearly erroneous *myk(ke)* and – depending on how the scribe formed *m, n, i,* and *u* – the potentially ambiguous *mik(ke).*

214 psidius, þe psidi: Some witnesses (GTSaSc CfCgBH) read *preidye/prey-dye* in place of *psidi* and change the Latin term to *preidius,* even though they retain the instruction to spell the word with *psi-* (a reasonable onomatopoetic initial sound for a word that means "to lisp").

224 as who seith: "that is, as if to say, as it were."

248–57 Gilbert seiþ expressely þat it is causede but in on maner ... in a hol cloude: Gilbertus discusses the origin of lividity in urine at some length in his Comment on Giles, beginning with the assertion that "qui[c]quid dicant moderni medici, dicemus quod liuor fit vna sola de causa, s. cum aliquid corpus peruium clarum lucidum aliqua occacione obfuscatur, et obfuscatio seu obumbracio iuncta splendori relinquit liuiditatem ut est uidere in flamma" (whatever modern physi-cians say, we would say that leaden colour happens from a single cause, namely when some clear bright shining body is darkened by some event, and the darkening or overshadowing, being joined to the brightness, leaves behind a lividity, as can be seen in a flame) (Wellcome 547, f. 111r–v). After the flame comparison, Gilbert continues with further detailed analogies to a candle, the rainbow, and the reflection of light on clouds, all of which Daniel evidently found too prolix for his audience.

257 hol cloude: "hollow cloud," rendering *nube concaua* in Gilbert.

269–70 if vryn aforn þat vryn aperede ... grenehede: "if the urine that was passed before the (present) urine had a greenish tinge." Compare 2.2.114–16n above.

295 *Febris cotidiana* ... : For a helpful introduction to the medieval understanding of fevers, see Demaitre 2013, 35–60. For a very thorough listing of Middle English names and definitions of many types of fever, see Norri 2016, s.vv. *febre, febris,* and *fever.*

304–5 *Terciana vera,* a verraie tercyene, ... 7 axces, as Ypocras seiþ: *Aph.* 4.59, "Tertiana uera si non iudicatur in septem periodis longissima erit" (An exact tertian reaches a crisis in seven periods at most) (*Articella* 1483, f. 29ra; trans. Jones, Loeb ed. 4: 151).

309 fro þe 3 dai to þe 3 day: "from the third day to the third day," i.e., every three days inclusive. As Demaitre notes (2013, 40), this means a forty-eight-hour cycle. In a double tertian, the fever spikes every day, but the first and third day of the inclusive count have more intense fevers, with a weaker fever on the intermediate days.

320 euery 4 day & 24 houres: This appears to mean that on the days when the fever appears, it lasts twenty-four hours, unlike false quartans (see lines 321–3), in which the fever *turmenteþ more or lesse þan 24 houres.*

347 And some of þat þat it draweþ: Witnesses other than RM7 make better sense here, reading either *And summe of that fume drawith inward* (CfCgBH) or *And þen some of þat fume is drawn inward* (SaSc M6G3 AG6EWSb; GT *with minor variants*). J omits the entire sentence.

350 vnkynd colde: Since Daniel is discussing febrile pathologies in this section (specifically *epiala* and *lipparia*), the interior cold characteristic of *lipparia* should be taken as unnatural, as in the alpha subgroup TGSaSc and all proto-alpha and beta witnesses. All of those witnesses also add the phrase "the innere parties of" before "þe body" at the end of the sentence. (The RM7 variant "kynd colde in þe body" also appears in CfCgHB W6J.)

As Daniel makes clear in the surrounding passage, *epiala* and *lipparia* were seen as related types of intermittent fever, both caused by corruption and imbalance in phlegm and choler or melancholy, with inner parts of the body unnaturally hot and external parts cold (*epiala*) or vice versa (*lipparia*). See Norri 2016, s.v. *epiala, lipparia* (quoting the unemended text of R in the latter entry).

403 se inward, lef {23}: Perhaps an error for *lef* {32}, as that leaf contains a description of the three types of hectic fever (modern f. 37rb–va, 2.3.521–40).

419–22 Now for to know ... i. of þe spiritual membres): This sentence fragment is atypical of Daniel's syntax, but is repeated in most alpha witnesses (RM7 GTSaSc CfCgBH). More regular expressions occur in M6G3 AEWSb J: ... *malum spirituale is sekeness of þe spiritualis, i. of spiritual membrys* (with minor variants).

433–4 or elles ... or elles: The second "or elles" (found in RM7 CfCgHB W6) is probably a redundancy introduced with "as Y saide ryȝt now." All other proto-alpha and alpha witnesses omit the repeated "or elles" and replace the self-reference with "it is taken" (G3M6 TGSaSc) or "it may be said" (J). The beta witnesses omit "or elles … or elles" entirely.

434–8   þe comentour … vppon Ypocras *Afforismys*, in þe 5 particule … noȝt longe after: See Galen's commentary on *Aph.* 5.9, "Hic hypocras dicens ptisis a xviii annis vsque ad. xxxv annum: non intendit spacium eorum esse equale: quid si perspicaciter intendamus verum esse inueniemus. Anni enim pueritie sunt a. xviii vsque ad. xxv & a. xxv vsque ad. xxxv sunt iuuentutis anni" (Here Hippocrates, saying consumption happens from eighteen years to age thirty-five, does not mean their space is equal [= that the years are equally likely?], which we will see to be true if we consider it carefully. For the years of youth are from eighteen to twenty-five, and the years of young adulthood from twenty-five to thirty-five) (*Articella* 1483, f. 31vb).

Cf. *Aph.* 5.9, "Ptisis fit maxime in etatibus a xviii annis usque ad xxxv annum" (Consumption occurs chiefly between the ages of eighteen and thirty-five) (*Articella* 1483, f. 31vb; trans. Jones, Loeb ed. 4: 159).

440–2   as Auicen seiþ, o skil … corrupte mater of blode: Source in Avicenna not yet identified.

451–5   seiþ þe same comentour … it seith deþ: Galen's commentary on *Aph.* 5.11, "Hic ptisim intelligit vulnera pulmonis: in quibus sputa proiecta monstrauit probare: si super carbones expuunt: & sputum putruerit: sicut dixit ante in vulneribus vesice: Si vrina fuerit &c. Dicit autem Si capilli a capite fluunt mortale. & verum est: quia significant nutrimentum ablatum esse: fetor vero corruptionem humorum: & consumptionem membrorum solidorum significat" (Here he takes consumption to be lesions of the lung and he has shown how to test the expelled sputa: if they are coughed up onto hot coals and the sputum stinks, as he said before for lesions in the bladder, "If the urine was, etc." In addition he says that if the hairs fall from the head, it is mortal. And this is true because it signifies that the nourishment has been taken away; the stink indicates the corruption of humours and wasting away of solid members) (*Articella* 1483, f. 32ra).

Cf. *Aph.* 5.11, "Qui a ptisi molestantur: si sputum qualecumque expuunt graue fetet super carbones effusum: & capilli a capite defluunt: mortale" (In patients troubled with consumption, should the sputa they cough up have a strong smell when poured over hot coals, and should the hair fall off from the head, it is a fatal symptom) (*Articella* 1483, f. 32ra; trans. Jones, Loeb ed. 4: 161).

524–5   and by þe powse, when þai … somtyme lesse: *Powse* should be read here as plural; most other witnesses spell the word with the usual plural *-is/-es* ending.

537–9   os Auicen seith … bifore mete as after: Avicenna discusses hectic fever in the *Canon* 4.1.3, chs. 1–11, with chs. 2–3 focused on signs of the fever, but we have not been able to find the specific symptoms of skin that does not fall back after being lifted up or discomfort both before and after eating in this tractate of the *Canon*. However, in the *Breviarius Ypocratis* (= *Breviarius medicine*), John of St Paul reports this sign: "Membris uero nimium consumptis, si cutis tracta manet tensa; ad proprium loccum \non/ reddiens; intelligimus esse [primam *canc.*] \terciam/ speciem ethice que est incurabilis" (The members are greatly wasted, and if the skin is drawn back, it remains stretched, not returning to its proper place: we understand this to be the third species of hectic fever, which is incurable) (Montreal, McGill University Library, Osler MS 7627, f. 56r).

562   **pays:** "weight." Expanded in the beta version to *a peyce* (varr. *peis, peys*) or *a charge or a baggyng* ("swelling"). Proto-alpha witnesses M6G3 do not include the explanatory phrase *os it were ... spirituales*; the late witness J changes *peys* to *peyne*.

562   **hese:** "his." A very unusual form in R's language, with only two appearances as *hese* (here and in 2.12.103) and one as *hes* (2.6.357). Aside from M7, all other witnesses with this phrase read *the*.

596   **in þe lef:** An atypical cross-reference, with no chapter name or number or leaf number, phrased thus only in RM7. Alpha and proto-alpha variants include *in þis cap'* (J), *in/of þe 9 lef* (CfCgBH), *in the 7 chapitre (de karopos)* (GT), omission of the entire *vena concaua* cross-reference (SaSc), and omission of the leaf reference (M6G3). The beta texts cross-reference bk. 2, ch. 8 (once or twice corrected from 3, once as an uncorrected 3); 8 is the correct chapter number in the best beta chapter numberings, and 3 is the correct chapter number for the alpha version.

645–51   **Ypocras seiþ ... mai noȝt be kept:** Cf. *Aph.* 5.44–6, "Que preter naturam tenues existentes concipiunt abortiunt antequam grossescant. Quecunque corpora moderat[a] habentes abortiunt secundo mense aut tertio sine omni occasione manifesta: his cottilidones mucilaginibus pleni sunt: & non possunt pre grauedine tenere fetum: sed abrumpuntur. Quecunque existentes preter naturam crasse non concipiunt: his pinguedo os matricis obturat: & priusquam extenuentur non concipiunt" (Women with child who are unnaturally thin miscarry before they grow large. Women who have average sized bodies miscarry without any obvious cause in the second or third month: for them, the cotyledons of the womb are full of mucus, and break, being unable to retain the unborn child because of its weight. When unnaturally fat women cannot conceive, it is because the fat presses the mouth of the womb, and conception is impossible until they grow thinner) (*Articella* 1483, f. 34ra–rb; our trans., modifying Jones, Loeb ed. 4: 169, 171). See also *Aph.* 59–63 for further discussion of fertility and conception.

654–8   **os techeþ *Liber geneciarum* ... ful of wormes:** This test (or *experimentum*, as it is labelled in the margins of many witnesses) for infertility and the preceding list of causes for failure to conceive translates the Trotula text titled *Liber de sinthomatibus mulierum* by Monica H. Green, §§ 74–5 (ed. and trans. Green 2001, 94–5).

657   17 daies or 15 daies: Only RM7J read *17* here; other alpha witnesses all have *7 dayes or 15 dayes*. In the *De sinthomatibus*, the waiting period is nine or ten days.

677–82   And if a man ... he is lepre: The fragmentary sentence (*And if a man ... to lecherie*) with which this passage begins occurs in RM7 GT CfCgBH. Other witnesses offer syntactically complete sentences in four different phrasings (J; SaSc; M6G3; AG6EWSb), but the general gist remains the same: women are exceptionally lecherous during their periods and are "made whole" by intercourse with men at that time, but the men are put at risk of death, lesions of the penis, or leprosy.

695–7   Þis matrice, os Galien seiþ in his *Bok of Anathomyes*, liþ on þe guttes ... byneþe is *uulua*: "Est autem posita matrix super intestina; et supra collum eius est vesica, et sub ea longaon est, et inferius est vulva" (The uterus is located above the intestine; above its neck is the bladder, and under it the *longaon*. Below is the vulva) (*Anatomia porci*, ed. and trans. Corner 1927, 50, 53).

The prepositions *super*, *supra*, *sub* and the adverb *inferius* refer to the organs of a body (whether human or porcine) lying supine for the process of dissection, as is the case with a number of other prepositions in the *Anatomia porci* that describe the positions of organs within the body.

705–7   þe mouþe of þe matrice closeth ... as Ypocras seiþ: *Aph.* 5.51, "Quecunque in utero habent: his concluditur os matricis" (When women are with child the mouth of the womb is closed) (*Articella* 1483, f. 34rb; trans. Jones, Loeb ed. 4: 171).

715   concepcioun is þus done: Although the reading in RM7 ("corrupcioun is þus gadrede") follows reasonably well from the preceding sentence, it makes less sense in the subsequent humoral discussion of the warming of the uterus upon conception. All other alpha and proto-alpha witnesses have some form of "concepcioun is þus doon" here; the beta texts all remove the phrase in a significant abridgment of the passage.

736–7   Of whiche cometh kindly swyche os þat is whos it is: "From which there naturally comes semen similar to the person/member to whom/which it belongs." If Daniel means the person from whom the semen comes, the pronoun *he* (instead of *þat*) might make this sentence a little smoother, but all alpha and most beta witnesses agree with R.

759–63   Seynt Austyn in a pistel ... to Seynt Jerom ... it is in waxing: This information does not appear to be in Augustine's epistles to Jerome, but can be found in the treatise *On Eighty-Three Different Questions* 56, "On the Forty-Six Years for the Building of the Temple" (Fathers of the Church, vol. 70, trans. Mosher 1982, 98). The relationship to embryology is numerological: the Temple is taken as a figure of Christ's body; the sum of 6, 9, 12, 18 and 1 (indicating a single sum) is 46, supposed to be the number of days it takes for a fetus to move through the stages of milk, blood, and solidity ("a sadde body") and achieve the "formes of membres"; multiplying 46 by 6 (the beginning of the series) yields 276, the number of inclusive days between Christ's conception and birth. The final point about gestational time is repeated in the *De Trinitate* 4.5, but not the four stages leading up to day 46.

Similar material on gestational periods and processes, citing Augustine, Constantine, and Galen, appears in Bartholomaeus Anglicus's *De proprietatibus rerum* 6.3.

764–7 *Conceptum semen sex ... producit ad ortum*: *Flos medicine* 1245–8, ed. De Renzi 1852–9, 1: 486; 1795–8, 5: 51. Not in Frutos González 2010b.

768–70 Aristotel, in þe *Boke of Kynd of Bestes*, þe 9 boke, þe 2 c., seiþ ... 80 day or þerabouten: Perhaps a reference to *History of Animals* 7.3 (despite the difference in book and chapter number), which gives the time of quickening for males as forty days and of females as ninety days. Daniel's "80 day or þerabouten" may be influenced by the biblical chapter that he cites in the next sentence, Leviticus 12 (see following note).

Daniel could have encountered Aristotle's work on animals in the translation of Michael Scot (Arabo-Latin, early thirteenth century) or that of the Dominican William of Moerbeke (Greco-Latin, second half of the thirteenth century).

770–1 Seynt Gregorie in þe glose vpon þe 3 boke ... vppon *Leuiticus*, þe 12 c.: We have not yet traced St Gregory's gloss on Leviticus 12 (Gregory did not write a commentary specifically on that book), but the chapter's concern with the forty or eighty days of purification after the birth of a male or female child makes it a likely text to generate comments about differential quickening of male and female embryos, as occurs in the *Glossa Ordinaria* (with attribution to "Isichius" or Hesychius): "*Triginta tribus diebus, &c.* [Isichius:] Septem additis xl. fiunt. Quadraginta diebus formari dicitur masculus ... Apertè hæc probantur per ea quæ de genere foeminæ sequuntur: Quia enim octogesima die in vtero formati foeminæ dicuntur, eundem numerum ad impletionem purgationis, vel purificationis earum quæ semen suscipiunt, præcepit sic: *Si foeminam peperit, immunda &c.*" (*Thirty three days, &c.* Isichius: Added to seven make forty. A male is said to be formed in forty days ... These matters are clearly proved by those which follow, concerning female nature. Because females are said to be formed in the womb by the eightieth day, the Lord commands the same number for fulfilling the purgation or purification of those who receive the seed, thus: *If she has borne a girl, she is unclean &c.*) (*Glossa Ordinaria* 1617, 1: 1017).

798–800 vnneþes shalt þou fynde eny distinccioun ... þat þai ne ar taken indifferently: Perhaps a double negative for emphasis = "There's hardly any distinction in medicine such that these terms ... are taken as indifferent [i.e., indistinct] from each other." It is interesting that after this apparent lumping together of medical understandings of prolapse/precipitation, oppression/suffocation, and distension, Daniel goes on to suggest that actually speaking to a sick female patient can help the *wyse & sliȝh* practitioner to know which she is actually suffering from.

844   ychon on oþer: "in each other." GSaSc add "& spekyth therof bytwene thaymselfe prively"; M6 replaces *ychon on oþer* with the same phrase. T adds "and speke þer of in here huþermoþere" (= *hudder-mudder* "huddled privacy"; *MED*, s.v. *heder-moder* [n.]); G3 replaces *ychon on oþer* with that phrase (including the form *hethyr moþyr*).

846–7   techeþ Aristotil ... Boke of Kynde of Bestes, by al þe 9 bok & þe 10 eke: Aristotle discusses the uterus at some length in books 6 (mainly on animals) and 7 (on humans) of the *History of Animals*. We have not determined the reason for the discrepancy in book numbers between Daniel and modern editions of the Greek text, but that divergence may be rooted in the scribal copy of whichever Latin translation Daniel was using. Faith Wallis notes (personal communication) that the discrepancy "does not seem to arise from Michael Scot's translation of *Generation of Animals*, *Parts of Animals*, and *History of Animals*, which he fused into a single 19-book work entitled *History of Animals*."

850–1   Of þe forsaide Greyns ... se in þe 3 boke: This cross-reference seems to be out of place – it might make better sense after the following material on livid Circles and Grains in the urine (signalling ascites) – but it occurs at this position in all witnesses. Perhaps Daniel was referring back to his introductory comments on the diseases signified by Blo urine (pulmonary, hectic, hepatic, and female reproductive maladies; 2.3.415–19), though that passage is at quite a distance from this cross-reference and makes no mention of the urinary Circle.

854   ierariolon: The beginning of this word, *iera-*, is a variant of *hiera-*, suggesting some reflex of the classical name for epilepsy, "the sacred disease" (ἱερὰ νόσος), which was familiar to Daniel's contemporaries. *DMLBS*, s.v. *hieros*, quotes a passage from John of Gaddesden explaining the Greek name for epilepsy: "dicitur hieranoson, de 'hiera,' i. sacra, et 'noceo.'" A misreading of *n* as *ri* and long *s* as *l* would explain corruption to *ierariolon*.

2.4

28   Yposarca & ydropisis Ypocras calleþ al on: Hippocrates does not distinguish the various types of dropsy identified in medieval texts (e.g., anasarca, ascites, leucophlegmatia, tympanites, and [h]yposarca). For a catalogue of words for dropsy in Middle English and distinctions among the subtypes, see Norri 2016, s.vv. *dropsy, ydropic(um), ydropisis, ydropsy; anasarca; ascites, asclitis; leucofleuma(nce), leucofleumancia, leucofleumancy, leucofleumansis, leucofleume; tympaniste(s), tympanites, tympanum, tympany; yposarca, yposarce.*

32–8   as techeþ Galien in his Anatomyes, epar ... fro epar to þe splen: "Ex dextra parte sub fundo stomachi est hepar positum, in cuius substantia est quaedam vesica, quae cystis fellis appelatur, et super hepar sunt duo panniculi, zirbus et siphac, qui sunt implicati velut rete. Quod apparet ibi pingue et grossum, dicitur zirbus; quod autem subtile est, siphac; quae procedunt usque ad splenem, per quos venae transeunt, per quas melancholia ab hepate ad splenem mittitur" (At the right side under the pouch of the stomach the liver is placed. In its substance there is a sac called the gall-bladder, and above the liver are two membranes, *zirbus* and *siphac*, which are folded together like a net. The one which appears thick and loaded with fat is called *zirbus*, but the one which is delicate is called *siphac*. These membranes reach as far as the spleen, and are traversed by veins through which black biliary humor (*melancholia*) is transmitted from the liver to the spleen) (*Anatomia porci*, ed. and trans. Corner 1927, 49, 52).

Following the ps.-Galenic *Anatomia porci*, Daniel applies the terms *zirbus* and *sifac* only to membranes around the liver, rather than taking them for the peritoneum as a whole, in line with other anatomical writers. For the membrane and fatty tissue enclosing the intestines, again emulating ps.-Galen, Daniel uses the terms *epigozontaymenon* and *omentum* (2.7.523 below).

41 Ypocras calleþ þis spice of *ydropisis* only *ydropisis*: See note to line 2.4.28 above.

47–8 þe leucofleume ... Ypocras calleþ it *fleuma album*, þe white *fleuma*: Hippocrates mentions white phlegm twice in the *Aphorisms* (7.29, 7.75), both times very briefly.

52–3 Ypocras calleþ þis maner of *ydropisis sicca*: Aph. 4.11, "Quibuscunque torsiones & circa umbilicum dolores & lumbos: & dolor non solutus sit: neque pharmacijs neque aliter in hydropem siccam perficitur" (Those who suffer from colic, pains about the navel, and ache in the loins, removed neither by purging nor in any other way, finish with a dry dropsy) (*Articella* 1483, f. 25rb; trans. Jones, Loeb ed. 4: 137; the Loeb footnote to this passage cites Francis Adams's identification of dry dropsy with tympanites).

74–5 And þerfor seiþ Ypocras in his *Afforismis* ... frenetik or nefretik: Aph. 4.72, "Quibus urine limpide aut albe: male: maxime si in phreniticis [*add.* & neufreticis Harley 3140] appareant" (When the urine is transparent and white, it is bad; it appears principally in cases of phrenitis [and nephritis]) (*Articella* 1483, f. 30rb; Harley 3140, f. 25r [c. 1300 *Ars medicinae*]; trans. Jones, Loeb ed. 4: 155, with minor modification). See also the Standard Commentary: "Et in hoc concordat Ypocras in *Afforismis*, dicens: vrine limpide et clare omnes male, et maxime in nefresi et frenesi" (And Hippocrates agrees with this in the *Aphorisms*, saying: Transparent and bright urines are all evil, and especially in nephritis and frenzy) (Sloane 282, f. 24v).

84, 87 leny pece ... lonye: "the loin part, lower back"; "the loin(s)." The spelling with -*ny*- may reflect the Old French etymon *loigne*, with a palatalized *n*. Cf. the form *loni* given in *MED*, s.v. *loine* (n.[1]). Other witnesses spell the word as *loyne* (CgHG) or *leyne* (Sc).

110–15 a reule þat Þeophil ȝeueþ in his *Boke of Vryns* ... he is but ded: Theophilus, *Liber urinarum*: "& siquidem frenesis quieuerit propter aliquam causam: ut in fluxu sanguinis per nares: aut propter sudorem multum in capite factum, urina subtili et alba ueniente, quietem significat. Si uero urina talis facta adest et frenesis permanens, ita dispositus moritur" (And if a frenzy should cease for any reason, such as bleeding from the nostrils or much sweating from the head, with the urine being thin and White, it signifies calm. For if such urine is made and the frenzy remains, someone so disposed will die) (ed. Dase 1999, 13; *Articella* 1483, f. 6ra).

150–1 *artetica passio ... os seiþ* **Gilbert:** Gilbert's Comment on Giles: "Nota quod si arthetica fiat ex solo frigore aut ex sola siccitate, non competit farmacia nec flebotomia, sed solum in illa que fit ex reumate humorum, et nota similiter quod in quadam ydropisi competit frigida, sicut quando fit ex multitudine humorum ut fit in crapulatis multociens, et regnum [*poss. error for* regimen?] suum inordinantibus, ut dictum est paulo ante" (Note that if joint pain come from cold alone or dryness alone, neither drugs nor bloodletting is effective, but only in the illness that comes from rheum of the humours; and note likewise that in a certain cold dropsy, as when it happens from many humours as often in drunkards and those who mismanage their rule, as was said a little before) (Wellcome 547, f. 114ra–rb).

161–2 *þe Comentour vpon Giles seyth ... 3 skiles ... vryn White:* The three reasons that urine is White are spread rather diffusely over the next few paragraphs, mainly because Daniel digresses into a discussion of *colica passio* (lines 168–206). They are 1) obstruction of humours, especially choler (lines 163–4); 2) ache and pain in the body, such as *colica passio* (lines 165–6); and 3) feeble digestion of the humours (lines 207–8).

Attributing the three reasons to the Standard Commentary is a bit odd, given that its author leads into his discussion of White and thin urine by warning readers that he will pass over the causes of White colour (Sloane 282, f. 24r). However, a variant reading later in this section of the commentary, following the gloss on *arthetica passio*, may be the source of Daniel's comment (which also follows *artetica*): "Dicit autem quod urine apparent intense iii casibus: s. ex dolore nimio, ut in colerica pasione; et ex debilitate digestiue, eo quod humores non possint depurari, unde admiscentur calidum humidum cum urina ut in ydropici; uel ex forti opilacione eo quod non euentatur eorum" (But he says that urines appear intense in three cases [*or* for three causes]: namely from great pain, as in *cholerica* [*lege* colica] *passio*; and from digestive weakness, on account of which the humours cannot be purified, whence hot [and] wet are mixed with the urine as in dropsy; or from strong obstruction, on account of which their [?wind ?humour] is not vented) (Wellcome 547, f. 150ra; not in Laud lat. 106 at this point).

189 *oyþer:* "either." The scribe of M7 does not distinguish *y* from *þ*, and uses an *-er* curl on this word, so the word actually looks like *oyy*[9] or *oy*[9]*y* in the manuscript. The spelling also occurs at line 2.4.275 (M7, f. 27v) and twice in R, at 2.11.45 and 47.

**196–200 & þerfor seiþ Ypocras ... Ypocras sawh a woman ... as Galien &
Ysaac rehersen:** This incident does not seem to appear in the *Aphorisms*, *Prognostics*, or *Epidemics*, but Gilbert mentions it in his Comment on Giles, citing
only Isaac as his authority: "Ypocras vero dicit quod vrina alba & tenuis in colica
pessima est & mortifera, vnde dicit Ysaac quod Ypocras de quadam muliere que
habebat vrinam talem in colica iudicauit ipsam mori in die vij, & sic euenit" (Hippocrates says that White and thin urine in colic is the worst and is fatal, whence
Isaac says that Hippocrates judged that a woman who had such urine with colic
would die in the seventh day, and so it happened) (Wellcome 547, f. 114rb). We
have not found a case history of a woman with colic and thin White urine who
died after seven days in Isaac.

201–2 if þe vryn apere ... os Auicen & Gilbert sein: Gilbert, Comment on
Giles: "In arthetica ergo est vrina alba et tenuis specificata per attomosa[s] resolutiones, sed si in arthetica fit talis propter deriuacionem materie ad locum doloris;
ergo a simili in colica vbi est dolor maximus vrina esset huiusmodi. Tamen dicit
Auicenna quod vrina in colica apparens tincta laudabilis est, quia spergitur colera
et incipit natura uincere supra materiam" (In gout, urine is White and thin, characterized by Mote-like particulates, but if such urine happens in gout, it is because
of the passage of the matter to the place of pain. Therefore from the like in colic,
where the pain is extreme, urine would be of this type. Nevertheless, Avicenna says
that coloured urine appearing in colic is laudable, because the choler is dispersed
and nature begins to overcome the matter of the illness) (Wellcome 547, f. 114rb,
with emendation from BAV, MS Vat. lat. 2459).

206 þe forsaide resoluciouns: A reference back to 2.4.144–5 ("resolucions
as smale as Motes in þe sonne"), but Daniel may have been reminded of that
line by Gilbert's mention of *attomosas resolutiones* in the commentary passage
just cited.

236–7 *albedo in vryna est filia frigiditatis*: In GTSaSc, M6G3, and all beta
witnesses, this quotation also appears, with attribution to Galen, early in the
chapter(s) on Albus, in connection with the streaky urine that indicates sickness of
the spleen. GTSaSc also give the quotation here, attributed only to *auctours*, but
M6G3 and the beta family omit this later occurrence.

**282–3 If þe vryn schew him so in wanysshyng of an acue ... tokne of saf.
Þus seiþ Giles:** Standard Commentary, commenting on Giles's *cum febre caumate*:
"Si in declinacione talis appareat, cretica determinacione precedente, signum est
salutare" (If [White urine] appears in the decline [of the fever], after the end of
the crisis, it is a sign of health) (Sloane 282, f. 25v). The possibility that Giles was
himself the author of the Standard Commentary was suggested by Sudhoff (1929,
132–3).

**284–7 Gilbert seiþ þat if þe vryn schew him White ... faileþ & sekenes may-
stre:** Gilbert comments on *Carmen de urinis* 56–9: "In al[go]re epatis [line 59]
aut a natura aut ab accidente est vrina alba & tenuis, ut dictum est; & distinguit

quod talis potest apparere in principio uel in augmento uel in statu uel in declinacione. In augmento uel statu frenesim signat. In principio cruditatem materie. In
declinacione similem, sed in declinacione, cum mala materia totaliter expulsa sit
et natura confortetur & ad se redierit, vrina non debet esse alba & tenuis. Vnde si
appareat talis in declinacione malum signat, quia morbi reuersionem ... Et hic est
malum signum, quia urina defecta est ex morbo precedente; male ergo dicit Egidius
quod concedo" (In cold of the liver, the urine is White and thin either by nature
or by accident, as is said; and he makes the distinction that such can appear in the
beginning or the increase or the state or the decline of the disease. In the increase
or state, it signifies frenzy. In the beginning, rawness of the matter. In the decline
it is similar, but in the decline, since the wicked matter is completely expelled and
nature would be comforted and return to itself, the urine should not be White and
thin. For this reason, if it should appear so in the decline, it signifies evil, because [it
signifies] the return of the disease ... And this is a bad sign, because the imperfect
urine is from the foregoing disease; therefore Giles speaks badly, which I concede)
(Wellcome 547, f. 114va; emendation from BAV, Vat. lat. 2459).

　　Although Gilbert explicitly criticizes Giles's claim that thin White urine at the
end of a fever is a good sign, Daniel argues that they are not really in conflict, perhaps because the sickness goes away before returning.

　　299　riste: "rises" (M7J's spelling). The CfCgBH variant *rysyth* makes better
sense here than GTSaSc's *resteth*.

　　303　dedisshe & made: "benumbed and stupefied"; cf. *MED*, s.v. *mad* (adj.),
sense 2.(b).

　　**331–9　But *fleuma vitreum* ... Herewiþ acordes Theophile in his *Vryns* &
Ypocras eke in his *Affurmis*, þe 4 particule:** Compare the Standard Commentary:
"Fleuma [uero] vitreum, cum adhuc crudum sit et compactu[m] resistebat nature
expellere volenti, et quia eius mala fiebat resolucio, pauca erat vrina; sed fleumate
digesto per caloris confortacionem, fit eius resolucio in partes minimas et disgregat,
unde multiplicatur urina et attenuatur. Et nota quod omnis materia in sui digestione
inspissat urinam, preter fleuma uitreum; huius regule concordanciam habemus apud
Ypocras in quarta parte *Afforismis*: quibus urine pauce et globose, non sine febre,
multitudo veniens tenuis iuuat; et apud Theophilum: urina alba et [multa & tenuis]
amphimer[in]am deficientem signat" (And vitreous phlegm, since it was still raw
and compacted, was resistant to nature's desire to expel it, and because its resolution
was bad, the urine was scanty. But once the phlegm was digested by the comfort of
heat, its resolution into small parts took place and it dissipated, on account of which
the phlegm was multiplied and attenuated. And note that all digested matter thickens the urine except for vitreous phlegm. We have concord with this rule from Hippocrates in *Aphorisms*, part 4: When the urine is thick, full of clots, and scanty, fever
being present, a copious discharge of (comparatively) thin urine coming afterwards
gives relief; and from Theophilus: Urine White and profuse and thin signifies a
receding ephemeral fever) (Sloane 282, ff. 25v–26r; emendation from Laud lat. 106).

The Commentator's quotation of Hippocrates is from *Aph.* 4.69. The quotation from Theophilus is a slightly abridged version of the original: "Urina tenuis et alba multum mincta in febribus anfimerinam deficientem significat per huiusmodi humorem" (Urine thin and White, profusely passed in fevers, signifies a receding ephemeral fever through this kind of humour) (ed. Dase 1999, 11; *Articella* 1483, f. 5vb).

339   Affurmis: Possibly an error for *Affurismes*, though some other alpha witnesses (CfCgBH) agree. Compare the OF form *Amforimes/Amphorimes* for another example of omitted medial *s*.

340–5   wiþ resoluciouns like fisshes scales ... Þo Scalis, os seith þe Comentour vpon Giles ... sperme: Standard Commentary: "Specifica si appareat cum squamis et nigris resolucionibus que signat retencionem melancolici sanguinis qui niger est et terrestris" (Namely if it appears with Scales and black resolutions that signify retention of melancholy blood, which is black and comes from earthy things) (Sloane 282, f. 26r). Neither Sloane 282 nor Laud lat. 106 mentions women's sperm in this passage, though Laud lat. 106 adds a clause that suggests the resolutions are caused by excoriation of the womb.

365   bosmyth: Cf. *OED*, s.v. *bosom* (v.), sense 1: "to form a bosom, to belly" (used of a sail, cited only from the *Scottish Troy Book*). Here, the sense appears to be something like "swells, inflates, opens up a space" (also as an effect of wind, though within the body). See also *MED*, s.vv. *bosom* (n.; esp. senses 3.c "the belly of a sail" and 4.a "an inner recess") and *bosoming* (ger.) "a hollow, concavity."

2.5

5   brighede: I.e., *brighthed* "brightness," with the R scribe's propensity to omit the letter *t* after *gh* or *ȝ*, and a collapsing of the *hh* sequence that follows that omission. See note to Prol.92 above.

30   mathe: "maketh" (a rare, contracted form). Compare *mathe* (2.13.87), *math* (3.16.346), *trethe* "treateth" (2.14.6), and *tath* "taketh" (2.14.27).

44–5   as techeþ Johannicius in his *Ysigogis* ... 5 maner of fleumes: *Isagoge in Techne Galieni*, §6 (ed. Maurach 1978, 152; trans. Wallis 2010, 141).

2.6

22–3   þis colour in vryn is euermore causede ... os Auicen techeþ: Avicenna discusses the colours of urine in *Canon* 1.2.3.2, ch. 2, distinguishing two main types of White urines (transparent vs non-transparent urine like milk or parchment) and then observing that "Album igitur secundum intentionem translucentis significat frigiditatem omnino & est auferens digestionis fiduciam . & si cum grossitudine fuerit significabit fleuma" (White in the sense of translucent signifies cold completely, and it takes away assurance of good digestion. And if it appears with grossness it signifies phlegm) (*Canon*, ed. 1522, f. 41rb). The chapter does not discuss the effect of cold interacting with humidity, and its only specific mention of *lactea* urine is to say that such urine is pernicious in acute illnesses (f. 41va).

146–9   Luna, the mone, is *frigida* & *humida* … os seiþ Ptholomeus in … *Almagisti*: Ptolemy's *Almagest* is heavily focused on astronomical and geometric observations and calculations, and does not appear to make the more general claims about the nature of the heavenly bodies seen here and below, which are more characteristic of the planetary discussions in Ptolemy's astrological work, the *Tetrabiblos* (e.g., bk. 1, chaps. 4–8).

160–9   A dai naturel is 24 houres … made at mydday: Daniel probably takes the different starting times for the day from Sacrobosco's *Computus ecclesiasticus*, composed c. 1232–5 (on the dating, see Pedersen 1985, 185): "Dies Naturalis secundum diuersos, diuersa habet principia. Romani enim diem Naturalem a media nocte incipiunt, & ibidem terminant, Quoniam legitur, quod Dominus natus fuerit in medio noctis diei Dominicae … Arabes uero a meridie incipiunt, qui dicunt Solem fuisse factum in meridie … Iudaei autem a Vespere, innitentes illi autoritati Genesis, Factum est Vespere & mane dies unus. Quidam etiam secundum sensum agentes, ut uulgus, diem Naturalem ab ortu Solis incipiunt, quia cum Sol sit causa diei, tunc merito debet dies incipere, cum Sol effertur supra nostrum horizontem" (The natural day has different beginnings according to different peoples. For the Romans begin the natural day at midnight and end it there, because it is read that the Lord was born in the middle of the night on a Sunday … The Arabs say that the Sun was made at noon, and they begin at noon … The Jews begin from evening, based on the authority of Genesis, "And evening and morning were made one day." And some who act according to their senses, such as the common people, begin the natural day from sunrise, because since the Sun is the cause of day, the day rightly ought to begin when the Sun is carried above our horizon) (*Computus ecclesiasticus*, ed. 1543, sigs. B2v–B3r; also in BL Harley 3647, f. 34ra, with the rubricated title *Compotus Iohannis de Sacrobosco*; cited in these notes by the title in the 1543 edition).

Much of Daniel's computistical information closely parallels material in the *Computus ecclesiasticus*, but the information could also be found, usually in less detail, in other computistical authors, such as Isidore of Seville, in *Etymologies* 5.28–36; Bede, *The Reckoning of Time*; Gerlandus the Computist; Roger of Hereford; Roger Bacon, *Opus maius*, part 4. For recent editions, studies, and translations, see Wallis, trans. 1999; Lohr, ed. 2013; Lohr, ed. 2015.

167–8   the first boke of Holy Writte seiþ … *dies vnus*: Gen. 1:5, quoted by Sacrobosco (see preceding note).

184–5   *Arabes meridie, Romani media nocte / Gens Judea sero, wlgus quoque solis ab ortu*: "The Arabs [begin the day] at noon, the Romans at midnight / The Jews in the evening, and the common folk from sunrise." The couplet is out of place in RM7; it should appear before the paragraph on the day quarters (at line 2.6.170 above), as it does in other alpha witnesses. The witnesses to Sacrobosco's *Computus ecclesiasticus* that we have consulted do not contain the couplet, but the verses could have circulated independently as a useful mnemonic for students of the computus (on the ubiquity of computistical verse mnemonics, see Thorndike 1955, 165–74). The beta version drops the verse entirely and offers an expanded biblical justification for the Christian practice of starting the day at midnight.

186–204   The units and relative proportions of time, both computistical and astronomical, correspond to Sacrobosco's discussion in the *Computus ecclesiasticus*, except for the erroneous ratio between *atomos* and *vncia* in RM7 (1:17 instead of the correct 1:47 found in the vast majority of witnesses to both versions). The 1:47 *atomus* to *vncia* ratio is found in the Harley 3647 copy of the *Computus* (f. 33v), though the 1543 print edition has 1:48 (sig. B2r).

217–20   Venus ... is neuermore ferrer fro þe sone þan 2 degres at þe moste: Something has gone wrong in the text here: the maximum elongation of Venus from the sun is between 45 and 47 degrees. The error occurs in all alpha witnesses; the proto-alpha texts M6G3 and beta texts AG6EW omit the reference to Venus's elongation. Venus has a wider orbit than Mercury, whose maximum elongation is between 18 and 28 degrees (so Daniel's figure of 30 degrees for Mercury is not far off the mark).

234   falleþ euermore on F lettre: 24 February (the Feast of St Matthias; also the sixth kalends of March) is the fifty-fifth day of the year, which always has the letter F in the seven-letter cycle that begins on 1 January (ABCDEFG, ABCDEFG, etc.). In medieval leap years, 24 February was repeated, still with the letter F and the date of the 24th, instead of the modern practice of inserting the extra day at the end of the month and giving it the date 29 February (see following note).

235   it schal be 2 saide sexte kalends: Two days in a row were called the sixth kalends of March in a medieval leap year.

243–6   þe 12 dai of the kalends ... laste day o þe fest: Daniel may be confused by the idea that *bis sexte* means twice six, as though two sixth kalends in a row would yield the twelfth kalends. The actual twelfth and eleventh days of the kalends of March are 18 and 19 February, neither of which is the feast of St Matthias (24 February). The comment about the last day of the feast seems to refer to the fact that, in a leap year, the saint's day is celebrated on the second of the two days numbered 24 February or sixth kalends of March.

263   and so euermore ... :   By stopping at eleven, Daniel leaves unclear how to deal with leap years ending in 2 and 6, such as 1392 and 1396, unless the phrase "fro þe laste j inclusif to his 10 inclusif" means the numbers in the last two places (01 to 99).

268–73 þer schulde no feste in þe ȝere be stedfaste ne certeyne ... *Boke of Compote,* **þe 4 c.:** Daniel appears to have misunderstood the calendrical calculation here: with no leap years for 364 years, 25 December would move *backward* through the solar year by ninety-one days, ending near the autumnal equinox in September, not the vernal equinox near the feast of the Annunciation.

Sacrobosco's original is more complex, but correct: "Notandum quod nisi bissextus obseruaretur in 364 annis, contingeret nathale domini celebrari in tam longis diebus, sicut nunc celebratur annunciatio beati iohannis babtiste. & natiuitas beati iohannis babtiste in tam breuibus diebus sicut nunc annunciatio Domini ... vel forte peius, scilicet, quod nathale celebraretur in tam longis diebus sicut nunc celebratur festum iohannis babtiste. Quod patet consideranti si duplicentur 364 anni" (It is to be noted that unless the leap day were observed, over a 364-year period, Christmas would be celebrated in days as long as now is celebrated the Annunciation of the blessed John the Baptist [i.e., around 24 September] and the Nativity of blessed John the Baptist [24 June] would be celebrated in days as short as the Annunciation of the Lord [25 March] ... or perhaps worse, namely, that Christmas would be celebrated in days as long as now is celebrated the Feast of John the Baptist [24 June]. Which is obvious to someone considering this if the 364 years were doubled) (BL, MS Harley 3647, f. 41va–vb).

Daniel's error may have arisen from the unusual reference to the "annunciation of John the Baptist," which is not a feast normally celebrated in the Church, leading to conflation with the more familiar Annunciation on 25 March. And the error may already have been present in the Latin manuscript tradition; certainly, by the 1543, 1549, and possibly other print editions, the same "Christmas in springtime" mistake occurs.

272–3 Maistre of þe Compote ... *Boke of Compote,* **þe 4 c.:** The Master of the Computus is most likely John of Sacrobosco, as suggested by the parallels already adduced to his *Computus ecclesiasticus.* Neither the manuscript copy in Harley 3647 nor the 1543 printed edition offers numbered chaptering systems. Perhaps Daniel had access to a copy of Sacrobosco's *Computus* that had been annotated with chapter numbers, in which the discussion of leap days occurred in the fourth chapter of the text, but until a modern critical edition of the text is published, such a suggestion must remain speculative.

278 þis figure þat stant on þe pacche: Referring to the small volvelle now attached to f. 51*/52, which aids in calculating dominical letters. Only R has such a device, and among full copies of the text, only RM7 mention the "pacche"; other witnesses refer to (and sometimes provide) a circular "figure" or "whele" that can be used for the same kind of reckoning. The *pacche* is also mentioned in the bk. 2.6 excerpt that appears in Cambridge, Magdalene College, Pepys Library MS 1661 (pp. 235–40), suggesting that it is closely related to RM7. Daniel's concern that his *figure* might be "loste or fordon" (2.6.301) was evidently warranted.

The "figure ... on þe pacche" (f. 51*/52) is related to the concentric sun-cycle diagram in Sacrobosco's *Computus ecclesiasticus* (Harley 3647, f. 42r; ed. 1543, sig. D5v), though with the information limited to 1) the dominical letters and 2) the numbers and dominical letters (1–2–3–DL repeated seven times) of the four-year leap-year cycle. Daniel's diagram omits the concurrents found in both Sacrobosco examples, and the twenty-eight year numbers and twenty-eight-syllable Latin verse in the outer rings of the Harley diagram.

287   Nos & Garlandus: This brief attribution attached to the instructional verses for the sun-cycle diagram may be an echo of Sacrobosco's *Computus*: Following the mnemonic Latin verse "Constans est genitor, bona donat, fertilis autor" (= letters CEGBDFA), Sacrobosco distinguishes himself and Gerlandus from Dionysius Exiguus in relation to the year in which they begin the solar cycle: "Cyclus uero solaris, secundum Dionysium, non incipit ab eo anno quem *nos cum Gerlando* [Harley: *nos & Gerlandus*] constituimus principium, sed a duodecimo illius" (*Computus ecclesiasticus*, ed. 1543, sig. D6v; BL Harley 3647, f. 42va; emphasis added). The phrase appears only in R and H, whose diagram appears on an otherwise blank parchment leaf in an otherwise paper MS; the figure in H and its concentric verses may have been added from some R-like exemplar. Faith Wallis notes (personal communication) that Sacrobosco follows Gerlandus in his analysis of the concurrents and the solar and leap year cycles, beginning the cycle of concurrents at the beginning of the four-year cycle of leap years (in which the leap year itself is year 4).

288   flite þrede forth, pryk to þe nere: "let the thread move outward, the pin being near to you," describing a thread anchored with a pin in the centre and moving around the circumference of the diagram. Leap year occurs *at þe ferþ* (letter), the thread *kenneþ* the user what letter *renneþ on* the Sunday, and what year of the sun-cycle it is (lines 289–91). Some scribes write *þrede/þrede/þridde* as *third*, either as an alternate spelling or a misunderstanding of the word, perhaps under the influence of *ferþ* "fourth." The beta group changes *pryk* to *hole*, which could refer to the small hole in the middle of a volvelle; GTSaSc have *prike to þe more* ("with the pin more toward you").

293   concurrantz: A cyclical numbering system for years, based on the number of the weekday for 24 March, with Sunday counted as 1. The number advances by one every year, except in leap years, when it advances by two. As Daniel notes, the Sunday letters run in tandem with the concurrents: F/1, E/2, D/3, C/4, etc.; both cycles skip forward an extra day in leap year.

294–300   þe verse ... the verses þat I haue writen aboute: I.e., the verses around the diagram on the *pacche* (2.6.287–92). Only R and H actually write the verses concentrically around a sun-cycle diagram. M7 refers to the figure and verses on the *pacche* but does not include it or any equivalent diagram. In GTSaSc and AG6EW the verses are incorporated in the text near the diagram or the space left for it. Other witnesses promise the verses and/or the figure but do not in fact provide them (CfCgB M7G3), omit the passage (J), or are missing leaves (Sb).

303–4   Fons . est . dans … ci . bus . glans: The usual form of this mnemonic couplet for dominical letters is as follows, with syllables separated by points:

Fons est dans bis a.gro, fun.dus ci.bat, au.fer e.da.cem

Au.gens fert es.cas, bos aut gens, e.da.ci.bus glans.

The bold letters that begin each syllable are the "Sunday letters" for each year, with leap years reflected by the omission of a letter in the *fedcbag* series. In leap years, the Sunday letter before the leap day is the omitted letter; after the leap day the Sunday letter is the next bold letter. For example, in 1381 the Sunday letter was F, in 1382 E, in 1383 D; in 1384, the letter was C before leap day and B after, in 1385 A, 1386 G, 1387 F, and in 1388, E before leap day and D after, and so on.

308–9   Vndur B … fro B exclusif: Daniel instructs his readers to "acompte" or tally each skipped letter underneath its following letter (C under the B of *bis*; E under the D of *fundum*; etc.), which would remind them that leap years have different Sunday letters before and after leap day. In the concentric circles of letters and numbers on the *pacche* (f. 51*/52), the "acompted" letters are written below their following letters to represent the leap years (see Plate 2). Thorndike gives other versified mnemonics for the calculation (1955, 170–1).

325   12 siþes 10 houres: Ten hours each month add up to 120 hours (five days) over a year; the readings *30 siþes* (RGSaScCfCgBH), *13 seþes* (M7J), and *10 syþes* (T) are all clearly mistaken. (Other witnesses omit the gloss.)

336–8   13 minutes & 45 2ᵉ … magnus bisextus: The superscript on the number 2 in RM7 is difficult to decipher, but must be equivalent to a Latin or English plural suffix (*-e* or *-es/-is*) for the word *secunda* or *seconde*. Daniel (and presumably his source, which we have not yet identified) is mistaken about the difference in the real length of the tropical year and the 365.25 days used in the Julian calendar: the tropical year is actually slightly shorter than 365.25 days, by about 11 minutes and 14 seconds, leading to the shortfall that was only compensated for with the Gregorian reform of the calendar. However, if the year were in fact 13 minutes and 45 seconds longer than 365.25 days, 100 years would add up to an additional 1375 minutes, fairly close to the 1440 minutes in a day. But the idea of a second leap day once a century was never put into practice, and we have not been able to trace a source for the term *magnus bisextus*.

350   a helply fader: An allusion to a traditional etymology of the name Jupiter as *iuvans pater* "helping father" (Isidore of Seville, *Etymologies* 8.11.34; ed. Lindsay 1911).

358–9   12 ʒer … in a gre aboute a 7 daies: Jupiter's orbital period is 11.86 years, so Daniel's *12 ʒer* is pretty close, as is the one year per sign ratio. To get the 7 days per degree result, Daniel may have been including Jupiter's retrograde motion, which carries the planet "backward" in the sign by about 10 degrees and then forward again, adding about 20 degrees to its path in each sign. Traversing a path of 50 degrees in 365 days (by this reckoning) would require 7.3 days for each degree, to which Daniel's figure of 7 is a reasonable approximation. Alternately, if one divides 365 days by 30 degrees (one sign), ignoring retrogradation (as Daniel does for Saturn and Mars), the days/degrees ratio would be just slightly over 12, raising the possibility that 7 is simply a scribal error for *12*.

362   wikedest of al in effect: The textual situation for this phrase in the alpha and proto-alpha traditions is somewhat vexed, with versions of "wickid/wikkedest (of alle) in effect" (G3M6 GTSASc), "werst of all in effect" (CfCgHB W6), and some form of corruption generating "proued soþ al in effecte" (RM7 J). The beta witnesses revise the passage completely.

376–88   The *rota celi* diagram on f. 49v (Plate 3) may have been inspired by a diagram in Sacrobosco's *Computus*, showing the concentric planetary spheres and, in the 1543 edition, the elemental and stellar spheres at the centre and circumference of the cosmos (Harley 3647, f. 34v, labelled *Figura 7 planetarum*; *Computus ecclesiasticus*, ed. 1543, sig. B4r, labelled *Figura ostendens distributionem & ordinem Sphærarum cœlestium*).

380–2   Þe dyametre of erþe … Ptholomeus *in libro Almagesti* **… þe 21 difference, is 11 hundred thousand mile:** In the *Planetary Hypotheses* (ed. and trans. Goldstein 1967), Ptolemy estimates the radius of the earth to be 28,667 stadia, which may be somewhere on the order of 5300 kilometres (using the estimate of 185 m./st. for the Ptolemaic stadium, though the measure varied throughout the classical period), about 17 per cent shy of the rough 6370-kilometre average radius by modern observations. Even with some of the higher values for the stadium (200 to 210 m.), Ptolemy's figure comes in 10 to 6 per cent lower than the modern figure.

However, the medieval West had no direct access to the *Planetary Hypotheses*. Instead, Latin astronomical writers relied on the figures of 3250 and 6500 miles for the earth's radius and diameter respectively, provided by the Arabic astronomer al-Farghānī (800/805–870; also referred to as Alfraganus) in his *Differentie scientie astrorum*, later known as the *Elements of Astronomy* (ed. Carmody 1943). These figures were usually taken over without worrying about differences in length between various Arabic and European "miles" (van Helden 1985, 38).

In this general context, Daniel's figure of "11 hundred thousand miles" for the diameter of the earth is wildly inaccurate, even though it is repeated consistently throughout the alpha tradition. In the beta tradition, the number is given as "600 M and 500 M mile," which would add up to "1100 thousand miles" and could conceivably be an error for "6 M and 500 mile," the number that al-Farghānī gives for the diameter. If this is the source of the error, it must have been made extremely early in the composition process, possibly even by Daniel himself, as the following instruction for calculating the circumference by adding twice as much again to the diameter (= multiplying by 3) is a crude rounding of the equation $C = \pi D$. The beta witnesses repeat that instruction and the resulting "33 C M" or 3,300,000 miles.

One clue that some distant echo of al-Farghānī's figure for the diameter of the earth lies behind Daniel's egregious error lies in the brief reference to "þe 21 difference," which is the correct section title and number for the chapter in the *Differentie* where the Earth's diameter is given (ed. Carmody 1943, 38). The citation of the *Almagest* is mistaken, though not surprising, given al-Farghānī's own acknowledged indebtedness to Ptolemy's work.

389–91   Luna, as techeþ Ptholomeus … 39 part of al erþe … & 36 myle: For the ratio of the volume of the moon to the earth as 1:39.25, see *Almagest* V 16, where Ptolemy also approximates the ratio of the sun's volume to the earth's as about 170:1 (ed. and trans. Toomer 1984, 257). We have interpreted R's use of a bar (or *vinculum*) above arabic numbers in this section as a multiplier of 1000 and signalled its use with double underlining in the text.

The distances between the planetary spheres and the planetary volumes in proportion to that of the earth are ultimately derived from Ptolemy's *Planetary Hypotheses* (ed. and trans. Goldstein 1967), a work not known directly in the Middle Ages, but whose content was transmitted by al-Farghānī in his *Differentie scientie astrorum*. Various Anglo-Latin writers on astronomy, including Roger Bacon and Robertus Anglicus, adopted al-Farghānī's calculations to a greater or lesser extent. Daniel himself knew of al-Farghānī's work and cites him as an authority in the beta version of the astronomical digression; see also the preceding note on "þe 21 difference."

Daniel's volume and distance figures – not to mention the variants introduced by his scribes – do not always correspond precisely to the Latin astronomical tradition, but are clearly related to it (see Appendix 4). He also seems to have misunderstood the "nearer distance" from Earth to a given planetary sphere (i.e., the inner surface of the concentric shell in which the planet moved) as the distance from the immediately lower sphere ("fro þe hidder partie of þe spere of þe mone to þe hidder partie of þe spere of Mercurie," etc.).

407–8   Þis firmament wiþ his sterres Ptholomeus diuiseþ into 6 ordres, i. into 6 speres: Although Daniel glosses "orders" as "spheres," they are in fact classes of stars based on brightness or magnitude. Ptolemy lists the magnitudes of stars in the tables of constellations in *Almagest* VII 5 and VIII 1 (trans. Toomer 1984, 341–99).

412   bach: An unusual spelling for *back*, glossing *retrograde*, but spelled thus in RM7H; variants include *bacche* (G), *bac/backe* (SaScCgB), *bryʒt* (T).

428–9   Þe 13 spere (þat Ptholome calleþ þe 10 spere): Daniel's count of spheres takes the empyrean heaven as the thirteenth, the *primum mobile* as the twelfth; below the *primum mobile* are eleven spheres from "erþe exclusif" to the "firmament inclusif," i.e., the elemental spheres of water, air, and fire, the seven planetary spheres, and the fixed stars or firmament. Omitting the three elemental, sublunary spheres leaves the ten spheres that Daniel attributes to Ptolemy: seven planets and three "heavens." For the various counts of the celestial spheres in the Middle Ages, see Grant 1994, 308–23.

472   *Tabula lune*: See Plate 4. For discussion of this type of lunar/zodiacal table, which can be traced as far back as the Carolingian era and is widespread throughout computistical literature, see Wallis 2015, 18–23.

479   *Tabula planetarum*: See Plate 5. Knowing which planet rules a given hour might have been seen as providing guidance as to the time of day for giving medicines or performing procedures related to limbs and organs governed by those planets (a point made in the beta version in connection with this table), though not as important as noting which zodiacal sign the moon was in, which could be determined from the *Tabula lune*. In Chaucer's Knight's Tale, lines 2209–2437, Palamon, Emily, and Arcite pray to their respective gods at the appropriate planetary hours (Venus, Luna, Mars). The table is made more compact by putting all recurring hours for a given planet on a given day (e.g., 1, 8, 15, 22 for the first planet of the day) in a single row, which causes the columns to run left-to-right through the downward planetary order Saturn, Jupiter, Mars, etc., instead of in their daily order (Sunday, Monday, Tuesday, etc.); this plan also generates the handsomely aligned, upward-slanting, single-planet diagonals in the table).

494   **Eluenden in his** *Kalender*: Walter Elvenden or Elveden (d. before 1360) was a Cambridge-educated astronomer and East Anglian churchman, who composed a calendar for the years 1330–86. His *Kalendarium* is an antecedent of the better-known calendars by John Somer and Nicholas Lynn for the years 1387–1462, which were probably compiled after Daniel's death and certainly after he had finished the *LU*. On Elveden, Lynn, and Somer, see the *Oxford Dictionary of National Biography Online*.

Some alpha witnesses (GSaSc) say that Elveden is *not* to blame for starting the day at noon, like the Saracens; agreeing with R are M7THCf; BCg say that Elveden is "foule for to blame." The beta version, G3M6, and J do not refer to Elveden, though G3 adds the peculiar comment "Falsum est quod tywel paremofay" after saying the day begins at midnight.

495–6   **Þogh I haue gone out of my waie, i. a litil fro my purpos, I þonk God I haue noȝt erryd:** Daniel acknowledges the digressive nature of his astronomical and calendric excursus, and may be attempting a small pun in claiming that he has not "erryd" (been mistaken/digressed) in discussing the "errande" (wandering) planets. The assertion that knowledge of astronomy was necessary for physicians is a commonplace that can be traced back to the Hippocratic Corpus (*Airs Waters Places* 2; trans. Jones, Loeb ed. 1: 73).

497   *lactea* **&** *subtenuis* **& mykel:** The transition back to uroscopic matters is handled differently in different versions of the *LU*. All alpha witnesses return to the Lacteus chapter with the phrase "Item *vrina lactea & subtenuis* & mykel ... ." The beta witnesses AG6EWSb introduce the transition with the phrase *Agayne to*

oure purpose and read *white and thynne and mikel* instead of *lactea & subtenuis & mykel*. The late and idiosyncratic witness J has features of both versions: *agayne to owre purpose* and *lactea & subtenuis & moche*.

The hybrid manuscripts M6 and G3 change allegiance from a proto-alpha to a beta* exemplar right at this return to Lacteus colour, in slightly different ways: M6 makes a smooth beta-style transition after noting that the day begins at midnight: *Now touchyng to our former mater of vryn whyte and þynne and myche* … . G3's transition is more turbulent, first continuing with about a page of the alpha version (with *lactea & subtenuis*) after noting the start of day at midnight, then breaking off (leaving a blank page), starting up again by repeating previous material on Lacteus colour, skipping over the planetary digression and leaving another blank page, and finally beginning again with the beta continuation: *Bote an vryn whyte & þynne & mykyl* … .

510–11   Auicen seiþ þat *frigus* is causede … hete, of mater corupte: Source in Avicenna not yet identified.

517   rasking: Probably related to the ME words *rasken, raxlen,* and *raxling,* all with senses that involve stretching and exhaling or yawning (esp. on awaking from sleep, but possibly in other circumstances, including shuddering and exhaling *for colde*), as opposed to the word *raskinge* "spitting, hawking."

520–1   difference is bitwene *rigor & frigus,* as seiþ Haly in his *Persectif*: Which author and which work Daniel intends here remains obscure. There are two principal Halys in Latin medical literature: 'Alī ibn 'Abbās al-Majūsī, author of the *Pantegni* (which Daniel normally ascribes to its first translator, Constantinus Africanus; translated more fully by Stephen of Pisa as the *Liber regalis dispositionis* [c. 1127]), and 'Alī ibn Ridwān, author of an influential commentary on Galen's *Ars parva* or *Tegni*. We have not found a discussion of *rigor* and *frigus* in ibn Ridwān's commentary, but the *Pantegni* has a chapter "De malis motibus" (Theorica, 6.22), in which *rigor* and *tremor* are compared, explained in humoral terms (including "fumous superfluities" in the *Liber regalis*), and associated with various "accidents" like piercing pain, internal and external etiologies, *calor* and *frigor*, and certain fevers. Daniel's comparison of *frigus* and *rigor* is not a perfect match to the *Pantegni* chapter, but his point may be the more general one that "Haly" and other medical authors differentiate among types of morbid shivering. We are grateful to Alasdair Watson for pointing us to this chapter in the *Pantegni/ Liber regalis*.

The title *Persectif* (RM7) is also problematic, as are its variants *Perspectif* (SaScG BHCfCg M6G3), *Prospectif* (AG6EW), *Prospectis* (T), and *Prospeculis* (Sb). A work titled *Perspectif/Prospectif* would normally be a work on optics, which seems an unlikely source in this context. However, the *Pantegni* is divided into two parts, the Theorica and the Practica, and the term *speculativa* could mean "theoretical," as Daniel knew: he uses *speculatyf* and *practyf* for the two aspects of medicine in the beta-version discussion of diuretic and styptic drinks in bk. 1. Perhaps Daniel or a very early copyist was confused by a source text that cited al-Majūsī's Theo-rica – whether in Constantine's or Stephen's translation – in a phrase like "Haly per speculativam suam," possibly in abbreviated form.

Whatever authority Daniel is citing here, he has a clear idea of *frigus*, *rigor*, and *oripilacio* as increasingly violent forms of chills, prickling, and shivering/shaking in response to different kinds of fever.

538   rasyng: Most manuscripts agree with R's reading here, but three (GSaSc) offer the reading *raysyng/reysing* ("spasm of coughing, belching"), which seems a more likely symptom of cold and shivering than *rasyng* "a shaving." The pos-sibility that *rasyng* is an error for *rasking* (seen above in connection with *rigor*, 2.6.516–17 is supported by only one witness (Sb).

2.7

4   Karopos: Except in cases where the indeclinable *karopos* is used in a Latin phrase (e.g., *De colore karopos* and *color karopos* in the title and opening words of this chapter), we treat this colour term as Middle English, capitalizing it as a tech-nical colour name and leaving it in roman font, and follow similar practice for the terms Inopos and Kyanos.

14   þe 3 c. biforne: "the three preceding chapters" (i.e., Albus, Glaucus, Lac-teus), based on spelled-out *chapitles/chapitris/capitulis* in GCgH.

24–5   Þe Comentour vppon Giles ... onych stone: Standard Commentary: "Et est karopos color flauus uelleribus camelorum similis, tanquam lapis onichi-nus" (And Karopos colour is yellow like to the skins of camels, like the onyx stone) (Sloane 282, f. 27r).

54–5   Dyuerse leches seyne his water ... deye he schulde: I.e., different doc-tors examined his urine, and always agreed that he would die.

58   herd he in mustryng ... þoght on þat word: The patient heard the doc-tors whispering (perhaps because they didn't want him to hear the diagnosis) and thought about what they said.

59   myes: Bread crumbs (*MED*, s.v. *mies* [n.pl.]), probably made up into a gruel or a dish of sops with some kind of liquid (water, broth, wine).

68–9   centorie, i. peti bugle ... grete bugle: Daniel's identification of *cento-rie* ("centaury," either the common centaury *C. umbellatum* or yellow centaury *Chlora perfoliata*, also known as the lesser and greater centaury) with *peti bugle* (which may be *Ajuga reptans*, some other *Ajuga* species, or bugloss) is unexpected. *Centorie* is found only in RM7SaSc; the remaining alpha witnesses read *centonie* (an otherwise unattested term or spelling); beta witnesses drop the reference to *centorie* or omit the case history altogether.

In his herbal, Daniel lists neither bugle nor centaury as a synonym of the other, but he does identify *peti bugle* and *þe more bugle* with the lesser and greater *cel-foile*, and says that the great *celfoile*/great bugle is "sovereyne erbe for þe grene jaundis and salves" (BL Add. 27329, 55va; see also Arundel 42, f. 53r, also mention-ing the great bugle [with synonyms *celfoile*/self-heal] as effective against jaundice).

75   kenet: A small hunting dog, here used metonymically for the colour of its coat.

76–80   And þerfore Karopos is wel likenede to þe stone þat is called onyx … **þe 5 boke of Albert *Of Preciouse Stones* and also þe coment vppon þe *Lapida-rie* … os Y said ryght now of Karopos:** See Albertus Magnus, *Mineralium libri V*, 2.2.13, s.vv. *onyx, onycha* (1890, 5: 42). Albertus describes the colour of the best onyx as black with white veins, but notes that there are several varieties, coloured black, white, reddish (*rubicundus*), or the colour of a human fingernail (the origi-nal sense of the Greek and Latin noun *onyx*). The citation of a commentary on the *Lapidary* may be too general to allow for a definitive identification.

Commentaries on Rev. 21:19–20 (on the foundation stones of the New Jeru-salem) typically describe and interpret the various precious stones listed there, including the *sardonix* and the *sardius*, stones often identified with or related to onyx. Riddle provides three brief symbolic lapidaries in his edition of Marbode of Rennes, *De lapidibus* (1977, 119–29).

158–60   loyn & meluede … ouer lowe: *loyn* is a form of *lain* (pa.ppl. of *lie*; cf. *leyn* CgSc, *leynt* H); fruit needs to have lain in straw or on some other surface in order to ripen (cf. *meluede to þe ful* "mellowed, ripened completely"). Ale that gets too low (*ouer lowe*) in the cask or other container will become stale and nox-ious, as will old, long-standing, and badly boiled ale.

163   schepes inward: Probably referring to a dish similar to tripe or haggis. The use of *inward* as a noun is not noted in *MED*, but *OED* records a few OE and ME instances of the usage, "usually *spec.* the internal parts or organs of the body, the entrails." The singular form is labelled "now rare," and was eventually replaced by the plural *inwards/innards*.

170   if it haue longe tyme so: "if it holds [the colour] thus for a long time"; see *MED*, s.v. *haven* (v.), sense 5b.(b). Some alpha witnesses (TSaSc) and all beta/beta* witnesses expand R's simple *haue* (also in M7 CfCgHB W6J) to "haue schewid him" or "have apperid"; these expanded sentences also revise the simple colour *Karopos* to some form of "lactea or karopos and/or thick."

180–1   Þis also techeþ Ypocras … 4 boke of *Afforismis*: Although Hippocrates does not describe urine as *karopos* in colour, cf. *Aph.* 4.70, "Quibus urine in febri-bus conturbate & conuerse uelut subiugalium: his capitis dolores aut adsunt: aut aderunt" (In cases of fever, when the urine is turbid, like that of cattle, headaches either are, or will be, present) (*Articella* 1483, f. 29vb; trans. Jones, Loeb ed. 4: 153).

The term *karopos* appears only as an eye colour in Hippocrates and Galen. It is used of urine by Caelius Aurelianus (?fifth century), but only really enters the uroscopic tradition with Theophilos (Maxwell-Stuart 1981, 2: 12–15, 69, 72–3). Perhaps some medieval commentary on the *Aphorisms* that used the term is Dan-iel's source here.

217–19   *Et þerfor seiþ* Ypocras ... mykel egestioun, litle vryn: Cf. *Aph.* 4.83, "Urina multa facta noctu: modicum secessum significat & econuerso" (When much urine is passed in the night, it means that the bowel-discharges are scanty) (*Articella* 1483, f. 31rb; trans. Jones, Loeb ed. 4: 157).

228–31   as Theophilus techeþ, it hath a maner of Fathede ... & in þe þerme: Theophilus only discusses Karopos urine briefly (chaps. 7, "De tenui urina et colorum commixtione," and 8, "De complexionibus pinguis substantiae"; ed. Dase 1999, 19, 23; *Articella* 1483, ff. 6rb, 6va) and does not appear to associate it with the collection of morbid matter in apostemes (if fatty) or the flux (if non-fatty). Again, the commentary tradition on Theophilus might have provided Daniel with a fuller discussion of the significance of different types of Karopos urine.

252–5   for þogh it so be ... more principaly in þe cerebre: Daniel's syntax is rather convoluted in these lines, with two clauses that are best taken as parenthetical asides and have been so punctuated. The first parenthetical comment may have originally ended with the phrase "for without the soul is no life," which is preserved (or added) in CfCgBH. The cancelled phrase "for wiþouten þe soule" in R appears without cancellation in GTSaSc, but is a *non sequitur* without "is no life" to complete it. In M7 and J, the cancelled phrase from R is omitted entirely. The beta witnesses contain versions of the full parenthetical comment.

259–63   þe *Boke of Anathomyes* ... *Inder Parties of Mannes Body* ... 3 kawates: Here Daniel again cites the *Boke of Anathomyes*, but then equates it with the *Boke of þe Exposisioun of þe Inder Parties of Mannes Body*. At first sight, the alternate title could be a translation of *De interioribus* (the medieval Latin title for Galen's *De locis affectis*). But the *De interioribus* is more focused on signs and cures for diseases than on anatomy *per se* and does not address the prime qualities of the organs, so the identification may simply be a misapprehension by Daniel.

270–2   Gilbert, in his Coment vpon Giles ... for þe same skil it is nesche: Perhaps Wellcome 547, f. 133va: "Aristoteles probat cerebrum esse frigidius et humidius omnibus aliis membris sicut omnes anathomici attestantur, vnde est molle liquidum & in se male terminabile" (Aristotle demonstrates that the brain is colder and more humid than all other members, as all anatomists attest, whence it is soft, liquid, and in itself poorly defined).

272–5   It is rounde for þis skil, os seiþ Constantyn in his coment ... sauede fro strokes & fro hurtinges: Compare *Pantegni*, Theorica 2.3, "De ossibus capitis": "Rotunda vt a passibilitate fit remotior" (Round so that it is less vulnerable); and 3.12, "De compositis membris interioribus: vt cerebro": "qui [ventriculus] ideo rotundatur vt maior quantitas spiritus suscipiatur & ne facile patiatur" (which is rounded so that a greater quantity of spirit may be received and that it may not easily suffer) (*Omnia opera Ysaac* 1515, 2: 5vb, 10vb).

We have not yet found a passage in the printed edition of the *Pantegni* that mentions the lack of angles in the head or cranium, but the *Second Salernitan Demonstration*, which draws extensively on the *Pantegni*, says that the head "is round in order that it may not be subject to injury; for if there were angles tending to retain superfluities, they would be a source of harm" (trans. Corner 1927, 65).

349–50   Galienus in *Libro anathomiarum suarum* calleþ it *cartilago gutturis*: "et est trachea arteria super oesophagum, super quam est quaedam cartilago, quae dicitur epiglottis" (The *trachea arteria* lies in front of the oesophagus, and upon it there is a certain cartilage known as epiglottis) (*Anatomia porci*, ed. and trans. Corner 1927, 48, 51).

In Corner's edition, the *Anatomia porci* does not add "gutturis" ["of the gullet/throat"] to "cartilago"; however, Daniel does define the epiglottis as *cartilago gutturis* in his Latin version of the *LU*, without citing the *Anatomia* (Glasgow, Hunterian MS 362, f. 41v).

361–3   as þe auctour of *Anathomyes* techeþ ... þorgh melancolie: We have not found a clear source for this assertion about *casus uvule* in the *Anatomia porci*.

368–9   hert colk: Daniel's gloss for this phrase, "the mouth of the stomach," should be added to the *MED* definition "the center or bottom (of the heart)," s.v. *colk* (n.), sense 1.(b).

374–6   as Galien seiþ ... & þe stroup: "In radicibus linguae oriuntur duo meatus, scilicet trachea arteria, per quam transit ad pulmonem aer, et oesophagus ... et est trachea arteria super oesophagum, super quam est quaedam cartilago, quae dicitur epiglottis" (At the base of the tongue arise two passages, namely, the *trachea arteria*, through which air passes to the lung, and the oesophagus ... The *trachea arteria* lies in front of the oesophagus, and upon it there is a certain cartilage known as epiglottis) (*Anatomia porci*, ed. and trans. Corner 1927, 48, 51).

393–4   Þus seieþ Galienus in his *Boke of Anathomyes*: "locus qui dicitur isthmon ... in quo aliquando humor colligitur et facit apostema quod dicitur angina; aliquando pars est intra et pars extra et dicitur squinantia; aliquando totus extra et dicitur synantia" (a space known as the isthmus ... in which humours may collect and cause an abscess called angina; sometimes this is partly internal and partly external and is called quinsy; sometimes it is wholly external and it is then called *synanche*) (*Anatomia porci*, ed. and trans. Corner 1927, 48, 51).

424   *antropos*, i. *arbor euersa*: A medieval commonplace that can be traced back at least as far as Lotario dei Segni's *De miseria condicionis humane* (1.8), written c. 1195, before his election to the papacy as Innocent III (ed. Lewis 1978, 107). It is often found in medieval homiletic writings, typically in connection with biblical comparisons of man to a tree planted by God or bearing good or bad fruit.

437   *mappa ventris*: Latin *mappa* here has its frequent sense "table-cloth" (= Daniel's *borde-cloþe*). The meaning "map" for *mappa* was also available in the Middle Ages (e.g., *mappamundi* "map of the world"), by extension from cloths on which maps were drawn, but the metaphor here is simply one of a horizontal membrane near the stomach and the respiratory organs.

501–2   *Splen*, þe mylt, os Galien seiþ … lifte side: "[Zirbus et siphac] procedunt usque ad splenem, per quos venae transeunt, per quas melancholia ab hepate ad splenem mittitur. Est autem splen membrum oblongum in sinistro latere positum" (These membranes reach as far as the spleen, and are traversed by veins through which black biliary humor (*melancholia*) is transmitted from the liver to the spleen. The spleen is an oblong organ located in the left side) (*Anatomia porci*, ed. and trans. Corner 1927, 49, 52).

520   os I saide in c. *de albo colore*, lef {j}: The marginal number here is incorrect; the chapter on Albus urine would have been in the missing leaves between modern folios 42 and 43 (old leaves 38–42 are missing). *Zirbus* and *sifac* are mentioned only at the beginning of this passage, so the cross-reference should be to old leaf 38.

522–3   Galienus, in his *Bok of Anathomyes*, calleþ it *epigozontaymenon*: "Nam [uritides] infiguntur vesicae qui etiam transeunt per quendam panniculum, quo omnia intestina praeter longaonem clauduntur, qui vocatur epigorontysmeon coli, quo rupto intestinum cadit in osceum" (through [the *uritides pori*] the urine oozes into the bladder, passing through a kind of membrane by which all the intestines are inclosed except the *longaon*, and which when broken allows the intestines to fall into the scrotum) (*Anatomia porci*, ed. and trans. Corner 1927, 49, 52).

Corner does not directly translate the difficult word **epigorontysmeon**, and it does not appear in any of the medieval Latin dictionaries. Different copies of the *Anatomia porci*, the Middle English *Anatomia Galieni* (a translation of the *Anatomia porci*), the *LU*, and later uses in late medieval and early modern medical English provide the following variants:

AnatP: *epigorontysmeon coli, epygosanta ysmenon coli, epigome cinctus menon*;
AnatG: *epygontanymoun*;
LU: *epigozonta(y)meno(u)n, ypigozontamen, epizontamenon, epigozontaymeon, epigozontaminon, epitazantaymeon, epizantaymenon, egipseontaymenon* corr. to *epigesontaymenon* (a remarkably stable set for nearly sixty occurrences in twenty witnesses);
Andrew Boorde, *The Breviary of Health* (1547): *epigozontaymenon*, defining the word as "rupture" = hernia)

Norri (2016) includes the term **epizotis/-os**, found three times in the ME translation of the pseudo-Galenic *De humana natura*, in his dictionary entry for **epigozontaymenon**, but in its original context, **epizotis** means "diaphragm," i.e., the "litel membranes [that] dividen spiritual membres … the lunges and the herte in the vpper cellis abidyng, to the norysshyng membris in the lower parties degestyng." According to the ME version of the *De humana natura*, the **epizotis** (understood as plural) are pierced by the esophagus en route to the stomach, and the stomach is suspended from them. See Carrillo Linares, ed. 2006, 264.

528–9   grees þat Galienus calleþ *omentum*: " … in osceum, supra quem est pinguedo quae vocatur omentum. Super omentum est siphac" (… into the scrotum. Above this is a fatty structure called omentum. Above the omentum is the *siphac*) (*Anatomia porci*, ed. and trans. Corner 1927, 49, 52).

540   Which by sekenes: "What are the diseases" (an unusual spelling of "be" as *by*).

546   As Holy Writ witnesseth & telleþ: The verses here are an adaptation of Prov. 30:15–16. See also Whiting 1968, T121.

575   or elles al: "or all of the previously named things."

577   & it be fulle: "if it is full." A relatively rare use by Daniel of the ME conjunction *an(d)* "if."

2.8

15   lachede: "paleness, dullness (of colour)"; a contracted form of *lachehede*, a derivative of *lache* "weary, slow, dull; slack, negligent."

38–9   in as mykel as fleume: "in as much as (it contains) phlegm."

60–1   Johannicius in his *Boke of Ysagogis*, **þe j c. …   4 maner of colre**: *Isagoge ad Techne Galieni*, §§7–9 (ed. Maurach 1978, 152–3; trans. Wallis 2010, 141). Johannitius actually says that there are five kinds of red choler (natural, citrine, vitelline "like egg yolks," prassine "light green," and rusty green) and two kinds of black choler. The following several paragraphs on kinds of choler (to line 2.8.98) expand on the compact list given in the *Isagoge*, including Daniel's division of *colera viridis* into prassine and rusty choler in accord with Johannitius's list of five kinds of red choler.

88–91   Galienus seiþ … colre vitellyn … a grenehede: Faith Wallis suggests (personal communication) that this claim may derive from some commentary on the *Isagoge* of Johannitius, but that "it is not from [the] Bartholomaeus or Digby commentaries."

116   ofolde: "onefold," i.e., "simple."

155–8   þerfor seiþ Ysodre in þe 4 boke of *Ethimologies*, **10 c. …   for to come**: *Etymologies* 4.10.2 (referring to types of medical books), "Prognostica praevisio aegritudinum, vocata a praenoscendo. Oportet enim medicum et praeterita agnoscere, et praesentia scire, et futura praevidere" (Prognostics are a foreseeing of illnesses, so called from *praenoscendo* "fore-knowing." For it behooves a doctor to recognize things past, to know things present, and to foresee things that are to come) (ed. Lindsay 1911). Isidore here adapts the opening of the Hippocratic *Prognostics*, "Videtur mihi ut sit ex melioribus rebus ut medicus utatur prouisione. Quod est: quia quando prescit: & antecedit: & indicat infirmis aliquod presens ex eis que habent: & que preterierunt: & que futura sunt: & interpretatur ab infirmis totum quod abbreuiauerunt a narratione sua: est dignus ut de eo credatur quia est potens scire res egrorum ita ut illud prouocet infirmos: uel sit fiducia ad confidendum: & committendum se in manibus medici" (I hold that it is an excellent thing for a physician to practise forecasting. For if he discover and declare unaided by the side of his patients the present, the past and the future, and fill in the gaps in the account given by the sick, he will be the more believed to understand the cases, so that men will confidently entrust themselves to him for treatment) (*Articella* 1483, f. 47ra; trans. Jones, Loeb ed. 2: 7).

188–90   Aristotel seiþ ... contrariouse in qualite: Perhaps an allusion to passages in the *Nicomachean Ethics* 8 in which Aristotle discusses the attraction between similar people as part of friendship, though he excludes physical similarities in this context (trans. Ross and Urmson, in Barnes, ed. 1984, 2: 1825–39).

209   hath his aspecte, i. is openonde þiderwarde: In Daniel's anatomy, the heart "looks toward" or "opens toward" the liver, being located more on the left side of the body but radiating heat toward the right.

227   Gilbert seiþ þus: þer be 2 principal membres of lif in man: Wellcome 547, f. 120va (commenting on lines 113–15 of Giles's *Carmen de urinis*): "Cum sint duo principia uite, vnum materiale, s. epar, aliud formale, s. cor; ydropisis vero corrumpit epar" (Since there are two sources of life, one material, namely the liver, and the other formal, namely the heart; dropsy, however, destroys the liver).

Daniel's entire discussion of the effects of fever following various ailments (2.8.186–260) is a relatively close paraphrase of Gilbert's commentary on lines 113–15 of Giles's poem, covering almost an entire folio (Wellcome 547, ff. 120r–v), though it omits Gilbert's list of seven Galenic changes caused by sickness and adds citations of Aristotle and Constantine.

241–3   os Constantinus seiþ in his *Boke of Vryns* ... of þe hert ... of þe lyuer: Perhaps a double error for Constantine's translation of Isaac's *De febribus*, which sometimes follows directly after Constantine's translation of Isaac's *De urinis* in manuscripts, and which defines fever as "calor preter naturam in initio petens cor per mediocritatem: deinde subito se diuidens cum calore naturali per totum corpus naturali nocet actioni" (a heat beyond nature in the beginning seeking the heart on account of its centrality, and then, suddenly distributing itself with the natural heat throughout the whole body, it harms the natural action) (1.3; *Omnia opera Ysaac* 1515, 1: 204rb), though there is no mention of dropsy or the liver in the subsequent text.

264–5   it seiþ *pthisicam* ... wombe flux: The emendation is necessary here to make sense of the contrast that Daniel is drawing between symptoms of phthisic/consumption (paleness, frothiness, ashiness, no diarrhea, etc.) and the less frothy and less ashy quality of urine caused by general humoral imbalance and little moisture reaching the liver. The error must have been caused by eyeskip in a copy leading to R.

Interestingly, the beta/beta* witnesses add a reference here to Hippocrates' aphorism on phthisic with diarrhea as a sign of death (e.g., Ashmole 1404, 2.50, f. 112r; quoted again at the end of the chapter on f. 114r); see *Aph.* 5.14: "Ptisi habito: diaria superueniente mortale" (If diarrhoea attack a consumptive patient it is a fatal symptom) (*Articella* 1483, f. 32ra; trans. Jones, Loeb ed. 4: 161).

305–9   Item, in þis malady … huge & grete inwarde: This somewhat puzzling paragraph appears to be an expansion of the immediately preceding explanation of why slow (*lent*) fevers may be relatively imperceptible (*noȝt mykel felte*) at the surface of the body but still very harmful deeper within, causing great wasting. In such fevers, only a weak heat can manifest itself in the dry outer parts of the body, emitting vapours that pass to the extremities but (apparently) little or no outwardly perceptible fever.

348–9   os seiþ Ypocras, who so haue þe pthisik … but deþ: *Aph.* 5.14, quoted above in note to lines 264–5.

2.9

56–7   fro þe 3 dai … to þe 5 daie: I.e., every three days, every four days, or every five days.

134   and þat but: "unless."

2.10

83–5   And þerfor as Ypocras seiþ in his *Boke of Pronostiks* … þan he is incurable: Compare *Prog.* 8: "Omnis ydrops in acuta egritudine malum. Infestat enim febre & grauedine membrorum & dolore" (Dropsies that result from acute diseases are all unfavourable, for they do not get rid of the fever and they are very painful and fatal) (*Articella* 1483, f. 56vb; trans. Jones, Loeb ed. 2: 19).

86–8   The same seiþ Theophilus in his *Bok of Vryns* … vryn Ruf is wickede in ydropsi, for þan is he incurable: Theophilus, *Liber urinarum*: "Urina talis [tenuis subrufa et rufa] ueniens in ydropicis periculosa, quemadmodum aquosa utilis" (And such [thin Subrufus and Rufus] urine coming in dropsical people is perilous, just as watery urine is good) (ed. Dase 1999, 19; *Articella* 1483, f. 6ra).

The mortal significance of Rufus urine for dropsical patients is also affirmed in the widely disseminated text *Urina Rufa* (found in both Latin and English): "Item vrina in ydropico rufa vel subrufa mortem significat" (Bodleian Library, MS Ashmole 391, Part V, f. 3ra; ed. Tavormina 2019, 7, 47).

88–9   Constantyn & Gilbert & Thade & alle autoures seie þe same: The fatal significance of Rufus urine in dropsy is noted by Giles ("Ydropico talis portenditur exitialis" [Such urine is predicted to be fatal to a dropsical patient]; line 162). Gilbert glosses each word in the line, explains why dropsy in an acute fever is so pernicious, and supports his commentary with the quotation from Theophilus mentioned in the preceding note (Wellcome 547, f. 124ra).

"Thade" is presumably Taddeo Alderotti (c. 1210–1295), the Italian physician who taught at the University of Bologna and wrote numerous texts, including commentaries on works in the *Articella, consilia*, and a regimen of health. Other Thade/Tadeus citations occur in bks. 2.14.94, 3.5.12, and 3.7.46.

The classic study of Alderotti is Siraisi 1981; Siraisi's list of works by Alderotti contains no commentaries on Theophilus, Giles, or Isaac, though his commentary on the *Articella* includes *expositiones* of Hippocrates' *Aphorisms*, part 4, which contains some of the most influential Hippocratic writing on urines. We are deeply grateful to Faith Wallis for alerting us (personal communication) to a commentary on Giles with a pseudo-Taddean connection in two French manuscripts: Paris, Bibliothèque de l'Arsenal, MS 1024, ff. 1ra–12va, and Université de Paris, Bibliothèque de la Sorbonne, MS 131, ff. 88r–96v (eTK 0956M and 0920H). The text is anonymous in the Arsenal MS, which titles it "Noua reportata super Egidium de vrinis" (f. 12va). In the Sorbonne MS, the text is titled "Glose versuum urinarum a m[agistro] T. collecte" (f. 88r) and "Glose versuum Egidii, secundum lecturam m[agistri]. T." (f. 96v); it is one of several short treatises on ff. 61r–108v that are collectively titled "Thadei expositiones" (f. 66r). Siraisi includes the Sorbonne manuscript in her Select List of Manuscripts, but describes the attribution as doubtful (424).

It is possible that Daniel had access to a copy of this collection of brief commentaries, or at least the glosses on Giles, with attribution to Taddeo. All four of the citations of Taddeo in the *LU* deal with commonplace uroscopic knowledge, so identifying the "Noua reportata" as Daniel's source must remain provisional. For Daniel's citation here, on Rufus urine in dropsy, the point is made in language that is very similar to both the Standard Commentary and Gilbert's Comment (Arsenal 1024, f. 6rb; Sloane 282, f. 32r; Wellcome 547, f. 124ra), though this is not the case for the later citations.

We have not yet identified analogous material in Constantine, but given the long-standing canonicity of the rule, it would be unsurprising to find it stated somewhere in his works.

155–9   os Maistre Ferare & Maistre Platearye & also Maistre Johan de Sancto Paulo ... wiþoute þe vesseiles. But Giles & Maistre of þe Mesondeu seyn *e contrario* ... fleume corrupt wiþin: Standard Commentary: "Nec vos lateat sentencia Ferrarii et Platearii et Mauri et [Laud lat. 106: & platearij & magistri] Johannis de Sancto Paulo, qui asserebant minorem emitriceum fieri de colera nigra [Laud lat. 106: intra] et fleumate extra; sed eorum sentencie supersedendo Petri Musandini auctoritatem prosequemur" (Nor should the opinion of Ferrarius and Platearius and Maurus and [Laud: and Platearius and Master] John of St Paul be overlooked, which claims that the lesser emitrice derives from black choler [Laud:

choler within] and phlegm without; but we will follow the authority of Petrus Musandinus in setting aside their opinion) (Sloane 282, f. 33r).

Daniel's text corresponds more closely to the better readings in Laud, omitting Maurus and having *colre in the vesseiles* = Laud's *colera intra*, rather than Sloane's *colera nigra*. He also explains more clearly how Musandinus differed from his Salernitan colleagues and predecessors (phlegm corrupt within the veins and choler outside them). Here, as in some other passages, Daniel conflates the author of the Standard Commentary with Giles himself, possibly correctly (see also 1.2.27–8n; 2.4.282–3n; 2.12.82; 3.7.5).

Daniel probably did not consult the Salernitan authors directly, but merely transmitted the Standard Commentary's citations. However, those citations that we have been able to trace are correctly reported in the Commentary: for Platearius (in his *Practica*), see Recio Muñoz, ed. and trans. 2016, 198; for John of St Paul (in his *Breviarius medicine*), see McGill University Library, Osler MS 7627 (f. 68v).

158 Maistre of þe Mesondeu: In the beta version of this passage, Petrus Musandinus's name is represented somewhat more accurately, as "Piers Massendoun."

2.11

44–7 Constantyn seiþ ... aboute the hert: We have not yet identified a Constantinian passage about the causes of continual fever that matches Daniel's statement here.

69–70 þat is þat semes os it were a grenehede: "that (i.e., choler) is what seems like a greenness."

81–3 Ypocras in his *Bok of Pronostikes* teches ... *non valde pleuretici sunt*: Not from the *Prognostics*, but rather *Aph.* 6.33, "Acidum ructuantes non ualde: pleuretici fiunt" (Those suffering from acid eructations are not very likely to be attacked by pleurisy) (*Articella* 1483, f. 39rb; trans. Jones, Loeb ed. 4: 187).

83 One of the key features distinguishing the alpha and the beta families, besides the renumbering of chapters, is the addition of a new chapter on leprosy (usually numbered 2.69) at the end of the section on Rubeus urine (in AG6EW G3M6 J, and partially in Sb). The text is taken *nerehond word for word* from the *Practica* of Roger de Barone, bk. 2, ch. 14, *de lepra* (in *Cyrurgia Guidonis ...* , 1519 ed., ff. 225vb–226va), whom Daniel calls Roger of Normandy. The transition to the beta* text in HBCfCg occurs just a few lines after the point at which the leprosy chapter would have occurred.

2.12

25 *choabens*: I.e., *cohabens*, "having together," a reading attested by GTSaSc AG6EW J M6. R's spelling may be an alternative spelling or a scribal error. Other witnesses read *choabeus* (M7), *choabens* Sb, *ceabens* (G3H); and *se habens* (CfCgB).

30–1   alle þise 3 causes ar in no maner febre so, namely os *in synocho*: "these 3 causes are in no (other) fever in the way they are in *synochus*."

33   *homothena*: "having the same tension, *unius tenoris*" (*DMLBS*, s.v. *homotonus*). On this and the related terms *augmastik* and *epamastik*, see Alonso Guardo 2001. See also Norri 2016, s.vv. *augmastica, epamastica, fever,* and *homothena,* citing Daniel and Andrew Boorde, *Breviary of Health* (1547).

60   dogg-leches: The qualifying prefix *dogg* is used here "as a term of abuse or contempt … wretch, cur" (*MED*, s.v. *dogge* [n.], sense 1.[b]). Daniel's characterization of unskilled, meddling, arrogant, loquacious, and greedy practitioners as "dogg-leches" is recorded only in RM7, though the reading "in þise days ben callid lechis" in T may be a corrupt copy of the RM7 reading. T and the rest of its group GSaSc all retain the phrase "as þise entermeters and þise bolde braggres þat stonde in chateryng and in clateryng and nought in connyng and þat only for moyney wynnyng," while the beta texts AG6EW Sb and the hybrid G3 only read "(an) vnwyse leche" (the late manuscript J reads "an vnwyse phisicien"). The remaining beta witnesses (CgCfB M6H) omit the sentence about physicians entirely. However, the beta version reintroduces a criticism of *dogg-leches* in bk. 3.23, in discussing Ypostasis:

> But ofte tymes whitehed in vryn or in Ypostasy is taken for yolowyshed and for very whitehed among thes dog leches and among them þat haue not parfyte vnderstondyng, that hath sen litel and speken mikel and wold be sen and mow not for pride and dulhed lerne, as many of my order. (Ashmole 1404, f. 173v)

78–82   *Et tak hede þat synochus is causede … filþe & corrupcioun. Þus seiþ Egidius*: The comparative etiologies given for *synochus* and *synocha* in this passage and in the following paragraph (*synochus* being caused by wicked qualities of corrupted blood, *synocha* by excessive quantities of blood) are stated somewhat circuitously in the Standard Commentary: "Sinochus est febris continua ex sanguine putrefacto in venis … vrina rubea uel rubicunda … sine liuiditate et fetore, sinocham inflatiuam signat. Sinocha de multo; sed sinochus ex putrefacto. Fit autem sinocha de sanguine peccante in quantitate et non in qualitate" (*Synochus* is a continual fever caused by rotten blood in the veins … Rubeus or Rubicund urine … without a leadish colour and a rotten odour, indicates *synocha inflativa*. *Synocha* from excess; but *synochus* from rot. For *synocha* comes from blood that goes wrong in quantity and not in quality) (Sloane 282, f. 35r).

Daniel zeroes in on the essential contrast between quality and quantity, though he goes on to note that some authorities think that *synochus* is defective in both.

Witnesses in the beta tradition read "the Comment on Giles" (AG6EWJ), "the Commentor on Giles" (M6G3H), or "the Commentors on Giles" (CfCgB), instead of "Egidius" (RM7 TGSaSc).

99–110   Constantinus seiþ ... & in þe 2 c. next byforn: Daniel draws this list of symptoms for *synocha* and the attribution to Constantine from the Standard Commentary on Giles, though with some expansion: "*Sinocham*: inflatiuam de sanguine puro penite sincero et superincenso secundum Constantinum. Sinoche accidenta sunt hec: dolor capitis infixiuus et emergens a profundo, dulcedo oris, genarum rubor, inflacio uenarum et maxime circa spiritualia" (*Synocha*: an inflative fever caused by very pure, unmixed, and superheated blood, according to Constantine. The symptoms of *synocha* are these: an unremitting headache coming from deep in the head, sweetness of the mouth, redness of the cheeks, swelling of the veins and especially around the respiratory organs) (Sloane 282, f. 35v).

This passage is omitted in the beta* texts CfCgB M6G3H.

101–2   bolnyng & beting, and stoppede at brest: "swelling and throbbing and (the patient is) congested in the breast." Alternatively, *stoppede* could be a form of *stophede* "the state of being stopped or blocked"; cf. the scribe's occasional interchange of the *-hede* suffix and *-ed(e)* past marker in other words (e.g., the past participles *dymhede and dulhede & al dismaihede* at 2.3.21–2; *dymhede* at 2.3.284; the abstract noun *myʒtyed* at 2.2.241).

155   ferrene: A difficult word, complicated by the fact that the medial *-re-* is an expanson of an *-er/-re* curl above the word in RM7. Variants include *ferene* (A), *ferne* (W), *frene* (E), and *feruente* (J), with added surrounding material related to heat, inflammation, and fire, so the best gloss appears to be "fiery" (cf. *MED*, s.v. *firen* [adj.], sense [a]).

2.13

8–10   Theophilus seiþ ... of hem comeþ *color ynopos*: Theophilus does not appear to describe Inopos in these terms, but compare his characterization of Kyanos: "Kianon uero ut sanguis putrefactus ex felle rubeo et superadustus, et colore ut garus et ut ictericorum urinae. Regula autem kiani coloris est secundum Galienum talis: albo splendidum adueniens et in nigrum plurimum incidens kianon facit" (Kyanos: like blood corrupted by red bile and overheated, and in colour like fish-sauce and like the urines of jaundiced patients. The rule of Kyanos colour, according to Galen, is that something bright, approaching white, and falling on something very black causes Kyanos) (ed. Dase 1999, 15; *Articella* 1483, f. 6ra).

17–20   Gilbertus seiþ ... þat Kyanos often tym haþ diuerse coloures ... Rubicund os feir ... swart rede ... bloysh ... wiþ a grenehede: Although Gilbert does not give a list of variable colours in Kyanos urine that matches this list exactly, his commentary on Inopos and Kyanos does discuss the contribution of multiple colours to those two types of urine, including white, red, black, and green, with brief mentions of saffron colour (*croceitas*) and lividity (Wellcome 547, ff. 129va–130va).

73–4   Þis forseide reule techeþ þe Comentour vpon Giles: Standard Commentary: "Item talis urina apparet in ruptura kilis uene, unde maximus sentitur dolor in vii spondili, facta computacione ab inferiori, et tunc feculencior apparet urina in fundo. Est autem medico maximus honor cum per talem vrinam dolorem in tali loco pronosticet" (And such urine appears in the rupture of the *kilis* vein, from which the greatest pain is felt in the seventh vertebra, counting from below, and then a more stinking urine appears in the bottom of the urinal. And there is very great honour to the physician when he predicts pain in such a place through such urine) (Sloane 282, f. 36r).

108–11   But if þow wilt knowe wel … os techeþ þe Comentour vpon Giles: Standard Commentary: "Nec tamen ex hoc temerarie precipitanda est sentencia de ydropisi, temeraria namque et preceps discrecio artificem deuenustat, et ei ruborem incutit et pudorem incitat. Item talis urina apostema epatis, vel pleuresim vel peripleumoniam, uel apostema renum signat. Sed distinguendum est per alia accidentia discernendum et etiam inquirendum utrum paciatur puncturam in dextro ypocundrio vel sinistro, angustia respirandi, pondus et grauedinem circa renes" (Nevertheless, the judgment of dropsy is not to be recklessly rushed into from these symptoms, for a reckless and precipitous judgment disfigures the practitioner, and inflicts blushing and incites shame. And such urine signifies aposteme of the liver, or pleurisy or peripleumonia, or aposteme of the kidneys. But one should distinguish among them, by discerning through other symptoms and also inquiring whether he feels pricking in the right or left hypochondrium, restriction in breathing, or weight and heaviness around the kidneys) (Sloane 282, f. 36r).

134–5   But in *pleuresis* … as techeþ þe *Tretee of Pouses* … perile: Giles of Corbeil, *Carmen de pulsibus*, lines 221–5: "Pulsus durities in pleuresi perniciosa, / Arida materies, terrestris, cruda probatur, / Solvi difficilis, ex quo discussio morbi / Protrahitur, vis opprimitur, natura fatiscit, / Victaque succumbit longo lassata duello" (Intensity of the pulse is pernicious in pleurisy, showing the matter of the disease to be dry, earthy, and undigested, difficult to resolve; on account of that, shaking off the disease is protracted, the life force is oppressed, nature breaks down and succumbs, conquered and exhausted, to the long battle) (ed. Choulant 1826, 37).

149–67   Galienus techeþ 5 dyfference … of þe ribbes … Þus seiþ he: Cf. Standard Commentary: "Hiis iiiior differenciis v superadduntur que habentur ex epistolis Galieni ad Glauconem" (To these four differences [between pleurisy and aposteme of the liver] are added five taken from the letters of Galen to Glaucon) (Sloane 282, f. 36r).

204–7   Ysaac in þe 4 boke *Of Febres* … o þe ribbes: Daniel's discussion from here to the end of 2.13 is drawn largely from Isaac's *De febribus* 4.8–9 and 4.11, the chapters "De synocha sine putredine: que inflatiua dicitur: et de pleuresi," "De sputo laudabili & illaudabili & mediocri," and "De differentia vere & non vere pleuresis" (*Omnia opera Ysaac* 1515, 1: 214vb–216ra). For the definition of pleurisy, see ch. 4.8: "pleuresis nihil aliud est nisi calidum apostema in diaphrag-mate ortum: & aliquando illa materia que a capite descendit venit ad lacertos & carnem: quibus coste sunt indute & faciunt apostema quid abusiue vocatur pleure-sis" (pleuresis is nothing but a hot aposteme arising in the diaphragm: and some-times the matter that descends from the head comes to the muscles and flesh that surround the ribs and they create an aposteme that is improperly called pleurisy) (*Omnia opera Ysaac* 1515, 1: 214va).

209   **but litel peyn os to reward:** "only a little pain in comparison (to other illnesses)" or "only a little pain as far as one notices it."

209–11   **for *pulmo* is a membre ... oght mykel:** I.e., the lungs are an organ in which one can suffer serious disease for a long time before realizing it or feeling it very much.

230   **Of whiche þou hast as Isaac techeþ:** The reference here is to Daniel's own discussion of nunciative days in bk. 2.2, which was largely drawn from the *De febribus* 4.6–4.7 (see notes to 2.2.191–257 above). The immediately preceding sentence, about scant, white, light, and viscous spittle that is produced in one or two coughs as a good sign, corresponds to passages in *De febribus* 4.8 (*Omnia opera Ysaac* 1515, 1: 214vb) and 4.4 (213rb), though Daniel is probably taking it from 4.8.

239   **þe more nere þat tokne of digestioun be þe bigynnyng:** "the closer the sign of digestion is to the beginning (of the sickness)." Most witnesses read "be þe bigynnyng" or "by/bi þe bigynnyng" (RM7 GTSaSc AEW G3H), leaving either a preposition (*by/bi/be*) or a verb (*be*) implicit; only three of the beta* witnesses (CfCgB) read "be to þe begynnyng."

245–6   **Wickede colour in spotle ar þise: grene, blo, & blak & bitwene grene & blak:** Daniel's colour terms translate the phrase *viride liuidum venetum* ("sea-green") *nigrum* in the *De febribus*, and the paragraph that follows corresponds, with some rearrangement, to the subsequent description of *illaudabile sputum* (4.9; *Omnia opera Ysaac* 1515, 1: 215ra–rb).

269–72   **But what tyme, seiþ Ysaac, ar we noȝt siker ... grete drede:** *De febri-bus* 4.9: "Unde non sumus securi propter temporis longinquitatem quando pec-cent infirmi: aut mutentur tempora vel aer in malas qualitates: & morbus mutetur: & timorem innuat ... Sed tamen si male significationes illud sequantur ... acutam significat materiam & timorem esse vicinum" (Because of which we are not sure, on account of the length of time when the sick may misbehave, or the weather or the air may change into bad qualities, and the disease may change, and hint at fear ... But nonetheless if evil signs follow ... it signals sharp matter and that fear is near) (*Omnia opera Ysaac* 1515, 1: 215rb).

288–302   **veray *pleuresis* ... os Ysaac seiþ ... donward agayn:** Daniel returns to the definition of pleurisy, near the beginning of *De febribus* 4.8, and continues with more of that chapter, including the comparison of rising and falling humours to a bath-house with an impervious roof (*Omnia opera Ysaac* 1515, 1: 214va–vb).

377   **at on plechching or at 2:** "in one or two hawkings, expectorations." Variants for *plechching* (derived from ME *plicchen* "to pull, pluck, or draw out") include *coghinges* (GTSaSc), *raysyng/reysingg(es)* (AG6Sb M6G3), *rysynge(s)* (CfCgBG3H), *receyuyng* (EW). Cf. *MED*, s.v. *reising(e* (ger.).

393–4   **Alle þise forsaide thinges seiþ Ysaac in the 4 *Bok of Febres*, nerhand worde for worde:** I.e., most of the material from line 2.13.204 above to here is taken from the *De febribus* 4.8–9, 4.11. See preceding notes.

397   **themself:** A highly unusual form in the R scribe's spelling system, which uses forms with initial *h-* for the third person plural almost everywhere else (*hem* 233x, *hemself* 3x, *hemselfe* 4x), and very rarely forms beginning with *þ* (*þam* 8x and *þaym* 1x, all in the Prologue, possibly suggesting an exemplar in a different dialect from the main text). See Appendix 5.

420–2   **For if woman haue swych vryn ... wommanes kynde ar different. Þus seiþ Giles:** Standard Commentary: "Huius autem vrine, magis suspecte in uiris quam in mulieribus, nisi sint tales in mulieribus cum acutis febribus, gratia ipsarum febrium et non propter menstruorum erupcionem; tunc enim summum nunciat periculum, magis etiam quam in uiris, quanto a natura ipsarum sunt remociores" (But of this urine [Kyanos/Inopos], more suspect in men than in women, unless they be such in women with acute fevers on account of the fevers themselves and not on account of the release of the menses; for then it announces the gravest danger, even more than in men, insofar as they [men] are more distant from their [women's] nature) (Sloane 282, f. 36r). Compare the sign given in the *Urina Rufa* treatise, widespread in both Latin and English, asserting that "Urina lactea et cum spissa substancia – et si accidit in mulieribus non est ita periculosum sicut in viris propter indispociciones matricis – tamen in acutis febribus est mortalis" (Middle English: *Vrina lactea* and with þikke substance: if hit bifalle in wymmen hit is nouȝt so perlous as in men for inordinances of matrices ... But neuerþelater in scharpe fyueres hit is mortel). Ed. Tavormina 2019, 7 (ME), 177 (Lat.).

Daniel's phrase "by cause of malady on here floures" seems to be a mistake, though it occurs in all witnesses: the wicked sign that is worse in women than men is caused by fever, *not* by the menses. Perhaps the difficulty reflects an early scribal error, repeating and slightly expanding on the phrase "be cause of floures" in the preceding sentence.

423–4   **Gilbert þus: os seiþ Ypocras in his *Pronostikes* ... warshing by bledyng at nose:** Gilbert does not cite the *Prognostics* in his comments on the colours Inopos and Kyanos (in Wellcome 547), but he does note that "in causone febre si appareat, signat crisim vel fluxum sanguinis a naribus cum capitis dolore, secundum quod dicit Theophilus" (if [Inopos] should appear in a fever causon, it signifies the crisis of the disease or a discharge of blood from the nose with headache, according to Theophilus) (f. 129rb). The relevant passage in Theophilus may be the paragraph on fat, Inopos-coloured urine: "et si uenerit in febribus causon capite dolente et circumdolente, fert crisin" (and if it appears in causon fevers, with the head aching all around, it brings the crisis) (ed. Dase 1999, 25; *Articella* 1483, f. 6va).

References in the *Prognostics* to nosebleed occur in parts 7, 21, and 24, associated with fevers in all three sections, with headache in 21 and 24, and noting the possibility of relief in 7 and 24, though the colour of urine is not mentioned in any of these contexts.

425–31   Theophilus seiþ þat þis warshing ... ake in the heuede ... colre and blode by myght of his owen kynde: The Theophilus citation properly applies only to the linkage of Inopos with headache (see preceding note). The rest of the explanation is Gilbert's: "Cum enim colera bulliat & aduritur multi uapores generantur in ista adustione, qui multi sunt & subtiles & calidi ualde, quod materia huius ad capud eleuata, trahit sanguinem et coleram propter uehemenciam uirtutis" (For when choler boils up and burns, many vapours are generated in this burning, which are many and subtle and very hot, so that when their matter is elevated to the head, it draws with it blood and choler on account of their power) (Wellcome 547, f. 129rb).

458–9   þat it is impossible kynde hem to ouercome or for to maistri: "that it is impossible for nature to overcome or control them."

460   Þus seiþ Gilbert: Only found in RM7 GTSaSc; all other witnesses read "þus techeth/seith Theophilus," though neither Gilbert's Comment nor Theophilus's *De urinis* contains a warning against treating patients with desperate prognoses.

2.14

6   trethe: A contracted form of *tretethe* "treats, discusses." Compare the forms *math(e)*, *tath* (see 2.5.30n).

15–18   oure leches and Grece and alle leches ... rubeus color is þe kynde coloure of colre: Adapting Gilbert's comment that "colera enim naturaliter est citrina, unde eius color secundum Grecos est citrinus, secundum Arabes est rubeus, licet Greci in hoc uerius sunt opinati sicut sunt in singulis" (for choler is naturally citrine, whence the Greeks say its colour is Citrine, whereas the Arabs say it is Rubeus, although the Greeks in this matter have judged more truly, as in [other] details) (Wellcome 547, f. 130ra). Similar lexical differences are found between the Greco-Latin and Arabo-Latin translations of the red colour known as *pyrron* in Greek medical texts: *rufus* in Theophilus's *De urinis* and *citrinus* in Isaac Israeli's *De urinis* (see Introduction, pp. 9–10).

19   to here site and to oure site: The ambiguously spelled word *site* seems to have been unclear to scribes as well: variants include *site* (RM7 EW), *cite(e)* (GTSaSc A), *syȝte* (SbJ), and *syȝt and cyte* (CfCgB M6G3H), though the gist of the passage remains the same – the differing locations and perspectives of Arab and English doctors shape their complexions, and thus their ideas about the natural colour of red choler.

46–7   a wesel of þe felde … noȝt *e contrario*: Daniel seems to have been a bit uncertain of the best gloss for *mustela agrestis*, and in the beta version, he adds the further qualifier *perauenture* to this statement, or perhaps to the following sentence (Ashmole 1404, f. 139v, and other beta/beta* witnesses).

91–4   os Gilbert seiþ … ar al on: Cf. Gilbert's comment: "Nota quod calor adurens sanguinem eius florem et splendorem obumbrat et destruit. Flos sanguinis est vnctuositas" (Note that heat burning blood overshadows and destroys its flower and splendour. The flower of blood is its oiliness) (Wellcome 547, f. 130ra).

94–6   and Thade also … but only þe j spice … : We have not found this point about the types of jaundice and their origin(s) in the Urina Viridis section of ps.-Taddeo's "Noua reportata" commentary, as preserved in Arsenal 1024.

99–100   wiþ hem accordeþ Gilbert … principaly but in the lyuer: "Non enim generatur humor nisi in epate" (For humour is generated only in the liver) (Wellcome 547, f. 131va).

107–10   Ysodre eke in þe 4 bok of *Ethimologyis*, **þe 6 c. …** *neruorum causata*: "Spasmus Latine contractio subita partium aut nervorum cum dolore vehementi … Fit autem duobus modis, aut ex repletione, aut ex inanitione" (Spasm in Latin is a sudden contraction of the members or the nerves with intense pain … It happens in two ways, either from eating to excess or from exhaustion due to lack of nourishment) (Isidore of Seville, *Etymologies* 4.6.11; ed. Lindsay 1911).

113–14   *Tetanus est maior spasmus … eadem causata*: "Tetanus maior est contractio nervorum a cervice ad dorsum" (Tetanus is a greater contraction of the nerves from the neck to the back) (*Etymologies* 4.6.12; ed. Lindsay 1911).

119–22   Constantyn in his first *Boke of Medycyns*, **þe last c. saue on, seiþ … substancial humidite:** "Oportet autem ut intelligamus quod si sano homini subito evenerit spasmus ex plenitudine necesse est quod efficiatur. Si post acutam febrem fiat labor et vigilie et similia antecedant ex inanitione esse intelligimus" (We must understand that if spasm suddenly comes upon a healthy man, it was necessarily caused by fullness; if it happens after an acute fever, [and] labour and waking and like things have preceded it, we recognize that it came from exhaustion) (*Viaticum* 1.24; *Omnia opera Ysaac* 1515, 2: 148ra–rb).

3.1

4–5   þorogh gift of him þat mannes ende haþ in hande: Alpha witnesses RM7 TGSaSc agree in reading *ende* in this phrase; SaSc read *goste* for *gift*. In the beta witnesses AG6EWSb, *ende* is changed to words for "breath": *onde* (AG6), *wynde* (EW), and *puf* (Sb); *gift* is changed in EW to *myȝt*. The beta* texts omit *gift of* entirely and change *ende* to *powce* (M6G3H) or *power* (CfCgB).

17   pores of þe veyns: I.e., the diameters of bodily ducts or vessels, possibly including vessels for blood and other fluids. The *waies of þe vryn* in line 3.1.19 are urinary ducts strictly speaking.

44   habit ... rotede: *Habit*, like *rotede*, should be read as a past participle with the sense "habituated, engrained over time," as Daniel's own gloss *so mykel broght in vse & in vsage* suggests. Daniel is drawing here on the Aristotelian notion of ἕξις (*hexis*), an acquired and stable disposition, familiar in the Middle Ages by way of works such as the *Nicomachean Ethics*, which Daniel cites as *The Boke of Thewis* in the beta version of the Ypostasis: Subrubea chapter.

56   cafuist: This abbreviation for *cassia fistula* (the seed pods or fruit of the cassia tree) may be Daniel's own; it is not included in Hunt's *Plant Names of Medieval England*, the *MED*, *OED*, or *A-ND*. Daniel glosses cassia fistula as *cafust* in the Arundel 42 copy of his herbal (f. 60v), but does not appear to use the abbreviation in the BL Add. 27329 copy. Most of the beta* witnesses (G3CfCbH and Sb at this point in the text) direct readers to "se in oure Practyke" for more information on cassia fistula and cassia lignea.

62–4   os techeþ Ypocras and al auctours ... membris of þe body: Probably a generic reference to medical writers across history.

67   for to vndo hem by and by: To gloss or explain them later in the text. In RM7, this "undoing" only occurs "by and by," as Daniel reaches the relevant chapter for each content. Three other witnesses (M6 SeJ) also give only the Latin verse with no English translation. But in the majority of manuscripts (GTSaSc AG6EW Sb CfCgB G3H), the Latin verse is followed by one or two English content-lists. Single lists appear in the alpha subgroup GTSaSc, the main beta group AG6EW, and the idiosyncratic beta text Sb, while the remainder offer two distinct English lists.

68–71   *Circulus ampulla ... octo decem*: Giles of Corbeil, *Carmen de urinis* 216–19. The verses given in RM7 vary slightly from those in Choulant and Vieillard, with *quoque nebula* replacing *nubecula*, *necnon attomique* replacing *partes atomosae*, and – most notably – *ypostasis octo decem* (glossing *sedimen*) instead of *spiritus alta petens* "the rising vapour." GTSaSc keep the word *spiritus* directly after *sedimen*, but still replace *alta petens* with *ypostasis octo decem* and *partes attomose* with *necnon attomique*.

The remaining witnesses follow Giles's diction more closely, retaining *partes attomose* and *spiritus alta petens*: AG6EW SeJ Sb CgCfB M6G3H. However, seven of them disorder the Latin verses, moving *crinoides ... alta petens* between *granum* and *nebula* (Sb CgCfB M6G3H).

3.2

31–4   os Gilbert seiþ ... noght sperplyn ne spreden ham as in men: "Et nota quod hec est cautela caloris naturalis qui congregat et coadunat et spergere non potest, sicut est in mulieribus: propter enim debilitatem caloris in eis non spergunt uapores, ut in eis barba generetur, unde calor naturalis debilis in eis congregat eos in capite uel capillis, et maxime in anteriori parte, et ideo non caluescunt quoniam materia capillorum ibi congregatur plus quam in uiris" (And note that this is a warning about the natural heat that gathers together and unites and cannot disperse, as happens in women. Because of the weakness of heat in them, the vapours do not disperse so that a beard might grow, whence their weak natural heat gathers in the head or the hair, and especially in the front part, and therefore they do not go bald because the material of the hair gathers there more than in men) (Wellcome 547, f. 130rb).

41–2   blode colde and moyst: Blood is by nature hot and moist in medieval humoral theory, but here Daniel seems to be suggesting a type of blood that is suited to feeding the humorally cold, wet brain.

49   *De rubeo circulo*: The order in which the text treats red and pale Circles is a distinguishing feature between textual subgroups of the *LU*, as is the order of black and tremulous Circles, as follows:

Red, then Pale; Black, then Tremulous: alpha texts RM7; mixed texts (all with beta* sections) CgCfB G3M6H

Pale, then Red; Tremulous, then Black: alpha texts GTSaSc; beta texts AG6EW Sb JSe

Note that this feature crosses the alpha/beta version line, suggesting some kind of organizational contamination between the versions but not within the subgroups inside the two versions.

56–7   it is causede: "there is caused … " (RM7TG); SaSc have *it is callid*.

66   dasthede: Possibly equivalent to an otherwise unattested word *dasedhede* "the quality of being dull, lethargic, or timid." See *MED*, s.v. *dasednesse* (n.) and *dasen* (v.); *OED*, s.v. *dastard* (n.), esp. the suggested etymology. Most other witnesses have some form of *gasthed* "fearfulness"; SaSc read *gastnos(e)*, probably an error for *gastnesse*; A has *wastehed*. The Latin version of the *LU* has *timorem et suspicionem et fantasiam in corde, multam vigiliam et avariciam* for the string of nouns (*drede & dasthede … grete aueryce*) in the English text.

73   afte: A rare form of *after*, attested in a few *LALME* profiles and the *Corpus of Middle English Prose and Verse*.

75–6   *Cerebrum* … mortificacion: The internal cross-references here have been reversed: *cerebrum* is discussed in the chapter on Karopos, bk. 2.7, but on old leaves 55–6; mortification is defined in bk. 2.1, on the verso of old leaf 17.

109   schagge menely mewand þe vrynal: "shake the urinal, moving it gently."

115   And fonden al þat in hem is: "And everything that is in them strives."

116–17   so fayn þai wolden … the hatrel: "so eagerly do they want to have their flowing in the back part of the head."

136–8   *Litargia* is causede … Constantyn in þe j *Bok of Medecynes*: *Viaticum* 1.14, "De lethargia": "ex multa phlegmatis frigiditate & humiditate cum in puppi cerebri superat: & animatum spiritum suffocat" (from great coldness and wetness of phlegm, when it overcomes and suffocates the animate spirit in the rear of the brain) (*Omnia opera Ysaac* 1515, 2: 146rb).

138–40 Frenesis, os seiþ the same auctour ... persand þe cerebre: *Viaticum* 1.18, "De frenesis": "Nascitur duobus modis: vel ex incensione cholere rubee cerebrum ascendentis: vel de sanguinis ebullitione in corde cuius fumus cum ascenderit cerebrum fit apostema" (It arises in two ways: either from burning of red choler rising to the brain or from the boiling of blood in the heart, whose vapour, once it rises to the brain, becomes an aposteme) (*Omnia opera Ysaac* 1515, 2: 146vb).

3.3

53–4 For as Gilbert seiþ ... kyndly to the reynes: Possibly paraphrasing Gilbert's remark that "ampulla signat nefresim propter grossos humores per uias urine descendentes in renibus, uiscositate sua adherentes et sua grossicie nocentes" (Bubbles signify kidney disease on account of gross humours descending into the kidney through the urinary vessels, adhering by their viscosity and causing harm by their grossness) (Wellcome 547, f. 136ra).

60 mewyng: "moving," with *w* used for the sound usually represented by *v*.

3.4

6 the cerebre, os Gilbert seiþ, is kyndly *frigidum & humidum*: Possibly a reference to Gilbert's comment, "Aristoteles probat cerebrum esse frigidius et humidius omnibus aliis membris sicut omnes anathomici attestantur" (Aristotle shows that the brain is colder and wetter than all other members, as all anatomists attest) (Wellcome 547, f. 133va).

7 acordeþ mykel toward in kynd grece and marie: "greatly corresponds with fat and bone-marrow in nature."

26 queynt swoyng: "a remarkable roaring or ringing (in the ears)" (*MED*, s.v. *swouen* [v.(1)]), a reading found only in RM7; other witnesses use forms of the more common sound-related words *sounen*, v., and *soun*, n.

44–7 Ypocras geueþ his reule in his *Afforismis* ... into the guttes: *Aph.* 7.30, "Quibuscunque spumose egestiones in diaria his a capite phlegma defluit" (In cases where frothy discharges occur in diarrhoea there are fluxes from the head) (*Articella* 1483, f. 42vb; trans. Jones, Loeb ed. 4: 199).

47 þe reye: A possibly dialectal term for lientery, a form of diarrhea, attested with application to sheep and cattle in the sixteenth to nineteenth centuries (see *OED*, s.v. *ray* [n.[10]]). Some witnesses gloss the Latin more fully: *the squyrte* (*squit* G6EWSb) *or the reye* (G6EWSb CfCgB M6G3H); A has only *the sqvyrte*.

66–8 riȝt vpon þat ... Greynes in the vryn: "depending on whether the members or places that the matter draws to are higher or lower, the Grains will hold themselves likewise in the urine."

3.5

The chapter on Sky or Cloud (*Nebula*) in urine shows substantial variation between the alpha and beta versions, with alpha texts opening as R does (comparing Sky to a spider web or powder strewn on the surface), and beta texts opening with some variant of A's "*Nebula vrine*, Sky in vryn, is noo thing els but an vmbre, a shadow, a swarte dymhed above on þe vryn in þe over party of þe vryn, toward þe colour of oyle or of multen talovgh ('tallow')" and with significant divergence throughout the chapter.

12–15   os Tadeus seiþ … like a cop-web … poudre or dust strewed þeron: Cf. ps.-Taddeo, "Noua reportata": "[nubes] petit superiorem partem urine que dicitur pars aerea & hoc uapor cum a corpore exierit propter frigiditatem aeris coadunatur & assimilatur quasi tele aranee siue subtilissimo pulueri ?supersperse superficiei urine" (*nubes* seeks the upper part of the urine, which is called the aerial part, and when this vapour goes out of the body, it coalesces on account of the frigidity of the air, and is likened to a spider web or the finest dust ?scattered on the surface of the urine) (Paris, Bibliothèque nationale de France, Arsenal 1024, f. 8vb).

14   sweyth: "moves, flows, floats." Only found in R; M7 reads *swich* (poss. error for *swith*), GTSaSc *scheweth*; *om.* all beta texts.

30   saffran chies: Cheese flavoured with saffron. The reading occurs only in RM7; GTSaSc have simply *safron*; *om.* all beta texts.

36   mykil toward as: "much like what."

38–9   os Isaac seiþ … malady hard & scharp: Source in Isaac not yet identified.

3.6

21–2   in alse mykel … saie os lastand: "insofar as *continuus* or *continua* is equivalent to saying 'lasting.'"

31–4   os Gilbert aleggeþ þat Galien seiþ … vnkynd hete … aboute the lyuer: Gilbert's commentary in Wellcome 547 does not describe the generation of Foam or Froth precisely as an *ebullicio caloris (unnaturalis)*, though the general metaphor of boiling within the body is mentioned and Galen is credited with other observations about Foam (ff. 135r–137v). Gilbert does note that Foam "signat passionem membrorum mediorum, cordis scilicet et epatis et adiacencium vicinorum" (indicates sickness of the middle members, namely of the heart and liver and those adjoining them nearby) (f. 135rb).

39–42   Gilbert seiþ … more high in colour: Gilbert: "Si autem debili calore sit, spuma est remissa; si forti, forcius est tincta. Si a debili calore, substantia spume est grossa; si forti, magis est tenuis" (But if it be [generated] from weak heat, the Foam is of a low colour; if from strong heat, it is higher in colour. If from weak heat, the substance of the Foam is gross; if from strong, it is thinner) (Wellcome 547, f. 137va).

42   **Wherfore ȝet:** "On account of which, indeed," with only minor force to *ȝet/indeed.* GTSaSc read merely *Wherfore.*

3.7

5–8   **Giles in þe Coment seiþ þus ... & þerabouten:** See the Standard Commentary: "In hoc capitulo agit auctor de sanie que cum urina effunditur. Signat vlceracionem vesice aut renum; signat et passionem epatis ex aliqua superflua materia in eius collecta regione" (In this chapter the author treats Pus that is emitted with the urine. It signifies ulceration of the bladder or the kidneys; it also signifies disease of the liver caused by some superfluous material gathered near it) (Sloane 282, f. 39v).

15–17   **Ypocras in the ende of þe 4 particule of *Afforismys* ... o þe vesie:** *Aph.* 4.81: "Si sanguinem aut pus minguntur: aut squamas: & odor grauis uesice ul[ce]-rationem significat" (If the urine contain blood, pus and scales, and its odour be strong, it means ulceration of the bladder) (*Articella* 1483, f. 31ra; trans. Jones, Loeb ed. 4: 157).

18–23   **Gilbert seiþ þus:** *sanies* ... & **musseleþ and falleth awaie ... drestish and modissh:** "Sanies fit ab epate et renibus et uesica: ab epate quandoque a corrupcione eius, quoniam corrumpitur calor naturalis ipsius et coroditur eius substancia; tunc est sanies ex corrupcione epatis et tunc est quasi amurca cum re mollita, sicut testatur Ypocras in *Amphorismis*" (Pus comes from the liver, the kidneys, and the bladder. It comes from the liver sometimes because of its corruption, because its natural heat is corrupted and its substance is corroded; then the Pus comes from the corruption of the liver, and then it is like the dregs of oil with something soft, as Hippocrates attests in the *Aphorisms*) (Wellcome 547, f. 138ra).

See *Aph.* 7.45: "Quicunque in capite [*error for* epate] propter saniem uruntur: siquidem sanies pura fluxerit & alba euadunt. In tunica enim illius sanies est. Si uero uelut amurca fluxerit: pereunt" (Whenever abscess of the liver is treated by cautery or the knife ["or the knife" *not in Latin text*], if the pus flow pure and white, the patient recovers, for in such cases the pus is in a membrane; but if it flows like as it were lees of oil, the patient dies) (*Articella* 1483, ff. 43vb–44ra; trans. Jones, Loeb ed. 4: 203).

21   **musseleþ:** "wears away, goes mouldy, mildews." Not in *MED*, but probably derived from Anglo-Norman *museler* (itself derived from Lat. *mucidus*); see *A-ND*, s.v. *museler²*. The word is not used in the GTSaSc parallel passage, but appears again (in the spelling *moseleþ/muslys*) in the beta and beta* texts AEW CfCgB M6G3H.

42–5   **Also euermore of whiche of alle 3 ... somtyme distroiþ him al fully:** Gilbert: "Cum aggregatur sanies in aliquo predictorum membrorum fit dolor uehemens qui prosternit uirtutem; vnde accio illius uirtutis minoratur & leditur, aut omnino prosternitur" (When Pus accumulates in any of the foresaid members, there occurs a powerful pain that overthrows the vital force; on account of which, the action of that force is diminished and damaged, or is entirely overthrown) (Wellcome 547, f. 138rb).

45   Þus techeþ he: Gilbert, referring to the preceding material.

46   Tadeus & eke dyuerse auctors thus: Ps.-Taddeo, "Noua reportata": "Tria sunt qui gerunt similitudinem in vrina s. humor . ypostasis . & sanies" (Three things in urine are like each other, namely Humour, Ypostasis, and Pus) (Arsenal 1024, f. 9ra), followed by criteria for distinguishing among these three contents. Cf. 3.9.2–3n below for the equivalent material in the Standard Commentary and Wellcome 547, f. 138va–vb, for Gilbert's take ("Sed inter ypostasim, saniem, et humorem crudum, hec est differentia ... ").

56   wit wil: "wite well" ("know well").

82   sanies goth more space: "the Pus goes further" (pus from the kidneys and liver is warmer than that from the bladder, and therefore spreads out more in the urine; pus from the cold bladder, as noted earlier, draws to the bottom of the urinal).

89   be cause os I seide: "for the reason I said."

98   the þin ... þe thik: The thinner, lighter, upper portion of the specimen and the thicker, pus-filled, lower portion respectively.

111   vnderstonde þat it is: Possibly an error for vnderstonde þat [if] it is or vnderstonde þat [when] it is, but there is no manuscript support for either emendation.

114   Gilbert seiþ þat only sanies of þe reyns is wiþouten eny blode: "Cum uero corroditur eius carnositas solum renum fit sine sanguine" (And only when the fleshiness of the kidneys is gnawed away does it happen without blood) (Wellcome 547, f. 138ra).

3.8

2–4   Pinguedo in vrina, os sciþ þe Comentour vppon Giles ... forth wiþ þe vryn: Standard Commentary: "Hic nomine pinguedinis intelligitur quedam pinguis et unctuosa substantia a membris resoluta, que cum urina emittitur" (By the term "Fat" is understood here a certain fat and greasy substance dissolved from the members, which is emitted with the urine) (Sloane 282, f. 40r).

25–6   bestes bodies þat ar opynd: Perhaps a reference to ordinary butchering, but the addition of the phrase and namely in swyne in CfCgB M6G3H may allude to medieval anatomical texts that are based on dissection of pigs, such as the Anatomia porci (see note to line 1.3.23–4 above).

36   louseþ: M7's spelling here is doubly ambiguous, thanks to the similarity of u/n in the scribe's hand here and his use of y for both y and þ, yielding four possible readings: loupes, lonþes, louyes, lonyes, none of which offers plausible sense. Almost all other witnesses read *lesseth/lassith*, aside from SbJ, which omit the word. We have assumed that the M7 form is *loupes*, an error for *lousep* "dissolves."

64–6   if þou poure þe vryn ... seiþ þe Coment of Gilis: Standard Commentary: "In tercia vero specie pinguedo est diffusa per totum, unde urina super lapidem infusa sonat ut oleum" (In the third type [of hectic fever], the Fat is diffused throughout the urine, whence the urine poured on a stone sounds like oil) (Sloane 282, f. 40r).

66   & diuerse oþer: See, for example, the much-copied *Dome of Uryne*: "The 3 spice [of hectic fever]: the vryne ys fat oueral aboute as oyle and ȝyf hit be cast on a ston of marbyl, hit sowneth as oylle. And this spice hit ys incurable" (Sloane 374, f. 7v, on Fat in urine; ed. Tavormina 2019, 33).

67–74   Gilbert seiþ þus: Fathede in vryn ... whitish ... ȝelowish ... citrin ... grenish ... caused a grenishede: "Et pinguedo quedam est alba, et a forciori calore crocea, quedam est citrina ut pectoris; et recens est alba, uetus autem magis citrina. Item a debili calore liquefacta est alba, et a forciori calore crocea, et a fortissimo, uiridis; quod patet in pinguidine suspensa in aere exeunti cuius calor aquositatem consumens citrinescere facit si sit fortis et diuturna, autem uirescere si forcior et diuturnior" (And some Fat is white, and with stronger heat saffron-coloured; some is citrine as that of the breast; and new Fat is white, old more citrine. And white Fat is melted by weak heat, and saffron by stronger heat, and green by the strongest heat, which is clear from fat that is hung in moving air. The heat thereof causes the fat to become citrine by consuming the wateriness, if the heat is strong and lasting, or to become green if it is stronger and longer lasting) (Wellcome 547, f. 138r).

111   ȝede: This archaic word for "went" (from OE *ēode*, the irregular past of *gān* "go") appears only in RM7; all other witnesses use more familiar verbs of movement, like *goth* and *passeth*.

3.9

2–3   os techeþ þe Comentour vppon Giles ... & *humor crudus*: Standard Commentary: "Et nota quod tria sunt que similitudinis mutacione speciem sediminis pretendunt: sedimen, putredo, crudus humor" (And note that there are three things that claim the appearance of similarity with variation: Sediment, Pus, Raw Humour) (Sloane 282, f. 40v). Like Daniel, the Commentator continues with motion tests to distinguish among these three similar contents.

28–31   If it ocupie þe neþer ... Þus seiþ Giles and þe Comentour eke: Standard Commentary: "Si infimam partem [optineat], passionem renum et lumborum et parcium adiacencium et thenasmon et nefresim et stranguriam, tibiarum et genuum dolorem declarat" (If it occupies the lowest part, it indicates diseases of the kidneys and loins and nearby parts, and tenesmus and nephritis and strangury, and pain of the legs and knees) (Sloane 282, f. 40v).

34–8 Gilbert seiþ þus: if Humor ... þe 3 reule aforn: "Post pinguedinem, agit actor de humore, qui si superiorem partem urine occupet & corpus sit sine febre, uicium declarat spiritualium; vnde asma uel disma uel arteria passio quandoque declaratur. Si in medio uasis fuerit uicium stomachi ex replecione superfluitatum, torcio uentris, inflacio, rugitus intestinorum quandoque portenditur. Si infimam optineat partem, sepius passio renum & lumborum parcium adiacencium indicatur" (After Fat, the author deals with Humour, which if it occupies the upper part of the urine and the body is without fever, announces an illness of the spiritual members, whence it announces asthma, dyspnea, or sometimes an ailment of the windpipe. If it should be in the middle of the urinal, it presages a stomach disorder from fullness of superfluous matter, twisting of the abdomen, gas, and sometimes intestinal rumbling. If it holds the lower part, it often indicates a disorder of the kidneys and loins and adjacent parts) (Wellcome 547, f. 138va).

43 if age ... be gode, gode hope of saf: If the patient is young or has a strong constitution, there is good hope for recovery.

52–90 Gilbert seiþ þus. But difference, seiþ he, is atwene *ypostasis* and *sanies* & *crudus humor* ... Þus seiþ he: This lengthy passage is a slightly expanded paraphrase of Gilbert's comments on the distinctions between Ypostasis, Sanies/Pus, and Raw Humour (Wellcome 547, 138va–vb).

118–19 and so is *tenasmoun* caused ... Þus techen þai: "Þai" may simply be a generic reference to medical authorities, or it may be a glance back at Giles and the Commentator, cited just before Gilbert at lines 3.9.30–1 above. Daniel's self-reference is a bit confused: he does not mention *t(h)enasmoun* (tenesmus) in bk. 1.3, in either the alpha or beta versions of the text, although the *longaoun* (the rectum) is introduced and defined in 1.3 and several earlier cross-references to the *longaoun* itself cite 1.3 and old leaf 3.

3.10

2–4 þus auctoures speken, þe Coment vpon Giles þus ... elles of the kil: This list of four sources for Blood in the urine is actually given by Giles himself, at lines 265–6 of the *Carmen de urinis*. The Standard Commentary refers first to blood from the liver and the bladder, and a few lines later mentions the *kilis* vein, but does not discuss blood from the kidneys (Sloane 282, f. 40v).

6 coldissh and clumish: So in RM7, but possibly an error for *cloddish and clumprish*: variants for *coldissh* include *cloddyssh* (GTSaSc AG6 Sb), *clowdyshe* (J), the verb phrase *it cluddys* (EW), and *coldysch* again (CfCgB G3H; *om.* M6); for *clumish* (only in RM7), we also find *crumpryssh* (G), *clomprissche* (TSc

AG6 CfB M6G3H), *clumpish* (Sa), *cluprysh* (Cg), the verb *clumprys* (EW), and omission (SbJ).

21–2   os Galien seiþ … a water leche: Quoted in the Standard Commentary: "Et ut refertur Galienus, talis sanguis per virgam quandoque per modum sansuge, siue sanguissuge, quod id est, emittitur" (And as Galen is reported to have said: such blood is sometimes emitted through the penis in the manner of a water-leech, or blood-sucker, which that is) (Sloane 282, f. 40v).

22–7   Ypocras techeþ … of þe vesie … when it was of the vesie: Several of the *Aphorisms* deal with pain and ulceration in the kidneys and bladder, and the associated discharges of blood, pus, and other contents, most notably 4.75–81 and 7.39. The Standard Commentary quotes *Aph*. 4.75, 4.78, 4.80, and 4.81 (Sloane 282, ff. 40v–41r).

28–34   If it be o þe lyuer, þe Blode … Þus seiþ Gilbert and þe Comentour: Standard Commentary: "Sanguis autem emissus cum urina, aut procedit ab epate, et tunc debet esse purus et sincerus et in dextro ypocundrio dolor sentitur, et talis sanguis cum sit calidus perfeccius urine permiscetur … Si ex ruptura kilis vene proueniat est similiter in septimo spondili, facta computacione ab inferiori parte superius, et tunc vehemens dolor occurrit" (But Blood that passes with the urine, it either proceeds from the liver, and then it should be pure and clean and the pain is felt in the right hypochondrium, and such Blood since it is hot is mingled perfectly with the urine … If it comes from the breaking of the *kilis* vein, it is [felt] similarly in the seventh vertebra counting upward from the lower part, and then intense pain occurs) (Sloane 282, f. 40v).

Gilbert: "Sanguis enim renum kilis uene & epatis magis colorat urine liquorem quam econtrario, quam propter sui multitudinem, sed a renibus minus est purus quam a kili uena & epate, quoniam renes minus habent de calore quam superiora, ideo sanguis eorum minus depuratur & coloratur, et sanguis epatis plus est purus quam kilis" (For the blood of the kidneys, the *kilis* vein, and the liver colours the urinary fluid more than not, on account of its quantity; but that from the kidneys is less pure than from the *kilis* vein and liver, because the kidneys have less heat than the higher members, and thus the kidneys' blood is less refined and coloured. And the blood of the liver is purer than that of the *kilis* vein) (Wellcome 547, f. 139ra).

35–8   Gilbert þus: Blode aperand … longe tyme or in exces: Compare Gilbert: "De sanguine et eius significacionibus quoniam prouenit quandoque ex epate, & hic fit duobus modis: s. quando uena rumpitur in eo uel crepatur aliqua de causa, vel cum aliquis exercitatur diu vel fortiter, postea uenit in quietem, quoniam sanguis qui per exercicium consumebatur concurrit ad epar, vel cum sangui[s] qui per exercitium consumebatur prius fluebat a naribus vel menstruis vel emoroydibus, & constringitur reuertitur ad epar" (Concerning Blood and its significance: because it comes sometimes from the liver, and this happens in two ways, namely when a vein is broken in the liver or it is ruptured from some other cause, either when someone has exerted himself long or hard, and afterwards comes to rest, because the blood that was expended by the exertion runs to the liver, or blood that was expended previously flowed out from the nose or via the menses or hemorrhoids, and is stopped [and] returns to the liver) (Wellcome 547, f. 138vb).

49   **som stryng of hem:** I.e., a ligament attached to the kidneys.

62–3   **Þus seiþ he. Som þus ... somtym of þe lyuer:** "He" is probably Gilbert, the most recently cited authority: cf. his comments quoted in the note to lines 28–34 above, with the surrounding remarks: "Vesica enim parum habet de sanguine; est enim membrum ualde frigidum et panniculosum. Sanguis enim renum kilis uene & epatis ... et sanguis epatis plus est purus quam kilis. Hac eadem ratione dicta facit *trumbosum* quia a debili calore sanguis coadunatur et quasi coagulatur vel congelatur. *Grauis* est quia calor debilis plus dissoluit quam consumit; *maculosus* racione primo assignat, *subsidens* propter grauitatem" (The bladder has little blood, for it is a very cold and sinewy organ. For the blood of the kidneys, the *kilis* vein, and the liver ... And the blood of the liver is purer than that of the *kilis* vein. For this reason, it makes clotted blood, because the blood is collected from a weak heat, and is almost coagulated and congealed. It is heavy because the weak heat dissolves more than it consumes; spotty he ascribes to the first reason, sinking down because of its weight) (Wellcome 547, f. 139ra). The generic "som" cited in the last sentence are presumably authors who do not analyse the sources of Blood in the urine as carefully as Gilbert does, following in the footsteps of both Giles and the Commentator.

87   **and skile whie ... seyn be poyntes þat ar saide:** "and you may well see the reason why it is so by the points made."

3.11

34–6   **as Alexandre telleþ of one þat had þe pthisik ... induracioun of humores:** Alexander of Tralles (Alexander Trallianus), *Therapeutica*, 2.11, "De lapide sputato": "Spuit quidam uir lapidem specialiter & hoc non forte pinguem humorem et glutinosum ... et postea proiecit lapidem, non post multum dies ut pthisici solent ita defunctus est" (A man spat up a stone, specifically that is to say, not just some thick and glutinous humour ... and after he threw up the stone, a few days later, as consumptives usually do, he died) (ed. and trans. Langslow 2006, 222–7).

54–63   *arena* **somtym seiþ þat þe stone ... Þus seiþ þe Coment vpon Giles; Gilbert þe same:** The closest passage in the Standard Commentary to Daniel's remarks on the "breeding" of kidney and bladder stones appears to be the following: "Et nota quod quandoque harene signant lapidem diuidendum (L: diminuendum), quandoque confirmandum, et quandoque confirmatum. Si prius non apparentes cotidie multiplicuntur magis ac magis, quousque minus appareant, signant lapidem diuidendum (L: diminuendum). Si diu multis apparentibus cotidie diminuantur magis ac magis signant lapidem confirmandum, quando enim penitus non apparent cum purgate non fuerint signant lapidem confirmatum" (And note that sometimes sandy particles indicate that the stone is going to be broken up (L: diminished), sometime that it is going to grow, and sometimes that it has grown. If after not appearing, they are multiplied daily more and more, until they appear to a lesser extent, they indicate that the stone is going to be broken up (L: diminished). If many grains have been appearing daily for a long time, and then they decrease more and more, they indicate that the stone is going to grow. For when they suddenly do not appear, since they were not passed, they indicate that the stone has grown) (Sloane 282, f. 41r–v; variants from Bodl., Laud lat. 106).

Gilbert limits his remarks on the generation of sandy particles to a brief cross-reference: "satis dictum est in predictis capitulis de urina alba & karopos" (Wellcome 547, f. 139rb), but the earlier passages do not discuss the three stages of stone formation.

66–72   experiment þat Gilbert techeþ in his Coment … Þus seiþ he: "Si uis scire utrum lapis sit in renibus facias vrinam in pelui colari per pannum lineum, mundum et subtilem, & si inueniantur quedam harenule subtilissime, est in renibus; si grossiores magis & albe, est in uesica. Hic expertum est" (If you want to know whether the stone is in the kidneys, you should cause the urine in a basin to be strained through a clean, fine linen cloth, and if some very fine tiny grains of sand are found therein, it is in the kidneys; if they are larger and white, it is in the bladder. This has been proved by experience) (Wellcome 547, f. 139rb).

80–1   ek os kynde skil gifeþ it: "also as natural reason demonstrates."

81–7   os techeþ Constantyn in þe 5 *Boke of Medicynes*, þe 16 c. … as in men … gros and viscouse: See Constantine's *Viaticum*, a translation of ibn al-Jazzār's *Zād al-musāfir*, 5.18: "In mulieribus vero raro [lapis] nascitur: quia materia vnde lapis concreatur: non adunatur multis ex causis in mulieribus: quia collum vesice earum curtum est & foramina sunt larga & non multum tortuosa sunt: & minus bibunt aquam quam pueri: lapis enim maxime nascitur quando aqua diuersa & turbida bibitur: ex qua humores grossi & viscosi ad concreandum lapidem coadunantur" (The stone rarely arises in women, because the material from which stone is generated does not coalesce in women, for many reasons: because the neck of their bladder is short, and the openings are large and not very twisting; and they drink less water than children do. For the stone most often appears when murky water of varying quality is drunk, out of which gross and viscous humours are combined to generate the stone) (*Omnia opera Ysaac* 1515, 2: 163ra–rb).

3.12

14–16 Þerof spekeþ Ypocras in *Afforismis* ... of þe reyns: *Aph.* 4.76, "Quibus in urina grossa: quasi carnium frusta: uel sicut pili sunt: his de renibus exeunt" (When the urine is thick, and small pieces of flesh-like hairs pass with it, it means a secretion from the kidneys) (*Articella* 1483, f. 30vb; trans. Jones, Loeb ed. 4: 155).

23 os wel more þan an here: "such as much more than a single hair (in size/diameter)."

28–9 giffen myght ... to oþer partis of the body: Unless they are obstructed, the vital spirits should carry power to the limbs.

34–6 whan *pili* apperen ... Þus seiþ þe Coment vpon Giles: Standard Commentary: "Et nota quod pili apparent in vrina aut cum febre, aut sine febre. Si cum febre tocius corporis dissolucio signat; si sine febre, de renum substantia decisio fieri particulariter indicatur" (And note that Hairs appear in urine either with a fever or without a fever. If with a fever it signifies dissolution of the entire body; if without fever, the substance of the kidneys is being lost by itself) (Sloane 282, f. 41v).

36–41 Gilbert seiþ þat *pili* come ... Þus seiþ he: "Uidetur quod a carne figura non fiat pili decisio [V: a carne non debeant fieri pili], quod bene concedimus, sed fit a membris lacertosis, neruosis, pilosis & panniculosis ... Ex hiis patet quod non sunt pili a substantia renum, sed magis propter humorem grossum uiscosum exeuntem in grossis uenis ipsorum vel aliorum membrorum, vel propter dissolucionem membrorum filosorum, lacertosorum, vel neruosorum, ut sunt & arterie & huiusmodi" (It is evident that the shedding of [the content] Hair does not come from flesh in shape, which we grant, but it comes from members that are sinewy, made up of nerves, hairy, and membranous ... From these points it is clear that the Hairs are not from the substance of the kidneys, but rather caused by the gross viscous humour going out in their great veins or those of other members, or on account of the dissolution of hairy, sinewy, or innervated members, such as the arteries and their like) (Wellcome 547, f. 139rb–va).

38 faxwax: The ligament at the back of the neck. Daniel or the scribe of R also uses the form *paxwax* (see 3.16.18, 3.20.102, and 3.20.306 below).

46–7 Isaac seiþ ... are alike: Source in Isaac not yet identified.

3.13

8 royns: "scabies, mange, scab" (OF *roigne*).

18–23 fatt vryn and wiþ *furfura* ... Þus seiþ þe Coment vppon Giles: Cf. Standard Commentary: "Vrina ergo furfureas habens resoluciones aut signat dissolucionem tocius corporis aut vesice tantum ... predicta corpora quandoque fiunt calore partes liquidas consumente vel frigiditate condensante" (Therefore urine with Branny resolutions signifies either the dissolution of the whole body or of the bladder alone ... the foresaid bodies sometimes occur through heat consuming or cold condensing the liquid parts) (Sloane 282, ff. 41v–42r).

3.14

4   **onely gronde:** The basic sense here is of coarsely ground wheat, "ground only once," or possibly an error for *euely gronde* "badly ground" (supported by variants in most other witnesses).

16–18   **An vryn wiþ** *crinoydes* **... os Ypocras seiþ:** *Aph.* 7.31, "Quibuscunque in febribus in urinis crinoides hypostases fiunt: longam egritudinem significant" (In fever cases, sediments like coarse meal forming in the urine signify that the disease will be protracted) (*Articella* 1483, f. 43ra; trans. Jones, Loeb ed. 4: 199).

3.15

3   **goiown:** *MED*, s.v. *gojoun* (n. [1]), "the European gudgeon (*Gobio gobio, G. fluviatilis*)."

27–8   **þe more del of auctours ... al vnder on:** "most authors discuss *squame* and *furfura* under the same heading."

32–4   **Theophilus (os Gilbert reherceth) seiþ ... os it is seid:** Theophilus distinguishes only two sources for scales (which he labels *petaloides*) and *furfura*, namely the whole body or the bladder, depending on whether the contents are accompanied by fever or not. His paragraph on *crinoides* speaks of three "dimensiones corporis ... longitudinem et latitudinem et profundum," but does not mention a specific part of the body as a point of origination for these large particulates (ed. Dase 1999, 51–5; *Articella* 1483, f. 7va–vb). Gilbert seems to have taken Theophilus's three-dimensional *corpus* to refer to a member rather than the body as a whole, commenting that "posuit Theophilus quod ab eodem membro poterant fieri squama, furfur & scrinium [*sic*; *lege* crinium]; & cum calor agit in superficie, laminam eius dissoluit, consumpta humiditate in superficie, tum fit squama non habens profunditatem notabilem; cum ergo plus profundatur calor et secundum plures dyametros agit in membro fit furfur, habens de parte membri grossioris plus quam squama; cum ergo calor agit secundum omnes dyametros membri fit crinium; ita ponit Theophilus" (Theophilus says that Scales, Bran, and Crinoids can be made from the same member: when heat acts on the surface, it dissolves its (upper) layer and consumes the surface humidity, (and) then a Scale with no great thickness is made; when heat is increased and acts in more dimensions in the member, Bran is made, taking from a thicker part of the member than a Scale does; when heat acts in all dimensions of the member, a Crinoid is made. So says Theophilus) (Wellcome 547, f. 139va).

34–6   Bot Ypocras and Galienus … þat ar carnouse: Continuing the comment in the preceding note, Gilbert says, "Sed Galienus & Ypocras qui plus senciunt de anathomia membrorum & forma & figura eorum posuerunt quod crinium fit magis a membris carnosis" (But Galen and Hippocrates, who understood more about the anatomy of the members and their form and figure, said that a Crinoid comes more from fleshy members) (Wellcome 547, f. 139va).

39   þing: Uninflected plural form.

3.16

20   sewen: "follow, reflect, correspond to."

30   in virown: This character-string can be interpreted as one word (*enviroun*) or as a phrase. We have read it as a phrase because Daniel glosses it with another phrase, *in rownde abouten*, but it could also be taken as a single word. See *MED*, s.vv. *enviroun* (adv.), *viroun* (n.).

51–2   water þat amydown were wasshen inne: Water in which crushed hulled wheat or grits have been washed or soaked. Cf. Avicenna's comparison of the urine of pregnant women to chick-pea water and to neat's-foot broth (*Canon* 1.2.3.2 c.10; ed. 1522, f. 43vb).

53–4   os Auicen seiþ, þan þer apereþ … mykel toward rawe silke: Cf. Gilbert, Comment on Giles: "Apparet super urinam quoddam subtile album ad modum bombacis sicut dicit Auicenna" ([In pregnant women] there appears on the urine a certain fine white thing like raw silk, as Avicenna says) (Wellcome 547, f. 140rb). The Latin text of the *Canon* describes this white cloud as being "sicut cottum carminatum" (like carded cotton fibres) (*Canon* 1.2.3.2 c.10; Lyons 1522, f. 43vb).

67–9   os Gilbert seiþ, when Motes betokne concepcioun, þai ar caused oþerwise þan when þai seyn þe gowte: After several paragraphs on the ways in which Motes signifying gout are generated, Gilbert continues, "Si uero significent conceptum, alio modo de illis est determinandum" (If, however, they signify conception, they must be understood in another way) (Wellcome 547, f. 140ra–rb).

91   seweand and faileand: Glossing *guttand*, this doublet must have the general sense of "dripping, falling in drops." More narrowly, *seweand* is probably a form of *seuen* "to follow," in the sense of following a path (through the body), and *faileand* is likely to be a variant spelling for *falland* "falling." Alpha variants GTSaSc offer a fuller and clearer version of the gloss: *guttyng i.* (var. *and*) *droppynge & sewyng & fallyng*; beta witnesses all omit *sewyng/seweand*, reading either *guttyng i. dropyng and* (var. *i.*) *fallyng* or *gowtyng i. fallyng and droppyng*.

94   and anguishand bolnyng: "and painful swelling."

95–7   somtyme it is causede of hote humor ... os Constantyn seyth in his *Antitodarie*, in þe 6 bok, þe 18 c.: From the *Viaticum*, Constantine's translation of ibn al-Jazzār's *Zād al-musāfir*, 6.18, *De sciatica passione*: "Fit ... aliquando ex humoribus sanguineis cum cholera rubea mixtis" (Sometimes [sciatica] comes from sanguine humours mixed with red choler) (in *Omnia opera Ysaac* 1515, 2: 166ra). As can be seen in line 3.16.151 below, Daniel understands sciatica as a form of gout.

103–10   Constantyn, in þe forsaide bok, þe 19 c. ... when none nedith: *Viaticum* 6.19: "Plurimum nascitur hec passio suauiter & quiete viuentibus et exercitia negligentibus: vel purgationes & mundificationes corporis nolentibus: maxime cum multum comedant atque bibant: he enim res in corpore creant humores ... Hec passio venit maxime principibus et suauiter viuentibus et corpora humida habentibus: maxime si multo coitu vtuntur: et cibis nimijs impleantur" (This malady mostly occurs in those who live comfortably and quietly and who neglect exercise, or who avoid purging and cleansing of the body, especially when they eat and drink a lot, for these things create humours in the body ... This malady comes especially to princes and those living comfortably and having moist bodies, especially if they have intercourse frequently and are fattened with too much food) (in *Omnia opera Ysaac* 1515, 2: 166rb).

120–2   as Constantyn seiþ ... and of wickede humores: *Viaticum* 6.19: "Vnde fit vt quia non coeunt eunuchi non patiuntur hunc morbum: et si habuerint tamen raro: quod fit eis ex multitudine humorum propter inordinationem diete" (Hence, because eunuchs do not have intercourse, they do not suffer from this disease, or they only have it rarely, which happens to them as a result of a multitude of humours on account of immoderate diet) (in *Omnia opera Ysaac* 1515, 2: 166rb).

162–4   Galien & Constantyn seyn þat podagre ... harde for to helen: *Viaticum* 6.19: "Galie[nus] podagra inquit est passio incipiens in vere vel in estate: et sanatur in quadraginta diebus vel antea. Si in autumno & vsque ad hyemem durauerit: durum est eam curare" (Galen says that podagra is a malady beginning in spring or in summer, and it is cured in forty days or sooner. If it should last into autumn and on to winter, it is hard to cure it) (in *Omnia opera Ysaac* 1515, 2: 166rb).

232–7   Gilbert techeþ and seiþ þat þe most axen ... oþer poyntes and circumstaunces: "& oportet similiter uidere etatem & uirtutem & condicionem mulieris, & si menstrua solet habere & retinentur non, & si habeat [V: *add* societatem] cum uiro qui potens est generare ... & uideas si sit priuacio doloris & in membris superioribus, aut mediis, aut inferioribus; & secundum hanc doctrinam poteris significare de conceptu si fit vel non" (And likewise it is necessary to consider the age and strength and condition of the woman, and if she is accustomed to have her periods and that they are not retained, and if she keeps company with a man who is reproductively potent ... And see if there is a lack of pain either in the upper or the middle or the lower parts; and according to this knowledge, you will be able to diagnose whether she has conceived or not) (Wellcome 547, f. 140rb).

232 þe most axen & weten: "you must ask and find out"; *þe most* is an impersonal construction, "it is necessary for thee (to ask and find out)." *MED*, s.v. *moten* (v. [2]), sense 8.(a).

240–1   os Holy Scripture techeþ, *Omnia munda mundis*: Titus 1:15.

244–5   os ... best on þe moder pappe: "like ... a beast on its mother's teat."

247   boketh noght ne bolketh: "neither *boketh* nor *bolketh*." In context, the two verbs appear to be related to the apparent "closure" of the mouth of the womb during pregnancy (cf. "ne openeth þe self"), which medieval medical writers took as a general symptom of pregnancy, the body's way of retaining both semen and menstrual blood for the nourishment of the fetus. Against this backdrop, *boketh* and *bolketh* may be specialized uses of *bouken* "to cleanse" and *bolken* "to produce bodily emissions (belching, vomiting, bleeding, etc.)," both in reference to the suspension of the menstrual cycle in pregnancy.

275–80   blowte ... engrosseþ & bloppeþ & blouteþ: Although the *MED* defines *blo(u)t* (adj.) as "soft, flexible, pliable," Daniel's explanation of the breasts swelling in pregnancy in response to diverted menstrual blood (another commonplace in medieval medicine) suggests that *blowte* and *blouteþ* here may mean something like "plumped up" and "plumps up, swells." His other uses of the word are linked to other terms for swelling or fullness of bodily parts (*bolne, puble, ful, step, grete*), confirming this non-*MED* sense. *Bloppeþ* is not found in the *MED* in its own right, but it too seems likely to refer to mammary enlargement in pregnancy. It may be related to *blober* "bubble; *med.* pustule"; *blobbed* "affected with pimples or swellings" (*OED*; used of a hawk's cheeks in 1486); and *blobber* "swollen, protruding" (*OED*; used of lips in 1593).

286–91   os techeþ Ypocras in his boke of *Afforismis*, **in þe 5 particule ... noght conceyuede:** *Aph.* 5.41, "Mulierem si uis scire si concepit: mellicratum quando dormitura est da ei bibere. & siquidem torsiones habuerit circa uentrem: concepit. si uero non: minime" (If you wish to know whether a woman is with child, give her hydromel to drink [without supper] when she is going to sleep. If she has colic in the stomach she is with child, otherwise she is not) (*Articella* 1483, f. 34ra; trans. Jones, Loeb ed. 4: 169).

302   rawe water: Only RM7 have this reading, which is probably an error for *raine water*, the reading of all other witnesses, though the phrase *rawe water* has been used earlier in connection with foods and drinks that are harmful to those who have the stone (2.7.159).

307–11   os techeþ Gilbert: for it causeth ... distourbling in here body: "Facit uentositatem multam in stomacho cum est conceptus, maxime si fetus magnificetur. Conprimuntur enim intestina, vnde uentositas illa non potest exire, que cum sit <in> intestinis & in uentre de loco suo uellet egredi, vnde fit perturbacio magna in uentre" (It causes great gassiness in the stomach when she has conceived, especially if the fetus grows larger. For the intestines are compressed, so that the gas – which wants to go out from its place when it is in the intestines and the stomach – cannot escape, and thus there develops a great disturbance in the stomach) (Wellcome 547, f. 140vb).

320–6   os Gilbert seiþ, þat by cause of gode hote mater ... brightnesse in the face: "*splendor faciei*: quoniam ex materia calida que ebullit in matrice eleuantur uapores calidi ad epar, & super ad cor, vnde calefiunt & materia ex hiis membris sic calefactis, eleuantur vapores calidi ad caput & ad faciem, vnde facies splendescit & rubor est ex flore sanguinis uirtute caloris depurati" (*brightness of the face*: because of hot matter that bubbles up in the womb, hot vapours are lifted up to the liver, and higher to the heart; and from there they and the matter heated up from those members are heated, and hot vapours are lifted to the head and to the face, and thus the face shines. And the redness is from the best blood purified by the power of the heat) (Wellcome 547, ff. 140vb–141ra).

331   excocte: Probably equivalent to *decocte* "digested," rather than "boiled away," the *MED*'s tentative definition of *excocte* (s.v. *excocten* [v.]). Cf. MLat *decoquere, decoctio*, with senses including "to digest" and "digestion" (*DMLBS*). Some witnesses (GTSaSc AJ) read *decocte* in place of *excocte* (found in RM7 and the remaining beta witnesses).

346   math: "makes"; see note to 2.5.30.

351–2   For os Aristotil seiþ, *Omnis virtus vnita forcior est se dispersa*: "Every virtue is stronger united than scattered in itself." This commonplace sentiment appears in a wide range of medieval works, sometimes but not always with a general attribution to Aristotle or "the Philosopher." Those works range from philosophy and theology (John Buridan, Peter of Auvergne, Augustinus de Ancona) to political theory and history (Giles of Rome, the author of the *Gesta Edwardi Tertii*) to literature (as a marginal Latin gloss on Chaucer's Summoner's Tale, lines 1968–9, in the Ellesmere MS: "Lo, ech thyng that is oned in himselve / Is moore strong than whan it is toscatered").

363–7   þis experiment techeþ Maistre Bartholome in his *Boke of Genecyes* ... in bothe þe vryn, both: See note to 2.3.654–8 above. Daniel may have had access to the book he calls *Boke of Genecyes* and *Liber Geneciarum* (in 2.3) in a manuscript of Salernitan texts that included an anonymous copy of the *Liber de sinthomatibus mulierum* (= *Liber geneciarum*) alongside one or more treatises or commentaries by Bartholomaeus of Salerno. We are grateful to Monica Green for confirming that there are no extant attributions of the *Liber de sinthomatibus* to any Bartholomaeus, whether of Salerno or elsewhere.

368–9   as þou schalt se in our *Medycynarie*: I.e., the book of remedies that Daniel promised to write after completing the *LU*; see note to Prol.85–6.

3.17

—

3.18

65–9   Wiþ þise forsaide signes accordeþ Gilbert ... dust or poudre of grauel:
"Huiusmodi resoluciones cinerose ualde sunt similes harenis, cum non tamen sint
terrestres siue lapidie & sunt quasi puluis harenosus" (Ashy resolutions of this
kind are very much like Sandy particulates, although they are not earthy or stony,
and they are like sandy dust) (Wellcome 547, f. 141rb).

78   þe stomp moste be brent: I.e., the "stump," or stub that remains after cutting off a blood-filled tumour, must be cauterized.

117   Þe Coment vpon Giles seiþ þus: *attrices sunt 3 collecciones:* Cf. Standard Commentary: "Atrici vero sunt a trice [*sic*; L: atre] collecciones facte circa
anum ex melancolico sanguine congesto in illis partibus, et trumbositatem [L:
tuberositatem] inducente" (Attrices are braided/tangled (*var.* black) gatherings
around the anus made from congested melancholy blood in those parts and leading to clotting [*var.* swelling]) (Sloane 282, f. 44r). Daniel's reference to *three*
"collections" may reflect some kind of confusion, possibly in his Latin copy
of the Standard Commentary, between *a trice* "from a tress (of hair), from a
tangle" or *atre* "black" (nom.pl.) and *tres/tria* "three," perhaps with some influence from the etymologies relating to *trica* that Daniel cites in the surrounding
material.

3.19

116–18   *eucrita ... eutrica ... Eutricus:* The expected forms would be *eucrita/
eucritus*, as Daniel's etymology (< *eu* "good" + *crisis* "recovery or judgment")
indicates, but the scribe of R clearly distinguishes his *c* and *t* forms in both *eucrita*
and the subsequent *eutricus/-a* spellings. Most witnesses opt for the spelling
eucric- (AG6J CfCgB G3H), though *eutric-* (T EW M6), *eucret-/encret-* (SaSc),
eucrytic- (G), and *entrit-* (M7, whose scribe usually distinguishes *n* and *u*) also
appear.

**148–53   Herewiþ accordiþ Gilbert in his Coment vppon Giles ... þe sen-
tence of Ysaac ... att laste it is white:** Gilbert's Comment on the *Carmen de
urinis* (lines 326–30, on red and reddish Ypostases) invokes Isaac's *De urinis* (*par-
ticulae* 8–9, *passim*; ed. Peine 1919, 49–51, 64, 68–9 = lines 1643–1721, 2265–71,
2425–60, etc.) in order to qualify Giles's remarks: "& Ysaac ponit tres colores in
ypostasi mediocres: s. ruffum, glaucum, & album; cum enim sanguis aliquantulum digeratur, respicit [V: recipit] colorem ruffum illo modo quo accepit Ysaac

in ypostasi, ruffum i. aliquantulum declinans a rubore versus albedinem" (And Isaac counts three colours in Ypostasis as middling: reddish, yellow, and white. For when blood is somewhat digested, it looks toward [V: takes on] the colour *rufus* as Isaac understands it in the Ypostasis, namely reddish declining somewhat from red to whiteness). By whiteness, Gilbert says, Isaac understands reddishness, yellow, and pure white, "& tunc rubedo illa, que est in sanguine, cum iam per ulteriorem coccionem declinet in albedinem, subrubeitas potest dici, que melior est quam ipse rubor, sed de illa non intellexit actor [i.e., Giles] iste" (And then that redness that is in blood, since it already would decline into whiteness through external coction, can be called sub-redness, which is better than redness itself. But this author [Giles] does not understand that) (Wellcome 547, f. 144vb)

155–6   os it semeth wel by Ysaac and by Gilbert, os Y saide riȝt now: See preceding note.

172–3   For þat þat is more answerand and more ner to best is bettre of þe 2: In witnesses other than RM7, this sentence is identified as a quotation from Aristotle's *Ethics*, a title that Daniel glosses as the *Boke of Þewys* (*thewes* "customs"), though spellings vary (*þewys/thewys*; *yewys*, reflecting an archetype with an identical grapheme for *þ/y*; and the errors *Jews* and *þᵉ wyse*).

We thank Faith Wallis for suggesting that Daniel may be remembering, somewhat loosely, a line in *Ethics* 1.7.8 (1097b), "of goods the greater is always more desirable" (trans. Ross and Urmson, in Barnes, ed. 1984). The medieval Latin translation of the *Ethics* by Robert Grosseteste reads "bonorum autem maius eligibilius semper" (ed. Gauthier 1972–4, 3: 150).

177   sang: Probably an abbreviated form of *sanguis* or *sanguine* "blood," or perhaps a direct borrowing of OF *sanc/sang*.

221–2   os Gilbert seiþ, *sedimen nigrum* is worse in himself þan *eneorima nigrum* or þan *nephilis nigra*: Gilbert comments at some length on Giles's observation that "Quod summum tenet [i.e., *nephilis*] aut medium [i.e., *eneorima*] minus est uiciosum [quam *sedimen*]" (What is above or in the middle is less harmful [than what is in the bottom]) (*Carmen de urinis* 333, expanded on in lines 334–8). See Wellcome 547, f. 145rb–va, glossing *quod summum*, etc. The Standard Commentary also explains this passage in Giles, in Sloane MS 282, f. 46r–v. Both commentaries agree that the problems in black *sedimen* are fewer but more grievous than those in black *eneorima* or black *nephilis*.

3.20

2–3   the reules þat Isaac ȝeueþ in þe laste ende of his *Bok of Vryn*: *Liber urinarum, particula* 10. This entire chapter is a close translation of the last section of Isaac's work, provided by Daniel (as also by Isaac) for readers seeking a convenient summary of urinary symptoms and diagnoses ("comune reules shortly ʒifen"), free of the conceptual frameworks in the rest of the two works. For the Latin original and sigils for witnesses to that text, see Appendix 2. In some witnesses, Daniel moves a few of the *reules* into chapters on the colours: for example, several signs from Isaac's Urina Nigra and Urina Oleagina sections are given at the end of the chapter(s) on Black urine in G3M6 GTSaSc AG6 EWSb and the Latin version of the *LU*. We have left Isaac's terms for colours and contents uncapitalized in this chapter, because his terminology is not an exact match for that used later by Giles of Corbeil and his successors.

Not all complete or near-complete copies of the *LU* contain the "Rules of Isaac": those that end with a beta* text (G3M6 CgCfHB and possibly J) conclude with the chapters on Ypostasis, followed directly by the Latin verse Epilogue.

6–8   As whoso may noʒt tochen … þe bynderes: "So that if someone cannot get to the good strong marrow inside the bone, let him be satisfied with that which is on the outside. And whoever cannot gather the sheaves of grain, let him glean after those who bind up the sheaves." Possibly an allusion to Ruth 2, in which Ruth gleans in the fields of Boaz after the reapers have passed through, or to Leviticus 19:9–10, the Mosaic law about leaving enough grain in the fields for the poor to glean.

30–1   Of creticacioun and of cretik daies os techeþ Isaac in þe 2 bok: *De febribus* 4.6–7, the primary source of information on critical days in *LU* 2.2.

55   oynyoun: "a pearl," Lat. *unio* (acc. *unionem*), a misinterpretation of *niueam* "snow" or some variant thereof (see Appendix 2, p. 290), presumably involving a confusion of minims.

87   Vryn crude in þe bigynnyng of a febre is gode: Note that the Latin original of this rule has *non laudabilis est* in most of the cited witnesses (Appendix 2, p. 291), but at least one Latin witness (O = Bodl. Laud lat. 106) omits the negative.

101–3   *Rubea* and stynkand … muselynges of paxwax … & deth: Lat. *Urina rubea & fetida cum hypostasi nigra: turbida quasi pili: vel in vnctuositate: pessima est & mortalis* (see Appendix 2, p. 292). The phrase *vel in vnctuositate* "or in oiliness" has a number of Latin variants that must arise at least partly from misinterpretations of minims and c/t characters: *vel mutationes* (P); *uel ?inuictiones uel* <blank> (O); *uel muccaciones \uel muscilagines/* (H); and *muscilagines* (V). Daniel's source may have had some form of the word *muscilagines*, generating his *muselynges* "?mouldy pieces, ?sloughings (off)" (see 3.7.21n above), but *paxwax* "tendon at the back of the neck, *nucha*" is harder to explain. It may be connected to the hair-like contents mentioned in this *regula*, since Daniel had earlier said that the content Hairs originated in stringy sinews like the *nucha* (*faxwax, paxwax*). See 3.12.36–41n, 3.12.38n above.

305–50   Vryn sandarik … : The following twenty-two signs, up to Ypostasis, are not in the Latin witnesses UOHVP consulted for Appendix 2, but do share a majority of items with the extra signs from Leipzig MS 1154 (L) given by Peine at the end of his edition based on U (1919, 74–5, lines 2668–96). See also Appendix 2, p. 296n2.

393–4   Þus fonde I in Ysaac, nerhand worde for worde in þe laste boke of his Vryns: *Liber urinarum, particula* 10.

395–410   Epilogue: For an English translation of the Latin verse epilogue, see Appendix 3.

General Glossary

The General Glossary contains important or obsolete technical terms, words whose meanings have changed significantly or become obsolete, unusual spellings, and forms of lexical or dialectal interest. Predictable plurals of nouns (-*s*, -*es*, and -*is*/-*ys*) are usually not distinguished in the entries, but the more complex accidence of glossed verbs is included as fully as Daniel's text allows, except for some of the more common forms of *ben* and *haue*. Definitions are intended to explain words and forms in their immediate context or to clarify points of potential difficulty.[1] Selected Latin and other foreign-origin words are also included in the Glossary, indicated by the symbol †, and usually listed in the nominative singular for nouns and adjectives, even when the form in the text appears in an oblique case. Passages of running Latin text, however, are normally left unglossed. Uncertain or conjectured senses, uncertain instances of a particular sense, and ambiguous grammatical functions are preceded by a question mark.

Headwords and cross-references to headwords are printed in bold type, with variant spellings and additional grammatical forms in italics. Phrases using the headword (or a form thereof) follow single-word senses and forms and are printed in italics. A tilde (~) represents recurrences of the headword a) within phrases; b) after variant spellings; or c) after intervening grammatical forms whose spelling differs from that of the headword.

References are by book, chapter, and line number; for words or phrases extending over more than one line, the reference is to the starting line. References usually include two or three early appearances of the word, with additional representative references as needed to illustrate additional forms or senses. Words or forms that result from emendation are indicated by a preceding asterisk on the word or

---

1 Important sources for determining senses of technical terms, in addition to the *MED*, include the *DMLBS;* Hunt 1989; Getz, ed. 1991; M.H. Green 2001; and Norri 2016. Despite our broad intention of glossing generously, the Glossary inevitably omits some words that readers may wish to look up; the MED and Norri 2016 should be particularly useful to anyone seeking definitions of words excluded from the following pages.

relevant line reference. The existence of an explanatory note for a particular word or sense is indicated by "(see n.)" after the line reference.

The order of entries is alphabetical (letter by letter), with thorn (þ) entered after *th* and yogh (ȝ) after *y*. Cross-references are given when the main headword is five or more entries away from the cross-referral. The following grammatical and lexicographic abbreviations are used in the Glossary:

abbrev.	abbreviation		*num.*	number
acc.	accusative		*obj.*	objective
adj.	adjective		*pa.*	past
adv.	adverb		*pa.ppl.*	past participle
art.	article		*phr.*	phrase
coll.	collective		*pl.*	plural
comp.	comparative		*poss.*	possessive
conj.	conjunction		*ppl.adj.*	participial adjective
corr.	correlative		*pr.*	present
def.	definite		*prep.*	preposition
dem.	demonstrative		*pron.*	pronoun
dep.	deponent		*pr.ppl.*	present participle
f.	feminine		*refl.*	reflexive
fig.	figurative(ly)		*rel.*	relative
ger.	gerund		*sb.*	somebody
impers.	impersonal		*sg.*	singular
impv.	imperative		*sth.*	something
inf.	infinitive		*subj.*	subjunctive
interj.	interjection		*sup.*	superlative
lit.	literal(ly)		*v.*	verb
nom.	nominative		*1 (2, 3)*	first (second, third) person
n.	noun			

A list of proper nouns in the *Liber Uricrisiarum* appears after the General Glossary.

able, *adj.* ~ *(for) to* capable of, able to, suitable for 1.4.46, 2.2.242

abouen, *adv. as n. at his* ~ in control 2.8.155

abstynence, *n.* abstinence (from food), fasting 1.4.665, 1.4.666, *abstinence* 1.4.361, *abstynance* 1.4.675

acces(se), *n.* an attack of fever 2.2.295, 2.6.123, *axces* 2.3.299, 2.3.302, *exces* 2.3.311

accidental(e), *adj.* unnatural, pathological 1.4.530; secondary, less essential 1.4.823

accion, *n.* operation, activity 2.4.88, 2.13.283

accompte, accomptede see **acompten**

ac(c)ordeþ, *v.pr.3sg.* agrees 1.4.784, ~ *to* agrees with 1.2.27, *acordiþ* 2.3.4, *acordes* 2.4.338; *pr.pl. acorden* 1.4.429; *pr.ppl. acordand (toward)* similar, corresponding (to) 2.3.266, *ac(c)ordyng* 2.2.3, 2.3.385

accreseþ, *v.pr.3sg.* of a disease: increases, becomes stronger 2.5.22

acetouse, *adj.* sour, vinegary 2.5.59, 2.8.100

achaufeþ, *v.pr.3sg.* heats, warms, inflames 1.4.527, 1.4.667; *pr.pl. achaufe* 1.4.716, 1.4.815; *pa.ppl. achaffid* 3.8.56, *achaufede* 1.4.560

acompten, *v.pr.pl.* consider, reckon 1.4.402; *impv. accompte* 2.6.313; *pa.ppl. ac(c)ompted(e)* counted (as) 2.2.246, 2.3.195, 2.6.309

actif, *adj.* active 1.4.35, *actyf* 1.4.39, †*actyue* 1.4.35

acu(e), *n.* an acute fever 2.2.143, 2.2.149, 2.4.260

†adolocencia, *n.* adolescence 1.4.395, *adolossencia* 1.4.398

adort, *n.* the aorta 2.3.105, †*adortus* 2.3.105

adust(e), *adj.* overheated, burned up, scorched, destroyed by heat 2.8.44, 2.8.45, 2.8.94, †*adustus* 2.8.53, 2.8.55, 2.8.57

adustio(u)n, *n.* corruption of humours, food, etc. within the body by heat 2.1.35, 2.2.15; ~ *complet(e)* total corruption of bodily humours, food, etc. by heat 2.1.21, 2.1.36, 2.1.52

aertrarie, *adj.* drawing air 2.1.76, *aertraharie* 2.1.76

affermeth, *v.pr.3sg.* asserts, states *(used collectively for pl.)* Prol.57

aforn(e), *adv.* before 1.4.232, 2.3.402; *þe next c. (ca., reule, nyght, etc.)* ~ the immediately preceding chapter (rule, night, etc.) 2.4.45, 2.4.346, 2.8.124, 2.10.190

afte, *prep.* after 3.2.73 (see n.)

after, *prep.* following, according to Prol.14, Prol.59, 2.6.495

agayn(e), *adv.* again, back 1.3.202, 1.3.204

agayn(e), *prep.* against 1.1.27, 1.4.650, *agayns* 3.20.303

agayn(e)ward, *adv.* back, in return 1.4.217, opposite, conversely 1.4.144, 1.4.350

agaynstanding, *v.pr.ppl.* withstanding, being opposed Prol.85

aggregen, *v.* to gather, collect 2.8.148; *pr.3sg. aggregeþ* 2.8.146

aggreueþ, *v.pr.3sg.* aggrieves, disturbs 2.4.365; *pa.ppl. agreuede* 1.4.691

agitate, *ppl.adj.* moved around violently 2.8.286

albowe, *n.* elbow 2.3.134, 3.16.87

†albus, *adj.* of urine: clear 1.4.283, 1.4.694; of face, hypostasis, phlegm, etc.: white 1.4.381, 2.3.338, 3.19.166

alchite, *n.* ascites, abdominal edema 2.10.207, †*alchita* 2.10.203, 2.10.205, †*alchites* 2.3.860

alday, *adv.* always, every day 1.4.269, 1.4.357

al(l)egeance, *n.* relief, alleviation 2.2.321, 2.2.325, *aleggawns* 2.9.141, *allegance* 2.2.329

al(le) maner, *phr.* every kind of, all kinds of, all 1.4.254, 1.4.644

al on(e), *phr.* all one, the same 1.3.144, 1.4.29; *ar ~ to say (seyn)* mean the same 1.2.29, 1.3.139

alse, *conj.* as 1.4.81, 2.4.451; *for (in) ~ mykil (mychyl, mykel)* in as much, for as much, insofar, just as 1.3.203, 1.3.209, 1.4.709

alþer- , *pref.* to the highest degree (prefix to superlative forms): *alþer-depest* the most intense 2.14.60; *alþer-longest* longest of all 3.10.89; *alþermost* the very most, most ... of all 2.14.60; *alþerwerste* the worst of all, the absolute worst 1.4.578

alwai(e), *adv.* always 1.3.62, 1.4.474

†amans, *ppl. adj.* loving 1.4.369

amydown, *n.* unground or coarsely ground husked grain, grits 3.16.51

an, *conj. (variant spelling)* and 2.10.74, 2.14.48

and, *conj.* if 2.2.324, *&* 2.7.577

anentes, *prep.* concerning 2.4.358, 3.18.55; *ouer ~* facing, next to 2.6.475; *os ~ (as anenþes, as aneþes)* as regards, with respect to 1.4.238, 1.4.451, 3.19.7, *anentys* 2.4.357, *anentz* Prol.91

anentisshede see **anyntissheþ**

†anglice, *adv.* in English 1.2.23, 1.3.20

anglis, *n. pl.* angles, corners 2.7.273

annex, *v.pa.ppl.* connected, adjoining, near (to) 2.3.506

anogh, *adv.* enough, sufficiently 2.6.300, 2.14.123, *inow* Prol.35, *ynow* 2.3.844, *ynogh* 2.7.342

anon(e), *adv.* immediately, soon, shortly 1.4.602, 1.4.797, 2.2.268; *~ as* as soon as 1.4.134

answereþ, *v.pr.3sg.* corresponds (to) 1.4.303, *answeriþ* 1.4.299, *onswereþ* 1.3.122; *pr.pl. answere* 1.4.298, 1.4.302; *pr.ppl. answerand(e)* 1.4.294, 1.3.141, *answerond(e)* 2.7.603, 2.9.22, *answerant* 2.3.33, *answering* 1.3.120, *answeryng* 1.3.17

†antraces, *n.pl.* malignant and purulent skin lesions 1.3.255, *antraxa* 1.3.259

anyntissheþ, *v.pr.3sg.* wastes, diminishes 2.4.191; *pr.sg.subj. anyntisshe* 2.8.299; *pr. ppl. anyntisshond* 2.3.513; *pa.ppl. anentisshede* 2.4.278

*anyntis(s)hing, *ger.* wasting, diminishing *2.3.455, 2.14.112, *anyntisshyng* 2.3.567, 3.20.262, *enyntisshing* 2.6.34

aperceyue, *v.* to perceive 2.3.240, 2.10.196; *pa.ppl. aperceyuede* 2.10.143, 2.10.169, *aparceyuede* 1.4.221

apert see **ap(p)ert**

apertly, *adv.* clearly 2.11.77

aperyn, *v.pr.sg.subj.* should appear 1.4.462, *apere* 2.11.77

apeyryng, *ger.* impairing 2.3.450

apostem(e), *n.* a swelling or tumour in or on the body 1.3.249, 2.3.410, 2.13.336, *eposteme* 2.7.226, *emposteme* 2.4.272 (no unambiguous instances of the aphetic form *postem(e)* occur in R)

apothecaries, *n.pl.* makers and sellers of medicines 1.4.761

appeireþ, *v.pr.3sg.* weakens, becomes impaired 1.4.329

ap(p)ert, *adj.* clear 2.4.11; visible 2.8.253

†aqua, *n.* water 1.4.292, 1.4.301

aquosite, *n.* liquidity, wateriness 1.4.800, 2.3.397

aquo(u)se, *adj.* watery 2.3.7, 3.19.177, 3.20.73, *†aquosa* 2.4.5, 3.20.69

arages, *n.pl.* oraches, orache-plants (*genus* Atriplex) 1.4.749

arectcdc, *v.pa.ppl.* considered, regarded Prol.28, ~ *into* regarded as (a matter of) Prol.12

areyn, *n.* spider; ~ *(arayne) web* spider web 3.5.4, 3.8.62

armehole, *n.* the armpit 2.10.217

†arratice, *adj.* wandering, erratic; *stelle* ~ the planets 2.6.411

arste, *sup.adj. at* ~ for the first time, first 2.8.32

article, *n.* a joint or small limb (of the body), *fig.* a small part of a larger whole, little bit Prol.34

†artus, *n.* a small limb of the body (e.g., finger or toe) 3.16.132

as, *conj.* as 1.1.30, 1.1.42; (only) as much as 2.2.324; ~ *mykel to* as much as to 1.2.14

askes, *n.pl.* ashes 2.3.363, 2.8.262, *asshen* Prol.146, 3.18.1

askish, *adj.* ashy, like ashes 3.18.58, 3.18.104

asky, *adj.* ashy, like ashes 2.8.268, 2.8.284

asma, *n.* difficulty in breathing, esp. in exhalation 2.3.119, 2.3.121

aspecte, *n.* a looking in a given direction, a facing or fronting in a direction 2.8.209 (see n.)

assimulacioun, *n.* assimilation, a becoming like (sth.) 3.19.19, 3.19.30

as(s)tonying, *ger.* confusion, bewilderment 2.3.363, 2.3.364

astonyed(e), *v.pa.ppl.* dulled, numbed 2.2.237, 2.3.507; bruised, crushed 2.13.67, 2.13.72

astromyens, *n.pl.* astronomers 2.6.467

†*astutus,* *adj.* sly, cunning 1.4.376

asundre, *adv.* apart, *knowe ~* distinguish 1.4.480; *a-sondry* 3.7.48

at, *conj.* that 2.9.103

atter, *n.* pus, rotten matter 1.4.102, *attre* 2.3.671, 3.7.2, *attir* 3.7.3

attomies, *n.pl.* dust-like particles in urine, motes 3.16.56, *attomys* 3.16.44, 3.16.59, †*att(h)ome,* Prol.144, 3.16.1, 3.16.2, 3.16.14, †*attomi(e)* 2.4.155, 3.1.70, 3.16.4, †*attomy(e)* 3.16.2, 3.16.231; *n.sg.* †*attomus* 3.16.4

attri(e), *adj.* purulent, poisonous, containing *atter* "pus" 2.3.584, 2.10.210, 3.9.10

attrikes, *n.pl.* inflamed or swollen hemorrhoids, piles 3.18.8, †*attrices* 3.18.7, †*attricis* 3.18.71

attrishe, *adj.* purulent, poisonous, containing *atter* "pus" 2.13.224

atwynnen, *v.* to separate, to divide 3.3.38; *pa.ppl. atwynnede* 1.2.41, 3.16.353

auburne, *adj.* of hair: auburn, reddish brown 1.4.310, 1.4.316

aucto(u)r(e), *n.* author Prol.52, 1.3.43, 1.4.123, 2.1.17

†*audax,* *adj.* daring, bold 1.4.371, 1.4.374

auelong, *adj.* oblong, elongated 2.4.85, 2.7.467, *euelong* 2.7.501

auenant, *adj.* seemly, appropriate 2.9.73

aueryce, *n.* avarice, greed 3.2.67

augmastik, *adj., adj. as n.* of fever: building up to a crisis (*DMLBS*, s.v. *acmasticus*) 2.12.37; †*augmastica* 2.12.33, 2.12.47

auisementes, *n.pl.* decisions 2.7.267

†*autumpnus,* *n.* the season of autumn 1.4.407, 1.4.413

auyseth, *v.pr.3sg. (refl.) ~ hym* (he) considers, takes thought 2.7.310; *pa.ppl. auysede þe* (you) … taken thought 1.4.224

awasshyn, *v.pa.ppl.* washed 1.1.43

awrang, *adv.* indirectly, not in a straight line 2.3.107

axces see **acces(se)**

axen, *v.* to ask 2.8.245, 3.16.232; *pr.3sg. axeþ* asks, requires 1.4.566, *axceþ* 2.3.694

aye see **ey(e),** *n.*[1]

aȝeyne, *prep.* against, in the direction of 3.8.13, 3.19.34

aȝeyn(e), *adv.* again 1.3.176, 3.4.72, *aȝein* 2.6.301, 3.20.345

aȝeyn(e)s, *prep.* toward 1.4.222; ~ *þe day* around daybreak 1.4.240; ~ *deþ* as death approaches 2.2.197

baas see **veyn(e)**

bach, *adj.* of planets: retrograde, turning back 2.6.412

bachiler, *n.* young man 1.4.396; *pl.poss. bachileres* young men's 2.7.22

bag(g)e, *n.* a lump, swelling, bulge 2.13.186, 2.13.285

baggeþ, *v.pr.3sg.* hangs loosely, bulges 2.4.17; *pr.ppl. baggand* 2.7.458, *baggond* 2.7.463

balled(e), *adj.* bald 3.2.29, 3.2.37

ballok, *n.* a testicle; *n.pl. ballokkes* 3.17.12; ~ *stones* the testicles 2.3.699; ~ *codde* the scrotum 2.7.527; ~ *purse* the scrotum 2.7.527; *moder (womanes) ~ (bollok, ballokes) stones* the ovaries 2.3.700, 2.7.544, 3.17.46

barcynhede, *n.* infertility 3.16.370

barkeþ, *v.pr.3sg.* makes (sth.) rough, forms a crust or scab 2.14.143; *pr.sg.subj. bark* 2.14.145

barking, *ger.* barking (*fig.*), harsh words Prol.10

barouful, *n.* barrowful, the amount that fills a barrow 2.7.99

†*basilica* see **veyn(e)**

bataile, *n.* battle, struggle (*fig.*) 2.2.196; *n.pl. batelles* 2.6.341

be, *prep.* by 1.1.20, 1.2.30, 1.3.18; ~ *cause (þat)* for the reason that, on account of the fact (that) 1.1.21, 1.1.23, 1.2.10; ~ *resoun (þat)* because, on account (of), for the reason (that) 1.1.20, 1.3.96, 1.3.225

bedene, *adv.* together; *al ~* all told, taken as a group 2.1.19

bederide, *adj.* bedridden 1.4.404, *bedred* 1.4.282, 1.4.397

befalleþ, *v.pr.3sg.* (it) happens 1.4.329

behaue, *v. (refl.)* ~ *him* to behave (himself) 1.4.2

behoueþ, *v.pr.3sg. (impers.)* it is proper, it is necessary 2.2.29, *behoueth* 3.20.288; *þe ~* it behooves you (sg.), you should 1.4.820; *it bihoueþ him* he should 2.8.156

beleueþ, *v.pr.3sg.* remains (to) 1.3.30, 1.3.117, 1.3.138, *beleueth* 2.8.294; *pr.pl. beleue(n)* 1.3.204, 2.7.128

bely, *n.* the belly 2.3.863, 2.7.437

ben, *v.* to be 3.19.92, 3.19.93; *pr.pl. ar(e)* Prol.39, 1.3.126, *arn(e)* 1.1.5, 1.3.49,
1.4.6, *ben(e)* Prol.24, 1.3.116, 1.4.1, 1.4.113; *pr.sg.subj. war* 2.4.34, *wor* 2.6.353;
pr.ppl. beand(e) 2.10.50, 3.12.40; *pa.ppl. bene* Prol.26; also the common forms
is, art, was, wer(e)

beneþe(n), *adv.* beneath, below 1.3.198, 1.4.183, 2.7.412, *benethe* 2.3.789,
bineþe(n) 2.4.390, 2.11.36; ~ on earth 1.3.103

benigne, *adj.* well-intentioned Prol.87; †*benignus* kind, benign 1.4.371

benomen, *ppl. adj.* taken away from (sb.) 2.3.816

benoþen, *adv.* beneath, below (poss. error for *beneþen*) 1.4.99

benymmyng, *ger.* a taking away, deprivation 2.1.45

bere, *v.* to bear, carry 1.4.324, 2.3.78; *pr.3sg. bereþ* 1.4.775, *bereth* 3.17.24, *beriþ*
2.8.237; *pr.ppl. berand* 2.3.144, 2.3.157, *beronde of* carrying a certain amount
of (sth.) 2.3.146; *pa.ppl. born(e)* carried 1.4.157, 2.3.155; *borne doune* afflicted
3.18.112; ~ *bode* to carry a message (to the soul) 2.7.324; ~ to carry, transmit (a
sound) 2.3.162; ~ to tolerate 2.2.324; *pr.3sg. bereth* lifts 2.7.442, *bereþ* 2.2.368

besie, *adj.* busy 2.4.89, 2.4.247, *besy* 1.4.248

besily, *adv.* insistently, repeatedly Prol.6

besines, *n.* preoccupation, worry, vexation 1.4.522, 1.4.657, *besynes(se)* 1.4.9,
1.4.658

besperde, *v.pa.ppl.* enclosed, shut (in) 1.4.640

best(e), *n.* a beast 1.3.96, 1.4.205, 2.3.183; *n.poss. bestes* beast's 1.4.509, 1.4.512

beting, *ger.* beating, throbbing 2.12.102, 2.13.134, *betyng* 2.13.131, 2.13.344

betyme(s), *adv.* in good time 2.7.110, 2.7.130

bewapande, *v.pr.ppl.* wrapping 2.7.519

biforn(e), *adv., prep., conj.* before 1.3.23, 1.4.93, 2.2.174, *beforn(e)* 1.3.82, 1.4.623,
byforn(e) 1.4.229, 2.12.110

bifor(n)hand, *adv.* before, beforehand 2.3.720, 3.2.101, *befornhond* 1.3.155

bigges, *n.pl.* teats (of an animal) 3.18.34

bihete, *v.pr.1sg. (refl.)* ~ *me* (I) promise Prol.85

biholdeþ, *v.pr.3sg.* looks (at), examines Prol.64; *impv. biholde* 1.4.161; *pa.ppl.
biholden* 1.4.149

bile, *n.* a boil, a sore 1.4.103

†*bina quartana* see **quarteyn(e)**

birdlym, *n.* sticky substance spread on twigs for catching birds 3.6.29

biseke, *v.pr.1sg.* pray for, seek Prol.87

bisext(e), *n.* the intercalary day in a leap year 2.6.239, 2.6.261, 2.6.282, *bysexte* (†*bisextus*) 2.6.236; *grete ~* (†*magnus bisextus*) a secondary intercalary day, said to be required every hundred years 2.6.338

bit, *v.pr.3sg.* bites (*fig.*), corrodes 1.3.71, 2.8.96; *pr.ppl. bitand* 1.1.24, 2.3.683; *pa. ppl. biten* bitten (with cold; cf. *frostbite*), stung (by cold) 2.3.26; *colde-biten* 2.3.603, *colde-byten* 2.2.23, 2.3.605

bla(c)khed(e), *n.* blackness 2.1.21, 2.1.22, 2.1.55, 2.2.32, *blachede* 2.1.19, 2.2.110

blake, *adj.* black in colour 1.4.507

blank, *adj.* white; *fleume ~* , *fleume blawnch* white phlegm 2.3.339, 2.9.182; *~ plum* white lead, basic lead carbonate 3.5.19

bleche, *adj.* pallid 2.10.208

blecheþ, *v.pr.3sg.* whitens, bleaches 2.9.88, 2.14.143, 3.19.14

bledder, *n.* the bladder 1.3.159, 2.7.536; a membrane containing an organ (e.g., the gall bladder) 2.7.511

bledyng, *ger.* bloodletting 2.3.82, 2.3.113

bleik, *adj.* white, pale, sallow, wan 2.13.158, 3.2.16, *bleke* 3.3.37

blemesshing, *ger.* injury, impairment, harm 1.4.104, *blemisshyng* 2.2.30, *blemys-(s)hing* 2.14.149, 3.7.24, *blemysshyng* 1.4.96, 2.3.432

blemest, *v.pa.ppl.* injured 3.10.30

bleredhede, *n.* of eyes: bleariness 1.3.147

bleuiþ, *v.pr.3sg.* remains 2.2.11; *pr.pl. bleue* 2.6.327; *pr.ppl. bleuand* 1.3.165

bleuynges, *ger.pl.* leavings, waste 1.3.146, 3.18.13; particles produced by the wasting of the lungs 2.8.290

blo, *adj.* of urine: lead-coloured Prol.115, 2.2.113; of the body or parts of the body: bruise-coloured, livid, black-and-blue 2.2.24, 2.2.331

blod(e), *n.* blood Prol.138, 1.3.124, 1.3.225, 1.4.308

blod(e)last, *n.* bloodletting 2.3.119, 2.3.125

blois(s)h(e), *adj.* somewhat livid in colour 2.3.383, 2.7.366, 2.7.505, *bloissch* 2.3.43, *bloys(s)h(e)* 2.3.612, 2.10.231, 2.12.96

blo(o)hed(e), *n.* lividness 2.3.8, 2.3.11, 2.3.267, 2.4.26

bloppeþ, *v.pr.3sg.* ?swells 3.16.279 (see n.)

blout(e), *adj.* swollen, plump 2.8.253, 3.2.47, *blowte* 3.16.275 (see n.)

blouteþ, *v.pr.3sg.* swells, becomes full 3.16.280; *pr.pl. blouten* 2.7.87

blouthede, *n.* plumpness, fullness, swollenness 2.12.101, *blowthed* 3.16.170

bloyshede, *n.* lividness 2.13.398

blyue, *adv.* quickly 1.4.136, 1.4.801

boche, *n.* morbid lesion or tumour, sore, ulcer 1.3.259, 2.3.83

bodely, *adj.* corporeal 1.4.22, 1.4.304, *bodily* 2.6.140, *bodyli* 2.6.378, *bodyly* 1.4.435

body, *n.* the human body 1.1.8, 1.1.17, 2.3.434; of urine: substance, the liquid base of urine produced in the liver 1.1.9, 1.4.55, 1.4.835; relative density, thickness Prol.100, 1.4.150; *n.pl.* particles in urine 1.4.111, 1.4.153; *bodi* (in similar senses) 1.4.495, 2.4.82, 2.7.206, 2.8.296

boketh, *v.pr.3sg.* ?cleanses 3.16.247 (see n.)

bole, *n.*[1] a boil, a sore 1.3.259

bole, *n.*[2] a bull 1.4.507

boliede see **bolyand**

bolketh, *v.pr.3sg.* ?emits 3.16.247 (see n.)

bolle see **þrote bolle**

bollying, *ger.* swelling, gassy inflation, intestinal disturbance 2.10.112

boln(e), *ppl.adj.* swollen 2.3.363, 2.10.206, *bolen* 3.3.22, *bollen* 3.3.20

bolnehede, *n.* swollenness 3.16.169

bolneþ, *v.pr.3sg.* swells 2.7.86, *bolnyth* 2.3.818; *pr.pl. bolne(n)* 2.7.86, 3.18.32; *pr. ppl. bolnand* 3.20.234

bolnyng, *ger.* swelling 1.4.89, 2.3.115, 2.3.362

bolyand, *v.pr.ppl.* boiling, heating up 3.2.43, *bulyand* 2.13.427; *pa.ppl. boliede* boiled, cooked 2.7.160; *bulede* heated up, digested 1.3.153, *bullyede* 2.11.55

bolying, *ger.* boiling, unnatural heating 1.4.524, 2.12.52, *bul(l)ying* 2.10.229, 2.12.28

bonere, *adj.* kind, benign 1.4.370

bor, *n.* boar 3.6.17

borde-cloþe, *n.* tablecloth 2.7.438, 2.7.439

born(e) see **bere**

***bosmyng,** *ger.* swelling, bulging outward 2.7.147

bosmyth, *v.pr.3sg.* causes a hollow or opens up a space 2.4.365

bost(o)use, *adj.* of motion: rough, vigorous 1.4.158; of an organ: rough-textured 1.3.42

boþen, *num. as n.* both 1.3.205, 2.7.497, *boþin* 3.2.106; *as adj., adv.* both 3.1.16, 3.10.23

bot(t)okes, *n.pl.* the buttocks 2.7.450, 3.18.49, *buttokes* 3.18.52

botum(e), *n.* bottom 1.3.19, 2.3.535, *botme* 2.13.444, 2.13.449, *botime* 1.3.110, *botome* 2.7.116, 2.7.134

bowede, *v.pa.ppl.* ~ *agayn* turned back toward 2.3.206

boylicioun, *n.* boiling, heating, disturbing (with heat) 1.4.524

boystyng, *ger.* drawing blood by cupping (creating a partial vacuum in a small container placed over the skin) 1.4.553

braken, *v.pr.pl.* vomit 1.4.91

braking, *ger.* vomiting 3.20.126, *brakyng* 1.3.197, 2.2.328

braune, *n.* (a) muscle 2.4.373, *brawne* 3.20.306

brayand, *v.pr.ppl.* sounding, making a noise 2.3.132

braynede, *ppl.adj.* of animals: brindled, spotted 1.4.507 (see n.)

brede, *n.* distance; ~ *ouerthwert* distance across, diameter (of a sphere) 2.6.380

bren(ne), *n.* bran 3.13.3, 3.16.364; bran-like contents in urine Prol.141, 1.4.110, 2.10.152

brenne, *v.* to burn 2.3.255, 2.14.22; *pr.ppl. brennand(e)* 1.1.22, 1.1.24, 1.4.440; *pa. ppl. brent(e)* of humours: burnt, overheated, destroyed by heat 2.8.44, 2.8.89

brennyng, *ger.* burning (*lit. and fig.*) 1.4.778, 2.1.57, *brynnyng* 2.6.341, 2.11.22

bresede, *v.pa.ppl.* bruised, crushed 2.13.71

breste(n), *v.* to burst, rupture 2.3.774. 2.7.511; *pr.3sg. brestep* bursts, ruptures 2.2.182, 2.3.336, *bristep* 2.2.183; *pr.pl. breste(n)* 3.18.99; *pr.ppl. brestand* 2.9.122; *pa.ppl. brosten* 3.10.29, 3.10.40; *pa.ppl. brusten* broken up 2.13.57

bresting, *ger.* bursting, rupture 2.13.57, 3.19.240, *brestyng* 2.13.444, 3.10.36, *brusting* 2.13.66, *bristing* 3.19.240

bresur(e), *n.* a wound, blow, bruising 2.3.472, 3.10.51, *bresour* 2.3.471

brigh, *adj.* bright 3.19.49, 3.20.195, *brygh* 1.4.312

brighthed(e), *n.* brightness 1.4.474, 2.4.259, 2.7.104, *brighede* 2.5.5

brunstoun, *n.* brimstone, sulfur 2.7.51

brusshing, *ger.* bruising, a bruise 2.13.66, 3.20.283, *brus(sh)yng* 3.10.36, 3.10.50

brusten-coddede, *adj.* herniated, suffering from scrotal or inguinal hernia 2.7.525

*bryȝttisch, *adj.* somewhat bright; *quyk* ~ ?lively and somewhat bright (in opposition to *wan wattry and dedish*) 3.19.194

bud, *v.pr.pl.* ~ *out* swell outward, form bud-like swellings 3.18.33

buddy, *adj.* having small bud-like projections 1.3.49 (see n.)

bugle, *n.*¹ ox 1.4.751

bugle, *n.*² *peti* ~ a low-growing form of *Ajuga* spp. 2.7.68; *grete* ~ a taller form of *Ajuga* spp. 2.7.69 (see n.)

bul(ly)ede see **bolyand**

burble, *n.* a bubble Prol.131, 2.9.82, 2.9.106, 3.3.1

burblisshe, *adj.* of urine: containing bubbles 3.6.16

busshel, *n.* a bushel, an eight-gallon container for produce Prol.49

byh, *adv.* near, close by 2.3.550

byndand, *v.pr.ppl.* binding, constricting, styptic 1.4.763, 2.7.472; glutinous, sticky 2.7.9, 3.6.31

bynderes, *n.pl.* those who bind sheaves of grains 3.20.8

bytyng, *ger.* caustic action or effect 1.3.70, 1.4.109

bywelden, *v.* to control 2.2.312

cac(c)heþ, *v.*¹*pr.3sg.* catches, attains, acquires 1.4.522, 1.4.717; *pr.pl. cachen* catch, be afflicted by (a disease) 1.1.34; *cachen deþ* die 2.9.123

cachen, *v.*² to chase (away), drive out 1.3.175, 2.7.104, *cachyn* 2.3.584, *kac(c)he* 1.4.75, 2.13.329; *pr.3sg. cacheþ* 2.6.513, 2.7.405; *pr.pl. cacchen* 1.3.229; *pr.ppl. cachand* 2.7.355; *pa.ppl. cac(c)hede* 2.2.369

caching, *ger.* driving, impelling 3.19.218

cafuist, *n.* cassia fistula fruit, the seed pods of the cassia fistula tree, pulp from the pods (*Cassia fistula*) 3.1.56 (see n.), 3.1.57

calculouse, *adj.* of persons: suffering from kidney or bladder stones 2.13.55; *as n.* someone suffering from kidney or bladder stones 2.13.58, †*calculosus* 2.13.57

†***calculus,*** *n.* bladder stone 1.4.113

calderon, *n.* cauldron 1.3.112

calefaccioun, *n.* inflammation caused by heat 2.10.46, 2.11.33

calefacte, *adj.* heated, warmed 1.4.560, 1.4.561, 1.4.719

calidite, *n.* heat; heat as a primary quality 1.4.17, 1.4.21; †*caliditas* 1.4.34, 1.4.295

†***calidus,*** *adj.* hot 1.4.272, 1.4.300, 1.4.727; *as n.pl.* hot things 1.4.633, 1.4.647

†***calor,*** *n.* heat; heat as a primary quality 1.4.335, 1.4.337

†***canalis,*** *n.* ~ *pulmonis* an airway in the lungs, bronchus 2.7.345; a bodily vessel 2.3.231; *n.pl. canales pulmo(nis)* the bronchi 2.3.229, 3.4.40

†***cancer,*** *n.* cancer 1.3.260, *n.pl. cancros* 1.3.256

cancre, *n.* a cancer, a tumour (internal or external) *1.3.261, 2.13.178

†***cantans,*** *v.pr.ppl.* singing 1.4.371

†*capillares*, *adj.* of veins: hair-like 1.3.131, 1.3.152

†*capillositas*, *n.* hairiness 1.4.105

†*capitarrus*, *adj.* flowing from the head 2.3.626, †*capiterus* 2.3.626

capitles, *n.pl.* chapters 1.4.476

carbuncle, *n.* a large, red precious stone 1.3.259, ~ *stone* 1.3.257

†*carbunculus*, *n.* a large, red, suppurating boil 1.3.255, 1.3.256

carnouse, *adj.* fleshy, plump 3.15.36, *charnouse* 2.7.474, †*carnosus* 1.4.371

cas, *n. in* ~ perhaps, perchance 1.4.328

†*cassia fistila*, *n.* cassia fistula fruit, the pods of the cassia fistula tree, pulp from the pods (*Cassia fistula*) 3.1.57

cassia ligne, *n.* the bark of the cassia fistula tree 3.1.59, †*cassia lignea* 3.1.58

cast, *v.pa.ppl.* envisioned, imagined 2.7.311

casting, *ger.* envisioning, considering 2.7.284, 2.7.288

†*catarrus*, *n.* catarrh, a cold with runny nose 2.3.418, 2.3.614

†*cauma*, *n.* intense heat 2.12.132

causand, *v.pr.ppl.* causing 1.4.56, 2.6.515

†*causonides*, *n.* a continual fever arising from red choler and blood, especially from choler 2.2.371, 2.12.112

causo(u)n, *n.* an intense continual fever 2.2.363, 2.2.364, 2.12.127, 2.12.147

celle, *n.* a ventricle or chamber within the brain 2.7.263, 2.7.289

celoure, *n.* canopy (over a bed) 2.7.444

centorie, *n.* common centaury (*Centaureum umbellatum*) or yellow centaury (*Chlora perfoliata*) 2.7.68

centyne see sentyne

cephalarge, *n.* headache 2.3.116, *sephalarge* 2.3.114, †*cephalargia* 2.3.116

cercle, *n.* the surface at the top of a urine sample Prol.130, 2.3.850, 2.4.241, 3.2.1

cerebre, *n.* the brain 2.3.150, 2.3.155, *cerrebre* 2.4.256, *n.pl. cerebris* ?lobes of the brain 2.7.338, †*cerebrum* 2.7.251

certeyn, *adj.* of symptoms: reliable, certain 2.2.206, 2.3.109

cessen, *v.* to cease, stop 3.16.251; *pr.3sg. seseth* 2.3.297; *pr.pl. cessen* 2.3.837, 2.3.840, *cesse* 3.16.271

cessing, *ger.* cessation, stopping 2.2.227, 2.6.139, *ces(s)yng* 2.2.187, 3.20.161, *ses(s)yng* 2.2.347, 2.10.196

charnouse see carnouse

chauel(le), *n.* the jaw 2.3.205, 2.3.206

chaufeþ, *v.pr.3sg.* heats, warms, inflames 1.4.167, 1.4.682, *chaufeth* 1.4.783; *pa.ppl.* *chaufed(e)* 3.16.111, 3.16.324, *chafed* 3.10.39, *chaffede* 1.4.175

chaufyng, *ger.* heating, warming, inflammation 1.4.179, 1.4.523, 1.4.717

chaumbres, *n.pl.* compartments, cells 2.3.659

chekeand, *v.pr.ppl.* checking, overwhelming 2.3.582

cheketh, *v.pr.3sg.* chokes, strangles, checks, stops 2.4.63; *pa.ppl.* *chekede* 1.4.267

chekyng, *ger.* a choking, strangling 2.3.786, 3.2.83

chese, *n.* cheese 1.2.35, 2.7.156

chesel, *n.* a small, coarse sandy precipitate in urine 2.4.67, 2.4.72, *chysel* 2.7.91

chesing, *ger.* choosing 2.7.292

chikes, *n.pl.* the cheeks 3.4.18, *chokes* 2.3.623, 2.3.624

childeberyng, *ger.* giving birth 2.3.788

childer, *n.pl.* children 1.4.262, 2.3.661, *childern(e)* *1.4.269, 1.4.619, 3.1.31; ~ *of* *þis worlde* worldly people Prol.24

chilland, *v.pr.ppl.* chilling, cooling 1.4.440

chilþe, *n.* childhood 1.4.396

chippeþ, *v.pr.3sg.* chips, breaks away in small pieces 3.13.8; *pr.ppl.* *chippand* 3.12.11; *pa.ppl.* *chippede* 1.4.207

chippinges, *ger.pl.* pieces, fragments, flakes, bits 3.6.9, *chippynges* 3.4.57

†choabens, *v.pr.ppl.* having at the same time 2.12.25 (see n.)

†choos, *n.* labour, travail 2.12.22

chyldyng, *ger.* childbirth 1.1.34

chyuering, *ger.* shivering, tremor 2.6.531, 2.6.533, *chyueryng* 2.6.529

†ciatica see **†sciatica**

†cibus calidus, *n.* hot food, food of a hot complexion 1.3.235

cicle, *n.* a recurring period of years 2.6.317, 2.6.322; *sol- ~* the twenty-eight-year cycle in which the leap day runs through all seven days of the week 2.6.278, *sol-sicle* 2.6.291, *†ciclus solaris* 2.6.279

†cinancya see **cynancie**

†ciraga, *n.* gout in the hand 3.16.150

†cista fellis, *n.* the gall bladder and its outer membrane 1.3.78

citrin(e), *adj.* (also as *n.*) of a yellowish colour Prol.121, 1.4.273, 1.4.731, *citryn(e)* 2.9.2, 3.20.10, *†citrinus* 2.1.11

citrin(e)hed(e), *n.* yellowishness 1.4.733, 2.9.14, 2.9.178

*citrinish, *adj.* of a dull yellow colour, somewhat citrine 2.8.364

clabbed(e), *v.pa.ppl.* clustered, clumped, coagulated 2.4.315, 2.6.58

clammeth, *v.pr.3sg.* clumps, sticks (together) 3.8.18; *pr.ppl.* **clammand* 2.3.586; *pa.ppl. clammed(e)* 2.4.315, 2.6.48, *clammyd(e)* 2.1.103, 2.6.58

clam(m)ysh, *adj.* sticky, slimy, viscous 3.3.27, 3.9.10

clatteþ, *v.pr.3sg.* gathers together, heaps up, clots 3.8.19, *clatiþ* 2.7.131; *pa.ppl. clattede* 3.16.373

clensyng, *ger.* a cleansing, a filtration 1.2.4, 1.2.16, 1.2.40, *clensing* 2.9.151

cleped(e), *v.pa.ppl.* called 1.3.31, 2.3.55, 2.3.352

clere, *v.pr.sg.subj.* make (sth.) clear 1.4.145

cler(e), *adj.* clear, translucent 1.2.15, 1.3.91, 2.12.63

clerehede, *n.* clearness, transparency 1.4.474, 1.4.705, *clerehode* 1.4.221

cletten, *v.pr.pl.* gather, clump 3.16.52

cleue, *v.* to cleave, stick, or cling to 2.3.578, 3.16.375; *pr.3sg. cleueþ* 2.7.134, *cleueth* 3.17.20; *pr.pl. cleue* 2.8.288; *pr.ppl. cleu(e)and* 2.3.586, 2.13.337

clippend, *v.pr.ppl.* causing small particles in the body to waste away 3.12.10

cloddres, *n.pl.* clots, lumps 1.2.19

clod(e), *n.* clot, lump 1.2.21, 3.19.57

clompre, *n.* clump, clot 1.2.19, 1.2.21, *n.pl. clumpris* 3.10.67

clompreþ, *v.pr.3sg.* ~ clumps, clots, congeals 2.7.123, 2.13.24, *clumpreþ* 2.7.106; *pr.pl. clompren* 2.10.40; *pa.ppl. clomprede* 2.2.25, *clomprid* 3.10.16, *clumprede* 1.2.24, *clumprid* 2.6.48; ~ causes (sth.) to congeal 2.2.65, *clumpreþ* 3.8.19

clomprish, *adj.* somewhat thick, somewhat congealed 3.10.23

clongen, *v.pa.ppl.* shrivelled up 2.3.816

close, *n.pl.* clothes 2.10.37

closed(e), *v.pa.ppl.* enclosed 1.3.231, 1.3.252; closed, not open 1.4.639, 2.3.742; *nyh ~ in* closely adjoining, abutting 2.7.493

cloude, *n.* a cloudy suspension in a urine sample Prol.133, 2.2.158, 3.20.387

cloudis(s)he, *adj.* cloudy 2.7.592, 3.20.309, *clowdisshe* 2.10.57

clout(e), *n.* cloth, rag 1.1.42, 3.3.32, 3.6.25, *clowte* 3.11.67

cluddeþ, *v.pr.3sg.* ~ *togeder* clots 2.13.24; *pr.pl. clodden* 2.10.40; *pa.ppl. clodded* 2.1.103

cluddyng, *ger.* thickening, coagulation 2.5.66

clumish, *adj.* ?lumpy, clotted (?error for *clomprish*) 3.10.6

coct(e), *v.pa.ppl.* decocted, digested 2.13.236, 3.20.195

cod(de), *n.* scrotum 2.7.527, 3.17.51

colde, *v.pr.sg.subj.* should become cold 3.20.178; *pa.ppl. coldid* made cold 3.10.16

colde, *n.* ~ *sittying* sitting in the cold 2.3.787; ~ *takyng (taking)* catching or being exposed to cold 1.3.238, 2.3.775

colde-byten, *ppl.adj.* stung with cold 2.2.23, 2.3.605, *colde-biten* 2.3.603

cold(e)hed(e), *n.* coldness 1.4.296, 2.4.212, 2.5.66

co(o)le, *n.*[1] a coal 1.3.258, 2.3.452, 3.16.262

cole, *n.*[2] cabbage, kale, a leafy vegetable (often distinguished by colour: black, red, green, white) 2.1.53, 2.1.54, 2.1.55, 2.14.30

cole, *adj.* cool, cold 1.4.687, 1.4.776

†*colera*, *n.* the humour (red) choler, bile 1.4.293, 1.4.300, †*colra* 2.8.53, 2.8.55

coleric, *adj.* choleric, characterized by red choler 1.4.463, *colrik* 1.3.237, 1.4.480; *adj. as n. colrik* 2.10.23, †*colericus* 1.4.311, 1.4.346, 1.4.372

coleþ, *v.pr.3sg.* cools, refreshes 1.4.681, *coliþ* 1.4.536; *pa.ppl. colide* 2.3.104; *pr.3sg. coleth* becomes cool 3.20.241

†*colica*, *adj. as n.* colic, abdominal pain that arises from the colon 2.4.172, 2.4.196; † ~ *passio* 1.3.74, 2.4.166

colk, *n.* the bottom (of the heart) 2.7.369

†*colon*, *n.* the colon 1.3.73, 1.3.74

colre, *n.* the humour red choler, bile 1.3.122, 1.3.142, 2.8.66; *rede* ~ bile 1.4.748; *blak* ~ the humour melancholy 1.3.143

comentour(e), *n.* commentator on a text Prol.53, Prol.59, 1.1.30, 2.3.435

comfort, *v.* to strengthen 2.13.328, *confort* 1.3.98; *pr.pl. confort(en)* strengthen, reinforce 1.3.240, 3.16.190; *pa.ppl. comforted(e)* 2.4.334, 2.7.330, *confortede* 1.3.250

comfortatif, *adj.* strengthening 2.13.41, 2.13.50

commixtioun, *n.* mixture, mingling 1.4.742

compaccio(u)n, *n.* compaction, a state of being compact or solid 2.6.41, 2.6.47, 2.8.181

compact(e), *adj.* compacted, solid 2.4.314, 2.6.31, 2.13.237

company, *n.* ~ *of woman,* ~ *of man* sexual intercourse 2.3.520, 2.3.790, 2.3.820

complexio(u)n, *n.* complexion, the specific mix of the four humours that comprise an individual's nature 1.3.18, 1.4.7, 1.4.307, *compleccioun* 1.4.329, *conplexion* 3.16.108, †*complexio* 1.4.468; the proportions of the four primary qualities in a substance or object 1.3.233

componed(e), *v.pa.ppl.* compounded, made up 1.4.23, 1.4.36, 1.4.39

compote, *n.* computus, the calculation of the calendar; *Boke of* ~ a book on calculating the calendar 2.6.272; *Maistre of* ~ master of calculating the calendar 2.6.272

compownde, *v.pa.ppl.* mixed, compounded (of) 2.6.9

comprehende, *v.* to take in, contain, enclose 2.8.142; *pr.3sg. comprehendeþ* 2.8.200, *comprehendiþ* 2.8.146, *comprehendith* 3.16.82; *comprehendiþ* understands 2.7.302; *pa.ppl. comprehendede* 2.8.24

comunate, *n.* community 1.4.394

comune, *n. the (þe)* ~ people in general 2.6.162, 2.10.52

comune, *adj.* everyday, ordinary Prol.8; ~ *course (vse)* common practice or experience 1.4.276, 2.6.161

conceytes, *n.pl.* ideas, perceptions, impressions 2.7.324

concluden, *v.* to deduce, infer 2.7.335; *pr.3sg.impers. it concludeþ* it is demonstrated, shown to be valid 2.14.102; *pr.3sg. concludiþ* encloses, holds 2.8.200

concurrant, *n.* the extra day or days in the year after fifty-two full weeks 2.6.281, 2.6.293

condescende, *v.pr.1sg.* accede (to), grant Prol.49

condicio(u)n, *n.* condition 1.4.366, 2.13.159, 3.19.103; a point to be considered in diagnosing a patient 1.4.12, 1.4.27, †*condicio* 2.3.636, *n.pl. condicyons* 1.4.5

†*condilomata*, *n.pl.* morbid swellings around the anus, hemorrhoids 2.4.348, †*condilomate* 3.18.102

condilon, *n.* a morbid swelling around the anus, hemorrhoid 3.18.8, 3.18.128

†*condilus*, *n.* the head of a bone, a joint 3.16.154, 3.18.51

confort(en) see comfort

congelacioun, *n.* congealing, thickening 2.2.20, 2.2.22

†*congelare*, *v.* to freeze, set, congeal 1.4.547

congelen, *v.* to freeze or chill, to thicken 1.4.547; *pr.3sg. congeleþ* 1.4.535, 1.4.546; *pa.ppl. congelede* 1.4.699

conseile, *n.* counsel, advice 1.1.18

constipat, *adj.* constipated, obstructed 2.8.338, 2.9.113

constreyneþ, *v.pr.3sg.* constricts, restricts 1.4.41, 1.4.535; *pa.ppl. constreyned(e)* thickened, hindered, slowed in flowing 1.4.95, 1.4.608

constrictif, *adj.* causing constriction *1.4.352, 1.4.765, 1.4.767

constrit, *v.pa.ppl.* constricted 2.7.140

consum(p)cio(u)n, *n.* wasting away (of humours, of the whole body), destruction 2.2.57, 2.8.337, 3.1.39, 3.8.6, *consumpsioun* 2.8.291

consum(p)t(e), *v.pa.ppl.* consumed, wasted away, destroyed 2.3.401, 2.3.571, 2.13.93, 3.1.42

consumptif, *adj.* consuming, wasting, destructive 2.3.499, 3.8.30

contagiouse, *adj.* purulent, poisonous 2.3.584, 2.3.585

†*contenta vrine*, *n.pl.* contents of the urine 1.4.196, 3.1.5

contentes, *n.pl.* things contained (within a urine sample) Prol.129, *contentez* Prol.101

contract(e), *v.pa.ppl.* contracted, shrunken 2.3.815, 2.8.316

contrarie, *n.* the opposite 1.4.534, 2.3.64

contrarious(e), *adj.* opposing, opposite 2.6.122, 2.6.137

contre, *n.* country, area Prol.90, 1.4.576, 2.7.26, *cuntre* 1.4.577

*contumelez, *n.pl.* abusive language Prol.31

conyn, *v.* to know, to understand 3.16.239, 3.20.3

conyng, *ger.* understanding 3.16.240

cop-web, *n.* cobweb 3.5.14

†*cor*, *n.* the heart 1.3.96, 1.3.113

corciouse, *adj.* corpulent 2.7.526

†*corexa*, *n.* catarrh, a cold with runny nose 3.4.21

corosif, *adj.* corrosive, caustic 2.3.683

†*corpus vryne*, *n.* the body or substance of urine 1.4.29

cor(r)upcio(u)n, *n.* rotting, putrefaction, infection 1.3.232, 1.3.253, 1.4.74, 1.4.489, 1.4.490, 1.4.494, 2.3.714, 2.12.40, *corrumpcioun* 3.9.4

cor(r)upt(e), *adj.* infected, rotten 1.4.101, 2.1.104, 2.3.331, 2.3.359, *corumpt* 3.9.12; ~ *in soule* depraved, evil Prol.32

†*costa*, *n.* a rib 2.3.578, 2.3.579

costrel, *n.* a bottle, flask 2.3.861, 2.3.863

coth(e), *n.* fainting, syncope, loss of consciousness 1.4.93, 2.3.814

cotidien, *adj.* of a fever: occurring daily; also as *n.* 1.4.653, 2.6.518, *cotidian(e)* 2.3.295; ~ *continuel* a fever with daily attacks and no full remission between attacks 2.3.292

couenable, *adj.* appropriate, suitable 2.2.243, *2.2.244

couenablie, *adv.* easily, without difficulty, suitably 3.19.179

couenant, *adj.* suitable 1.3.210, 2.2.242; *as n.* the suitable, desirable thing(s) 1.2.42

couer, *v.* to recover 2.2.337; *pr.3sg.* couerith 2.8.129; *pr.pl.* ~ 2.6.71

couertoure, *n.* a cover, canopy 2.13.299

coueryng, *ger.* recovery (?or error for *v.pr.pl. coueryn*) 3.2.81

couetouse, *n.* avarice, greed Prol.23

coueyteþ, *v.pr.3sg.* desires, covets Prol.25; *sg. used for pl.*, couaiteþ Prol.42, coueteþ Prol.51

course, *n.*[1] *be comune* ~ in the usual way of things, normally 2.4.276

course, *n.*[2] movement, motion along a path 1.3.204, 1.4.447, 1.4.609

couþe, *adj.* knowledgeable 2.1.5

cowh, *n.* cough 2.3.508, *cogh(e)* 3.4.38, 3.20.215, *kogh* 2.10.125, *kowh* 2.10.198, 2.13.144, *kuowh* 2.13.348; **coghe* syncope 2.3.813

cowhynges, *ger.pl.* coughings, fits of coughs 2.13.338

cracchyng, *ger.* scratching 3.16.213

craft(e), *n.* an occupation or art Prol.62, Prol.66, Prol.92

crakkyng, *ger.* farting, breaking wind 1.3.197

crekede see crokede

crepines see cripyns

crepyng, *ger.* constriction 1.4.115

cresses, *n.pl.* watercresses (*Nasturtium officinale*) 2.8.84, *crescis* 1.4.751

creticacio(u)n, *n.* crisis, turning point in a sickness 2.2.201, 2.2.242, 2.2.244; *day (dai) of* ~ the day an illness leaves a patient, either by recovery or death 2.2.184, 2.2.202, 2.2.240

cretik(e), *adj.* pertaining to a crisis, the turning point in a sickness 2.2.251; ~ *day (dai, daie)* the day of crisis (of an illness) 2.2.212, 2.2.213, 2.2.229, 2.2.274; *as n.* 2.2.209, 2.2.215; †*creticus* 2.2.184

cretyng, *ger.* ?error for crecyng (translation of Lat. *augmentate*) 3.20.277

cribracioun, *n.* sifting, filtering 1.2.39

cribre, *n.* sieve 1.2.41

criceland, *v.pr.ppl.* of sound: crackling 3.8.65

†*crinium*, *n.* a flake in the urine, thicker than bran or scales 3.14.4, 3.14.8

†*crin(n)oydes*, *n.pl.* flakes in the urine, thicker than bran or scales 2.10.223, 3.1.70, 3.14.2, †*crin(n)oides* 2.10.225, 3.14.3, †*cryn(n)oydes* 3.14.18, 3.15.19

cripyns, *n.pl.* flakes in the urine, thicker than bran or scales 3.14.7, *crypyn(e)s* 3.15.17, 3.15.26, †*cripine* 3.14.7, crepines Prol.142, †*cripina* 3.14.7; *n.sg.* †*cripinum* 3.14.8

crise, *n.* the turning point of a disease 3.20.187, †*crisis* 2.2.185, 2.2.195

†*croceique coloris*, *phr.* and of saffron colour 1.4.376

crodede, *v.pa.ppl.* crowded, pushed aside (by other organs) 2.13.167, *croden* 2.3.564

crokede, *v.pa.ppl.* crooked, curved, not straight 2.3.111, 2.3.170, 2.3.174; *crekede* decrepit, crippled with old age 1.4.397

crom, *n.* a crumb 2.7.383

cronclide, *v.pa.ppl.* contracted, crinkled, wrinkled 2.8.316

cropen, *v.pa.ppl.* ~ *togeder* crept together, shrunk 2.8.317

croteles, *n.pl.* small grains 3.8.80

croudyng, *ger.* crowding, pushing, bearing down 3.9.33, *crowding* pushing or pressing (down) 2.3.780

croupe, *n.* the buttocks 2.4.83

crowlyng, *ger.* intestinal growling, rumbling 3.9.27, 3.16.290

cruddes, *n.pl.* curds, coagulated material 1.2.19

cruddeþ, *v.pr.3sg.* coagulates, clots 2.2.65; *pa.ppl. cruddede* coagulated, clotted 1.2.24

crud(e), *adj.* raw, undigested 1.4.545, 1.4.673, 2.3.34, †*cruda* 1.4.695

†*cruditas humorum*, *n.* rawness of the humours, undigested humours 1.3.206

crudite, *n.* lack of digestion, non-digestion, rawness 1.4.176, 1.4.177, 2.4.265

crumblend, *v.pr.ppl.* contracting, shrinking, causing to shrivel 3.13.21

crushil, *n.* cartilage, gristle 2.7.350

crushilbone, *n.* cartilage, gristle 2.7.351

crusshede, *v.pa.ppl.* crushed, squashed 2.3.784

cunt, *n.* vulva 2.7.558

†*cupidus*, *adj.* covetous 1.4.384

cure, *n.* care, worry, anxiety 1.4.657, 1.4.662

curede, *v.pa.sg.* recovered (from an illness) 2.7.69

curteis, *adj.* courteous 1.4.368

cynancie, *n.* a form of quinsy 3.4.33, †*cinancya* 3.4.33, †*sinancia* 3.4.35

†*cynoca* see †*sinoc(h)a*

†*dampnaleoun*, *adj. vnguentum* ~ oil of laurel, daphnelaeon 1.4.815

dampnede, *v.pa.ppl.* damned 2.6.379

dappede, *v.pa.ppl.* dipped lightly 1.1.29

dase, *n.* daze, dizziness 2.4.254, *daswe* 2.4.255, *daswie* 2.4.257

dasowyng, *ger.* dimming (of the eyes) 2.3.368

dasthede, *n.* timidity, dullness 3.2.66 (see n.)

deceueren, *v.* to separate one thing from another, dissever 3.10.98; *pa.ppl.* *deceuered* 3.16.221

deceyued(e), *v.pa.ppl.* led astray, misled 1.4.159, 1.4.214

decisede, *v.pa.ppl.* sloughed off, cut away, shed 2.3.735, 3.20.228, *desisede* 1.4.197, 3.16.70, *desicede* 3.16.21, *desicyd* 3.16.26, **desised* 3.19.141

decisions, *n.pl.* small pieces, fragments, bits that have been sloughed away 1.4.207, *desicions* 3.4.57, 3.6.9

declaring, *ger.* explanation 2.8.113

declinacioun, *n.* of a sickness: the end (by recovery or death) of an illness 2.2.289, †*declinacio* 2.2.283

declynond, *v.pr.ppl.* of the sun: setting, going down 2.10.172

decoccio(u)n, *n.* digestion as the "cooking" of food in the body 1.3.223, 1.3.225, 1.4.253, 2.2.304

decocte, *v.pa.ppl.* cooked down, boiled down; *physiol.* digested, metabolized, transformed by a bodily organ 1.1.11, 1.2.8

†*decrepita,* *adj. as n.* old age 1.4.388 (see n.), 1.4.391

dede see **doþ**

dede, *n.*[1] death 1.4.401

dede, *n.*[2] deed 1.4.248, 3.16.253

dedisch, *adj.* lacking sensation, somewhat dead, numb 3.8.39, *dedis(s)h(e)* 2.3.569, 2.4.374, 2.10.207

defaut(e), *n.* defect, lack, fault 2.3.483, 2.4.156, 2.10.116, 3.19.205

defendant, *v.pr.ppl.* defending 2.7.343; fending off 2.7.356

defhed(e), *n.* deafness 3.4.27, 3.20.108

defien, *v.* to digest 2.3.583, 2.6.48, *defie* 2.4.118, *defiei* 2.2.210; *pr.3sg.* *defieþ* digests, breaks down 1.4.629, 2.2.317; *pr.pl.* *defyen* 1.3.211, *defie* 2.3.441; *pa.ppl.* *defiede* 1.1.12, 1.3.4

def(i)ying, *ger.* digestion 2.2.316, 2.13.183, 3.19.86

defoulede, *v.pa.ppl.* be ~ has had sexual intercourse 2.7.560

delateþ, *v.pr.3sg.* dilates, spreads (out) 1.4.345

dele, *n.* a part, a share; *more* ~ greater number, greater part 2.14.98; *most* ~ greatest number 2.4.40

delyte, *n.* a culinary delicacy 1.4.715 (see n.)

deme(n), *v.* to judge 1.4.166, 2.2.255; *pr.3sg. demeþ* 2.8.116; *pa.1sg. demede*
Prol.62; *pa.3sg. dempte* 2.7.54, 2.7.315; *pa.ppl. demede* Prol.40, *dempt(e)* 1.4.82,
1.4.129; ~ *of* to make a judgment about, to interpret 2.3.109

demyng, *ger.* judging, interpreting Prol.43, Prol.63, Prol.98, *demeng* 2.8.116

deneyin, *v.* to refuse, to deny 2.3.583

departed(e), *v.pa.ppl.* divided, partitioned, separated 1.2.41, 1.4.197, 2.6.186,
2.6.374

depe, *adj.* intense, dark (in colour) 1.4.18, 1.4.273; *comp. depper* 1.4.56, 1.4.808

depede, *v.pa.ppl.* deepened 1.2.9

deperdicioun, *n.* ruin, destruction 2.8.354

deppede, *v.pa.ppl.* ?blocked, ?impeded 2.3.404

depurede, *v.pa.ppl.* purified 2.3.27, 2.4.209, 2.7.286

dere, *n.* harm, injury 2.2.339

dere, *adj.* dear, beloved Prol.42, Prol.82; costly 2.2.338

derkehede, *n.* darkness 2.2.53, 2.3.254

derki(s)sh, *adj.* somewhat dark 1.4.486, 3.9.69

descernede, *v.pa.ppl.* discerned, judged 2.7.315

descryuede, *v.pa.ppl.* described 2.2.187, 2.7.259

desiccacioun, *n.* drying out 1.1.28, 2.8.330

desiccatif, *adj.* drying, desiccating 1.1.21, 1.4.806

desisede, *ppl.adj.* sick, diseased 2.8.273

desturbleþ, *v.pr.3sg.* disturbs 1.4.660, *distourbleþ* 2.4.176; *pr.pl. desturbleyn*
1.4.659; *pr.ppl. destourband* 3.2.39; *pa.ppl. dest(o)urbled(e)* 1.4.837, 2.12.54,
desturblid 3.19.79, *distourbled(e)* 2.3.388, 2.3.396, *distourblide* 2.13.31

determinacioun, *n.* of a disease: conclusion, final outcome 2.2.222; a definite
decision or interpretation 2.2.186, †*determinacio* 2.2.185

deuquarteyn, *n.* a duoquartan fever: a quartan fever with two attacks on the
fourth day 2.3.325, †*duoquartana* 2.3.319, 2.3.325

deutercien(e), *n.* a duotertian fever: a tertian fever with two attacks on the third
day 2.3.309, 3.2.325, †*duoterciana* 2.3.304, 2.3.309

†*dextroque tenax*, *phr.* and tenacious, holding fast 1.4.384

deynte, *n.* delight, pleasure 2.3.709

diabet(e), *n.* diabetes 2.4.123, 2.8.342; *diabeth* 2.4.127; †*diabetes* 2.4.122, 2.8.341;
†*diabeta* 3.12.17

†*diafragma*, *n.* diaphragm 2.3.98, 2.3.101

diarie, *n.* 2.8.349, *dyarie* 2.3.465, 2.8.350, *dyary* 2.3.466, †*diaria* 2.3.466, 2.8.350

diete, *n.* regimen, management of food, drink, and behaviour for health 1.4.9, 1.4.266

diete, *v.* to feed 1.4.598

diffundeþ, *v.pr.3sg.* spreads, diffuses 1.4.45, 2.3.348, *diffundiþ* 2.3.337, 2.3.346

diffusioun, *n.* spreading 2.3.349

digestede, *v.pa.ppl.* digested, metabolized, transformed by a bodily organ 1.1.11

digestioun, *n.* the digestive process, metabolism of food 1.3.4, 2.2.316; *first (second, third) ~ stages in the digestive process* 1.3.6, 1.3.7, 1.3.8

dilacioun, *n.* spreading 1.4.171

dilate, *v.* to spread, disseminate 2.8.327; *pr.3sg. dilateþ* 1.4.349, *dilatiþ* 1.4.45; *pr.3sg. (refl.) dilateþ him (here)* spreads itself (herself) 2.3.346, 3.2.804, *pr.pl. (refl.) dilaten hem* 1.4.606

diriuiede, *v.pa.ppl.* derived, passed on 3.19.28, *diriuyede* 3.18.15, *dyryuede* 3.16.278, *dyryuyed* 3.19.23

dirked(e), *v.pa.ppl.* darkened 2.3.284, 2.3.412

dirk(e)hede, *n.* darkness 2.3.266, 2.3.385, *dirkehode* 2.2.3

discatereþ, *v.pr.3sg.* scatters 2.14.125; *pa.ppl. discatered(e)*, scattered 1.4.836, 2.4.203, 3.16.351

discraseþ, *v.pr.3sg.* unbalances 1.4.530; *pa.ppl. discrasede* 2.8.107, 2.8.127

discrasioun, *n.* imbalance of humours 3.19.121, *discracioun* 3.11.28

discresioun, *n.* judgment, ability to distinguish between two things 1.4.503

dises(s)e, *n.* discomfort, distress 2.3.520, 2.4.302, 2.10.125

disgregate, *v.pa.ppl.* disintegrated, separated 2.4.336

†*disma*, *n.* difficulty in breathing, dyspnea 2.3.120, 2.3.235

dismai(h)ede, *v.pa.ppl.* dismayed, perturbed 2.2.237, 2.3.21

dismaying, *ger.* lethargy, mental inactivity 2.10.188

disperpleþ, *v.pr.3sg.* scatters 2.3.348, 2.5.24, *disperpliþ* 2.3.512, *disparpliþ* 2.3.337; *pa.ppl. disperpled(e)* dissipated, scattered 1.4.219, 1.4.836, *3.8.59, *disperplide* 2.13.409, *disperpled* 3.8.63

disperplyng, *ger.* scattering 2.3.349, 2.6.44

disposeth, *v.pr.3sg.* inclines (sth., sb.) to, leads to, arranges 1.4.194, 2.4.229, 2.6.211, *disposeþ* 2.6.341; *pa.ppl. disposede* 2.2.25, 2.2.173

disposicio(u)n, *n.* constitution, temperament, mixture of humours in the body or a body part 1.1.16, 1.4.305, 1.4.829, *dispocisioun* 2.4.358, *disposisioun* 2.7.592; ordering, arrangement 2.3.212

disquasseþ, *v.pr.3sg.* squashes, smashes, destroys 2.13.324; *pa.ppl. disquasht* 3.19.100

dissenterie, *n.* dysentery 3.20.336, 3.20.347, *dissentarie* 2.3.465, †*dissenteria* 2.3.467

†*dissuria*, *n.* dysuria, painful urination 1.4.85, 1.4.114

distempereþ, *v.pr.3sg.* unbalances, throws the humoral balances out of alignment 1.4.531, *distemperiþ* 2.3.334, *destempereþ* 1.4.661; *pr.ppl. distemperand* 2.12.137; *pa.ppl. distemp(e)red(e)* 1.4.562, 1.4.837, 2.1.37, *destemprede* 2.3.17

distemper(o)ur(e), *n.* a state of humoral imbalance 2.1.101, 2.3.345, 2.8.294, *destemper(o)ur(e)* 1.4.170, 2.1.93, 2.2.83

distencio(u)n, *n.* stretching, swelling, expansion 2.3.796, 2.3.841, 2.10.131

distendiþ, *v.pr.3sg.* extends, stretches, reaches 2.4.365; *pa.ppl. distent* 2.3.807

distillacioun, *n.* falling in drops or parts from one part of the body to another 3.4.51, 3.16.16

distincte, *v.pa.ppl.* divided (into parts) 2.7.263, 2.7.277

distourbleþ, **distourbled(e)** see **desturbleþ**

disturblyng, *ger.* disturbing, disordering (of the soul) 2.4.103; unbalancing, troubling 2.7.205, 2.10.13, *distourbling* 3.16.311

†*diu*, *adv.* long, for a long time 1.4.771

diuersite, *n.* distinction (between two or more things) 1.4.710, 1.4.712, *dyuerste* 2.7.46

diuinite, *n.* theology 1.4.393

diuise(n), *v.* to divide 1.3.99, ~ *hem* separate (themselves) 1.3.48; *pr.3sg. diuiseþ* divides, breaks (sth.) into pieces 1.4.198, *diuiseþ him* divides itself, splits, separates 2.3.74, 2.3.106; *pr.pl. diuisen* 2.1.40, *diuisen hem* divide (themselves), split, separate 2.3.72, 2.3.152; *pr.sg.subj. diuise hym* should divide itself 1.4.230; *pa.ppl. diuisede* 1.2.41, 1.4.219; *pr.3sg. diuiseþ* divides, defines 1.4.392

diuisioun, *n.* separation into different parts 1.2.44, 1.2.45

diuretik, *adj.* able to induce urination 1.4.760, *diuritik* 1.4.757, *diurytik* 1.4.757, †*diureticum* 1.4.786

dogg-leches, *n.pl.* quacks, medical charlatans 2.12.60

dome, *n.* judgment Prol.7, Prol.99, 1.4.159

domesman, *n.* judge Prol.65

†*dominatur*, *v.pr.dep.3sg.* has dominion, reigns 1.4.57, 1.4.455, 2.1.86

donward(e), *adv.* downward 1.4.491, 2.2.123

doþ, *v.pr.3sg.* does, acts 1.4.40; *pr.pl. done* 1.4.37; *pa.sg. dede* 2.6.331, 2.6.489, *dede make* caused to make 2.7.59; *pa.pl. dede* Prol.72; *pr.ppl. doand* 1.4.248

douce, *adj.* fresh, sweet; ~ *fleume* sweet phlegm, phlegm mixed with blood 2.10.95

doutously, *adv.* doubtfully, in doubt Prol.46

dowh, *n.* dough 3.17.17

dra(u)ght, *n.* draw, pull 2.4.149; ~ *of lede* a mark made by lead on paper 2.3.264

drawing, *ger.* ~ *of honde* drawing breath 2.10.195

dreggy, *adj.* full of dregs 3.20.330

drencheþ, *v.pr.3sg.* penetrates, soaks 1.4.793; *pa.ppl. drenchede* dissolved, soaked 2.5.81, 2.8.262

drestes, *n.pl.* dregs, lees 1.3.64, 2.2.136

drestish, *adj.* full of dregs 3.7.22, 3.9.9

dresty, *adj.* full of dregs *2.7.598, 2.8.279, 2.10.11

drilliþ, *v.pr.3sg.* flows in drops, trickles, drips 2.2.43; *pa.ppl. dryllede* ?absorbed by drops or sips 1.3.12

drogger(i)s, *n.pl.* druggists, apothecaries 1.4.761, 1.4.763

droppyng, *ger.* exudation (from the ears) 1.3.148; dripping 3.4.52

droubleþ, *v.pr.3sg.* makes turbid or muddy in consistency 2.9.162

droublihede, *n.* turbidity, murkiness 2.3.381, *droublehede* 2.2.54, *droblyhede* 1.4.159, *droblyhode* 1.4.220

droublis(s)h(e), *adj.* somewhat turbid 2.3.395, 3.16.66, *droblysh* 2.11.15, *drublish* 3.7.22

dro(u)bly, *adj.* turbid, murky 1.4.151, 2.1.95, 2.4.325, 2.7.575, *droubli(e)* 2.7.223, 3.20.229

drowonde, *v.pr.ppl.* drawing, pulling 2.7.386; *pa.sg. drowe* drew in, pulled 3.16.244, 3.16.246

druryhede, *n.* sadness, fearfulness 2.3.487

dryand, *v.pr.ppl.* drying 1.1.21, 1.1.22

dryhed(e), *n.* dryness, desiccation, dehydration 1.1.21, 1.4.34, 1.4.280, 1.4.704

drylle, *n.* a drop; *now a ~ and now a ~* drop by drop 2.3.406

dryllede see drilliþ

dryt, *n.* feces 1.3.64

duelleþ, *v.pr.3sg.* dwells, stays 1.3.153, 1.4.641; *pr.sg.subj. duelle* 2.3.742; *pr.ppl. duellond* of a planet in a zodiacal sign: remaining 2.6.152

duellyng, *ger.* dwelling place 2.3.481, *duelleng* 1.3.223; *maken (mak, makeþ) ~* take up residence, stay in a place 1.3.238, 2.3.482, 2.7.125

dulhed(e), *n.* dullness 2.4.356, 2.10.188

dunne, *adj.* brownish-grey 2.7.27, *don* 1.4.507

duoden(e), *n.* the duodenum 1.3.26, 1.3.30, †*duodenum* 1.3.25

†*duoquartana* see **deuquarteyn**

†*duoterciana* see **deutercien(e)**

dwynen, *v.* to waste away 2.3.446; *pr.3sg. dwyneþ* 2.3.572; *pr.pl. dwynen* 2.3.549; *pr.sg.subj. dwyne* 3.7.101; *pa.ppl. dwynede* 2.4.276, 3.16.113

dwynyng, *ger.* wasting 2.3.433, 3.8.46; shrinking, contracting (together) 3.16.371

dyametre, *n.* diameter 2.6.380

dyede, *v.pa.ppl.* dyed, coloured 1.2.9, 2.7.53

dymhed(e), *n.* dimness 2.2.3, 2.2.9, 2.6.356, 3.5.18

dymhede, *v.pa.ppl.* dimmed, darkened (influenced by spelling of abstract noun *dymhede*) 2.3.284, 2.3.413

dymmyshede, *n.* the state of being somewhat dim 2.11.33

dymmyssh(e), *adj.* somewhat dim 1.4.486, 2.7.86, 3.20.389

†*ebes,* *adj.* dull 1.4.381

ebulicioun, *n.* boiling, disturbance (of humours) through heat 3.6.32

†*e contrario,* *phr.* conversely, in the opposite manner 1.4.143, 1.4.162

†*e conuerso,* *phr.* the opposite 1.4.349

†*effimera,* *n.* a worm or insect that lives only for a day 2.3.354

†*effimerina,* *n.* an ephemeral fever, a fever lasting only a day 2.3.352

†*effimeron,* *n.* Greek term for sth. "little and subtle" 2.3.356

effimeryne, *n.* an ephemeral fever, a fever lasting only a day 2.3.352

eft(e)sones, *adv.* again, another time 1.4.161, 1.4.162, 2.10.182; back(wards) 2.3.205

egestio(u)n, *n.* defecation 1.3.197, 2.2.313, 2.2.315

egre, *adj.* sour 2.5.44, 2.5.59

†*eirratica,* *adj. febris ~* an intermittent fever of unpredictable periods 2.9.61

eke, *v.pr.1sg.* add to Prol.50; *pa.ppl. ekede* Prol.75

ek(e), *adv.* also, likewise 1.4.508, 1.4.693, 2.3.580

†*elcosis,* *n.* ulceration in the bladder 1.4.85, †*helcosis* 1.4.96

elde, *n.* old age 1.4.260, 1.4.282, *elþe* 1.4.389, *olde* 1.4.397

elde, *adj.* old 1.4.743, 2.8.320, 3.20.331

elde, *adv.* ~ *baken* baked a long time ago 1.4.743

elles, *adv.* else, otherwise 1.1.38, 1.2.21, *ellez* 1.3.215, 1.4.240, *ellis* 2.3.461, 2.3.565, *elle* Prol.95, 2.8.81, *helles* 2.6.91

†ema(c), *n.* blood 1.4.119, 2.3.88, 2.3.223, *emak* 2.3.88, *emath* 2.7.587, 3.18.23

†emanacio, *n.* emanation, production 1.4.118

†emathasia, *n.* bleeding from the mouth 2.7.586, **†emathasis** 2.7.586, **†emothois** 2.7.586, **†emothoia** 2.7.586, *omothoye* 2.13.400, **†omothoia** 2.13.400

†emfraxis, *n.* obstruction, blockage 2.8.343, **†enfrasis** 2.8.311

emitrice, *n.* a compound fever that causes lethargy, "semitertian fever" 2.3.290, 2.14.135, *emytrice* 2.10.154, 2.10.156, 2.11.53; *lesse* ~ , *petit (pety)* ~ minor emitrice, compounded of a cotidian continual fever and a tertian interpolate fever 2.3.291, 2.10.153; *mydde(s)* ~ middle emitrice, compounded of a tertian continual fever and a cotidian interpolate fever 2.3.294, 2.11.54; *more* ~ major emitrice, compounded of a quartan continual fever and a tertian interpolate fever 2.3.293, 2.14.133

emorayde(s), *n.pl.* hemorrhoids 3.18.23, 3.18.95; *emoraide(s)* 2.3.87, 2.13.445, **†emoraidas** 3.18.7, *emorai(e)s* 2.3.93, 2.3.382, *emoray(e)s* 3.18.22, *emoroide(s)* 2.3.88, 2.3.91, *emoroys* 2.3.91, **†emeraidas** 2.4.348

†emorogia, *n.* hematuria 1.4.85, 1.4.117

†emothoia, †emothois see **†emathasia**

†emoys, *n.* blood 2.7.587

empime, *n.* bleeding at the mouth 2.10.208, **†empima** 2.7.585, 2.7.586

emplastre, *n.* poultice, medical plaster 1.1.41

emptihede, *n.* emptiness 2.4.363

enchaufen, *v.pr.pl.* heat 1.3.244; *pa.ppl. enchaufede* 1.3.245

enchaufyng, *ger.* heating 1.3.245

encheso(u)n, *n.* reason, explanation 1.3.48, 1.4.357, 2.7.490

encorperacioun see **incorporacio(u)n**

encresce, *v.pr.1sg.* increase Prol.50; *pr.3sg. encreseþ* 1.4.330, *encreceþ* 1.4.725, *encrecit* 2.12.46; *pr.sg.subj. encre(s)ce* 3.16.117, 3.20.80; *pa.ppl. encresede* Prol.75

encresing, *ger.* growing, growth, increasing 1.4.270, 2.6.91, *encresyng* Prol.77

ende, *n. ouer* ~ upper end 1.3.59, *neþer* ~ lower end 1.3.19, *tayle (tail)* ~ rump, buttocks 1.3.77

†eneorima, *n.* hypostasis suspended in the middle of the urine flask 2.2.353, 2.2.363

enfeccio(u)n, *n.* infection 2.3.47, 2.8.278

enfecteþ, *v.pr.3sg.* infects, afflicts 2.2.43, 2.3.573, *enfecteth* 2.3.596, *enfectiþ* 2.8.280, *enfectis* 2.13.409; *pa.ppl. enfecte* 2.3.21, 2.3.413

enflammeþ, *v.pr.3sg.* inflames, heats morbidly 2.1.98; *pr.pl. enflamme* 2.3.501; *pr. ppl. enflammand* 2.11.48, *enflaumand* 2.12.95, *enflawmand* 2.12.87, *enflawm-yng* 2.12.20

enflawmyng, *ger.* morbid heating, inflammation 2.10.131

enformede, *v.pa.ppl.* taught 1.4.164

†*enfrasis* see †*emfraxis*

engros(s)eþ, *v.pr.3sg.* thickens, becomes thick 2.13.373, 3.16.279; *pr.pl. engrosen* 2.10.39; *pa.ppl. engros(s)ede* 2.5.32, 2.9.53

enoyntyng, *ger.* anointing with therapeutic oils 1.4.10, 1.4.813

entermetours, *n.pl.* meddlers, interlopers 2.4.179, *entremetoures* 2.12.60

envenymeth, *v.pr.3sg.* envenoms, infects 2.8.281, *envenymyth* 2.3.596

enyntisshing see anyntis(s)hing

epamastik, *adj.* "of fever: following after on the crisis" (i.e., declining) (*DMLBS*, s.v. *epacmasticus*) 2.12.39, *adj. as n.* †*epamastica* 2.12.34, 2.12.41

†*epar, n.* the liver 1.2.22, 1.2.46, 1.3.85

†*epatica passio, n.* liver disease 2.3.127, 2.3.418

epial, *n.* a cold fever caused by putrefied phlegm and melancholy in the stomach, with hot internal organs and cold extremities of the body 2.3.343, †*epiala* 2.3.327, 2.3.329

epiglot(e), *n.* the epiglottis, cartilage at the opening of the larynx 2.3.426, 2.7.245, †*epiglotum* 2.7.345

†*epigozontaymenon, n.* visceral peritoneum 2.7.523; *ypigozontamen* 2.7.528

epilence, *n.* epilepsy 2.4.242, 2.4.245; †*epilencia* 2.3.852

†*equaliter, adv.* equally 1.4.336

ere, *n.* the ear 2.6.140; *n.pl. e(e)res* the ears 1.3.148, 2.2.179, *eeris* 2.3.157, 3.20.46

erkesom, adj. painful 2.4.374

erkhed, *n.* pain, irksomeness 2.4.356

erse-bubbe, *n.* the rectum 1.3.78

erse-þerme, *n.* the rectum 1.3.77

ers hole, *phr.* the anus 3.18.21

erþihede, *n.* earthiness, characteristics relating to the element earth 2.2.67

erþis(s)h(e), *adj.* having qualities of the element earth 2.2.11, 2.3.7, 2.4.343, 3.18.17

eschewe(n), *v.* to avoid, to escape Prol.30, Prol.35

ese, *n.* ease, comfort 1.4.359; *at male* ~ in distress, feeling discomfort, ill 3.2.120

esie, *adj.* easy, not difficult 2.3.241, 2.13.40, *esy(e)* 2.10.196, 2.14.41, 3.16.46, *ese* 3.9.45

essues see **issu(e)**

†*estas*, *n.* summer 1.4.407, 1.4.411

†*ethica*, *n.* hectic fever 2.3.417, 2.3.474, †*etica* 2.3.473

†*ethicus*, *n.* one suffering from hectic fever 2.3.478, *eticus* 2.3.474

ethimologies, *n.* etymologies; *bok(e) of* ~ *(Ethimologyis)* Isidore of Seville's *Liber etymologiarum* (c. 600–25) 2.8.155, 2.14.107

eþe, *adj.* easy 1.4.514, 2.2.214, *eþi* 2.13.327, 3.19.124; *sup. eþiest* 2.13.257, 3.11.24

etik(e), *n.* hectic fever, a wasting fever 2.3.402, 2.8.337, 3.5.21, 3.13.16, *febre* ~ 1.3.245, 1.3.246

etyng, *ger.* the act of eating 1.4.9, 1.4.269

eucratik, *adj.* of complexion: balanced, having even proportions of hot, cold, wet, and dry 2.10.4, †*eucraticum* 2.10.4

euelong see **auelong**

euen, *n.* evening 2.6.167, 2.6.221, 2.7.68; the evening or day before a feast, eve 1.4.422, 1.4.423, *euyn* 1.4.424, 1.4.425

euen, *adv.* evenly, equally 2.6.249, 2.6.259; ~ *streiʒt* directly, in a straight line 2.3.107, 2.3.108; ~ *vnder* directly under 1.3.110

euen(e), *adj.* even, equal 1.4.327, 2.2.105; ~ *with* equal to 1.3.27; ~ divisible by two 2.2.243, 2.2.244

euerych, *pron.* each, each one 1.4.587, 2.3.172

euerych, *adj.* each, every 1.4.129

euydent, *adj.* clear 2.4.11

euyl, *n.* an evil, illness Prol.39; *euel* 3.18.101; *n.pl. eueles* Prol.27; *womannes* ~ , *moneth* ~ menstruation 1.4.78, 2.3.673; *falland (fallend)* ~ epilepsy 2.3.738, 2.3.853

eventede, *v.pa.ppl.* vented, released 2.4.164

ewe, *n. as adj.* ~ *fleume* watery phlegm 2.5.65; *n.* ~ *citrin* a citrine-coloured urine or fluid 3.20.72

exces see **acces(se)**

exclusif, *adj.* of an item at the beginning or end of a series: not including 2.6.172, 2.6.175

excocte, *v.pa.ppl.* digested 3.16.331 (see n.)

experiment, *n.* a recipe or set of instructions 2.3.459, 3.11.66, 3.16.363, *expery-ment* 2.3.654

expositour, *n.pl.* expounder, commentator 1.4.6, 2.3.435

expo(u)ned(e), *v.pa.sg.* explained, defined (terms) 2.2.110, 2.4.225; *pa.ppl.* 2.3.428

†**texta,** *n.pl.* the intestines (esp. when removed from the body) 2.7.516

extencioun, *n.* extension, stretching 2.4.354

extremite(e)s, *n.pl.* the outer parts of the body (e.g., hands, feet, legs, arms) or of parts of the body 1.3.88, 2.10.171, *extremyte(e)s* 2.2.21, 3.20.152; ~ *of þe ribbes* 2.13.317; ~ *of þe veynes* 3.18.91

ey(e), *n.*[1] an egg 2.8.70, 3.7.4, 3.7.61, *aye* 2.8.71; *n.pl. eyren* 2.7.157

ey(e), *n.*[2] the eye 1.1.33, 1.1.34, 2.2.333, *eyhe* 2.6.378; *n.pl. eyen* 2.3.155, 2.3.362, *eyȝen* 1.3.147, 2.3.115, *eyne* 2.10.185; *at* ~ to the eye, visually 2.7.28, 2.7.70

eye-bryen, *n.pl.* the eyelids 3.4.24

eyr(e), *n.* air (the element or the substance), atmosphere 1.4.292, 1.4.605, 2.3.103, *air(e)* 1.3.238, 2.7.377, *ayre* 1.4.156, 1.4.220, *eir(e)* 1.4.308, 2.13.270, †*aier* 1.4.292, 1.4.300

eyrissh(e), *adj.* having the qualities of the element air 2.2.10, 3.5.9

eysel, *n.* vinegar 2.5.61

face, *n.* of urine: the surface 3.5.14, 3.8.3

†*facies,* *n.* the human face 1.4.381

faculte, *n.* field of knowledge, discipline Prol.16, Prol.35, 3.16.289

fadiþ, *v.pr.3sg.* weakens, enfeebles 2.8.281, 3.1.11; *pr.pl. fade* grow weak 2.7.86; *pa.ppl. fadede* 2.3.357, *fadid* 3.10.45

faile(n), *v.* to decrease, fail, be lacking (in) 1.4.279, 2.6.248; *pr.3sg. faileþ* 1.4.699; *pr.pl. faile* 2.5.67; *pr.sg.subj.* 2.13.46; *pr.ppl. failand* 1.4.282, *failend* 1.4.259

falland, *v.pr.ppl.* falling 2.4.146, 3.16.35, *faileand* 3.16.91 (see n.); ~ *euyl* epilepsy 2.3.114, 2.3.738

†*fallax,* *adj.* false, deceitful 1.4.374

falleþ, *v.pr.3sg.* belongs (to), pertains (to) 1.3.34

fallyng, *ger.* of a sickness: dissipation or relief (trans. Latin *declinatio*) 2.2.284, 2.6.81

false, *adj.* deceitful 1.4.373, *faws* 2.3.322; of fevers: seeming, not genuine 2.3.322, 2.4.319, 2.4.320

fantasie, *n.* the mental faculty of fantasy, the formation of mental images 2.7.283

fantasiede, *v.pa.ppl.* formed in the image-producing part of the brain 2.7.311

fantastik, *adj. as n.* the first cell of the brain, the site of the mental faculty of fantasy 2.7.281, †*fantastica* 2.7.280

fastand(e), *v.pr.ppl.* of urine: produced while fasting 1.1.35, 1.1.43; of a person or of the body: abstaining from food 1.1.36, 1.3.40; ~ *gut* the jejunum 1.3.32

fast(e), *adv.* near, close 2.3.234, 2.3.744, 2.4.170; immediately, quickly 2.2.220, 2.7.58

fathed(e), *n.* oiliness, greasiness 2.2.154, 2.3.646, *fathode* 2.2.152

fatnesse, *n.* oiliness, greasiness Prol.136

fat(t)(e), *adj.* oily, greasy 1.4.746, 2.2.148, 2.3.394, 3.12.16; of persons: fat, corpulent 1.4.343, 1.4.351, 2.3.839; of soil: sticky, glutinous 1.4.580

fattis(s)h(e), *adj.* somewhat fat, somewhat greasy 2.8.262, 3.5.3

fauour, *n.* patronage Prol.23, Prol.37

faxwax see **paxwax**

fayn, *adv.* eagerly 3.2.116

febliss(c)heþ, *v.pr.3sg.* becomes feeble, weakens 1.4.329, 2.7.137; *pa.ppl. febliss(c)hed(e)* 2.3.413, 2.3.536, 3.10.45, *feblysshede* 2.4.15

feblisshede, *n.* weakness 2.4.207

febre, *n.* fever; ~ *seke* sick with fever 1.4.646; *brennand* ~ an intense fever 2.3.342, 2.6.92; *continuel* ~ an unrelenting fever, a fever without intermission 2.8.160; see also **augmastik,** †*causonides,* **causo(u)n, cotidien, effimeryne,** †*eirratica,* **emitrice, epamastik, epial, etik, homoto(u)n, interpolate, lippiarie, nothe, planetik, quarteyn(e), sinoch,** †*sinoc(h)a,* †*sinochides,* **tercien(e)**

fecche, *n.* vetch 3.20.84; *n.pl. fechis* 1.4.750

feiȝit see **fiȝt**

feiȝteþ, *v.pr.3sg.* fights, struggles 2.6.59; *pr.pl. f(e)iȝten* 2.2.288, 2.2.288; *pa.ppl. foȝten* 2.8.154

†fel, *n.* the gall bladder 1.3.142, 2.4.218, *felle* 1.3.121; *sista (cista, sistis) fellis* the membrane that encloses the gall bladder 1.3.70, 1.3.78, 2.7.512

felawe, *n.* fellow, counterpart 2.3.173, *felow* 2.3.175; *felowe* friend, colleague Prol.4, Prol.6

fele, *adj.* many 1.4.7, 1.4.79

feloun, *n.* a suppurating sore 1.3.260

felying, *ger.* feeling, sensory experience 2.3.177, 2.3.566; ~ *synowes, synowes of* ~ sensory nerves 2.3.175, 2.3.179

fenestrede, *v.pa.ppl.* of urine: having alternating dark and light stripes, "windowed" 2.9.109, †*fenestrata* 2.4.22

fennyche, *adj.* like a fen or swamp 1.4.578

ferde, *adj.* fearful, timid 1.4.383

fer(re), *adj.* far 1.1.41, 1.1.44; *comp. ferrer* 2.6.220; *sup. ferrest* 2.6.209, 2.6.378; *alse ~ forþ* as much 1.4.81

ferrene, *adj.* fiery 2.12.155 (see n.)

fers, *adj.* bold, fierce 2.9.47

ferþ, *v.pr.3sg.* fares, happens 2.3.43

feruent, *adj.* hot, intense 1.4.241

feruour(e), *n.* fervour, heat 1.4.734, 2.2.176

fesiciens, *n.pl.* physicians 2.8.219

fest(e), *n.* feast day 2.6.246, 2.6.268

festenede, *v.pa.ppl.* connected 1.3.60

fetour(e), *n.* stink, stench 3.7.94, †*fetor* 2.2.153

feynten, *v.* to weaken, to dissipate 2.2.292; *pa.ppl. feyntede* 2.3.358, 2.4.368; *pr.3sg. feyntiþ* grows faint 1.4.329; *pr.3sg. feyntiþ* cause (a colour) to fade 1.4.681

feyntesse, *n.* faintness, weakness 3.6.68

feynthede, *n.* faintness, weakness 3.16.59; *~ of hert* timidity 3.2.67

feyntish, *v.pr.3pl.* make weak 2.10.185

fibres, *n.pl.* the vocal cords or ligaments 2.3.132, 2.3.133, *fibris* 2.3.835, †*fibra* 2.3.132, †*fibre* 2.3.132

fier, *n.* fire 1.4.292, 1.4.311, *fyur* 2.6.343

fike, *n.* a fig 3.18.53, 3.18.102; *n.pl. fikes* morbid swellings around the anus, hemorrhoids 3.18.54, *fikis* 3.18.9, †*ficus* 3.18.8

filþe, *n.* foul matter 1.4.489, 1.4.494, 2.3.662, *filth(e)* 1.4.499, 3.17.22; nasal mucus 1.3.148, 3.17.28

†**fistule**, *n.pl. ~ pulmonis* the airways in the lungs, the bronchi 2.3.229, 2.3.553

fiȝt, *n.* a fight, a struggle 2.2.196, 2.6.72, 2.6.341, *fiȝit* 2.4.267, *feiȝit* 2.4.286

flabbes, *n.pl.* lobes (of the liver) 2.7.459

flauouse, *adj.* yellowish, blond 2.7.25, †*flauus* 2.7.23

flawand, *v.pr.ppl.* an effect of rheum in the mouth, ?salivation 3.4.28

flawmand, *v.pr.ppl.* inflaming, heating morbidly 2.11.46

flegmo(u)n(e), *n.* swelling in the neck of the bladder 1.4.89, 1.4.94; cold that precedes syncope 1.4.91; a tumour caused by excess of blood 2.13.174; †*flegmon* 1.4.85, 2.13.175 (Latin and English forms not always distinct)

fleishede, *n.* fleshiness 3.12.19

fleishi, *adj.* fleshy 2.7.468

fleis(s)(c)h(e), *n.* flesh 1.3.49, 1.3.255, 1.3.163; ~, *flesch(e), flaish* meat 1.4.741, 1.4.744, 2.13.92, 3.19.13

fleten, *v.* to cause (sth.) to flow or move 2.2.36; *pr.3sg. fleteþ* moves (sth.) 2.8.201; *pr.pl.subj. (refl.) flete hem* move themselves 3.2.130; *pr.pl. fleten* flow, move 3.2.127

fl(e)umatik(e), *adj.* phlegmatic, characterized by phlegm 1.4.466, 2.6.98, 3.4.46, *fleumatic* 1.3.236, †*fleumaticus* 1.4.468, 3.19.114; *adj. as n.* †*fleumaticus* a phlegmatic person 1.4.315, 1.4.333, 1.4.351

fl(e)ume, *n.* the humour phlegm 1.3.121, 2.5.44, †*fl(e)uma* 1.3.120, 2.4.321; ~ *acetouse* sour phlegm 2.5.59; ~ *blank (blawnch)* vitreous phlegm, glassy phlegm 3.2.339, 2.9.182; *ewe* ~ watery phlegm, vitreous phlegm 2.5.65; ~ *naturel* natural phlegm 2.3.339, 2.7.183; *salse (salt)* ~ salt phlegm, salty phlegm 2.5.54, 2.10.51; ~ *vitre* vitreous phlegm, glassy phlegm 2.3.337

fleyþ, *v.pr.3sg.* flees (from) 2.3.793

flite, *v.impv.* move (sth.) 2.6.288

flode, *n.* an overflow 1.4.119, 2.4.219; *n.pl.* floods 2.6.363

floures, *n.pl.* menstrual flow 1.4.72, 1.4.73

flux, *n.* excessive flow of a bodily fluid 2.3.13, 2.3.15, †*fluxus* 2.3.89; *wombe* ~ diarrhea, dysentery, or lientery 2.3.12, 2.3.382; ~ *of blode (þe emoraies)* in men: blood flow from hemorrhoids 2.3.90, 2.3.382

fode, *n.* food 1.2.44, 1.3.3

fode, *v.* to feed 2.3.31, 2.9.79; *pr.3sg. fodeþ* 1.4.641, *fodiþ* 1.4.707; *pa.ppl. foded(e)* 1.4.202, 2.3.721, *fodit* 2.9.98

fodyng, *ger.* feeding, food, nutriment 1.3.92, 2.3.145

foldynges, *ger.pl.* the cells or ventricles of the brain 2.7.278

fol(o)wend(e), *v.pr.ppl.* following 1.2.47, 1.4.847, 2.3.865, *folw(e)and* 1.2.26, 2.2.371, *folowing* 1.4.452

fonde, *v.pa.sg.* found, discovered Prol.72, 3.20.393; *pa.ppl. fonden* Prol.74, Prol.76

fondeþ, *v.pr.3sg.* strives, endeavours 2.13.328, 3.4.12; *pr.pl. fonden* 2.3.449, 3.2.115

for, *conj., prep.* because, on account of 1.3.132; ~ *alse mychil (mykel, mykil)* in as much 1.3.209, 1.4.265, 1.4.328; ~ *to blame* in the wrong 2.6.495; ~ *whie* for the reason that, because Prol.16, Prol.90

forbarreþ, *v.pr.3sg.* blocks, prevents 3.7.43

fordo(n), *v.* to destroy 2.5.5, 3.16.22; *pr.3sg. fordoþ* 1.1.31, 1.1.32, *fordoth* 3.10.81; *pr.ppl. fordoand* 2.3.41; *pa.ppl. fordon(e)* 2.1.108, 2.6.142

fordoyng, *ger.* destruction 1.4.138, 1.4.664, *fordoing* 3.16.112

fordwynede, *v.pa.ppl.* caused (sth.) to waste away 2.3.537

forheuede, *n.* the forehead 2.3.152

formal(e), *adj.* providing form, providing the essential nature 2.8.228, 2.8.229, †*formale* 2.8.228

forme, *n.* essence, formal principle (of a thing), colour of urine 1.3.156, †*forma* 3.14.5

forme, *adj.* front, in a forward position 2.4.390, 2.13.432; *comp. former(e)* 2.3.619, 3.2.122

formely, *adv.* in (its) essential nature 1.1.6

fornymyng, *ger.* privation, taking away 2.1.46

forparty, *n.* forward part, front part 2.3.151, 2.7.282

forsc(h)alt, *v.pa.ppl.* burned up, scorched 2.13.428, 2.14.67

forskalkerede, *v.pa.ppl.* completely burned up 2.2.151, *forscolkerede* 2.1.104

fortrauailed(e), *v.pa.ppl.* worn out by labour 2.2.236, 2.8.164, 2.12.104

forwaried, *v.pa.ppl.* accursed, sinful 3.17.35

forȝetel, *adj.* forgetful 2.7.336

forȝetilhede, *n.* forgetfulness 2.12.68

fote, *n.* foot; *euery* ~ at each step (of a path), continual(ly) 3.16.17, 3.16.35

foule, *n.* fowl, bird (*sg. and coll.*) 1.4.745

freis(s)h(e), *adj.* fresh 2.7.156, 2.9.100; of water: not salt 1.4.680, 3.20.243; ~ (*fresshe*) *fleume* sweet phlegm, douce phlegm 2.5.51, 2.10.96, 2.10.124

fren(e)sy, *n.* madness, insanity, delirium 2.4.76, 2.4.102, 2.9.138, *frenesi(e)* 2.4.115, 2.6.33, †*frenesis* 2.4.102, 2.4.103

frenetik, *adj., adj. as n.* (someone) afflicted with delirium 2.4.75, †*freneticus* 2.12.69

frere, *n.* friar Prol.3, †*frater* 3.20.411; *n.pl. frerez prechoures* Dominicans, the Order of Preachers Prol.3, †*fratres* 3.20.411

freschyng, *ger.* refreshment, refreshing 2.3.71

fresen, *v.* to freeze 1.4.548

frete, *v.pr.3sg.* corrodes, poisons 2.8.96; *pr.ppl. fretand* 2.3.683

frety(i)ng, *ger.* corrosion, gnawing, sharp pain 1.3.70, 2.3.469

frigidite, *n.* coldness, cold 1.4.17, 1.4.21, †*frigiditas* 1.4.34, 1.4.295

†*frigidus,* *adj.* cold, frigid 1.2.33, 1.3.236, 1.4.276

†*frigus, n.* cold 1.4.94, 2.6.510

frikehede, *n.* strength, lustiness 3.20.391

fro, *prep.* from 1.3.13, 1.3.129; ~ *wiþinward* from within, intrinsic, essential 1.4.560, 1.4.822; ~ *wiþout(e)ward(e)* from the outside, external, externally 1.4.252, 1.4.527

front, *n.* forehead; *endys of þe* ~ the ends of the forehead (?the temples, ?the part of the head above the ears) 2.3.157

frotede, *v.pa.ppl.* rubbed or worn 2.3.643

froth, *n.* foam 2.10.220, 3.4.3, *froþ* Prol.134

froþi, *adj.* foamy 2.8.261, *2.8.273

*froþihed, *n.* frothiness, foaminess 2.8.274

fryke, *adj.* vigorous 2.8.344

ful, *adv.* fully, very, entirely Prol.26, Prol.45, 1.4.479

fullik(e), *adv.* fully, entirely, completely 2.1.58, 2.1.85, 2.10.96

fumosite, *n.* vapour, gas, windiness 1.3.149, 1.3.170, 1.4.540, 2.2.177, *fumasite* 3.2.125

fying, *ger.* digestion 2.3.489

fynal, *adj.* ~ *coloure* the ultimate colour of urine, toward which the digestive process is directed 1.3.154; ~ *forme* ultimate nature, the form toward which a process is directed 1.1.12

fyngerbrede, *n.* finger's width, the thickness of a finger 1.3.26

fysting, *ger.* farting 1.3.197

gad(e)re(n), *v.* to gather, to collect Prol.7, 2.3.608, 2.7.274, *gader* 2.7.211, *gedre* 2.7.228; *pr.3sg. gad(e)reþ* 1.4.491, 2.7.123, *gadriþ* 3.2.35, *gadrith* 2.4.364, *gaderet* 2.7.105; *pr.pl. gad(e)ren* 3.9.110, 3.10.12, 3.16.52, *gader* 2.3.665, 2.6.324, *gedren* 2.13.297; *pr.ppl. gaderand* 2.3.332, *gedrand* 2.13.171; *pa.ppl. gad(e)red(e)* Prol.51, 1.4.80, 1.4.186, *gadrad(e)* Prol.39, 1.4.131, *gadrid* 3.1.54

galle, *n.* the gall bladder (of humans or animals) 1.1.31, 1.3.70, 1.3.121; bile, the secretion of the gall bladder 2.11.7, ~ *of a nete, netes* ~ bile from a cow's gall bladder 2.8.17, 2.11.5; *blak* ~ the humour melancholy, black bile 2.4.222

†*gallice, adv.* in French 3.4.2

gastly, *adj.* ghastly, hideous 2.2.335

gauelles, *n.pl.* sheaves (of grain) 3.20.8

gend(e)ryng, *ger.* production 1.2.38, 2.7.133

gendre(n), *v.* to generate, to produce 2.3.145, 2.3.652; *pr.3sg. gend(e)reþ* 1.3.90, 1.3.248, *gend(e)rith* 2.3.449, 2.4.364; *pr.pl. gendre* 2.3.391; *pa.ppl. gend(e)red(e)* generated, produced, formed Prol.97, 1.3.2, 1.3.121; ~ to grow 2.3.608; *pr.pl. gendren* grow, are produced 1.4.539; ~ to produce offspring 2.3.652, 3.16.235, 3.16.362; ~ *into* become, develop into 3.2.94

genecyis, *n.pl.* women's matters; *Bok(e) of ~ (Genecyes), Liber geneciarum* The Book on the Conditions of Women 2.3.654, 2.3.655, 3.16.363

generac(c)io(u)n, *n.* production Prol.108, 1.3.1; reproduction 2.3.202, 2.3.652, 3.16.383

giffyng, *ger.* imparting, conveying (information) Prol.59

glade, *adj.* cheerful, joyful (in personality) 1.4.368

†glaucus, *adj.* (also as *n.*) of a whitish-yellow colour (similar to translucent horn) Prol.117, 2.1.11, 2.4.322

glet(t), *n.* phlegm, slimy matter 2.13.91, 3.7.4

glettissh, *adj.* viscous, slimy 2.13.224

gleyme, *n.* a sticky, phlegm-like substance 3.7.61

gleymouse, *adj.* slimy, sticky, viscous 2.7.9, 3.3.27

gleymousehede, *n.* stickiness, viscosity 2.13.332

glit(t), *v.pr.3sg.* glides, slides 3.16.380, 3.17.48; *pr.ppl. glidand* (easily) flowing 1.4.790, *glidond* 1.4.793

globbede, *v.pa.ppl.* ?lumpy 1.3.42

glotons, *n.pl.* gluttons, gluttonous people 1.4.696

glyrand, *v.pr.ppl.* shining brightly, gleaming 2.4.10

gnawen chalke, *phr.* to eat chalk (because of *pica* in pregnancy) 3.16.262

gobat, *n.* a lump, clump 2.3.761, 3.8.80

gode, *n.coll.* goods, property Prol.66, 1.4.383

goiown, *n.* the European gudgeon (*Gobio gobio, G. fluviatilis*) 3.15.3

golpyng, *ger.* yawning 1.3.196

gomes, *n.pl.* the gums 2.3.624, 3.4.37

gong, *n.* a privy or gutter 1.4.498

gonyng, *ger.* gaping 2.3.373

gorry, *adj.* muddy 1.4.579

goter see **guter**

gotes, *n.poss.* goat's 1.4.744, 2.7.157

goþ, *v.pr.3sg.* ~ *on brode* spreads out widely 1.4.345

goute, *n.* gout 3.16.6, 3.16.10, *gowt(e)* 2.3.738, 3.16.61; *colde (hote)* ~ gout characterized or caused by coldness (heat) 1.1.38, 3.16.100, †*gutta* 3.16.49; †*gutta artetica* arthritis 2.4.155, 3.16.131; †*gutta rubea (rosata, rosacea)* rosacea 3.16.200

gownd, *n.* secretions from the eyes 1.3.147

†*gracilis*, *adj.* thin, slender 1.4.360, 1.4.376

gramerly, *adv.* with respect to a word's form or etymology 1.4.770

granelouse, *adj.* of urine: granulous, full of grains 2.9.104, 2.10.216

grauel, *n.* a sandy precipitate in urine Prol.139, 2.3.535, *grayuel* 2.3.527

grauely, *adj.* of urine: containing small gritty particulates 2.7.599

gre, *n.* a degree of arc 2.6.196, 2.6.198; degree of kind (e.g., hot in the third degree) 3.1.59

grecihede, *n.* greasiness, oiliness 3.8.3, *grecyhede* 3.8.11

gren(e)hed(e), *n.* greenness 2.3.269, 2.9.16, 2.14.69

grenyshede, *n.* greenishness, the state of being somewhat green 2.8.44, 2.11.52, *grenishede* 2.4.251

gresie, *adj.* greasy, oily, fatty 2.3.394

greuance, *n.* injury, disease, pain 1.3.239, 2.2.223

greueþ, *v.pr.3sg.* causes pain to, harms 1.4.542, 2.3.334, *greueth* 3.16.173; *pr.ppl.* *greuand* painful, pain-causing 2.3.353

greuousely, *adv.* painfully, harshly Prol.26

greyn(e)s, *n.pl.* grains, small bits of foam dispersed in a urine sample Prol.132, 2.3.568; †*spume de greyne*, †*greyn de spume* grainy foam (French) 3.6.13, 3.6.13

gristeles, *n.pl.* cartilage, cartilaginous structures 2.3.166

gronten, *v.pr.pl.* grunt, groan 2.13.122

gros(se), *adj.* thick, heavy 2.2.11, 2.2.210, 2.3.331, *groos* 3.20.62

gros(se)hed(e), *n.* heaviness, thickness 2.13.267, 2.13.332, 3.9.41

grosseþ, *v.pr.3sg.* thickens 2.5.32

gro(u)nd(e), *n.* the lowest part of a urine sample 2.7.92, 2.13.451, *grownde* 3.9.104; ~ basis, foundation 3.2.72, 3.2.118, 3.7.102, 3.17.9; ~, *grownd* the base, bottom, or lowest part (of a body part, of a vessel) 2.6.314, 2.7.478, 3.11.69; ~ soil, earth 1.4.640, ~ font, origin (of a spring or well) 1.3.97, 3.2.74

gro(u)nde-soppes, *n.pl.* sediments, residues, dregs 1.3.64, 2.2.136, *grounde-sopis* 2.9.69

grusshing, *ger.* of teeth: grinding, grating, pressing together 2.6.518, *grosshyng* 2.3.817

grut(te), *n.* mud, slime 2.3.670, 3.9.78

gruttish, *adj.* muddy, slimy 3.9.69

gusshing, *ger.* outpouring 3.20.221, 3.20.223

guter, *n.* gutter or channel for waste (of a ship, of a kitchen, of the female body) 1.4.498, *goter* 1.4.500, 2.3.671

gut(t), *n.* a section of the intestines 1.3.31, 1.3.65; *n.pl. guttes* the intestines, the guts 1.3.73, 1.3.198

†*guttatim*, *adv.* by drops 1.4.87

gutteþ, *v.pr.3sg.* drains in drops, drips 1.4.87; *pr.ppl. guttand* of humours: falling away and dripping through the vessels of the body 3.16.91

guttouse, *adj.* afflicted with gout 3.16.123, 3.16.126, *guttowse* 3.16.121

gyle, *adj.* guileful 1.4.385 (see n.)

habit, *ppl.adj.* habituated, engrained 3.1.44

hac(c)he, *n.* pain, ache 2.2.296, 3.20.361

hale, *v.* to draw in 2.7.427; *pr.pl. hale* 2.7.581, 2.13.314

halkes, *n.pl.* chambers, compartments 2.3.660

halt(e), *v.pr.3sg. (refl.)* ~ *him* holds, keeps (himself, itself), remains 2.2.359, 2.3.287, 2.9.76; ~ *togeder (togedre)* coheres 1.4.41, 3.6.18, *haldeþ himself togedre* coheres 3.6.23, ~ *togedre* holds (sth.) together 3.16.161; ~ carries, holds (sth.) 3.10.13

ham see **hem**

hame, *n.* ?a membrane 3.7.4, 3.7.61

hames, *n.pl.* the hams, the backs of the legs behind the knees 2.6.465

hangond see **hongand**

happ, *n.* (good) fortune 2.13.89

haraiouse, *adj.* violent 3.20.97, *haragiouse* 3.20.136

haraioushede, *n.* violence 2.4.103

harde, *v.pa.ppl.* heard Prol.13

hard(e)hede, *n.* hardness 2.13.267, 2.13.332, 3.9.42

hardines, *n.* recklessness Prol.88

hastilik, *adv.* quickly, soon 1.4.634

hatrel, *n.* nape of the neck, back of the head 2.3.53, 2.3.183

haue, *v.* to have; *pr.2sg. hast(e)* (you) have Prol.9, 1.4.453; *pr.ppl. hauand(e)* having 2.2.130, 2.8.117; *hauond togedre* having together (glossing Latin *choabens = cohabens*) 2.12.25; *pa. and pa.ppl. had(e), hadde* had; *had of* taken from (a source) Prol.15; also the common forms and senses for *haþ*, *haue(n)*, *had(e)*, *hadde*

haue, *v.²* *(refl.)* to behave, to comport (oneself) Prol.98, Prol.110

haukes, *n.poss.* hawk's 1.1.31

haunten, *v.* to use, to fulfil 2.4.247

hede, *n.* heed; *take ~* note, pay attention (to the fact) 1.4.20, 1.4.28

he(e)r(e), *n.* hair 1.3.131, 1.4.310, 3.6.68

heil(e), *adj.* healthy 1.4.570, 2.1.87, *heyle* 1.4.467, 1.4.632

†*helcosis* see **†*elcosis***

helles see **elles**

help(e)and(e), *v.pr.ppl.* helpful, helping 2.8.205; *~ kynde hete (þe myʒt of kynde)* with the help of natural heat (nature's might) 1.2.25, 2.8.199; *God helping* with God's help Prol.84

helply, *adj.* helpful 2.6.350, 2.9.72, *helplich* 1.4.599

hem, *pron.3pl.obj.* them Prol.24, 1.1.26, 1.1.40, *ham* 1.3.245, 1.4.62

hemself(e), *pron.3pl.refl.* themselves 1.3.183, 1.4.519

hender, *adj.* *~ partie* of planetary spheres: near side (as opposed to the yonder or far side) 2.6.351; of the head: the posterior part (as opposed to the anterior part) 2.7.296, 3.2.11, *hendre* 2.7.185

hendreþ, *v.pr.3sg.* hinders, hurts 2.4.376

hendryng, *ger.* hindering, harming 2.3.450; *in ~ of* to the detriment of 1.3.217

hent, *v.pa.ppl.* taken 2.4.117, 2.6.42

hepe, *n.* the hip 2.3.81, 2.7.449, 3.16.152

hepe-bone, *n.* the hip joint (the ilium and/or the head of the femur) 3.16.152

herdes, *n.pl.* hards, the coarse part of flax 3.3.32, 3.6.25

her(e), *pron.3sg.f.poss.* her 1.4.72, 1.4.493, *hir(e)* 2.2.125, 3.20.388, *heir* 3.20.380

her(e) see **he(e)r(e)**, **þai**

her(e)selfe, *pron.3sg.f.refl.* herself 2.3.805, 3.16.253, 3.16.256

herihede, *n.* hair-like particles in urine, hairiness 1.4.105

hering, *ger.* hearing 2.2.175, *heryng* 2.7.137, *hereyng* 2.2.160

†*herisipula*, *n.* erysipelas and diseases of similar choleric origin 2.13.176

hernes, *n.pl.* angles, corners (in the brain or skull) 2.7.273

hert(e), *n.* the heart, 1.3.96, 1.3.102

hes(e), *pron.3sg.m.poss.* his 2.3.562, 2.6.357, 2.12.103

het(e), *n.* heat 1.4.273, 1.4.296, 2.8.232; *kynd(e)* ~ the heat that gives life to the body 1.1.10, 2.8.229; *vnkynd(e)* ~ unnatural, morbid heat in the body 1.4.530, 1.4.532

heþi, *adj.* like a heath, uncultivated 1.4.577

hetith, *v.pr.3sg.* heats 1.4.707, *hetiþ* 1.4.728; *pr.pl. heten* 1.3.244, 1.4.523

heued(e), *n.* the head 1.3.101, 2.3.465, 2.7.22, *hede* 2.2.178, 2.2.183; ~ *pan, hede panne* the cranium, the skull 2.3.150, 2.7.343; *heuedes of þe (þo) veyns* the ends of the veins near the anus, at which hemorrhoids develop 3.18.33, 3.18.75

heuy, *adj.* heavy, burdensome, inclining downward 2.2.333, 2.4.314, 2.4.374; of food: hard to digest 1.4.745, 1.4.747

heuyhede, *n.* heaviness, pain, or numbness 3.20.266

heuynes(se), *n.* heaviness, pain, or numbness 2.3.561, 2.4.356, 3.18.34

hewh, *n.* hue, colour 2.14.94

heyle see heil(e)

hide, *n.* skin 1.3.149, 1.3.201, *hyde* 1.3.169

hide, *v.pa.ppl.* hidden Prol.48

high, *adj.* of colour: deep, intense 1.4.264, 2.3.527, *hygh* 1.4.816; of position: high 1.4.581, 3.15.13, *hyh* 2.3.781; *comp. higher* 3.8.106, *hier* 2.2.359, 3.4.77, *hyer* 2.12.47, *heyer* 2.12.47; *sup. adj. as n. hiest(e) (higheste)* highest point, peak 2.2.226, 2.2.276, 2.2.279

†hillaris, *adj.* cheerful 1.4.369

hilly, *adj.* characterized by hills 1.4.577

†hinc, *adv.* hence, on account of which 1.4.381

†hirsutus, *adj.* rough, shaggy 1.4.374

hissingz, *ger.pl.* hissings (as a sign of disapproval) Prol.33

hole, *n.* opening, hole 1.3.19, 1.3.20, 1.3.68

hol(e), *adj.*[1] hollow 2.3.257, 2.4.86, 2.7.369, *holle* 2.7.377

hol(e), *adj.*[2] see ho(o)l(e)

holpen, *v.pa.ppl.* helped, taken care of 2.9.134

holwe, *adj.* hollow 2.2.335, 2.3.97; ~ *veyne* the vena cava 2.3.96

homoto(u)n, *adj. febre* ~ a variety of fever synochus 2.12.38, 2.12.40 (*DMLBS*, s.v. *homotonus* "having the same tension, unius tenoris"), *febre homotetica* 2.12.38; *adj. as n. homoten* 2.12.44, †*homothena* 2.12.33, 2.12.34

honde see o(o)nde

hongand, *v.pr.ppl.* hanging (down), drooping 2.10.183, 3.19.72 (glossing Latin *dependens*), *hangond* 3.17.67; ~ *togeder* holding together, cohering 2.2.326, 2.13.226

ho(o)l(e), *adj.*[2] healthy 1.3.181, 1.4.456, 1.4.467; whole, unbroken 3.3.11, 3.20.176

hopen, *v.* to anticipate a good outcome 2.2.263

horhoune, *n.* horehound (*Marrubium vulgare*) 2.14.35, *harhoune* 2.14.32, *horhow* 2.8.81

hos(e)hede, *n.* hoarseness 2.12.134, 3.4.29

hostiel, *n.* hostel, inn 2.7.49

houeþ, *v.pr.3sg.* floats 3.6.2, *houeth* 3.8.85; *pr.sg.subj.* *houe* should float 2.3.460; *houand* hovering, floating 2.2.159, 2.2.171; *pr.3sg.* *houeth* overflows 2.4.17

humectif, *adj.* moistening, increasing moisture 1.4.807

†*humidus*, *adj.* wet, moist 1.4.282, 1.4.300; *adj. as n.pl.* †*humida* moist things 1.4.633

humorosite, *n.* moistness 3.16.67

humo(u)r(e), *n.* a bodily fluid, esp. one of the four humours of medieval medicine (blood, phlegm, red choler, black choler) 1.2.4, 1.4.59, 1.3.139, 2.2.84

humydite, *n.* moistness as a prime quality 1.4.34, 1.4.42, *humidite* 1.4.284, †*humiditas* 1.4.37, 1.4.295; moisture, liquid 1.3.35, 1.3.90

hurlond, *v.pr.ppl.* of a liquid: tossing, surging, disturbing 2.11.55, 2.13.427

hurlyng, *ger.* a commotion, disturbance, roiling (of the humours or other bodily fluids) 1.4.524, 2.10.112, *hurling* 2.2.89

hurre, *n.* of planetary motion: whir, buzz (loud but inaudible to human ears) 2.6.140

†*hyems*, *n.* winter 1.4.639, *yeme* 2.13.290, †*hyemps* 1.4.415, †*yemps* 1.4.407, †*yems* 3.16.165

hylonde, *v.pr.ppl.* covering 2.7.343; *pa.ppl.* *hylde* 2.7.339, *hilede* 1.4.154

himself(e), *pron.3sg.m/n.refl.* himself, itself 1.2.13, 1.3.22, 1.4.75

hynder, *adj.* at the back, posterior 2.3.189, 3.2.127, *hyndur* 2.4.393, *hynner* 2.3.184

i., *abbrev. id est*, that is Prol.8, Prol.31

iaw(e)nys see **jawnys**

ic(c)he, *n.* the itch, an itching skin disease 1.3.253, 3.20.49, *(ȝ)yche* 1.1.27, 2.4.183

†*ictericia*, *n.* jaundice 2.13.405, 2.14.40

†*iecur*, *n.* the liver 3.10.44, *jecur* 3.10.43; *jecur* (in beasts) the stomach 2.7.466

ieiun(e), *n.* the jejunum 1.3.31, 1.3.42, 1.3.62, †*ieiunum* 1.3.31, 1.3.37

†*ierariolon*, *n.* epilepsy 2.3.854 (see n.)

if, *conj.* if Prol.11, Prol.29; *neuerþeles* ~ but only if Prol.67

†*ignis*, *n.* fire 1.4.292, 1.4.300

†*iliaca* see †*yli(a)ca*

iliale see yliale

ilk, *pron.* each one 2.6.260

ilk(e), *pron. as adj.* same, aforementioned 1.2.36, 1.3.51, 1.4.671, 2.2.274

†*immediate*, *adv.* without an intermediary, directly 2.3.185, 2.3.186, †*inmediate* 1.3.105

immutacioun, *n.* changing 2.3.484

†*imperium*, *adj.* empyrean (heaven) 2.6.429, 2.6.433

impotent, *adj.* powerless 2.4.90, 3.19.229

impulsioun, *n.* driving upward 3.19.218

inanicioun, *n.* depletion of natural moisture 2.14.122, †*inanicio* 2.14.109

incencio(u)n, *n.* burning 2.9.26, 2.9.34, *incensioun* 2.2.63, 2.11.72

inclusioun, *n.* enclosure, inclusion 2.4.361, *enclusioun* 2.4.354

incorporacio(u)n, *n.* incorporation 3.7.66, 3.8.89, *encorperacioun* 3.7.85

incorporat(e), *ppl.adj.* incorporated 3.7.88, 3.8.93, *incorperat* 3.7.89

inder, *adj.* interior 1.4.545, 2.3.346, *indre* 2.8.292

indifferently, *adv.* equally, as equivalents 2.3.800

indisposeþ, *v.pr.3sg.* unsettles, disorders 2.4.377

indisposicioun, *n.* imbalance 1.4.305

induracioun, *n.* hardening 3.11.36

indurat(e), *adj.* hardened 2.13.263, 3.11.42

inequal, *adj.* of urine: having an uneven quality (esp. density) 1.4.151, 2.2.79, 2.2.104

†*infancia*, *n.* infancy 1.4.394, 1.4.397

inflacioun, *n.* inflation, swelling 2.4.366, 2.7.147

ingestioun, *n.* taking in of food, eating 2.2.314, 2.2.315

†*inmediate* see †*immediate*

innatural, *adj.* unnatural, against nature; *melancolie (melancoly)* ~ an excess of the humour melancholy 2.8.49, †*melancolia innaturalis* 2.8.53, 2.8.55; †*ypostasis innaturalis* hypostasis that lacks at least one of the five conditions of ideal hypostasis 3.19.104

inobedient, *adj.* resistant 2.13.237, 2.13.263

inopos, *adj.* (also as *n.*) of a dark red colour, similar to the colour of dark wine or muddy water 2.8.13, 2.13.6, *ynopos* 2.1.13, 2.1.52

inow see anogh

inspissacioun, *n.* thickness, thickening 2.6.45, 2.8.218

inspissede, *v.pa.ppl.* thickened 2.7.195

instrument, *n.* an organ, humour, or quality that performs a specific function 2.3.15, 2.3.179, 2.4.375, 2.13.214, †*instrumentum* 2.8.230

intencio(u)n, *n.* deepness of colour 2.8.14, 2.8.15; *intensioun* strengthening 1.4.260

intens(e), *adj.* of colour: deep, intense 1.4.264, 1.4.816, 2.5.9

interclusioun, *n.* enclosure 3.3.25

interpol(l)acioun, *n.* a period of relief between episodes of fever 2.3.320, 2.10.196, 2.10.199

interpol(l)ate, *adj.* of fever: intermittent 2.3.293, 2.3.312, 2.3.351, †*interpolatus* 2.3.312; *simple (double, treble)* ~ intermittent fever with one (two, three) episodes per day 2.3.313, 2.3.315, 2.3.316; *veray (vnueray)* ~ intermittent fever with predictable (unpredictable) episodes 2.6.113, 2.6.112

interpretacions, *n.pl.* translations Prol.20

interpretate, *v.* to understand by interpretation Prol.93

†*inuidus, adj.* envious 1.4.384

inward(e), *adv.* inwardly 1.4.250, 2.8.309; of texts: below, later in the work 2.3.121, 2.3.127, *inwart* 2.4.280; ~ of diseases: later in the course of the illness 2.2.343, 2.5.27

iolle, *n.* the back of the head 2.7.297

iourne, *n.* journey, way 2.7.56

ious(e), *n.* liquid matter produced in the stomach (chyme) and the intestines (chyle) 1.3.37, 1.3.51, *iows(e)* 1.3.12, 1.3.33; ~ urine 2.3.78; ~ ?juice or sap of a plant, ?broth 3.8.61; *iows* essential quality, medicinal virtue 1.4.817

iowis, iowys see jowis

ioynt(e), *n.* a joint 2.6.315, 3.16.76, ~ *of (in) þe rigebon(e)* 3.10.32, 3.10.91; *n.pl. ioyntz* 2.6.313

ioyntour(e), *n.* a joint 2.3.195, 3.16.87; ~ *of þe bak (rigebone)* a vertebra 2.3.196, 2.13.70, 3.2.113; *n.pl. iountours of þe ryge* 2.3.193

ioyouse, *adj.* joyous 2.7.33

†*ipsa vrina, phr.* the urine itself 1.4.30

†*irascens, adj.* angry, easy to anger 1.4.374

†*ismon, n.* the space between the trachea and the esophagus 2.7.388

ismonie, *n.* ailment caused by something caught in the throat 3.4.31, †*ismonia* 3.4.31, †*ysmonia* 3.4.34; †*ismonia* an aposteme in the ismon (between trachea and esophagus), either *squinancia* (if within the *ismon*) or *cynancia* (if entirely outside the *ismon*) 2.7.394

issu(e), *n.* exit, place at which sth. or sb. leaves 1.3.19, 1.3.147, 1.4.498, 3.2.117, *essues* 1.3.201

iuggede, *v.pa.ppl.* judged 2.7.315

†iuuenes, *n.pl.* young people 1.4.624, 1.4.646

†iuuentus, *n.* youth 1.4.388, 1.4.390

jawnys, *n.* jaundice 2.7.61, 2.7.68, *jaunys* 2.14.40, *iawnys* 3.6.47, *jawenys* 3.20.109

jowis, *n.pl.* the jaws or jowls 3.4.18, *iowis* 3.4.37, *iowys* 2.3.623

kacheþ, *v.pr.3sg.* acquires, takes on 1.4.563; *pr.pl. kachen* 1.4.523

kalender, *n.* calendar 2.6.268, 2.6.277, 2.6.494

kalends, *n.* the first day of a month 2.6.233, 2.6.235, *abbrev. Kal.* 1.4.409, 1.4.411

kamel, *n.* camel 2.7.25; *n.pl. kamailes* 2.7.27, *kamayles* 2.7.26

kane, *v.pr.pl.* know, understand Prol.19, *can* 3.6.11

kare, *n.* care, concern, worry 1.4.558, 1.4.659

karopos, *adj.* (also as *n.*) of a colour like camel's hair 2.1.44, 2.7.1, *karapos* 2.1.11, 2.13.101

kawates, *n.pl.* cavities, cells, compartments 2.3.659, 2.7.263

kene, *adj.* of choler or phlegm: sharp, sour, bitter 2.9.156

kenet, *n.* a hunting dog 2.7.75

kenneþ, *v.pr.3sg.* teaches 2.6.290

kepe(n), *v.* to keep, preserve 1.4.154, 2.2.100, 3.16.257; *v.pr.3sg. kepeþ* keeps, observes, holds 1.4.147, 2.6.109; *kepeþ hym* retains for itself 1.3.92; *pr.pl. kepe(n)* 1.4.266, 2.4.35; *pr.sg.subj. kepe* should preserve, retain Prol.89, 2.4.112; *impv. kepe* 1.4.686; *pa.ppl. kepede* 2.3.193, *kept(e)* 1.4.203, 2.3.651

kepyng, *ger.* care of oneself or others 1.4.365, 1.4.553; *keping* retention 2.7.298

keste, *v.pa.sg.* cast, threw 2.7.53

kichyn, *n.* a kitchen 1.4.498, *kychyne* 2.3.671

kiker, *n.* the clitoris (poss. with some confusion with the hymen) 2.7.558

kil(e), *n.* the *kilis* vein, the inferior vena cava (?or the renal veins) 2.3.76, 3.10.4, 3.10.29, *kyl* 3.10.58, *†kilis* 2.3.76, *kiles* 2.13.67, 2.13.68

kiles, *n.pl.* sores 3.18.73

†kilos, *n.* juice, sap 2.3.77

kirnelles, *n.pl.* granulous particles in urine 3.4.2; ~ *of a fike* seeds of a fig 3.18.102

knarles, *n.pl.* small grains (like the seeds of a fig), lumps (like acorns) 3.18.48, 3.18.101, 3.18.103

knarlish, *adj.* lumpy 3.18.33

knarres, *n.pl.* swellings, lumps 3.18.115

knoddes, *n.pl.* swellings, lumps 3.18.47, 3.18.122

knoddishe, *adj.* lumpy 3.18.33

knoden, *v.pa.ppl.* kneaded, combined, thickened 3.17.17, *knoddede* 3.18.75

knokel, *n.* the knuckle, a joint 2.3.82, 3.16.153

knoppes, *n.pl.* swellings, lumps 3.18.122

knorles, *n.pl.* swellings, lumps 3.18.129

knottes, *n.pl.* knots, lumps 3.18.94, 3.18.115

knotty, *adj.* lumpy 3.18.109

knowlich, *n.* knowledge Prol.50

knyt(e), *v.pa.ppl.* knit, connected 1.3.25, 1.3.58, *knet* 2.3.102

kogh see **cowh**

koghing, *ger.* coughing 2.7.384, *kow(h)yng* 2.13.141, 2.13.380, *kuoghing* 2.13.143

konne, *v.* to know 2.6.302

konnyng, *ppl.adj.* knowledgeable, learned Prol.17

kowe, *n.* a cow 1.4.506; *poss. kowes* cow's 1.3.55, 3.16.277

kowh, kuowh see **cowh**

kowhing, kow(h)yng, kuoghing see **koghing**

kraskehede, *n.* vigour 3.17.33

kyanos, *adj.* (also as *n.*) of a dark reddish-purple colour, similar to rotten blood or Tyrian purple 2.1.13, 2.1.52, *kianos* 2.13.55, 3.10.33

kychyne see **kichyn**

kyde-lambes, *n.poss.* a young goat's, a kid's 1.4.741

kyl see **kil(e)**

kynd(e), *n.* nature, constitution (of an individual) 1.3.94, 1.3.154, 1.4.289; nature in general 2.2.273, *kind(e)* 1.4.573, 2.2.232; gender, sex 1.4.8; *way of* ~ the course of nature 1.1.20

kynd(e), *adj.* natural, *kind(e)* 1.3.97, 1.4.155, 2.2.216

kynd(e)ly, *adv.* naturally 1.1.6, 1.1.23, 1.2.10, 1.3.10, *kind(e)ly* 2.3.737, 2.8.39, *kindeli* 1.4.714

kyner, *n.* the *kilis* vein in women 2.3.141, †*kynirz* 2.3.141

kyns, *n.pl.* cracks in the skin, chapping of the skin 1.1.28

labored, *v.pa.ppl.* (that have been) accomplished, done Prol.74

lache, *adj.* of colour: dull, faded 2.8.36

lachede, *n.* of colour: dimness, dullness 2.8.15

†*lacteus,* *adj.* (also as *n.*) of the colour of milk or whey Prol.118, 1.3.52, 2.1.10

langer, *comp.adj.* ~ *or* for a greater period of time before 2.8.122

languishand, *v.pr.ppl.* suffering Prol.45

lappates, *n.pl.* lobes (of the lungs or liver) 2.7.399, 2.7.459, *lappatz* 2.13.187, *lip-petes* 2.13.180

large, *adj.* generous 1.4.368, †*largus* 1.4.369

largehed(e), *n.* largeness 2.2.97, 3.1.18

laste, *adj.* ~ *colour* ultimate colour, final stage of colour development 1.1.13

late, *adj.* slow, gradual 1.2.4; *of* ~ *tyme* recently 2.10.190

late, *adv.* recently Prol.80, 2.3.483

lateþ, *v.pr.3sg.* lets, allows 1.3.18, *late* 1.4.41; *impv. late* 1.4.162, 2.3.276

†*laurinum* see **†*oleum laurinum***

leche, *n.*[1] physician, healer Prol.68, Prol.98, Prol.110

lech(e), *n.*[2] *water* ~ the water leech (*Hirudo medicinalis*) 2.3.692, 3.16.244

lechecraft(e), *n.* the science or practice of medicine 2.4.179, 2.6.468

lechery(e), *n.* (lustful) sexual intercourse 2.3.491, 2.4.125, *lecherie* 2.3.679

ledit, *v.pr.3sg.* returns, guides, leads 1.3.176

lekes, *n.pl.* leeks 2.8.84, *likes* 1.4.751

lele, *adj.* loyal, reliable, faithful Prol.87

lende, *n.* kidney 2.4.69; *n.pl. lendes* the loins or kidneys (distinction not always clear in context) 1.1.4, 2.2.156

lene, *adj.* lean, thin 1.4.674, 2.3.838

lenehede, *n.* leanness 2.3.511, 2.3.646

lent(e), *adj.* of heat or fever (rarely of other symptoms): gentle, slow, easy 2.3.361, 2.3.375, 2.6.535, 2.8.161

lentlyes, *n.pl.* lentils 1.4.750

leny see **lonye**

lenysh, *adj.* somewhat lean, somewhat thin 3.8.39

lep(e), *adj.* ~ *ʒere* leap year 2.6.237, 2.6.243

lepre, *n.* leprosy 2.3.739; rosacea, which is called "lepre" when it afflicts women 3.16.203

lepre, *adj.* afflicted with leprosy 2.3.682

lerede, *v.pa.ppl.* learned Prol.20, 2.7.25

lernyng, *ger.* learning 2.8.215

lesingez, *ger.pl.* lies Prol.68

lesnend, *v.pr.ppl.* loosening 1.4.766

lest(e), *adj., adv., adj. as n.* least Prol.34, 1.4.134, 2.3.353

lesteth, *v.pr.3sg.* lasts, extends 2.7.447; *pr.sg.subj. leste* should last, should continue to exist 2.2.345

leþi, *adj.* weak 2.6.183

letres, *n.pl.* (knowledge of) writing; *wiþouten* ~ illiterate Prol.29

letteþ, *v.pr.3sg.* hinders 1.4.550, *letteth* 3.2.17; *pa.ppl. letted(e)* Prol.53, 1.3.47, 1.4.252; *lettede of* blocked with respect to 2.2.175

leucofleume, *n.* leucophlegmasia, a form of dropsy 2.4.27, †*leucofleuma* 2.4.27, †*leucofleumancia* 2.4.46

leue, *v.*[1] to believe in (God) 1.4.676

leuen, *v.*[2]*pr.pl.* remain 1.3.216

leuest, *v.*[3]*pr.2sg.* live 2.6.289; *pr.3sg. leueþ* 2.2.199, 2.7.410; *pr.pl. leuen* 3.16.104, 3.16.121

leueþ, *v.*[4]*pr.3sg.* leaves, takes leave of 2.2.190

leuing, *ger.* leaving, abandoning 2.7.293

leuyng, *ger.* living, life 1.4.565

lewede, *adj.* unlearned, not literate 1.3.72

liciouse, *adj.* delicious, sweet 2.9.100

liciouste, *n.* sweetness, tastiness 1.4.782

†*lienteria,* *n.* diarrhea that includes undigested pieces of food 3.4.44, 3.4.47

ligges, *n.pl.* the legs 1.3.89, 2.6.465

lik-pot, *n.* the index finger 2.6.314, 2.6.315

lippiarie, *n.* a hot fever caused by putrefied choler beneath the skin, with cold internal organs and hot extremities of the body 2.3.342, †*lipparia* 2.3.341

lippotomie, *n.* fainting 2.4.296, †*lip(p)otomia* 2.4.296, *lipitomia* 2.4.298

liquidite, *n.* liquidness 2.3.13

liquo(u)r, *n.* a liquid, a fluid 2.2.40, 2.3.226; of urine: the liquid base, fluid portion (excluding suspended contents) 1.4.30, *lycoure* 1.3.186, †*liquor vrine* 1.4.29

*listen, *v.pr.pl.* want, desire (to do sth.) 1.4.98

litarge, *n.* lethargy, stupor 3.2.133, *litargi* 2.12.67, *litargy* 2.12.59, †*litargia* 2.12.67

†*litargicus,* *adj. as n.* someone suffering from *litargia* 2.12.69

liteþ, *v.pr.3sg.* relieves, lightens (of a burden) 2.3.137

lith, *n.* a joint; *oute of* ~ out of joint 3.2.116

lit(i)asi, *n.* bladder stone 2.8.312, 3.11.37, *litiasy* 2.7.600, †*litiasis* 2.7.602, *3.11.3, †*lytiasis* 3.11.2, †*lityasis* 1.4.113

litil, *adv.* but ~ *goand o partie* only tending slightly 2.5.78

litilhede, *n.* smallness, scantiness 1.4.363, *litilhode* 1.4.363, *litlehede* 2.12.79

†*liuidus*, *adj.* (also as *n.*) of a bluish-grey colour, similar to lead Prol.115, 1.4.501, 2.1.10

liȝtede, *v.pa.ppl.* lighted, lit Prol.48

liȝthede, *n.* lightness, agility 2.2.311, 2.11.80

liȝtly, *adv.* easily, lightly, gently Prol.48, 1.4.226; *comp. liȝtlier* 1.3.46

liȝtsom(e)nes(se), *n.* lightness, ease 2.2.325, 2.4.367

liȝtsomhede, *n.* lightness, ease 2.13.228

loke, *v.pr.sg.subj.* examine 2.7.78, 3.8.13; *impv.* 1.4.136; *pa.ppl. lokede* 1.4.81, 1.4.134; *pr.ppl. lokand* appearing 2.2.335

lombes, *n.poss.* lamb's 1.4.748, *one-ȝeres* ~ a one-year-old lamb's 1.4.741

†*longao(u)n*, *n.* the rectum 1.3.73, 1.3.76, 1.4.89

longe see **lunge**

longeþ, *v.pr.3sg.* belongs, is proper (to) 1.3.138

lonye, *n.* the loins, upper part of the loins 2.4.87 (see n.); *leny pece* the lower back 2.4.84

lorn, *v.pa.ppl.* lost 2.1.109, 3.20.193

*louseþ, *v.pr.3sg.* dissolves 3.8.36 (see n.)

louyng, *ger.* loving, kind 1.4.368

louȝhyng, *ger.* laughing 1.4.368

lowh, *adj.* dull, dim, faded 1.4.816

loyn, *adj.* of fruit: ripened by lying for a period of time 2.7.158 (see n.)

lucre, *n.* wealth Prol.23, ~ *of fauour* wealth acquired through patronage Prol.37

lunge, *n.* the lung 1.3.140, 2.3.230, *longe* 1.3.115; *n.pl. lunges* 2.1.75, 2.1.78, *lungez* 2.7.377, 2.8.277, *longes* 2.6.461, 2.13.206

†*luteique coloris*, *phr.* and of muddy colour 1.4.386

lym(e), *n.* a bodily limb 1.3.6, 1.3.88, 1.3.201, 3.10.47

lymouse, *adj.* slippery 2.3.648

lymyng, *ger.* radiance, glow 1.4.513

lyueraunce, *n.* deliverance, emission 2.7.219

mader, *n.* common madder (*Rubia tinctorum*), a plant used for dyeing 3.20.305

magnete, *n.* ~ *stone* lode-stone 1.3.33

maistre, *n.* master 1.4.63, 2.1.97, 2.8.112, *mayster* 2.6.481, *maystre* 2.1.111, 2.4.389

maistri(e), *n.* mastery, power over, dominance 2.4.267, 2.6.83, *maystrie* 2.7.35, **maystry* 1.4.58

maistri(e), *v.* to overcome 2.2.214, 2.7.122, *maystry* 2.7.179, *maistre* 2.2.83; *pr.3sg.* *maistrieþ* 2.7.16, *maystrieþ* 2.6.513; *pr.sg.subj.* *maistri* 1.4.574, *maystre* 2.4.287; *pr.ppl.* *maistriand* 2.2.238; *pa.ppl.* *maistriede* 2.7.174, *maystried* 2.5.23, *maystriede* 2.5.56

makyng, *ger.pl.* production (of urine) 1.3.199, 1.4.128

malanchima see *melanchyme*

malancolie see **melancoli(e)**

mal(e), *adj. as n.* male 2.3.638, 3.16.336

maliciouse, *adj.* perilous, dangerous, bad 2.3.262, 2.3.683

manant, *n.* the rest, remaining amount 2.7.303

manye, *n.* madness 2.12.66, †*mania* 2.12.66, †*manya* 2.12.58

†*mappa spiritualis*, *phr.* the diaphragm 2.7.438

†*mappa ventris*, *phr.* the diaphragm 2.7.437

marchandise, *n.* trade, the mercantile profession 2.6.213

marow(e), *n.* marrow (*lit. and fig.*), essence Prol.81, 2.3.189, 2.7.325, *marrow* 2.7.325, *marie* 3.4.7

†*marubium*, *n.* horehound (*Marrubium vulgare*) 2.8.81

mas(e)ing, *ger.* confusion, bewilderment 2.3.364, 3.20.196

mater(e), *n.* a morbid substance in the body 1.3.232, 1.4.242, *materie* 2.3.192, *matier* 2.3.672; *n.pl.* 1.3.238, *materies* 2.2.37, 2.2.72, *materijs* 2.3.821; ~ matter in general 1.2.42, 1.3.64

materiale, *adj.* ~ *membre of lif* the organ that produces the material basis of life, the liver 2.8.234, †*membrum materiale* 2.8.233

math(e), *v.* makes, causes (abbrev. form of *maketh*) 2.5.30, 2.5.32, 2.13.87, 3.16.346

matrice, *n.* the uterus 1.4.363, 1.4.492, 2.3.634, †*matrix* 2.3.634

maw(e), *n.* the stomach 1.3.20, 1.3.29; the liver (in animals) 2.7.466

maw(e) ȝate, *n.* the pylorus, the opening from the stomach into the duodenum 1.3.20, 1.3.29

mayn, *n.* strength, essence 1.4.817, 2.13.103

mayste see **mowe**

mede, *n. mellicratum*, a drink of honey and water 3.16.289, †*medo* 3.16.289, †*meldo* 3.16.289

medeleþ, *v.pr.3sg.* mixes, mingles, blends 2.3.14, *medelith* 2.3.389; *pa.ppl.* *medelede* 2.5.5

†*mediana*, *adj.* the median vein, the median cubital vein (see **veyn(e)**) 2.3.118

†*mediate*, *adv.* by way of an intermediary 1.3.107

medwy, *adj.* meadowy 1.4.577

medycynable, *adj.* therapeutic, useful as a medicine 1.1.26

mees, *n.pl.* mice 2.14.49

melanchyme, *n.* black jaundice 2.14.56, *†melanchima* 2.14.55, *†melanchimon* 2.14.55, *†malanchima* 2.14.56

melancolic, *adj.* melancholic, characterized by black choler 1.3.237, 1.4.472, *melancolik* 1.4.506, *†melancolicus* 1.4.317, 1.4.354

melancoli(e), *n.* the humour melancholy, black choler, black bile 1.3.124, 1.3.143, 1.4.622, *melancoly(e)* 1.4.632, 2.4.255, *malancolie* 2.7.41, *†melanc(h)olia* 1.4.301, 1.4.433

mele, *n.* flour, meal 3.20.91, 3.20.352

†*mellicratum*, *n.* a drink of honey and water 3.16.289, 3.16.299

meltandhede, *n.* meltedness, the state of being dissolved 2.3.13

melteþ, *v.pr.3sg.* melts, dissolves 3.7.27, 3.8.84, *meltiþ* 2.3.394, *melteth* 3.8.26; *pr. pl. melten* 1.4.44, 2.3.549, 3.12.20; *pr.ppl. meltand(e)* 1.4.43, 3.8.32

meltyng(e), *ger.* liquefaction, dissolving 1.2.4, 1.2.16, *melting* 2.2.152; *ger.pl. meltingz* particles produced through consumption in the lungs 2.8.289

meluede, *v.pa.ppl.* ripened 2.7.158

membre, *n.* an organ, limb, or other bodily member Prol.61, 1.4.492, *menbre* 1.3.88, 1.3.96; *womennes membres* female genitalia 1.1.32

memoratif, *adj.* pertaining to memory 2.7.295, *†memoratiua* 2.7.294

memore, *n.* memory 2.7.295

memorial, *adj.* pertaining to memory 2.7.295, *†memoralis* 2.7.294

mene, *n.*[1] a means, a way (of doing sth.) 1.3.107

mene, *n.*[2] temperance, moderation 1.4.542

mene, *v.* to mean, to signify 1.4.297, 2.2.114; *pr.3sg. meneþ* 1.4.56

mene, *adj.* moderate, average, in a middle state 1.4.69, 1.4.141, 1.4.706, *meine* 2.8.11

men(e)ly, *adv.* gently, lightly 3.2.109; moderately 1.4.457, 2.6.19

mengeþ, *v.pr.3sg.* mixes 2.3.14; *pr.pl. mengen* 3.9.112; *impv. menge* 1.1.40; *pa.ppl. menged(e)* 1.4.517, 2.3.420, *menkede* 2.3.40, *menk(e)t* 2.3.290, 2.9.19

meng(e)yng, *ger.* mixing 1.4.742, 2.2.40

†*menstruum*, *n.* menstruation 1.4.496; *n.pl. menstrua* 1.4.77

†*menstruus*, *adj.* †*sanguis* ~ menstrual blood 2.2.41

meny, *n.* retinue, followers, meinie 2.6.225

meserays, *n.pl.* the mesenteric veins 1.3.36, *meseraices* 1.3.58, *meserayces* 1.3.63, *miseraices* 2.3.60, †*meseraice* 1.3.36

mete, *n.* food 1.3.3, 1.3.10; *grene metes* green vegetables 3.16.261

meuyng, *ger.* moving, motion, activities (of soul, of organs) 1.4.678, 2.4.378, *mevyng* 3.2.119, *mewing* 2.7.199, *mewyng* 3.3.60; agitation of urine to separate the contents 1.4.226

mewand, *v.pr.ppl.* moving 3.2.109

minucioun, *n.* bloodletting 2.3.125

minusheþ, *v.pr.3sg.* diminishes, reduces 3.4.14, *mynus(h)eþ* 1.4.531, 3.16.332; *pr.ppl. mynusshand* 3.8.112; *pa.ppl. minussede* 1.4.699, *menusede* 2.3.252, *mynus(s)hede* 3.8.117, 3.11.40

mischeif, *n.* disease, harm 2.4.302

mixtioun, *n.* mixture 2.2.39, 2.2.47

miӡtes, *n.pl.* physical powers, strength 2.2.303

mo see mo(o)

moder, *n.* mother Prol.4, 1.4.364; *modres* mother's 2.3.725; ~ *childe* mother's child 1.4.642; *tendre (softe)* ~ the *pia mater* membrane in the brain 2.7.340; *hard modir* the *dura mater* membrane in the brain 2.7.341

modie, *adj.* muddy, clay-like 1.4.385, *mody* 1.4.580, 2.13.3

modissh, *adj.* muddy, like mud in consistency 3.7.23

modur, *n.* the uterus 2.3.419, 2.3.797, *moder* 2.3.634, 2.3.841; *moder ballok stones* the ovaries 2.7.544

moisthede see moyst(e)hed(e)

mollisshede, *v.pa.ppl.* softened, weakened 2.8.323

†*monoculus*, *n.* the blind gut or caecum 1.3.68

monyth, *n.* month 2.3.667, 2.3.674, *moneth* 2.3.673, 3.16.270, *monyþ* 2.6.372; *n.pl. moneþes* 2.6.267

mo(o), *adj.* more Prol.48, 2.1.6, 2.3.306

mordicacioun, *n.* corrosiveness, gnawing 1.3.69

mordificatif, *adj.* corrosive, caustic 1.1.24

morisshe, *adj.* like a moor, boggy, marshy 1.4.578

morphe, *n.* the skin disease morphea 1.3.254

mortificacio(u)n, *n.* extinction of natural heat through excess of cold, destruction through excess cold 2.1.19, 2.1.30, †*mortificacio* 2.1.56

mosse, *n.* moss on a tree 1.3.174

most(e), *v.pr.2sg.* must 1.4.55; *pr.3sg.* ~ 1.3.69, 2.8.244; *pr.3sg.impers.* þe ~ it is necessary for you, you must 1.4.4; *pr.pl. mosten* 3.11.10

mote, *n.* a tiny particle, a mote 3.16.4; *n.pl.* dust particles (in the sun) 2.4.144, 3.9.15; dust-like particles in urine Prol.144, 3.16.1

motif, *n.* reason, explanation 2.4.180

moute, *v.pr.sg.subj.* should lose hair, should moult 2.3.454, 2.3.464

mouþe, *n. ouer* ~ upper entrance 1.3.58

mowe, *v. shal* ~ will be able (to) Prol.65; *pr.2sg. mayste* may, can, are able to 1.4.19; *pr.3sg. mai(e)* Prol.16, 2.13.162; *pr.pl. mow(e)* 1.4.126, 1.4.609, *mai* 2.3.814, 2.13.182; *pa.sg. and pl. myƷt* might, could, was/were able Prol.30, Prol.51, 1.2.14

mowlede, *v.pa.ppl.* mouldy 1.4.743

moyst(e)hed(e), *n.* moistness 1.4.296, 1.4.435, 1.4.800, *moisthede* 1.4.34

moysten, *v.* to moisten, to make (sth.) moist 2.9.118; *pr.3sg. moysteþ* 1.4.681; *pr. ppl. moystand* 1.4.808

moyst(o)ur(e), *n.* moisture, liquid 1.3.33, 1.3.40, 1.4.604, 2.9.117, 3.16.248

multrith, *v.pr.3sg.* crumbles, as by rubbing between the fingers 3.8.84; *impv. multre* 3.8.83

†multus, *adj.* prolific 1.4.379

mundefie(n), *v.* to cleanse *2.6.514, 2.9.80; *pr.3sg. mundefieþ* 1.3.124; *pa.sg. mundefiede* 1.3.128

muselynges, *ger.pl.* ?mouldy pieces 3.20.102 (see n.)

musseleþ, *v.pr.3sg.* ?becomes mouldy, sloughs off 3.7.21 (see n.)

mustryng, *ger.* muttering, whispering 2.7.58

mych(e), *adj.* much, great Prol.38, 2.13.76; *in how mich, in alse* ~ in as much (as) Prol.47, 2.2.75

mych(e), *adv.* very, greatly Prol.44, 1.4.576

myche(l), mychyl see **mykel**

myd, *n.* the middle part (of the body) 1.4.199

myd(de), *adj.* middle 1.4.205, 2.3.152; the second of three 2.3.291, 2.7.548; ~ *veyn* the median cubital vein (see **veyn(e)**) 2.3.118

myddes, *n.* the middle part (of an organ, a urine sample, etc.) 1.3.133, 1.4.183, *myddis* 2.7.572, *myddys* 2.2.171

myd(d)red(d)(e), *n.* the diaphragm 2.3.98, 2.3.782, 2.8.162, 3.20.186

mydpoynt, *n.* the centre 2.6.376

mydsomer, *n.* ~ *day* midsummer day, possibly also the summer solstice 2.6.271

myes, *n.* a dish made with bread crumbs 2.7.59, 2.7.60

mygh see myȝt(e)

mykel, *n.* a great amount 1.4.490

mykel, *adj.* much, great 1.4.54, 1.4.68, *mykil* 1.4.7, *mikel* 2.3.44, *mychel* 3.18.28, *mychil* 1.4.265, *mychyl* 1.3.203; *is as ~ for to say* means, is the same as 1.1.3; *in as ~ as (for alse ~ as, etc.)* insofar as 1.4.41, 3.18.28

mykel, *adv.* much, greatly, very 1.3.185, *mykyl* 1.4.222

mykel-man, *n.* the middle finger 2.6.316

mylt(e), *n.* the spleen 1.1.27, 1.3.123, 2.4.12

mynde, *n.* mind; *haue ~* remember, be aware of Prol.12; *makeþ ~* mentions Prol.28

myskepyng, *ger.* faulty care, misgovernance 1.3.239, 2.2.224

myslikyng, *ger.* suffering, discomfort 2.3.456, 2.3.531

mysreuleþ, *v.pr.3sg.* takes poor care (of oneself) 2.13.270

myssayingz, *n.pl.* abusive language Prol.31

mystisshe, *adj.* misty 2.7.591

mystrauailede, *v.pa.ppl.* strained through over-exertion, overworked 2.13.67, *mystraualid* 3.10.39

mystrauailyng, *ger.* harmful exertion, straining, suffering 2.4.141, 2.13.77

mysvse, *v.pr.sg.subj.* use improperly; *~ lif* live badly Prol.67

myswrenkt, *v.pa.ppl.* of veins: twisted, misplaced 3.10.30

myswriste, *n.* wrenching, torsion 2.13.77

myȝt see mowe

myȝt, *adj.* mighty, powerful, able 2.8.357

myȝt(e), *n.* power, might, force 1.3.70, 1.4.74, *myȝght* 2.3.285, *mygh* 2.14.85; *n.pl.* physical or mental powers 2.2.302, 2.3.154, *myȝtz* 2.3.158; *~ of þe skyn* power of the skin (to exude morbid matter) 1.3.251; *of ~* strong enough, of sufficient power 1.3.250; *with ~* powerfully 2.3.132

myȝtihede, *n.* strength, physical power 2.2.308, 2.9.10, *myȝtyed* 2.2.241

myȝt(t)ely, *adv.* greatly 1.1.36, 1.4.253

myȝt(t)en, *v.* to strengthen 1.4.650, 2.5.28, 2.9.118

myȝty, *adj.* powerful 1.3.168, 1.3.175, *myȝti* 2.1.72

namelik, *adv.* namely, especially 2.4.114

namen, *n.pl.* names (a rare plural form) 3.16.130

narowen, *v.pr.pl.* make (sth.) narrow 2.2.73

nase, *n.* nose 2.2.312, 3.16.204

natiuite, *n.* birth; ~ *of oure Lorde* the birth of Jesus, Christmas Day 2.6.251

†*naturaliter*, *adv.* naturally 1.4.263, 1.4.332

nauel(e), *n.* the navel 2.3.758, 2.7.93

nebulouse, *adj.* cloudy 2.7.591, 3.20.54

nedes, *adv.* necessarily 2.8.244, 2.8.359

nediþ, *v.pr.3sg.* needs 2.13.276; *pr.3sg.impers. nedeþ* (it) is necessary 1.4.235, *nedith* 3.16.110; *pr.3sg.impers. him nedeþ* (it) is necessary for him 1.3.29

nedyng, *ger.* a need, being in need 1.4.666

nefresi(e), *n.* nephritis, inflammation of the kidneys, kidney stone 2.4.69, 2.7.600, *nefresy* 2.13.61, *†nefresia* 2.4.76, *†nefresis* 2.4.76, *†nefrisis* 2.4.69

nefretik, *adj.* nephritic, affected by nephritis 2.4.75

neihen, *v.pr.pl.* move nearer 2.3.251, 2.3.807, *neʒhen* 2.4.300

†*nephilis*, *n.* hypostasis that rises to the top of the urine sample 2.2.354, 3.19.75

neres, *n.pl.* the kidneys 2.4.81, 2.4.139

nerhand(e), *adv.* almost, nearly 2.2.257, 2.6.394, *nerehond(e)* 1.3.262, *2.7.572

nerþeles, *adv.* nevertheless 1.4.437, 1.4.573

†*nerui petrosi*, *phr.* auditory nerves (*lit.* stony nerves) 2.3.161

neruosite, *n.* the state of being full of nerves or sinews 2.10.219

neruo(u)se, *adj.* ful of nerves or sinews 2.13.147, 2.13.211

†*neruus audibilis*, *n.* auditory nerve 2.3.159

nesch(e), *adj.* soft 1.4.43, 3.11.16, *nesshe* 2.6.36, *neysshe* 2.7.262

nesen, *v.* to sneeze 2.3.633; *pr.3sg. nesith amonge* sneezes at intervals 2.3.632

nes(she)hed(e), *n.* softness 2.3.14, 3.16.78

nessheþ, *v.pr.3sg.* softens, melts 2.8.252; *pa.ppl. neisshede* 2.8.323

nesyng, *ger.* sneezing; ~ *amonge* sneezing at intervals 3.4.22

nete, *n.* cow, ox 2.8.17, 3.20.377, *n.poss. netes* 2.11.5, *netis* 1.4.744

neþer, *adj.comp.* lower 1.3.19, 1.3.61; *sup. nederest* lowest 2.4.36, *nedrerest* 2.7.449; ~ *hole* lower opening 1.3.196; ~ *membre* a lower organ, in particular the genitals 2.3.774; ~ *pece* the lower part (of the back) 2.4.83

nettys, *n.pl.* thin skins or membranes 2.4.34

neuerthemore, *adv.* not at all, not entirely; ~ *hote* not entirely hot 1.4.441

newely, *adv.* in a new way Prol.79; recently 2.7.171, 2.7.177

neȝhede, *n.* nearness, proximity 1.4.600

†*niger*, *adj.* black 2.1.10, 2.4.221, 2.14.57

noble, *adj.* important, high-ranking, of high quality 1.3.96, 1.4.783; *sup. noblist* 2.6.224; of symptoms, etc.: of high quality, excellent, positive 2.2.309

noblete, *n.* excellence, importance 2.2.35

nocyf, *adj.* noxious, harmful 2.7.153

none, *n.* noon, midday 2.6.160, 2.6.161

†*non expers fraudis*, *phr.* not innocent of fraud, not without guile 1.4.386

norisch, *v.* to nourish, sustain, maintain 1.3.10, *norisshe* 1.3.135, *norsche* 2.3.31, *noryssch* 1.3.99; *pr.3sg. norischeþ* 1.4.641, *norissheþ* 1.4.708, *nursheþ* 3.19.20; *pr. pl. norisshe* 2.7.22; *pr.ppl. nurishand* 2.8.235, *nurishonde* 2.8.235; *pa.ppl. norisshede* 1.4.203, 2.3.721, *nurshede* 3.19.20

noris(s)chyng, *ger.* the act of nourishing, nutriment 1.3.17, 1.3.130, *noris(sc)hing* 1.3.95, 3.16.329, *norisshing* 2.3.27, *noriss(h)yng* 1.3.92, 2.3.743, *noryschyng* 1.3.116, *norysshyng* 1.3.215, *nurisshing* 2.1.88, 3.10.75

noselyng, *adv. liggen* ~ to lie face down 2.13.218

nosethirle, *n.* nostril 3.4.20, *noseþirle* 1.3.148, 2.7.358

notable, *adj.* noteworthy Prol.61

noteful, *adj.* needful, useful 1.3.210, 1.4.650, 2.9.72

nothe, *adj.* a type of quartan fever caused by corrupt humours 2.11.38, *†not(h)a* 2.4.318, 2.11.37

noþer, *pron. non* ~ no other 1.3.106

no(u)þer ... ne, *corr.conj.* neither ... nor Prol.14, 1.2.8, 1.4.502, *neiþer ... ne* 3.6.15, 3.18.68, *neþer ... ne* 1.4.643

noy, *n.* harm, injury 1.4.558

noyeþ, *v.pr.3sg.* harms, injures 1.4.541, 1.4.542, *noyeth* 3.16.198; *pr.pl. noyen* 3.16.184, *noyȝen* 1.4.812; *pa.ppl. noyede* 2.9.101

noyouse, *adj.* harmful, dangerous, noxious 2.6.340, 2.7.154

noȝt, *adv.* not Prol.12, Prol.48, *noght* 1.3.106, 1.4.349, *nouȝt* 1.4.173, *nogh* 2.14.102, 3.8.5, *noȝ* 1.3.216, 2.10.200, *noȝht* 2.6.259

noȝtforþan, *adv.* nonetheless, nevertheless, despite that 1.3.82, 1.4.22, *nogh(t)-forþan* 2.3.462, 2.3.515

nuk, *n.* (top of) the spinal cord or spine, the nape of the neck 2.3.188 (see n.), 2.3.189, *†nuca* 2.3.188

nunciatif, *adj.* forecasting (the future course of an illness) 2.2.206, 2.2.209, *nunciatyues* (modifying n.pl.) 2.13.229, **nunciatiuus* 2.13.243

nurish- see **norisch, noris(s)chyng**

nutrityues, *adj. as n.pl.* the digestive organs 2.3.127, 2.8.271

nygh, *prep.* near 2.3.503, *nyȝh* 2.6.210

nygheþ, *v.pr.3sg.* draws near 2.6.355, 2.6.367; *pr.ppl. nyghonde* 1.4.636

nygh(h)and, *adv.* nearly 2.1.17, 2.14.130

ny(ȝ), *adv.* near, nearly, almost 1.3.262, 1.4.5, 2.4.85, *nyh(e)* 1.4.511, 1.4.637, *nygh* 1.4.634, 2.13.146

nyȝhede, *n.* nearness 1.4.601, 2.3.253

o, *num.* one 1.4.257, 2.3.379

o, *prep.* of 2.3.115, 2.4.112; on 2.3.562, 2.3.692 (the two senses not always distinguishable)

obediens, *n.* obedience Prol.54

†octomia, *n.* orthopnoea; difficulty in breathing, esp. while lying down 2.3.119 (see n.), 2.3.121

octomyk, *adj. as n.* someone suffering from *octomia* (orthopnoea; difficulty in breathing, esp. while lying down) 2.13.399, *†octomicus* 2.3.243, 2.13.399

ocupacions, *n.pl.* activities 1.4.252

ocupiede, *v.pa.ppl.* engaged, kept busy 1.4.248, 1.4.249

od(de), *adj.* of integers: not divisible by two, odd 2.2.242, 2.2.243

oder, *adj.* other 3.4.52

office, *n.* function 2.4.65, 2.4.247, 2.7.143

ofolde, *adj.* simple, "one-fold" 2.8.116

of(te)tym(e), *adv.* often, oft-times 1.4.356, 2.7.491, 2.8.86, *oftymez* Prol.6, *ofte-tymes* Prol.53

oght, *pron.* anything, to any extent 2.11.65, 2.13.210

olde see **elde,** *n.*

†oleum laurinum, *n.* oil of laurel 1.4.814

†omentum, *n.* fatty tissue surrounding the intestines and other abdominal organs 2.7.529; a sausage 2.7.530

omothoye, †omothoia see **†emathasia**

oncomen, *v.pr.pl.* come upon, attack 1.1.31

onde see **o(o)nde**

ondede, *adj. schorte* ~ short of breath 2.7.580

ondoyng, *ger.* undoing, wasting away 2.7.237

ondyng, *ger.* breathing 2.3.242, 2.3.244

onelik, *adv.* only, simply, with no qualification 2.14.42

on-eyede, *adj.* the blind gut or caecum, a section of the intestines 1.3.68

one-ȝeres, *adj.* one-year-old, yearling 1.4.741

onid, *v.pa.ppl.* combined, coagulated 2.6.58

on(n)eþes see vn(n)eþe(s)

onreste, *n.* unrest, disturbance 2.2.178

onych, *n.* onyx 2.7.25, *onix* 2.7.79, *onyx* 2.7.77

onys, *adv.* once, at one time 2.3.667, *ones* 3.16.128; *at ~ (ones, ons)* in a single act 1.4.81, 1.4.127, 1.4.131

o(o)nde, *n.* breathing, breath 2.2.303, 2.2.310, 2.13.361, *honde* 2.10.195

openeþ, *v.pr.3sg.* opens 1.4.612, *openeth* 3.16.247, *open(n)yþ* 2.7.381, 2.7.431, *openyth* 2.3.201; *pr.ppl.* *op(e)nand* 2.7.404, 2.7.405; ~ expands (toward sth.), ~ faces or looks (toward sth.) 2.8.210; *pr.ppl.* *openonde* 2.8.209; *pa.ppl.* *opynd* of animal carcasses: cut open 3.8.26

†op(i)talmia, *n.* inflammation of the eye 3.4.22, 3.4.23

opne, *adj.* open, subject (to) Prol.9

opne, *adv.* openly Prol.16

op(p)ilacio(u)n, *n.* blockage, obstruction in an organ or bodily vessel 2.3.408, 2.3.603, 3.12.25, 3.18.72, *opylacioun* 3.12.23

optik, *adj. as n.* the optic nerve 2.3.154, †*opticus* 2.3.153

or, *conj.* before 2.2.234, 2.9.77, 2.13.280

†orbus, *n.* the blind gut or caecum, a part of the intestine 1.3.67

ordeyneþ, *v.pr.3sg.* brings about, arranges 1.4.194; *pa.ppl.* *ordeynede* 1.4.804, 3.16.224

ordre, *n.* a religious order Prol.54; ~ a class of stellar magnitude 2.6.407, 2.6.412

oripilacioun, *n.* a tremor or shivering associated with fevers, more severe than *rigor* and caused by cold 2.6.537, †*oripilacio* 2.6.517, 2.6.537

or ... or (... or), *corr.conj.* either ... or (... or) 1.4.560, 2.2.57, 2.2.264

or ... oþer, *corr.conj.* either ... or 2.2.190

ortographie, *n.* spelling Prol.92

†osceum, *n.* the scrotum 2.7.524, 2.7.526

†ossa petrosa, *n.* auditory nerves (*lit.* stony bones) 2.3.160

oste, *n.* a retinue, a large group, host 2.6.226

oþer, *adj.* next, following 2.3.300

oþer ... or see o(u)þer ... or

oþerwhile, *adv.* sometimes, occasionally 1.4.97, 1.4.137, *otherwhile* 3.4.63

ouercharged(e), *v.pa.ppl.* overburdened 1.4.691, 2.10.134

ouerdon(e), *v.pa.ppl.* done to excess, excessive 1.4.212, 1.4.535, 1.4.698

ouerdon(e), *pa.ppl. as adv.* excessively, overly 1.4.784, 2.2.303, 2.3.703

ouerest(e), *sup.adj.* uppermost 1.4.200, 2.14.86

ouergoþ, *v.pr.3sg.* overcomes, overwhelms 2.1.98, *ouergoth* 3.7.92; *pr.sg.subj. ouergo* 2.3.526; *pr.ppl. ouergoand* 2.2.80, 2.2.237; *pa.ppl. ouergon(e)* 2.5.81, 2.8.65

ouerstreyt, *adj.* of breathing: overly restricted, excessively difficult 2.2.310

ouerswymmand, *v.pr.ppl.* overflowing, drenching 3.2.15

ouerthwert, *adj.* across, crosswise 2.6.380

oute-castes, *n.pl.* wastes, things cast out or left behind 1.3.146

o(u)þer ... or, *corr.conj.* either ... or Prol.18, 1.4.502, 3.16.5, 3.17.31, *oyþer ... or* 2.4.275, 2.11.45

outtak(e), *prep.* except, with the exception of 2.4.329, 2.5.14, 2.14.16

owen, *adj.* own, belonging to a specified person 1.1.35, 1.1.43; *myne (his, here)* ~ my (his, its, their) own things, possessions, words, ideas Prol.56, 1.3.193, 1.4.476

oweþ, *v.pr.3sg.* ought (to), should 1.4.127, 1.4.187, *ow(e)* Prol.98, 1.2.7, 1.4.80, *owen* 1.2.6; *pr.pl. owen* 2.9.74

oylish, *adj.* oily, greasy 3.8.10, 3.20.226

oynyoun, *n.* a pearl 3.20.55 (see n.); *n.pl. oynons* onions (*Allium cepa*) 1.4.751, 2.8.84

oyþer, *adv.* either 2.4.189; see also **o(u)ther ... or**

pacche, *n.* a patch, a piece of vellum or paper inserted in a manuscript 2.6.278 (see n.)

pacient, *n.* a patient, sick person, person under medical care 2.2.302, 2.4.278, *pasient* 2.13.335

pagil floure, *n.* cowslip (*Primula veris*) 2.7.51

palate, *n.* the roof of the mouth 2.3.370

palehede, *n.* paleness 2.6.357, 2.8.29

palis(s)h(e), *adj.* somewhat pale 1.4.278, 2.8.16, 2.10.29, 3.8.108, *palesch* 1.4.262, *palesshe* 2.4.308

pal(le)sie, *n.* palsy, loss of control over the muscles, esp. with involuntary urination or ejaculation 1.4.121, 2.8.246, 2.8.247, *palasye* 1.4.124

†pallidus, *adj.* pale, wan Prol.120, 2.1.11

pankakes, *n.pl.* pancakes 2.7.165

pappe, *n.* breast, teat 3.16.245; *n.pl. pappes* 3.16.274, *pappis* 2.3.146

paralisis, *n.* palsy 1.4.86, 1.4.121

paralitik, *adj.* suffering from palsy 3.20.24

parbraken, *v.* to break, rupture 3.2.115; *pr.3sg. parbrakeþ* disrupts, imbalances 1.4.530; *pa.ppl. parbraked* 3.10.37

parbrakyng, *ger.* rupture 2.14.149

parfit(e), *adj.* perfect, complete Prol.65, Prol.92, 1.3.225

parfit(e)ly, *adv.* perfectly, completely Prol.19, Prol.64, 1.3.208

part, *n. half or 3* ~ to a half or a third (of an original measure) 1.1.46

particule, *n.* a division or section of a work Prol.96, 2.3.435, 2.4.339

particuler, *adj.* pertaining only to a part (of sth.) 2.3.273, 2.3.416, †*particularis* 2.3.427, 3.8.43

partie, *n.* a part, a component 1.3.7, 1.3.94, 2.3.166, *party* 1.1.16, 1.3.98; *a (o)* ~ partially, in part, somewhat 2.2.76, 2.8.337, 2.13.353; *neþer parties* lower parts, reproductive and excretory organs 1.4.206, 2.4.146; *inder parties (partyes)* interior parts 1.4.545, 2.3.346

passand, *v.* passing, issuing 1.4.637, 3.4.21

passio(u)n, *n.* disease, malady 1.3.233, 1.4.84, 2.1.69

passyue, *adj.* passive, acted upon 1.4.38, †*passiue* 1.4.38, *passif* 1.4.40

pawnche, *n.* the stomach 2.7.443

paxwax, *n.* a ligament at the back of the neck, the *ligamentum nuchae* 3.16.18, 3.20.102 (see n.), 3.20.306, *faxwax* 3.12.38

pays, *n.* weight, heaviness 2.3.562

pena(u)nce, *n.* pain, suffering 1.4.675, 2.13.115; penitential practices, self-mortification 3.17.54

penitratif, *adj.* penetrating, piercing 2.2.181

†*per accidens, phr.* by chance, incidentally, accidentally 1.4.356, 1.4.528, *per accidence* 2.2.251, 2.2.258

perauentur(e), *adv.* perhaps 1.4.327, 1.4.330, 3.7.59, *parauentur* 3.19.139

perchemyne, *n.* parchment 2.3.264

pere, *n.* a pear 1.4.764, 2.7.412

per(i)louse, *adj.* dangerous, perilous 1.3.241, 1.4.625, 1.4.633

*†*peripleumonia, n.* pleurisy 2.3.588

peripulmonie, *n.* an inflammation of the lungs 2.3.556, 2.10.213, †*peripulmonia* 2.3.119, 2.3.121

perisch, *v.* to pierce, penetrate 2.13.301; *v.pr.3sg. pers(h)eþ* pierces, penetrates 2.8.252, 2.8.256, *perissheþ* 1.4.546; *pr.ppl. pers(c)hond(e)* 2.2.181, 2.6.530, *persand* 3.2.140, *pirsonde* 2.2.181; *pa.ppl. pershede* 2.7.342, 3.5.26, *perchede* 2.7.340

persour(e), *n.* a pointed instrument, a piercer 2.7.113, 2.12.136

perturbacion, *n.* disturbance 2.8.266

peskes, *n.pl.* peaches 2.7.158

pestilence, *n.* epidemic disease 2.6.364

†*petala*, *n.pl.* scale-like particles in urine 3.15.2

†*petaloydes*, *n.pl.* scale-like particles in urine 3.15.2

peti, *adj.* small, minor, lesser 2.7.68, 2.10.197, *pety* 2.10.153, 2.10.156, *petit* 2.10.170

peynand, *v.pr.ppl.* causing pain 2.12.92, *peynant* 2.12.88

Peyto salt, *n.* sea salt from Poitou 1.1.45

philosophi(e), *n.* a reason, an explanation 1.3.53, 1.3.182, 1.4.246; natural philosophy, science 1.4.417

phisik, *n.* the study or art of medicine 1.3.20, 1.4.392, *phisic* 1.3.113, 1.4.502

†*piger*, *adj.* slow, lazy 1.4.379

piked, *v.pa.ppl.* picked over, cleaned 1.1.40

†*pingwse*, *adj.* fat 3.20.319, **†*pinguis*** 1.4.381, 3.8.9

pipes, *n.pl.* vessels 2.3.234; ~ *of þe (the) lunges, lunge* ~ airways, bronchi 2.1.75, 2.3.229, 2.3.230, *lunge pipis* 3.4.38, *pypes of þe lunges* 2.1.84

pirnale, *adj.* northeast 1.4.594 (see n.)

pistel, *n.* epistle 2.3.760

pith, *n.* essence 2.13.103, 2.13.105

†*pitiriasis*, *n.* a disease that causes bran-like particles in urine 1.4.85

pitte, *n.* grave, burial pit 2.6.70

planetik, *adj.* of a fever: intermittent at unpredictable intervals 2.6.118, 2.9.54, **†*planetica*** 2.6.101

plawen, *v.pr.pl.* surge around, boil (up) 1.4.616; *pr.ppl. plawand* 2.11.55

plawyng, *ger.* a surging, a boiling 1.4.524

plechching, *ger.* an act of coughing, expulsion of phlegm 2.13.377

plectoric, *adj.* plethoric, having an excess of a bodily humour or substance (e.g., blood, flesh, etc.) 2.7.525, 2.8.321; *adj. as n.* **†*plectoricus*** someone who is plethoric 2.7.525

plenerly, *adv.* fully 1.4.192, *pleynerly* 2.7.481

†*pleumo*, *n.* the membrane surrounding the lung 2.3.589

†*pleumonia*, *n.* pleurisy 2.3.587, 2.3.592

†*pleumoniasis, n.* pleurisy 2.3.592

†*pleura, n.* the membrane surrounding the lungs 2.3.578, 2.3.579, *pleuris* 2.3.578, 2.3.579

pleuresi(e), *n.* pleurisy, an inflammation of the pleura, the membrane around the lungs 2.3.580, 2.10.191, *pleuresy* 2.3.126, 2.3.128, †*pleuresis* 2.3.128, 2.3.418, †*pleuresia* 2.3.587

pleuretik, *adj.* afflicted with pleurisy 2.11.82; †*pleuretici* 2.11.83

†*pleuria, n.* pleurisy, an inflammation of the pleura 2.3.588, 2.3.591

pleyn, *adj.*[1] complete, total 1.4.142

pleyn, *adv.* fully, completely 2.3.538

pleyn(e), *adj.*[2] smooth, unwrinkled 1.3.45, 2.7.373, 3.9.66, *playn* 2.7.369

plie, *n.* one of three regions of the brain, understood as foldings or convolutions 2.7.278, 2.7.289, *plyes* 2.7.278

plot, *n.* clump 1.4.518, 13.18.3, 3.20.170

plum, *n.* lead; a plummet, a stick of lead used for writing 2.3.264, *blank* ~ white lead, basic lead carbonate 3.5.19

poble, *adj.* plump, fleshy 1.4.370, *puble* 2.14.75

podagre, *n.* gout in the feet 2.3.738, 3.16.104, †*podagra* 3.16.151

podagre, *adj.* afflicted with gout in the feet 3.16.121, 3.16.123

poddynges, *n.pl.* sausages 2.7.162, 2.7.531

pokete, *n.* a pocket, a hanging sack or bag 2.13.180

pompouse, *adj.* ostentatious Prol.67

pomys, *n.pl.* apples, fruits 3.5.19

ponde-fisshe, *n.* fish raised in ponds, farmed fish 2.7.164

pores, *n.pl.* minute openings (in the skin, sinews, etc.) 1.3.44, 1.3.71, 2.8.250, *poris* 1.3.169, 1.4.549, *porus* 2.3.832

†*pori,* †*pory* see †*vrythides*

poritz, *n.pl.* leeks and similar culinary plants (spring onions, shallots, scallions, etc.) 2.8.84

portonarie, *n.* the outlet from the stomach to the small intestine, the pylorus 1.3.24, 1.3.25; the duodenum 1.3.28, †*portonarium* 1.3.24

pose, *n.* head cold 2.3.631, 3.17.28

†*posticius, n.* postern, posterior 2.3.159

potacions, *n.pl.* drinks 2.3.490

potel, *n.* half of a gallon measure 1.1.44

poudre, *n.* powder, dust 2.2.74, 2.7.358, 2.8.288, *powdre* 3.5.19, 3.9.74

poudrish(e), *adj.* powdery 3.10.23, 3.18.13, 3.18.58

pouse, *n.* the pulse 2.13.131, 2.13.135, *pouce* 2.1.80, 2.2.304, 2.3.108; *n.pl. powcis* 2.3.814, †*pulsus* 2.1.81; the pulse point on the wrist 2.1.81

powdrowse, *adj.* powdery 3.18.16

poynt, *n.* topic, subject, something to be considered 1.4.10, 1.4.239, 2.13.73; position 2.6.166; a quarter-hour 2.6.188, 2.6.192; *in gode* ~ healthy, well 1.4.618, 1.4.645; *in* ~ *(for) to* about to, at the point of 2.3.607, 2.3.773; *in* ~ *of* on the brink of 2.3.680; *nedeles* ~ the tip of a needle 2.3.707

†*prassium color*, *phr.* the colour of horehound 2.14.61

†*prass(i)us*, *n.* horehound (*Marrubium vulgare*) 2.8.81, 2.14.31

prassyn, *n.* horehound (*Marrubium vulgare*) 2.8.81, 2.14.31

prassyn, *adj.* of urine or of choler: green 2.8.80, 2.14.33, †*prassina* 2.8.79, 2.14.32

pressing, *ger.* compression, pressure 2.13.164, 3.9.22, *pressyng* 2.4.184

pressour, *n.* a press (for wine, oil, etc.) 1.3.30

prest, *adj.* ready, active 2.6.127

priching, *ger.* prickling, a pricking or stinging sensation, pain 2.6.523, 2.13.145, *prichyng* 2.4.182, 2.6.521

pricking, *ger.* prickling, a pricking or stinging sensation, pain 2.4.294, *prickyng* 3.10.31, *preking* 2.4.166, *prykyng* 2.13.307

priuacio(u)n, *n.* lack, absence 2.1.44, 2.1.45, 2.8.3

priue, *adj.* private; ~ *membres* private parts, the genitals 1.4.124, 1.4.494

priued, *v.pa.ppl.* ~ *fro* deprived of, reft of 2.7.213

proces, *n.* explanation, exposition 2.1.23, 2.4.225, 2.6.502; procedure, series of events 2.10.139; *by (be)* ~ *of tyme* over a period of time, in the course of time 2.3.495, 2.4.58

†*prodigus*, *adj.* wasteful, extravagant 1.4.374

profundet, *v.pa.ppl.* of colour: deepened 1.2.9, 1.2.13

prolixite, *n.* long-windedness (in writing) 2.3.847, *prolixte* 2.3.257; long duration (of a sickness) 2.9.132

prolongacioun, *n.* distance 1.4.645

†*proporcionaliter*, *adv.* proportionally, in correspondence with 1.4.209

proporcionede, *v.pa.ppl.* balanced 2.7.319

proporcio(u)n, *n.* balance 1.4.339, 2.10.5, 2.10.15; *vppon þe* ~ in proportion to (sth.) 1.3.26; *euen in* ~ , *in euen* ~ in a 1 to 1 ratio 1.4.336, 1.4.337

propurlik, *adv.* properly, correctly 2.2.355, 2.2.357

prore, *n.* forepart of the head 3.2.45, 3.2.52; ~ *of þe hed(e)* 3.2.21, †*prora capitis* 3.2.21

prynging, *ger.* prickling sensation 3.16.182

psidi, *n.* vocal nerve 2.3.214

†*psidiare*, *v.* to lisp 2.3.219

†*psidius*, *n.* vocal nerve 2.3.214; someone who lisps 2.3.215

†*pthiphia*, *n.* an intermittent fever with unpredictable intervals 2.6.100

†*pthiphis*, *n.* an intermittent fever with unpredictable intervals 2.6.100

†*pthiphus*, *n.* a revolution, returning, repetition 2.6.107

†*pthipica*, *adj.* ~ *febris* an intermittent fever with unpredictable intervals 2.6.111, *pthphica febris* 2.6.101, *typik* 2.6.96

pthisan, *n.* a medical infusion of water and barley, barley gruel 1.3.13

†*pthisicus*, *adj. as n.* someone afflicted with consumption 2.3.429, 2.3.477

pthisik, *n.* phthisic, a wasting disease of the lungs, consumption 2.3.429, 2.3.430, †*pthisica* 2.3.429, †*pthisis* 2.3.430, 2.3.475

†*pueri*, *n.pl.* children 1.4.631

†*puericia*, *n.* childhood 1.4.388, 1.4.389

*****pullettes**, *n.pl.* young chickens, pullets 1.4.745

†*pulmo*, *n.* the lungs 1.3.115, 1.3.140

†*pulmonica*, *adj.* ~ *passio, passio* ~ a sickness of the lungs 2.3.417, 2.3.541

†*pulmonicus*, *adj. as n.* someone afflicted by a sickness of the lungs 2.3.246, 2.13.117

pulmonie, *n.* a sickness of the lungs 2.3.546, 2.3.556, †*pulmonia* 2.3.543, 2.3.545

pulse, †*pulsus* see **pouse**

purgacio(u)n, *n.* purging, excretion, elimination of excess or morbid humours 1.3.194, 2.2.81, 2.3.93

purge(n), *v.* to purge, to evacuate 1.3.194, 1.4.75, 1.4.99; *pa.sg.* purged 1.3.128; *pa. ppl.* purged(e) cleansed, purified 1.3.136, 2.7.287, 3.11.62

purgeyng, *ger.* purging, excretion, elimination of excess or morbid humours 1.3.198

purpos(e), *n.* function 2.8.169, 3.19.27; intention, aim 2.1.2; *in þis* ~ for the present purpose, in the present context 1.4.14, 2.3.779

purpre, *adj.* purple in colour 2.2.167, 2.7.458, *purpur* 2.1.100, 3.2.20

†*purus sanguis*, *n.* pure blood 1.3.138

pusshes, *n.pl.* pustules, boils 1.1.27, 1.4.253, 3.18.73

†*putredo*, *n.* pus 3.9.5, 3.9.11

putrifaccioun, *n.* corruption, decay 2.10.179

putrifacte, *ppl.adj.* corrupt, decayed, rotten 2.10.175, 2.10.179, *putrefact* 2.10.172

puttok, *n.* the European kite (*Milvus milvus*) 2.14.74

pyment, *n.* spiced and sweetened wine 1.4.782

pyn, *n.* a growth in the eye 1.1.33

pynote, *n.* pine cone 2.7.415, 3.9.65

†*quadra*, *n.* six hours, a quarter of a day 2.6.186, 2.6.190

†*quadrans*, *n.* six hours, a quarter of a day 2.6.190

quadre, *n.* six hours, a quarter of a day 2.6.171, 2.6.188; a quarter-year 1.4.421

qualite, *n.* quality, property, nature 1.4.17, 1.4.33; of urine: the colour 1.4.14, 1.4.20, *qualyte* 1.4.13; †*qualitas vrine* the quality of the urine, colour of the urine 1.4.14; †*qualitates prime* the primary qualities hot, cold, wet, and dry 1.4.25, 1.4.442; †*qualitates actyue* the primary qualities hot and cold, which act on matter 1.4.35; †*qualitates passiue* the primary qualities dry and wet, which are acted upon 1.4.37

qualmysh, *adj.* ?boiling, ?steaming 2.4.368

quart(e), *n.* a division of arc: 1/60th of a *terce*, 1/3600th of a second 2.6.202; a fourth of a gallon 2.7.60

quarteyn(e), *n.* a quartan fever, a twenty-four-hour-long fever that recurs every fourth day (inclusive), i.e., every seventy-two hours, 2.2.79, 2.2.112, 2.4.312, 2.11.42, *quartayn* 2.4.317, *febre ~* 2.2.79, †*simplex quartana* 2.3.317, *verray ~* 2.4.306, †*quartana vera* 32.3.319; *false (faws) ~* a quartan fever whose attack lasts more or less than twenty-four hours 2.3.322, 2.4.319, †*quartana non vera* 2.3.318, *nothe ~* 2.11.38, †*quartana not(h)a* 2.4.318, 2.11.37; *dubul ~* a quartan fever that includes an attack of fever on the second day after the fourth day 2.3.324, †*duplex quartana* 2.3.318, *twey ~* 2.3.323, †*bina quartana* 2.3.318; see also **deuquarteyn**

quauiþ, *v.pr.3sg.* shakes, quakes 3.7.60, *quauyþ* 3.2.122; *pr.sg.subj. quaue* 3.2.110; *pr.ppl. quauand* 3.2.108

quayste, *v.pa.ppl.* squashed, crushed 3.20.132

quench, *v.* to quench, to extinguish 2.12.139; *pr.3sg. quencheþ* 2.3.45, *qwencheþ* 2.4.64, *quenches* 2.4.62; *pr.ppl. quenchand* 2.3.40; *pa.ppl. quenched(e)* 1.3.258, 2.9.50, 3.19.199, 3.19.246

quenchyng, *ger.* extinction, destruction 2.1.26, 2.2.59

queynt, *adj.* remarkable, strange 3.4.26

quint, *n.* a division of arc: 1/60th of a *quarte*, 1/3600th of a *terce* 2.6.203, *quynt* 2.6.202

quytter, *n.* pus, putrid matter Prol.135, 1.4.102, *quyttre* 3.7.2, *quyt(t)ur(e)* 3.7.1, 3.16.215

qwobbeth, *v.pr.3sg.* shakes, quakes 3.7.60

racheþ, *v.pr.3sg.* stretches (out), swells outward 2.3.805, 2.4.365; *pr.pl. rechen* reach, extend 2.3.187; *pa.ppl. rachede* 2.7.99, *rawght* 2.7.443

rach(e)yng, *ger.* stretching, swelling outward 2.3.797, 2.4.354

racionatif, *adj. as n.* the middle cell of the brain, which controls reasoning 2.7.289, 2.7.308, †*racionatiua* 2.7.289

†*radiata* see **rayed(e)**

radigownd, *n.* rosacea in children 3.16.202, *redegownd* 3.16.201

radiouse, *adj.* of light: bright, brilliant, radiant 1.4.216, *radyouse* 1.4.219, †*radiosa* 2.4.23

rammys, *n.poss.* ram's 1.4.744

†*ramosa,* *adj.* branching, branched; *vena* ~ the portal vein 2.3.55, 2.3.56

rank, *adj.* abundant, copious 3.17.41

rarefacte, *adj.* of the veins: thin, sheer, permeable 2.13.83

rasking, *ger.* ?stretching 2.6.517 (see n.)

rasyng, *ger.* ?coughing, ?error for *rasking* 2.6.538 (see n.)

rasynges, *ger.pl.* scrapings, shavings, material sloughed off from skin or scabs 1.4.103

ratelith, *v.pr.3sg.* rattles, makes a rattling sound 2.3.242

raþer, *comp. adv.* sooner 2.8.189, 2.8.221; rather (than), in preference (to an alternative) 1.4.349, 2.3.843 (these two senses not always easily distinguished); *sup. adv. raþest(e)* most often, soonest 2.3.487, 2.13.290

rauyng, *ger.* raving, madness 2.4.103, 2.12.67, 3.20.147, *rav(e)yng* 3.20.79, 3.20.141

raw(e), *adj.* of humours, urine, food: undigested 1.3.217, 1.4.545, 1.4.695, 2.4.213; ~ *ey(e)* uncooked egg 3.7.4, 3.7.61; ~ *humour (humores, humors)* undigested humour(s) Prol.137, 1.3.207, 3.9.38; ~ *water* ?unboiled water, ?unstrained water 2.7.159; ?error for *raine water* 3.16.302 (see n.)

rawght see **racheþ**

rawhed(e), *n.* rawness 1.3.206, 2.8.85

rayede, *ppl.adj.* streaked, full of bright rays 2.4.23, †*radiata* 2.4.23

*rayes, *n.pl.* rays of light 2.6.210

rechen see **racheþ**

recidiuacioun, *n.* return, recurrence (of a fever) 2.9.150

recleym, *n. broght to* ~ brought into submission, subdued 2.6.87

rede, *n.* advice 1.1.18

red(e)hede, *n.* redness 1.4.459, 1.4.526, 2.9.13

redilik, *adv.* readily, easily 2.7.265, *redely* 3.11.64

redish(e), *adj.* somewhat red 2.13.3, 2.13.343, *redissh(e)* 1.4.456, 2.13.154, 2.14.66, *redysshe* 2.3.534, *redisse* 3.16.56

redished(e), *n.* reddishness, the state of being somewhat red 2.5.79, 2.4.84, 2.8.58

reflecte, *v.pa.ppl.* turned back, bent back 2.3.206, 2.3.211

refreiþ, *v.pr.3sg.* cools 1.4.536

refreteþ, *v.pr.3sg.* cools, refreshes 1.4.683, *refreteth* 1.4.681

refte, *v.pa.ppl.* ~ *fro (of)* deprived of, reft of 2.1.28, 2.4.94, 2.4.117

refus, *n.* leavings, waste 1.3.146

regebon see **rigebon(e)**

regio(u)n, *n.* one of four layers (circle, *corpus aereum* or *regio spiritualis*, middle, ground or *fundus*) in a urine sample 2.7.564, 2.7.566, 2.13.48; one of four regions of the body (containing sensory and intellectual organs, respiratory organs, digestive organs, and reproductive and excretory organs) 2.7.242, 2.7.344, 2.7.564; †*regio* 2.7.241, 2.7.584

regne(n), *v.* to dominate 1.4.279; *pr.3sg. regneþ* 1.4.17, 1.4.58, *regneth* 1.4.656, *regnyth* 2.4.388, †*regnat* 1.4.57, 2.1.67; *pr.pl.* ~ 2.1.111, 2.6.128; *pr.sg.subj. regne* 2.10.173; *pa.sg. regnede* 2.7.173

reherceth, *v.pr.3sg.* repeats, reports 3.15.32; *pr.pl. rehersen* teach, explain 2.4.200

relef, *n.* remnant, that which is left over 1.3.66

reles, *n.* relief, alleviation 3.20.145

releseth, *v.pr.3sg.* alleviates, mitigates 2.6.352

remena(u)nt, *n.* residue, what remains, remnant 1.3.18, 2.2.234, *remanant* 1.3.164

remissio(u)n, *n.* weakening, reduction of intensity, dullness 1.4.260, 2.8.14

remys, *adj.* dull, dim, faded 2.8.36, 3.2.15, 3.6.40, *remis* 1.4.816, 2.9.179

remytteþ, *v.pr.3sg.* abates, cools 1.4.668

renably, *adv.* fluently 2.6.200

reneyng, *ger.* deprivation, forsaking, abandoning 2.1.45, 2.1.46

renneþ, *v.pr.3sg.* flows, runs, passes 2.3.16, 2.3.393, *rynneþ* 1.4.121; *pr.pl. renne(n)* 1.4.285, 1.4.616, 2.3.388

replecioun, *n.* fullness or overabundance 2.3.559, 2.3.561; †*replecio* 2.14.109

repleisshynd, *v.pr.ppl.* filling fully, sating 2.8.219

replete, *ppl.adj.* full 1.4.668, 1.4.672

reprouabli, *adv.* negatively, with reproof Prol.28

repugnen, *v.pr.pl.* attack, do battle 2.2.288

resceyuyng, *ger.* receiving 2.3.729

residence, *n.* of urine: material that sinks to the bottom of the urinal 2.2.124, 2.2.131, *residens* 2.2.124; ~ resting place, settling 1.4.155, 2.12.50; *pr.ppl.* †*residens,* †*residence* permanent, abiding 3.3.7, 3.3.8

residu, *n.* residue, what remains 1.3.164

resolub(i)le, *adj.* easily dissolved, dissolvable 3.19.123, 3.19.124

resolucio(u)n, *n.* sediment, particulates (in urine, other bodily humours), material that has been broken down within the body by various natural or morbid processes 1.4.206, 2.4.206, 2.6.44, 2.10.117, 2.13.60

resoluen, *v.* to reduce, melt, dissolve, cause to break down (into liquid or gas) 2.4.362, 2.6.99; *pr.3sg. resolueþ* 3.8.18; *pr.ppl. resoluand* 3.8.32; *pa.ppl. resolued(e)* 2.2.176, 2.4.336

restyng, *v.pr.ppl.* resting, at rest 1.4.617; *resting place* dwelling, home 2.6.430

restyng, *ger.* place of rest 1.4.155, *resting* 3.3.12; act of resting, rest 1.4.228, 2.3.310

resudacioun, *n.* sweating out 2.13.155

retencioun, *n.* holding, retention 2.7.471

retentif, *adj.* retentive, able to hold 2.7.298, 2.7.472

†retinere, *v.* to retain, to withhold 1.4.771

†retrograde, *adj.* of planets: moving backward (from east to west) through the Zodiac 2.6.411

reule, *n.* rule, principle Prol.102, 1.4.503, *rewle* Prol.58, 2.4.70

reulers, *n.pl.* rulers 2.8.112

reulesse, *adj.* lacking restraint, unregulated 1.4.266

reumatik, *adj.* characterized by rheum, an internal watery flow from the head 2.4.146, 3.4.52

reume, *n.* humoral flux, a bodily humour that flows from the head to other organs 2.3.20; †*reuma* 2.3.621

reuolucio(u)n, *n.* turning, returning, cycle 2.6.279, 2.6.280, †*reuolucio* 2.6.108

reward(e), *n.* regard 2.2.130, 2.2.207, *but litel peyn os to* ~ only slightly noticeable pain 2.13.209 (see n.)

reye, *n.* þe ~ violent diarrhea, lientery 3.4.47

reynbowe, *n.* rainbow 2.3.256

reyn(e)s, *n.pl.* the kidneys 1.1.3, 1.3.130, 1.3.135, 2.3.79, *reines* 3.8.5, *rynes* 2.4.93, †*renes* 1.1.4, 2.2.147; *n.sg. reyn* 2.4.79, †*ren* 2.4.80

reyny, *adj.* rainy 1.4.600

reysyng, *ger.* a spasm or fit of coughing 2.3.374, *reysing* 2.13.227

reyuede, *v.pa.ppl.* robbed, deprived 2.6.32

†*ridens*, *v.pr.ppl.* laughing 1.4.369

rig, *n.* the back 3.10.31, *ryge* 2.3.194

rigebon(e), *n.* the backbone, the spine 1.3.133, 2.3.74, 2.3.78, 2.3.189, 2.6.540

†*rigor*, *n.* stiffness, cold, and prickling associated with fevers, stronger than *frigus* and weaker than *oripilacioun* 2.6.516, 2.6.519

rikelith, *v.pr.3sg.* clatters, rattles 2.3.242

rikelyng, *ger.* a rattling 2.3.244

riste, *v.pr.3sg.* arises, occurs 2.4.299, 2.6.285

riȝt, *adv.* very, most Prol.22, Prol.81; just, exactly 1.2.19, 1.2.40, 1.3.103, *ryȝt* 1.2.17, 1.2.43, *ryght* 1.4.33, 2.7.80, *riȝ* 1.4.678, 2.14.37

rodehede, *n.* redness, ruddiness 1.3.258, *rodihede* 3.16.325

rody see **rudy**

rod(y)ish, *adj.* somewhat ruddy 2.13.343, 3.16.57

rof(e), *n.* a roof 2.13.299, 2.13.300

rok(e), *n.* mist, cloudy substance 2.2.358, 2.2.366

rokis(s)h(e), *adj.* smoky, misty 2.4.369, 2.7.591

rollyede, *v.pa.ppl.* rolled, turned over, agitated 2.8.287

rolying, *ger.* agitation, disturbance, churning 2.12.28, *rollyng* 2.1.95, *roulyng* 3.9.26, *rulyng* 2.2.89, *rullyng* 1.4.524, *rulyyng* 3.6.35

ropand, *v.pr.ppl. as adj.* ropy, stringy, viscous 2.13.90, 2.13.224

rope, *n.* an intestine, a gut 2.3.61, 2.7.97, *n.pl. ropis* the intestines collectively 1.3.198, *ropes* 2.9.117; *smale ropes* the small intestines 1.3.72, 2.7.100

rore, *n.* a tumultuous state 2.3.17

roryng, *ger.* tumult, agitation 2.2.89, 2.10.112

rospyng, *ger.* belching 1.3.196

rote, *n.* root, origin, foundation 2.4.248, 2.4.302

roted(e), *v.pa.ppl.* rooted, established 2.3.462, 3.3.36; ~ habituated 3.1.44

rotel, *n.* rattling in the throat, a malady of the uvula 3.4.34

rotenhede, *n.* rottenness, crude or infected matter 3.9.4, 3.9.12

roþer, *n.* ox, cow 1.4.750

rotyng, *ger.* rotting, decay, putrefaction 2.2.153, 2.10.180

roust, *n.* rust 3.20.189, 3.20.253

rousty, *adj.* rusty in colour 2.8.95, 2.14.33

routoures, *n.pl.* belchers 2.11.82

rouus, *n.pl.* flakes or scabs in urine 1.4.111

ro(w)gh, *adj.* rough, not smooth 1.4.373, 2.3.640, *rowh* 2.7.467

roynes, *n.pl.* flakes or scabs in urine 3.13.22

rube, *adj.* of urine: red, between golden-red and blood-red 3.19.183, 3.19.190;
    †*rubeus* 2.1.13, 2.4.274

†*rubeique coloris,* *phr.* and of red colour 1.4.369

rubicund(e), *adj.* of urine: blood-red or red as fire 2.9.137, 2.12.9, 2.13.19,
    rubecund(e) 2.1.99, 2.12.6; †*rubicundus* Prol.124, 2.4.274, †*rubecundus* 2.1.13,
    2.2.167

rubie, *adj.* red, of the uroscopic colour *rubeus* 2.4.98

rudieþ, *v.pr.3sg.* reddens, makes sth. appear ruddy 2.9.161

rudihede, *n.* ruddiness, golden-redness 1.4.313, 1.4.459, *rudyhede* 1.3.134, 1.4.714

rudy, *adj.* ruddy, of a golden-red colour Prol.122, 2.10.1, *rody* 1.4.702, 2.10.2

ruf, *adj.* of urine: golden-red, ruddy 2.8.131, 2.10.3; †*rufus* 2.1.12, 2.4.310

ruggedhede, *n.* hairiness, shagginess 1.3.172

ruhhed, *n.* roughness or irritation of the tongue 3.20.126

rullyng, rulyng, rulyyng see **rolying**

ryge see **rig**

ryme, *n.* skin or membrane 2.4.34, 2.7.511

rymmyshe, *adj.* membranous 2.7.536

rynde, *n.* bark 1.3.174

rynes see **reyn(e)s**

rynnyng, *ger.* running, flowing 1.4.120

ryped, *v.pa.ppl.* of an aposteme: ripened (*fig.*), brought to a head 2.8.202

s., *abbrev.* scilicet, namely Prol.17, 1.3.3, 1.3.59

†*saccus infantis,* *n.* the afterbirth, comprising the amniotic sac, placenta, and
    umbilical cord 2.3.754

†*saccus ventris,* *n.* the caecum 1.3.65

sad(de), *adj.* solid, hard, dense 2.3.164; sober, prudent 1.4.396; ~ *schaggyng* firm
    shaking 3.9.73; ~ *body* a small, dense piece of flesh 2.3.761, 2.7.412

sad(de)hede, *n.* firmness, denseness 3.12.6, 3.12.19

saddeth, *v.pr.3sg.* hardens 3.16.346

saf, *n.* safety, health 2.4.283, 3.9.43

saggand, *v.pr.ppl.* sagging, descending 3.10.6

saiingez, *ger.pl.* sayings, oral teachings Prol.26, *sayingz* Prol.53

saloȝwy, *adj.* sallow 1.4.318

saltis(ch)hede, *n.* saltiness 1.1.23, 2.4.30

salt waterishede, *n.* salty wateriness 2.4.31

sandarik, *adj.* of a red or red-orange colour, like the dyes produced from madder root 3.20.305

sang, *n.* blood 3.19.177, 3.19.178

sanguine, *adj. and adj. as n.* having a temperament dominated by blood 1.4.337, 1.4.456, *sanguyne* 1.4.307, †*sanguineus* 1.4.307, 1.4.331

†*sanguis,* *n.* blood 1.2.23, 1.3.138

†*sanies,* *n.* pus Prol.135, 3.7.2

saniouse, *adj.* purulent 3.20.281, *sanyouse* 2.10.209, 2.13.223

†*sansugenicus,* *adj. as n.* one afflicted with *sansugium* 2.3.245

sansugiouse, *adj.* afflicted with *sansugium* 2.13.399, †*sansugiosus* (also as *n.*) 2.13.399, 2.13.401

†*sansugium,* *n.* difficulty in breathing, especially in inhaling 2.3.234, 2.3.238

sap, *n.* earwax 1.3.148

†*satis,* *adv.* sufficiently 1.4.371

satlede, *v.pa.ppl.* settled, fixed 2.9.51

sauacioun, *n.* recovery, health 2.2.262

saundres, *n.pl.* powdered sandalwood 3.5.31

sauour(e), *n.* a smell 2.2.155, 3.7.12; *wickede (euel)* ~ disagreeable odour 1.4.233, 2.2.148; *grete* ~ strong smell 3.7.10

sawcestres, *n.pl.* sausages 2.7.162

saws(e)fleume, *n.* salty phlegm 2.5.55, 2.10.52, *sausfleume* 3.19.161

scabbe, *n.* a skin disease characterized by itching, sores, and formation of scabs 1.1.27, 2.10.67; *n.pl. scabbes* scabs 1.3.254

scabbede, *adj.* of people or organs: having scabs, scabby, suffering from the *scabbe* 3.10.99, 3.13.18, *scabbid* 2.13.37

scabbyhede, *n.* scabbiness 1.4.112, *scabihede* 1.4.104

scaldeþ, *v.pr.3sg.* burns, scalds 2.4.109, *scaldiþ* 2.2.12; *pr.ppl. scaldand* 2.2.54; *pa. ppl. scalt* 2.8.89, 2.13.27

scaldyng, *ger.* burning, destroying through heat 2.12.7, 2.13.428

scales, *n.pl.* scaly flakes in urine, the content *squamae* Prol.143, 3.7.16, *scalis* 2.4.344, *shales* 3.15.17, *shalis* 3.15.2

scape, *v.* to escape, recover from (an illness) 2.2.343, 2.3.461, *skape* 2.4.199; *pr.3sg.* *scapeþ* 2.4.115, 2.8.97; *pr.pl.* *scape(n)* 2.3.437, 3.20.331; *pr.sg.subj.* *scape* 2.12.149; *pa.ppl.* *scapede* 2.2.293; *inf.* *scapen* of an illness: to abate, to come to an end 3.19.117; *pr.3sg.* *scapeþ* issues, emerges 2.2.73

scaply see **schaply**

scapyng, *ger.* recovery, healing 2.4.271, *scaping* 2.12.51

scarp, *adj.* sharp, piercing 2.6.523

scarsenes, *n.* insufficiency, limitation Prol.56

schadewand, *v.pr.ppl.* obscuring, concealing 3.1.11

s(c)hagge, *v.impv.* shake 1.4.225, 3.9.6; *pr.sg.subj.* ~ 3.2.109; *pa.ppl.* *s(c)hagged(e)* 1.4.157, 3.7.52, 3.7.59

schag(g)yng, *ger.* shaking 1.4.158, 3.4.75, 3.9.72

schalt, *v.pr.2sg.* shall 1.4.16, 1.4.153

schapen, *v.pa.ppl.* shaped 1.4.188, 2.3.699

schaply, *adj.* suitable for a given purpose 2.2.173, 2.6.214, *scaply* 2.4.134

schar, *n.* the pubic region, the groin 2.4.177, *sc(h)ore* 1.4.91, 2.4.182, *schere* 2.6.463

scharper, *comp.adj.* sharper 3.19.96, 3.19.97

scharphed(e), *n.* sharpness, intensity 1.4.779, 2.2.176, 2.8.86

schedant, *v.pr.ppl.* dispersing, scattering 1.4.223

schent, *v.pa.ppl.* damaged, destroyed 2.6.39

schere see **schar**

schet, *v.pr.3sg.* shoots, squirts, streams out suddenly 3.4.47

schetteþ, *v.pr.3sg.* shuts, closes 1.3.22; *pa.ppl.* *schet* 1.3.230, **shote* 1.3.21

schewe(n), *v.* to show, to reveal, to appear 1.4.191; *pr.pl.* 1.3.168, *schew* 2.6.62; *pr.1sg.* *sewe* Prol.83; *pr.3sg.* *scheweþ* 1.1.16, 1.3.184; *pr.sg.subj.* *schew* 2.8.26; *pa. ppl.* *schewede* Prol.16; *reflexive forms: schewe hym* to show itself, to appear 2.2.71; *pr.3sg.* *scheweþ him* 1.4.111; *pr.pl.* *schewen hem* 1.4.208; *pr.sg.subj.* *schew(e) him (hym, himself)* 1.4.842, 2.2.170, 2.4.264; *pr.pl.subj.* *schew(e) hem (him)* 1.4.153, 2.2.272; *pr.ppl.* *schewand him* 2.10.203, 2.10.223

schewyng, *ger.* a showing, a demonstration 1.1.15

schire, *adj.* clear, bright 1.4.690, *scher* 1.4.789, *shiere* 3.20.192, *shir* 2.4.74, *sheir* 3.20.392

schirisshe, *adj.* somewhat clear 1.4.695, *s(c)heris(s)h* 1.4.701, 2.4.198

schite, *v.pr.3sg.* defecates 2.2.318

schityng, *ger.* defecation 2.2.315, *schytyng* 1.3.197

sc(h)ore see **schar**

schote, *n.* muscular spasm or rigidity, tetanus 2.14.105, 2.14.123

schouen, *v.* to push (out) 1.3.251; *pr.3.sg. schoffeþ* 2.6.513, *shouyt* 2.3.781; *pa.ppl.* ~ 2.13.166, *schouyn* 2.3.564

schouyng, *ger.* ~ *doun* pressing down 2.3.780, 2.13.163

schrankeland, schronclid, schronkelede see **shronklyn**

schrewede, *adj.* wicked, savage Prol.41, 3.18.126

schronk(k)(e)lyng see **shronkelyng**

schrynkand, *v.pr.ppl.* shrinking, constricting 1.4.352

schrynkyng, *ger.* the act of shrinking 1.4.115

s(c)hynand, *v.* shining, gleaming 2.1.20, 2.4.20, 2.12.127

†*scia*, *n.* the hip-joint 3.16.153, *cia* 3.16.151

†*sciatica*, *n.* pain in the hip, sciatica 3.16.151; ~ *passio* sciatica 3.16.151, †*ciatica passio* 3.16.129

sciatik, *adj.* afflicted with sciatica 3.20.121

science, *n.* a body of knowledge, area of study Prol.13, *sciens* Prol.59; *sciences of interpretacions* forms of expertise in translating Prol.20

sclendre, *adj.* slender 1.4.347, 1.4.354, *sklendir* 1.4.375, *sklendre 1.4.346

scolkeriþ, *v.pr.3sg.* scalds, burns, destroys by heat 2.2.12; *pa.ppl. scolcret* scalded, burnt, destroyed by heat 2.10.76, *scolcrid* 2.14.67

scolkeryng, *ger.* scalding, burning *2.2.58, *skolkeryng* 2.1.106

scorclid(e), *v.pa.ppl.* burnt, scorched 2.13.27, 2.13.428, 3.18.90

scotomie, *n.* dizziness and dimness of vision 2.4.252, †*scotomia* 2.4.252

†*scrophula*, *n.* scrofula, swelling of the lymph nodes in the neck 1.3.256, 1.3.260

scuddes, *n.pl.* dandruff-like or bran-like flakes in the urine Prol.141, 3.13.2, *scuddis* 1.4.111

scuruyhede, *n.* scurfiness 1.4.112

†*secundarie*, *adv.* secondarily 1.3.107

secundyn(e), *n.* the afterbirth, comprising the amniotic sac, placenta, and umbilical cord 2.3.754, 2.3.755, †*secundina* 2.3.754, †*secunda* 2.3.754

†*sedimen*, *n.* the hypostasis when it appears in the bottom of the urinal 3.1.71, 3.9.3, 3.19.69

se(e), *n.* seat, dwelling place 2.3.747, 3.7.40, 3.7.92

seiþ(e), *v.pr.3sg.* says, means, signifies Prol.93, 1.4.56, 1.4.70, 2.2.88, *seieþ* 2.7.393, *saiþ* 1.1.30, 1.2.2., *seyt* 1.4.845; *as who seith (saie, sai, say, seie)* as people say, that is to say 2.3.224, 2.3.551, 2.9.68, 2.12.22, 3.6.8

seken, *v.pr.pl.* sicken, grow ill 1.4.602

sekenes(se), *n.* sickness Prol.60, 1.4.482

sekenessede, *v.pa.ppl.* sickened, made ill (?error for *sekenede*) 2.13.215

sekis(s)h(e), *adj.* somewhat sick 1.4.632, 3.17.53, *sekeisch* 1.4.631

selden, *adv.* seldom, rarely 2.6.211, 2.13.322

self(e), *adj.* same, very (referring to following noun) Prol.28, 1.3.186, 2.4.139

semeþ, *v.pr.3sg.* seems 1.3.62, 1.4.348

sen, *conj.* since, because 3.3.55

se(n)(e), *v.* to see 1.4.16, 2.1.56, 3.1.66; *pr.2sg. sest(e)* 1.2.40, 2.2.161; *pr.pl. sen(e)* 3.19.183; *pa.2sg. seye* 1.4.163; *impv.* ~ 1.1.5; *pr.ppl. seand* Prol.45; *pa.ppl. sene* 1.3.41, 2.8.309, *seyn(e)* 1.3.132, 1.4.82, 1.4.129, 1.4.221

†*senectus, n.* maturity, old age 1.4.388, 1.4.390

†*senes, n.pl.* old people 1.4.619, 1.4.632

seneuey, *n.* mustard 1.4.751

†*sensus, n.* sense, intellect 1.4.381

sentence, *n.* meaning, position, view 1.4.784, 3.19.149

sentyne, *n.* of a ship: bilge, lowest part of the hull, refuse that collects in the bilge (also, waste outlets of other locations) 2.3.635, *centyne* 1.4.497, †*sentina* 14.497, 2.3.635

sephalarge see cephalarge

sequestracioun, *n.* separation 1.2.44, 1.2.45

seruit, *v.pr.3sg.* serves, contributes to, pertains to 3.2.6; *pa.ppl. seruede* copulated with 3.16.62, 3.16.243

sesen, seseth, ses(s)yng see cessen, cessing

sethen, *v.pr.pl.* boil, heat, cook 1.3.208; *pa.ppl. sod(d)en* 13.16.343, 3.19.13; digested 1.1.12, 1.3.87

sette, *v.pa.ppl.* ~ *in þi soule* considered, pondered 1.4.149

setting, *ger.* ~ *at noȝt* treating as worthless Prol.32

sewe, *v.* to follow, to take the same course 2.4.66; *pr.3sg. seweþ* 2.3.794, 2.10.175; *pr.ppl. sewand* 2.6.478, *sewyng* 1.2.31; *pr.3sg. seweþ* of bodily fluids: moves through the ways of the body, goes, proceeds 2.2.42, 2.13.84, *seweth* 2.3.394 3.17.42; *pr.ppl. seweand* 3.16.91, *sewond* 3.17.38; *pa.ppl. sewede* 1.3.12; *pr.3sg. suyth* accords with, follows logically 3.19.156; *pr.pl. sewen* reflect, correspond to 3.16.20

sexte, *n.* 1/60th of a quint 2.6.198, 2.6.203

shales, shalis see **scales**

shalish, *adj.* scale-like, flaky 3.10.23, 3.10.24

*sheuedys, *n.pl.* particles like bran or bits of straw or tow (Lat. *furfurea*) 3.20.250

*shote see **schetteþ**

shronkelyng, *ger.* contraction, constriction 3.16.371, *schronkkelyng* 2.3.361, *schronklyng* 2.14.117

shronklyn, *v.pr.pl.* shrink, contract 3.16.309; *pr.ppl. schrankeland* 3.13.22; *pa.ppl. shronkelide* 2.8.316, *schronkelede* 2.3.816, *schronclid* 2.8.317

shryue, *v.pr.pl. (refl.)* ~ *hem* confess, make confession 3.17.36

shynand see **s(c)hynand**

siccite, *n.* dryness 1.4.274, 1.4.348, *siccyte* 1.4.34, †*siccitas* 1.4.37, 1.4.40

†*siccus,* *adj.* dry 1.3.236, 1.4.272, 1.4.311

†*sifac,* *n.* the lowermost of two membranes around the liver 2.4.37 (see n.), 2.7.519, †*syfac* 2.4.32, 2.7.454

significacio(u)n, *n.* meaning, interpretation, understanding Prol.99, Prol.101, 1.1.1, 1.4.179

siker, *adj.* secure, reliable, certain 2.2.253, 2.2.255; of persons: sure, certain (of sth.) 2.2.270

sikerhede, *n.* security, certainty 2.13.393

sikerly, *adv.* certainly, surely 2.6.247, *sekirly* 3.1.64

sikernes, *n.* certainty, surety 2.2.338

sikeþ, *v.pr.3sg.* sighs, draws air in or out 2.13.189

sillabe, *n.* syllable 2.6.306; *n.pl. sillablis* 2.6.312

similitude, *n.* simile, comparison, likeness 1.2.38, 2.13.435

†*sinancia* see **cynancie**

†*sincopis,* *n.* loss of consciouness, fainting 1.4.92

†*sinoc(h)a,* *n.* an unrelenting fever caused by excess quantity of blood in the veins 2.12.87, 2.12.87, †*synoc(h)a* 2.12.86, 2.12.94, †*cynoca* 3.20.349

†*sinochides,* *n.* an unrelenting fever arising from blood and choler, especially from blood 2.12.117, †*synochides* 2.12.117

†*sinochus* see **synoch**

sinow, *n.* sinew, tendon, ligament 1.3.163, 2.3.199, *synow(e)* 1.4.818, 3.16.161; a nerve or fibre by which sensation or motor instructions are transmitted

2.3.204, 2.3.214; *synowes motiues* the motor nerves 2.3.183; *synow of heryng* auditory nerve 2.3.159

sirurgie, *n.* surgery 3.16.86

†*sista fellis,* *n.* the gall bladder 1.3.70, 2.7.512, †*sistis fellis* 2.7.512

site, *n.* sight 1.4.193; ?sight, ?city, ?site 2.14.19 (see n.)

siþen, *adv.* after, afterward 2.3.495, 3.16.242, *syþen* 1.1.8; ~ because 2.2.29, 2.10.59

siþer, *n.* cider 1.4.769, *syþer* 1.4.768, 1.4.780

siþes, *n.pl.* times, occasions 1.4.7, 1.4.79, *syþes* 1.4.255; ~ times (expressing multiplication) 2.6.325; times (expressing comparison) 2.6.402, *syþes* 2.6.404

skalide, *v.pa.ppl.* scaled, full of scales 1.4.746

skape see **scape**

skateryn, *v.* to scatter, break up, disperse 2.8.33; *pr.3sg. skatereþ* 2.5.29, *scatereþ* 3.16.125; *pa.ppl. scaterede* 3.16.341

skil(e), *n.* reason, explanation 1.3.21, 1.4.64, 1.4.690, 3.10.87, *skyl* 1.2.5, 1.3.45

skilful, *adj.* reasonable, appropriate 1.4.706; of a pulse or breathing: orderly, even 2.2.304, 2.2.344; of sleep: comfortable, proper 2.2.310; of spittle: normal, proper 2.13.337

skilful(l)y, *adv.* appropriately, suitably 1.4.312, 2.6.379, 2.13.132

skippyng, *ger.* leaping, hopping, skipping 2.4.125, 2.13.79

skirwhittes, *n.pl.* parsnips 1.4.749

skolkeryng see **scolkeryng**

sky(e), *n.* cloudiness in urine 2.2.166, 2.10.50, *skie* 3.20.29

skyisshe, *adj.* somewhat cloudy 2.7.591, 2.10.57

skyn, *n.* the skin 1.3.147, 1.3.244; a membrane 1.3.49, 1.3.79; ~ *of þe galle* the membrane around the gall bladder 1.3.78

skynny, *adj.* membranous 3.12.38, 3.15.37

skynnys(s)h(e), *adj.* membranous 2.7.536, 3.10.56

slake, *adj.* slow 3.10.65

slakely, *adv.* slowly 3.10.85

slake(n), *v.* to ease, to mitigate 2.7.406, 3.20.97; *pr.3sg. slakeþ* eases, mitigates 2.6.219, 2.6.351; *pr.sg.subj. slake* 3.20.356

slakked, *v.pa.ppl.* weakened 3.16.113

sleand, *v.pr.ppl.* destroying 2.2.55

slely, *adv.* carefully, discreetly 1.4.451

slepand, *v.pr.ppl.* of limbs: numb, asleep 2.7.136

slepy, *adj.* prone to falling asleep 1.4.378

slit, *v.pr.3sg.* slides, slips 2.7.334, 3.16.379

sliʒh, *adj.* wise, sly 2.3.803, *slygh* 1.4.375

slombrihede, *n.* sleepiness 2.7.188

slowhede, *n.* slowness 2.7.187

slyper, *adj.* slimy, slippery 3.16.379, *slypir* 2.3.648

smalehode, *n. for* ~ because of smallness 1.3.132

smeke, *n.* smoke, fumes 2.2.177

smert(e), *adj.* quick, sudden 2.13.347, 2.13.371

smerthede, *n.* severity 2.6.534

smokishede, *n.* smokiness 1.3.171

smoþe, *adj.* smooth 1.3.45, *smethe* 3.11.61

smoþer, *n.* smoke, smouldering fumes 2.2.177

smoþerhede, *n.* dense, smouldering smokiness 1.3.171

smyte(n), *v.* to strike 2.3.162; *pr.3sg. smyteþ* 2.3.244, *smyt(e)* 2.3.336, 3.2.133, *smet* 2.3.511; *pr.pl. smyten* 2.3.500; *pr.ppl. smytand* 2.3.344, 2.12.137; *pa.ppl. smyten* 1.4.124, 2.3.506, *smyt(e)* 2.8.239, 3.14.23; ~ to fall (into illness) 3.20.91, 3.20.153

smyting, *ger.* hitting, striking 2.7.384, 2.13.170, *smytyng* 3.2.84

snyke, *n.* catarrh, a cold in the head 2.3.630

so, *adv.* such Prol.29

softely, *adv.* gently 1.4.154, 1.4.226

sokeþ, *v.pr.3sg.* sucks, takes in fluid from, absorbs 2.3.692; *pa.sg. sok(e)* 3.16.244, 3.16.246; *pa.ppl. soken* 1.3.12, 1.3.37; *pr.3sg.* moistens, soaks, steeps 1.4.45, 2.8.252

sol-cicle, *n.* the twenty-eight-year cycle of dominical letters and leap years 2.6.278, *sol-sicle* 2.6.291

solucioun, *n.* loosening 2.4.100, 2.7.236; release (from illness), healing 3.20.160

somdel(e), *adv.* somewhat 2.1.71, 2.3.19, 2.4.85, *sumdel* 2.1.85

†sompnolentus, *adj.* sleepy, lazy, prone to fall asleep 1.4.379

sondisshe, *adj.* sandy, like sand 1.4.581

sone, *adv.* soon 1.2.6, 1.2.8

son(ne), *n.* the sun 1.3.103, 1.4.409, 1.4.611, *sone* 1.4.412

sophene, *n.* one of the saphenous veins in the leg 2.3.84, *†sophena* 2.3.84

soppes see **gro(u)nde-soppes**

sorehede, *n.* soreness 2.7.227, 3.20.266; ulceration 3.7.6, 3.7.112

sothfastnesse, *n.* truthfulness, reliability Prol.46

soþerne, *adj.* southern 1.4.584

souereynly, *adv.* above all others, supremely 1.1.26

soueriþ, *v.pr.3sg.* suffers, is susceptible to 3.16.248

sounde, *n.* a tone, a sound 2.3.862

sounde, *adj.* healthy 2.1.87; *sowne* 1.4.570

soune, *v.* to produce a sound, resound 2.3.214; *pr.3sg. soun(n)eþ* sounds, resounds, makes a noise 2.3.164, 2.4.52; *pa.ppl. souned* 1.4.786

sounyng, *ger.* sounding, production of sound or speech 2.3.212

sour(e), *adj.* sour 3.20.225, 2.5.60, *sowre* 2.5.59

sourhede, *n.* sourness 2.8.86, *sowrehede* 3.16.197

sowne see **sounde** *adj.*

spak(e), *v.pa.sg.* spoke 1.2.32, 2.1.66

sparcle, *n.* a spark, a small amount 2.6.73

sparcle, *pr.pl.* sparkle, flicker 2.6.344, 2.6.346; *pr.ppl. sparkelond* 2.6.344

sparplyn, *v.* to scatter, to break up (humours), to spread (through the body or part of the body) 2.8.33, *sperplyn* 3.2.33; *pr.3sg. sparpleþ* 3.16.228; *pa.ppl. sparplede* 2.8.34

spasme, *n.* pathological muscular spasm 2.8.216, 2.8.224, †*spasmus* 2.8.226, 2.14.104

spatlyng, *ger.* spitting, production of spit or phlegm 2.13.191, 2.13.330

spawd, *n.* the shoulder 2.3.502; *n.pl. spaudes* 2.4.295

speking, *ger.* speech, words Prol.36, 2.7.379

spere, *n.* a sphere of the Ptolemaic cosmos 2.6.159, 2.6.384

speren, *v.*[1] to investigate 2.2.268

spereþ, *v.*[2]*pr.3sg.* closes, shuts (in), constricts 1.4.42, 2.7.381, *speriþ* 2.3.201; *pr.ppl. sperand* 2.7.404, 2.7.426, *speronde* 2.7.404; *pa.ppl. spered(e)* 1.4.639, 2.13.298, *sper(i)de* 1.3.252, 1.4.613, *sparede* 1.3.204

sperme, *n.* semen, male or female seed Prol.145, 2.3.705, *sparme* 2.3.717, 2.13.88, †*sperma* 1.4.365, 2.3.734

spice, *n.* a type or kind 1.4.65, 2.3.36, 2.2.129, *spise* 2.3.474

spiren, *v.pr.pl.* breathe, respire 2.7.581

spirit(e), *n.* vital fluid, vital force, a tenuous bodily substance carrying sensation and sensory power to and from the brain 1.4.135, 2.7.330; *n.pl. spiritz* 1.4.218, 1.4.718, †*spiritus* 1.4.559, 1.4.723

spiritual(e), *adj.* pertaining to the respiratory system; ~ *membres, membres* ~ respiratory organs, esp. the lungs and heart 1.3.115, 2.7.407; *malum* ~ sickness of the respiratory system 2.3.416, 2.3.421; ~ relating to the soul 2.7.328, 2.7.329

spirituales, *n.pl.* the respiratory organs 1.4.798, 2.3.120, *spiritualis* 3.8.74

spishede, *n.* thickness 2.10.104

spis(se), *adj.* thick 1.4.758, 1.4.759, 1.4.795, *spise* 2.10.103, †*spissa* 1.4.283

splen(e), *n.* the spleen 1.1.27, 1.1.35, 1.3.123

†**spleneticus**, *adj. as n.* a person suffering from an ailment of the spleen 1.1.34; †*splenetica passio* sickness of the spleen 2.4.12, 2.9.110; †*splenetica vena* a vein in the little finger believed to connect to the spleen 2.3.137

spolied, *v.pa.ppl.* despoiled, stripped (of colour) 2.4.94

spongiouse, *adj.* spongy, porous 3.16.277, 3.16.285

spotle, *n.* spittle, sputum 2.13.245, 2.13.254, *spotel* 2.3.452, 2.3.455, *spatle* 2.2.328, *spatel* 2.2.326

spotleþ, *v.pr.3sg.* spits, coughs up spittle or phlegm 2.13.326

spottish, *adj.* spotted 3.10.60

sp(o)umo(u)se, *adj.* frothy, foamy 2.8.273, 3.20.26, 3.20.321

sprai, *v.* ~ *him* to disperse itself 2.8.327

spryngond, *v.pr.ppl.* springing, arising 2.3.105

spume, *n.* foam, froth 3.4.57, 3.6.4, †*spuma* Prol.134, 3.6.1

†**sputamen**, *n.* spit, sputum 1.4.379

sputyng, *ger.* spitting; sputum 1.3.149

squalprede, *v.pa.ppl.* disturbed, roiled 2.12.53

squalpryng, *ger.* disturbance 2.2.91

†**squame**, *n.pl.* scale-like or flaky particles in urine Prol.143, 3.1.70

squamouse, *adj.* scaly, full of scales or scale-like particles 1.4.746

squaterith, *v.pr.3sg.* scatters, disperses 2.14.151

squob(be), *adj.* flat, squat 2.13.177, 3.16.189

squobbish, *adj.* of a squat form 3.9.10

squynancy, *n.* quinsy, a disease of the throat 2.7.390, 3.4.32, †*squynancia* 2.7.390, 3.4.32

stamerer, *n.* a nerve ending in the tongue that affects speech (*lit.*, one who stammers) 2.3.218

stanccy, *n.* a stammer, ?one who stammers 2.3.218

†*stancitare,* *v.* to stammer 2.3.219

†*stancus,* *n.* one who stammers 2.3.218

stant see **stond(e)**

starkehede, *n.* stiffness, rigidity 2.3.374

starkyng, *ger.* stiffening, stiffness 2.6.517

stere(n), *v.* to move, to stir 2.2.311, 2.6.424; *pr.3sg. stereþ* 2.6.425, *stereth* 2.6.427; *pr.pl. styreyn* 1.4.659; *pr.sg.subj. stere* 3.6.24; *pr.ppl. stiring* 2.11.66; *pa.ppl. sterede* 2.6.426, *stirred* 2.6.426

stering, *ger.* stirring, motion, activity 2.3.182, *steryng* 1.4.522, 2.7.399

steynede, *v.pa.sg.* stained, discoloured 2.7.51

stie(n), *v.* to move upward, to climb, to rise 2.6.32, 2.9.139; *pr.3sg. stieþ* moves upward, climbs, rises 2.2.180, 2.4.108, *styeþ* 2.3.783; *pr.pl. ~* 2.7.176, 2.8.307, *styen* 2.3.833, 2.4.256; *pr.sg.subj. sty(e)* 3.7.49, 3.9.6; *pr.ppl. st(e)yand* 2.13.296, 3.2.140, *stiand* 2.6.523, *styond* 2.4.104

stifhede, *n.* stiffness, rigidity 2.3.374

stil(le), *adj.* unchanged 1.4.138, 1.4.147, *still* 3.3.57

†*stipes,* *n.* the stem or trunk of a plant 1.4.773, 1.4.774

stiptik, *adj.* astringent, constricting 1.4.757, 1.4.758, *†stipticum* 1.4.781; of persons: constipated 3.20.24

stirting, *ger.* the action of starting or springing up 3.16.169

stodie, *n.* study, brooding over 1.4.520, 1.4.662

stok(e), *n.* the stem or trunk of a plant 1.4.774, 1.4.778

stokfissh, *n.* stockfish, unsalted dried fish (often cod) 2.7.157

stomp, *n.* the stub that remains after removing an anal wart or other swelling 3.18.78

stond(e) *v.* to stand, to reside, to hold firm 2.3.657, 3.16.365; *pr.3sg. stant* 1.4.305, 1.4.565, 3.19.68, *standeth* 2.7.429; *pr.pl. ~* 2.12.61, 3.3.35; *impv. ~* 1.4.686; *pr. ppl. standond* standing, placed 1.3.112, *stondand* 2.7.160; *pa.ppl. stonden* stood, remained undisturbed, (something that has) stood 1.1.45, 1.3.182; *pr.3sg. stant* of a sickness: reaches a peak, reaches the *status* phase 2.2.218, *pr.sg.subj. stonde* 2.2.212; *pr.3sg. stant ... by (be)* consists of, corresponds to, is based on 1.4.59, 1.4.323, *pr.sg.subj. stonde by* 1.4.455; *pr.ppl. stondand by* holding (more) to, tending toward 2.7.7

stondyng, *ger.* of a sickness: the peak phase of the illness (Lat. *status*) 2.2.279, 2.2.284, *stonding* 2.2.216, 2.2.225

ston(e), *n.* kidney or bladder stone 2.4.191, 2.3.409, 2.7.117

stones, *n.pl.* ovaries or testicles 2.3.699, 2.3.699

stony(i)ng, *ger.* confusing, dulling (the mind or brain) 2.12.68, 3.20.196; bruising, crushing 2.13.66

stoupand, *v.pr.ppl.* stooping, bent over 3.19.227

strangeleþ, *v.pr.3sg.* quenches, chokes 2.4.63, 3.16.374; *pa.ppl. strangeled* 3.18.11, *stranglide* 1.4.266

strangelyng, *ger.* choking, stifling 2.3.786, 3.2.83

stranguirie, *n.* difficulty in passing urine, painful urination 2.3.414, 2.7.600, *stranguyrie* 2.3.407; †*stranguiria* 1.4.85, 3.9.31, †*stranguyria* 2.7.602

strawght, *ppl.adj.* stretched, made taut 2.7.443

streit(e), *adj.* narrow, constricted 2.3.440, 3.1.34, *streyt(e)* 1.4.648, 2.3.647, *strite* 3.16.376; of breathing: tight, constricted, short 2.2.304, 2.3.239; *streite-ondede* afflicted with shortness of breath 2.13.190, *strete-onded* 2.13.115; ~ *breste* a constricted breast 3.8.21

streithed(e), *n.* constriction, tightness (of breath) 2.13.279, 2.13.306, *streythede* 2.3.548; ~ narrowness, narrowing (of vessels) 2.12.152, 3.11.45, *strey(t)t(e)hede* 1.4.270, *2.7.121, 3.1.17

strekyng, *ger.* stretching 2.3.797

strengh, *n.* strength 2.2.237, 2.3.449, 2.13.281

strenghen, *v.pr.pl.* strengthen 1.3.240, *strenhen* 2.13.50; *pa.ppl. strenghede* 2.4.58, 1.3.250

strite see **streit(e)**

stroke, *n.* a blow 2.3.163, 2.3.863; ~ visual impact (of brightness) 1.4.223

stroup, *n.* the epiglottis 2.7.374, 2.7.376, *strowp(e)* 2.7.349, 2.7.373

stryng, *n.* ligament 3.10.49 (see n.)

stuffeþ, *v.pr.3sg.* obstructs, blocks, stifles 2.7.106, 3.16.374; *pr.pl. stuffen* 3.9.116; *pa.ppl. stuffed(e)* 1.4.692, 2.4.174

stuffing, *ger.* obstruction, blockage (of organs, vessels, etc.) 3.9.22, *stuffyng* 2.4.163

stying, *ger.* climbing, rising 2.12.57

stymede, *v.pa.ppl.* inflated, filled with vapours 3.2.124

subcitrin(e), *adj.* (also as *n.*) of a dull citrine or light yellow colour 2.8.6, 2.9.9, *subcitryn* 2.9.168; †*subcitrinus* 2.1.12, 2.8.11

subcitrinysshe, *adj.* somewhat subcitrine, somewhat pale yellowish 1.4.277

subpale, *adj.* (also as *n.*) of a faintly pale colour 2.8.35, 2.8.160, †*subpallidus* 2.1.11, 2.4.307

subrube, *adj.* (also as *n.*) of a dull reddish colour 3.19.182, 3.19.189, †*subrubeus* 2.1.12, 2.4.98, †*subrubia* 2.4.274

subrubecund, *adj.* (also as *n.*) of a dull blood-red or fire-red colour 2.12.6, *subrubicund* 2.9.137, †*subrubecundus* 2.1.13, 2.4.99, †*subrubicundus* 1.4.274, 2.4.274

subruf, *adj.* (also as *n.*) of a dull reddish-gold colour 2.10.3, †*subrufus* 2.1.12, 2.4.310

substancial, *adj.* essential, intrinsic 1.4.822; ~ *humidite* the natural moisture proper to the body 1.3.51, 2.2.57

substancialhede, *n.* of urine: the liquid substrate of the urine produced in the liver 1.3.155

substa(u)nce, *n.* material, the material of which something consists 1.2.36, 1.3.216; of urine: the liquid substrate of the urine produced in the liver 1.1.9, 1.3.129, 1.4.33, †*substancia* 1.4.29, 1.4.49

†**subtenuis**, *adj.* somewhat thin, thinnish 2.6.28, 2.6.30

subtil(e), *adj.* fine, thin, not thick, weak 1.2.4, 1.2.12, 1.4.44, *suptil(e)* 1.4.757, 3.9.45; ~ *abstruse* Prol.73

subtilede, subtileþ see **suptilen**

subtiliacioun, *n.* the process of making sth. thin, less dense 2.6.500

subtilte, *n.* thinness, fineness 1.4.789

succosite, *n.* moisture 2.7.215, 2.9.117

†**succus**, *n.* juice, sap 2.3.77

suffocacioun, *n.* of the uterus: an ailment thought to involve the uterus rising and compressing the lungs and heart 2.3.785, 2.3.786, †*suffocacio* 2.3.785, 2.3.799

superficial, *adj.* peripheral, non-essential 2.8.258; transient 3.1.11

superfluite, *n.* excess, residue, waste 1.3.166, 1.3.173, *superfluyte* 1.3.145, 1.3.175, †*superfluitas* 1.3.165; *n.pl. superfluities* 1.3.178

suptilen, *v.* to thin, cause (sth.) to become thin 3.19.223; *pr.3sg. subtileþ* 1.4.525; *pa.ppl. subtilede* 2.6.87, *suptilede* 2.8.153, *suptilide* 2.4.336

suspeciousehede, *n.* suspiciousness 3.2.66

suspecte, *adj.* dangerous 2.6.52

susteyneþ, *v.pr.3sg.* sustains, nourishes 1.4.707; *pr.pl. sustene* 3.17.55; *pr.ppl. sustenande* 2.8.235; *pa.ppl. sustened* 1.3.3

suyth see **sewe**

swageþ, *v.pr.3sg.* reduces, moderates 1.4.734; *pr.sg.subj. swage out* should ease, should decline 2.2.322

swagyng, *ger.* alleviation, relief, assuaging 2.2.289, 2.13.361, *swageing* 3.20.145

swart(e), *adj.* of colour: dark 1.4.151, 1.4.795, 2.2.166, *sward* 2.14.30, *swert* 1.4.810; ~ *rede* deep or dark red Prol.125, 1.4.795, 1.4.809, 2.13.1

swarthed(e), *n.* darkness 2.2.12, 3.8.14, *swerthode* 2.2.2

swartis(s)he, *adj.* somewhat dark 1.4.486, 2.4.341, 3.5.3

swche see **s(w)ich(e)**

sweltiþ, *v.pr.3sg.* transpires (through organs or pores or walls of vessels), is exuded 1.3.54, 1.3.55, *swelteþ* 3.7.27, *swelt* 3.18.64; *pr.pl. swelten* 1.4.44, 2.7.127

sweltyng, *ger.* exudation 2.13.155

swet(e), *n.* sweat, perspiration 1.3.39, 1.3.169, 2.2.319

swete, *v.* to sweat, to perspire 1.3.44; *pr.3sg. sweteþ* 1.3.54, *swetiþ* 1.3.55; *pa.sg. swette* 2.7.63, 2.7.65

swetehed(e), *n.* sweetness 1.4.782, 1.4.797

swetesh, *adj.* somewhat sweet 2.12.125

swetishede, *n.* sweetishness, the state of being somewhat sweet 3.16.170

swetyng(e), *ger.* perspiration 1.3.150, 3.20.172

sweyth, *v.pr.3sg.* flows, moves 3.5.14

s(w)ich(e), *adj.* such Prol.44, 1.3.254, 1.4.57, 1.4.127, *swych(e)* 1.3.238, 1.3.256, *swhich* 1.4.685, *swche* 2.4.312

swolwyng, *ger.* swallowing 2.7.380

swong(e), *adj.* lean, thin 1.4.667, 2.3.439

swongen, *v.pa.ppl.* beaten, stirred 3.17.16

swounyng, *ger.* syncope, loss of consciousness 2.4.304

swoyng, *ger.* ringing of the ears 3.4.26

swymmeth, *v.pr.3sg.* moves or flows through a bodily vessel 2.3.628, 3.16.78, *swym(m)eþ* *2.4.136, 2.10.136; *pr.ppl. swymmand* 2.9.82, 3.8.4

swymyng, *ger.* flowing 2.3.628

syf see **syue**

†syfac see **†sifac**

synacy, *n.* a type of quinsy 2.7.393

synerouse, *adj.* ashy 2.8.284

syngand, *v.pr.ppl.* singing 1.4.370

synoch, *n.* an unrelenting fever caused by corruption of blood within the veins 2.12.16, †*sinochus* 2.12.16, †*synoc(h)us* 2.12.15, 2.12.23, 2.12.25; see also †*sinoc(h)a*, †*sinochides*

synopre, *n.* a red pigment 2.13.120

synowy, *adj.* relating to or characterized by sinews 2.7.468, 3.12.37; relating to or characterized by nerves 2.3.161

syue, *n.* sieve 1.2.41, *syf* 1.2.40

table, *n.* a table of information, a chart 2.6.471, 2.6.473, †*tabula* 2.6.472, 2.6.479

tail(e) end(e), *n.* the anus, the buttocks 1.3.77, 1.3.196, *tayl(e) end(e)* 1.3.77, 1.4.107

takyng, *ger.* apprehension, understanding 3.2.122; *colde (hete)* ~ being affected by cold or heat, catching cold or being overcome by heat 1.3.238, 2.9.115

talow, *n.* tallow, animal fat 2.7.529, 3.8.18

tarried, *v.pa.ppl.* delayed 3.18.124

tarying, *ger.* delaying 3.18.107, *tariing* 3.18.123

tath, *v.pr.3sg.* takes (contracted form) 2.14.27

taubre, *n.* a drum 2.4.52, *tawbre* 2.4.50

taȝght, *v.pa.sg.* taught 1.4.762; *pa.sg.* taght 2.2.133; *pa.pl.* taght Prol.71; *pa.ppl.* taght(e) Prol.47, 2.7.68, *taught* Prol.96, *taugh* Prol.92

temperur(e), *n.* balance, esp. of humours 1.4.304, 2.1.92, *temperour* 2.1.87

temples, *n.pl.* the temples 2.2.313

temporal, *adj.* worldly Prol.23

tempre, *v.* to make temperate, to moderate 2.7.406; *pr.3sg.* tempreþ 1.4.707, 2.6.141; *pa.ppl.* temp(e)red(e) 2.3.104, 2.7.319

ten, *n.* pain, suffering 1.4.558

tenasmon see **t(h)enasmo(u)n**

tentif, *adj.* attentive 2.4.246

†***tentigo***, *n.* the hymen (poss. confused with the clitoris) 2.7.534, 2.7.558

terce, *n.* 1/60th of a second of arc (= 1/3600th of a minute of arc) 2.6.201, 2.6.202

tercien(e), *adj. and adj. as n.* of a fever: recurring every third day inclusive (i.e., every forty-eight hours) 2.6.115, 2.10.56, 2.11.41, 3.2.90, †*terciana* 2.3.298; *simple* ~ a normal tertian fever 2.3.301, 2.9.22, †*simplex terciana* 2.3.300; *verraie tercyene* a tertian fever that lasts for only seven attacks 2.3.304, †*terciana vera* 2.3.303, *kynd* ~ 2.3.306, †*terciana naturalis* 2.3.303; *false* ~ a tertian fever that continues for longer than nine days 2.4.319, †*terciana non vera* 2.3.303,

vnkynde ~ 2.3.307, †*terciana non naturalis* 2.3.303; *double* ~ a tertian fever
with less intense attacks on the second day 2.3.308, 2.9.37, †*duplex terciana*
2.3.304; *terciane interpollate* a tertian fever with intermissions 2.3.293; see also
deutercien

term(e), *n.* of an illness: period of time until resolution, duration 2.2.216, 2.2.218

†***terra***, *n.* the element earth 1.4.292, 1.4.432

terrestre, *adj.* earth-like, having qualities of the element earth 2.2.11, 2.3.7; *adj. as*
n. þe ~ earthiness, earthy quality 2.2.66

terrestrete, *n.* earthiness 2.3.397, 2.6.541

terrestrihede, *n.* earthiness 3.19.208

†***tetanus***, *n.* tetanus, muscle spasms or rigidity 2.14.105, 2.14.113

†***t(h)enasmo(u)n***, *n.* tenesmus, the urge to defecate with little or no actual production of stool 3.9.30, 3.9.32, 3.9.118

then(ne), *adj.* thin 1.4.144, 1.4.464, 1.4.803, *thene* 2.9.61, *þen(ne)* 1.2.14, 1.4.138,
þinne 1.4.730, *þyn* 1.4.44, *thyn(n)e* 3.6.56, 3.9.68; *comp. þenner* 2.3.373; *adj. as*
n. þin thin material 1.3.137

therfe, *adj.* (of bread) unleavened 2.7.165; *therue* pure, like unleavened bread
(*fig.*) 3.20.392

therme, *n.* a part of the intestines, a gut 1.3.25, *þerme* 2.7.231, 2.7.454; *n.pl.*
tharmes 2.7.145

thikkish, *adj.* somewhat thick 2.10.230, 3.9.66, *thickesh* 2.7.206

thirle, thirlede see **þirleþ**

this(e), *adj./dem.pl.* these 1.4.10, 1.4.342, 1.4.366, 1.4.429

tholen, *v.* to suffer, to endure 3.18.125; *pr.3sg. þoles* 1.4.40; *pr.pl. thole* 1.4.39

tholyng, *ger.* suffering, enduring 1.4.38

thonewenges, *n.pl.* the temples (of the head) 2.2.313, *þonewynges* 3.20.108

thorog(h), *prep.* through, by means of 1.3.148, 1.3.173, *thorow(h)* 2.7.477, 2.8.76,
thorgh 1.4.219, *þorgh* 1.3.69, *þorʒ* 1.3.245, *þorou* 1.2.41, *throgh* 2.1.38, *þrogh*
1.2.18, 2.4.125, *throuʒ* 2.1.27, *þrouʒ* 1.3.15, *þrough* 2.13.169, *þrugh* 3.18.88

throte golle see **þrot(e) golle**

tiede, *v.pa.ppl.* tied, connected 1.3.62, 2.3.78, *tyed(e)* 1.3.25, 1.3.31

†***timidus***, *adj.* fearful, timid 1.4.386

tinct, *ppl.adj.* (deeply) coloured 2.9.86, 2.9.164, *tynct* 1.4.661

tisanarie, *n.* chyle, the milky fluid sent to the liver from the stomach 2.3.59,
tysanare 2.4.44, †*tisanaria* 2.3.59, †*tysanaria* 2.4.44

tobreste(n), *v.* to burst open, burst apart 2.3.783, 2.6.540, *tobrest* 2.13.123, *tobristen* 2.3.375; *pr.pl.* ~ 2.13.441

tochen, *v.* to touch (on), deal with, discuss 3.20.6; *pr.pl.* ~ 2.3.808; *pa.ppl.* *toched(e)* Prol.84, 2.13.395

tocleue, *v.* to split open 2.12.100, 2.12.135; *as who* ~ *it* as if someone were splitting it open 2.12.135

tokne, *n.* sign, symptom, evidence 2.2.81, 2.2.96, 2.4.268, *token* 1.4.313, 2.2.161

tolde, *v.pa.ppl.* counted, counted as a part of 2.6.172, 2.6.173

ton(e), *adj. as pron.* the one (of two) 2.2.289, 2.6.318, 3.7.99

too, *n.* a toe 3.16.133; *n.pl.* *toos(e)* 1.3.89, 2.3.81

tormentede see **turmenteþ**

torneth, *v.pr.3sg.* turns, changes (into a different colour) 3.19.14; *turneyt* changes 1.3.123

toschaken, *v.* to shake (sb.) violently 3.20.118

toscorclede, *v.pa.ppl.* of blood: completely burnt, scorched 2.13.8

toþer, *adj. and adj. as pron.* other, the other (one) 1.3.115, 1.4.506, *toder* 2.6.318, *todre* 2.13.16

to(u)gh, *adj.* strong, tenacious 1.4.383; thick, sticky 1.4.580, *towȝ* 3.20.181

trachearterie, *n.* the windpipe, the larynx and trachea as a unit 2.7.371, 3.4.38, *tracheartarie* 2.3.426 *trachiarterie* 2.7.384, *trachiartery* 2.7.383, †*trachearteria* 2.7.344

trachel, *n.* the windpipe, the larynx and trachea as a unit 2.7.371

trauail(e), *n.* labour, work, travel 1.4.568, 2.3.776, *trauayl* 1.4.8, *traiuail* 2.4.125; the term "travail" 1.4.534; affliction, suffering 1.4.521, 1.4.657, *trauel* 2.10.178

trauailen, *v.* to afflict, to burden 3.20.118; *pa.ppl.* *trauail(l)ede* 2.3.784, 2.6.38, *traualede* 3.16.191, *trauayled(e)* 2.1.37, 2.3.530; *pr.3sg.* *trauaileþ* of a person: suffers, is afflicted 1.4.72, 1.4.76; *pr.pl.* *trauaile* labour, exert (themselves) 3.16.126

trauailouse, *adj.* painful, causing distress 3.20.22, 3.20.118, *trauaylouse* 2.12.23

trauailyng, *ger.* labouring, working, exertion 1.4.361, *trauailing* 2.10.187, *trauaylyng* 1.2.18, *trauayling* 3.17.17

tremeþ, *v.pr.3sg.* trembles 3.2.121

trendelen, *v.pr.pl.* roll, trundle 3.16.35

trendelyng, *ger.* rolling, trundling 3.16.36

treteþ, *v.pr.3sg.* treats, discusses 2.5.11, *tretiþ* 3.3.18, *trethe* (contracted form) 2.14.6; *pr.pl. trete(n)* 2.3.4, 2.5.6; *pa.ppl. tretede* Prol.102

tretyng, *ger.* handling, examining, considering 1.4.158

†trichiasis, *n.* a disease characterized by hair-like particles in the urine 1.4.85, 1.4.105

†tristis, *adj.* fearful, timid 1.4.384

trompe, *n.* trumpet (*fig.*) Prol.93

trowe, *v.pr.1sg.* believe Prol.18, Prol.35

trumbid, *v.pa.ppl.* clotted 3.10.16

trumb(o)use, *adj.* full of clots or lumps 3.10.6, 3.10.25, 3.10.68, *trumbowse* 3.10.10

tuo, *num.* two 1.3.158, 1.3.159

turbacio(u)n, *n.* turbulence, disturbance, violent movement (of the humours) 2.3.12, 2.7.205

turmenteþ, *v.pr.3sg.* torments, causes pain 2.3.296, *turmentes* 2.3.298, *turmentz* 2.3.324, *turmentiþ* 2.6.106, *turmentith* 2.3.311; *pr.pl. turmenten* 2.9.55; *pa.sg. turmentede* 2.2.296; *pr.ppl. turmentand* 2.12.93; *pa.ppl. turmentede* 2.10.177, *tormentede* 2.8.168

turneyt see **torneth**

twycheþ, *v.pr.3sg.* draws (away) 3.4.14

twyn(e), *num.* two 2.7.37, 2.14.89

twynneþ, *v.pr.3sg.* separates 1.3.91; *pa.ppl. twynnede* separated into equal parts 2.6.260, 2.6.261

tyede see **tiede**

tykelyng, *ger.* a tickling sensation 1.4.109

tyme, *n. in what ~* in whatever time 1.4.654

†tympanites, *n.* a form of dropsy 2.4.50

*tynnyng, *ger.* ringing of the ears 3.4.25

typik see **†pthipica**

tysanare see **tisanarie**

þai, *pron.3pl.* they Prol.37, 1.2.39, *þaie* 1.4.209, *þay* 2.3.651, 2.13.123, *þei* 1.4.606, 2.3.33; *her(e)* their 1.1.34, 1.3.94, 1.4.269, 1.4.403, *þair* Prol.26 (*Prol. only*); *hem* them Prol.24, 1.1.26, *ham* 1.3.245, 1.4.62, *þam* Prol.50, Prol.51 (*Prol. only*), *þaym* Prol.71 (*Prol. only*)

þen(ne) see **then(ne)**

þen(ne)hede, *n.* thinness 1.4.51, 2.4.330, *þynhede* 1.4.526

þennyshede, *n.* the state of being somewhat thin 2.6.99

þennys(s)ch, *adj.* somewhat thin 1.4.262, 1.4.268, *þennys(s)h(e)* 2.5.14, 2.6.15, 2.6.30, *þinnysshe* 1.4.271

þenward, *adv.* thence, from that place 2.3.210

þerfro, *adv.* thence, from there, from that (place) Prol.53, 1.3.48

þerste, *n.* thirst 1.4.9, 2.3.525, *þriste* 2.13.198, *threste* 2.9.116

þerweþ, *adv.* therewith, with that 1.3.122

þi(c)k(e)hede, *n.* thickness 1.4.159, 1.4.286, 1.4.475, 1.4.729, *þicked* 2.5.34

þider, *adv.* thither, there, in that direction 1.4.500, 2.3.665

þiderwarde, *adv.* in that direction 2.8.209, *þidirward* 2.8.211

þies, *n.pl.* the thighs 2.3.81, 2.6.464

þik(e), *adj.* thick 1.2.19, 1.3.64, *þikk(e)* 1.4.51, 3.20.358, *þyk* 1.3.91

þink, *v.*[1]*pr.pl.* think 3.17.39; *pa.sg. þoght* 2.7.58, 3.16.245

þinkeþ, *v.*[2]*pr.3sg.impers.* him ~ it seems to him 2.4.374, 2.7.307; *pr.sg.subj.* him þink 2.2.323, 2.13.227; *pa.sg.* him þoght 2.7.65

þirleþ, *v.pr.3sg.* penetrates, pierces, enters 2.8.252, *þrilleþ* 1.4.817; *pr.sg.subj. thirle* 2.12.136; *pa.sg.subj. thirlede* 2.7.112

þirsteþ, *v.pr.3sg.* compresses 2.4.18; *pa.ppl. þristede* 2.4.19

þise, *dem.pl.* these 1.3.145, 1.3.159, 1.4.3

þit, *conj.* that (*introducing object clause*) 2.6.376, 2.10.35

þo, *def.art, dem.pl.* those Prol.73, Prol.74

þo, *pron.pl.* they, those 1.3.239, 1.4.358

þogh, *conj.* although, though 1.3.81, 1.4.20, *þoʒ* 1.4.262, 3.20.154, *þou* 2.7.341, *þow* 1.4.573, 1.4.574, *þowh* 2.2.302, *þough* 1.4.841, *þoght* 3.20.390; *þow* nevertheless 2.7.99; *as *þow* as if 2.8.262; *al be it so* ~ although 1.3.154

þoght, *n.* thought, brooding 1.4.248, 1.4.658, 3.17.32, *þouʒt* 1.4.663

þoght see þink, þinkeþ, þogh

þoles, *v.pr.3sg.* suffers, is acted upon 1.4.40

þombe, *n.* the thumb 2.6.314, 3.16.88

þonewynges see thonewenges

þor(o)ghout(e), *prep.* throughout 2.3.274, 2.6.322, 2.8.43

þou, *pron.2sg.* thou, you (*nom.*) Prol.6, Prol.9, *þow* 1.4.213, 2.6.307, *þowh* 2.8.245; *þi(ne)* thy, thine, your (*poss.*) Prol.49, 1.4.149; *þe* thee, you, thyself, yourself (*obj.*) Prol.8, Prol.50, 1.4.216, 1.4.686

þrede, *n.* thread 2.6.288

þrid(d)(e), *num.* third 1.3.60, 1.3.162, 1.3.181, 1.4.52

þrilleþ see þirleþ

þristede see þirsteþ

þristyng, *ger.* pressing, thrusting 1.2.18, *þristing* 2.4.184

þrote bolle, *n.* the epiglottis 2.7.348

þrot(e) golle, *n.* the epiglottis 2.7.348, 2.7.353, *throte golle* 3.4.17

þrowes, *n.pl.* by ~ by turns, at certain times 2.11.49

value, *n.* the vagina or vulva 1.4.493, 3.17.21, †*vulua* 2.7.534, †*uulua* 2.3.697, *wlua* 2.7.544; †*valua ventris* 2.3.697

vanisshe, *v.* to vanish, (cause to) dissipate 3.11.55, *vanysshyn* 2.3.445; *pr.3sg.* *vanys(s)heþ* 2.3.295, 3.7.21, *vanis(s)heþ* 1.4.330, 2.14.125, *vanessheþ* 2.2.10, *vanysseth* 3.9.56; *pr.pl.* *vanysh* 3.12.20; *pr.ppl.* *vanishand* 3.11.61; *pa.ppl.* *vanysch* 3.10.45

vanysshyng, *ger.* disappearance, dissipating 2.3.284, *vanysshing* 2.2.284, *vanis-(s)hing* 2.1.47, 3.8.47, *vanissching* 2.6.499

vaporeþ, *v.pr.3sg.* evaporates, gasses (out) 1.4.628

vaporouse, *adj.* gassy, full of fumes 2.7.175, 3.5.2, *vaporows* 13.16.37

vapurne, *v.* to evaporate, to exit as a vapour 1.4.641

ventosite, *n.* accumulation of gas in the body, swelling caused by such gas 1.4.170, 1.4.171

venymouse, *adj.* poisonous, diseased 2.3.584, 2.3.682

venymoushed, *n.* virulence 2.14.98

†*verbi gratia*, *phr.* for example 1.3.219, 1.4.40

ver(e), *n.* the season spring 1.4.599, 1.4.618, †*ver* 1.4.407

verged(e), *ppl.adj.* streaked, full of bright rays 2.4.22, 2.9.109, †*virgulata* 2.4.21

verges, *n.pl.* streaks, rays 2.4.10

vermylon, *adj.* vermilion, bright red 2.13.345

verrai(e), *adj.* true 2.3.304, 2.3.365, *verray* 2.1.61, *verrei(e)* 2.2.253, 2.2.286, *ver-rey* 2.12.64

verreyly, *adv.* truly, accurately 1.1.15, *verreily* 2.2.164, *verayly* 1.4.132, 1.4.824

†*vertebrum*, *n.* the head of a bone that fits into a socket in another bone 3.16.153

†*vertigo*, *n.* dizziness 2.4.253

vertu(e), *n.* strength, power 1.2.24, 1.4.175, 1.4.811, *virtue* 3.16.353, †*virtus* 3.16.352

vesie, *n.* the bladder 1.3.160, 1.4.84, *ves(s)y* 1.4.104, 1.4.801, *vesye* 1.3.158, 1.4.112, †*vesica* 1.4.96, 2.7.533

vesse(i)l(e), *n.* a container 1.4.129, 1.4.156, 1.4.188, 2.2.133; *n.pl. vessailes* 1.4.128; *vesseiles of (þe) blode* blood vessels, veins 2.3.227, 2.3.360; *vesseles of þe sede* seminal ducts 3.17.46

vexacioun, *n.* disturbance in the body, affliction 2.3.498, 2.3.505

veyn(e), *n.* a blood vessel (both venous and arterial) 1.2.8, 1.3.36, 1.3.48, 2.3.48, †*vena* 2.3.222, 2.3.224; a nerve: *~ of siȝt* the optic nerve 2.3.154, †*vena visibilis* 2.3.154, poss. also *n.pl. veynes* 2.10.186, 2.12.138; *n.pl.* ducts, vessels 2.7.538, 2.8.312, 3.16.277, *weynes* 1.3.177; *~ blode* bloodletting 1.4.686; *baas ~* the basilic vein 2.3.124, 2.3.134, †*vena basilica* 2.3.124; *braunche ~* the portal vein 2.3.55, 2.3.68, †*vena ramosa* 2.3.55; *heuede ~* the cephalic vein 2.3.113, †*vena cephalica* 2.3.113; *holwe ~* the vena cava 2.3.96, †*vena concaua* 2.3.96; *lyuer ~* the basilic vein 2.3.124, †*vena epatica* 2.3.123; *myd ~* the median cubital vein 2.3.118, 2.3.123; *pouse ~* a pulsing vein, an artery 2.13.131; *spiritual ~* the median cubital vein 2.3.139; *splene ~* a vein from the spleen to the little finger 2.3.138, *†*splenetica vena* 2.3.137; †*vene capillares* capillary veins 1.3.131

†*vibrans, v.pr.ppl.* vibrating 2.3.132

villouse, *adj.* shaggy, hairy, rough 2.3.640

violent(e), *adj.* forceful, powerful 2.2.181, 2.6.145, †*violentus* 2.6.144

†*virgulata* see **verged(e)**

†*viridis, adj., n.* green 2.1.14, 2.1.107

†*virilitas, n.* adulthood, manhood 1.4.395, 1.4.399

virown, *n. in ~ (abowten)* around, near, in that vicinity 3.16.30, 3.16.83

†*virtus* see **vertu(e)**

viscosite, *n.* stickiness 3.3.27, 3.3.59

viscouse, *adj.* glutinous, sticky 2.7.41, 2.7.102, †*viscosus* 3.6.29

vitellyn, *adj.* of choler or urine: having the consistency or colour of an egg yolk 2.8.88, 2.13.350, †*vitellinus* 2.8.71

vitre, *adj. fleume ~* vitreous or glassy phlegm 2.3.337, 2.3.339, †*fleuma vitrium (vitreum, vitrum)* 2.3.338, 2.5.64, 2.4.329; *adj. as n. vitre* 2.4.335

vlceracio(u)n, *n.* an injury characterized by sores 3.7.6, 3.7.17, 3.10.24

†*vlcus, n.* an ulcer, a sore 1.3.259; *n.pl. vlcera* 1.3.255

vmbrede, *v.pa.ppl.* shadowed, darkened 2.3.284

vnable, *adj. ~ (to)* incapable (of) 2.3.704, 2.3.708, 2.13.262

vnablete, *n.* inability, incapacity 3.19.208

vnbynden, *v.* ?to interpret (signs of illness), ?to alleviate (an illness) 2.2.263; *pr.3sg. vnbynt* dissolves, melts 1.4.612; *pr.ppl. vnbyndand* unbinding, loosening 1.4.766

vnche, *n.*[1] 1/12th of a moment (= 1/480th of an hour) 2.6.189, 2.6.193, *vnce* 2.6.189, †*vncia* 2.6.187

vnche, *n.*[2] 1/12th of a foot, an inch 3.12.22

vnclat, *v.pa.ppl.* unclumped, no longer clumped together 2.4.337

vncouenant, *adj. as n. þe* ~ that which is unsuitable, undesirable 1.2.43

vnctuosite, *n.* viscosity, oiliness, greasiness 2.13.29, 2.14.79, †*vnctuositas* 2.14.91

vnderfonge(n), *v.* to receive 2.3.201, 2.6.6; *pr.3sg. vnderfongeþ* 1.3.32; *pr.pl. vnderfongeþ* 1.3.215; *pa.ppl. vnderfongede* 2.3.641, 2.7.478, *vnderfongen* 1.3.28, 1.3.85

†*vnde versus, phr.* whence (i.e., from which comes) the verse 1.4.418, 1.4.426

vndisposeþ, *v.pr.3sg.* unsettles, puts out of balance, makes indisposed 1.4.531

vnduþ, *v.pr.3sg.* releases 1.4.612

vneuenhede, *n.* unevenness, inequality, imbalance 1.4.339

vnhele, *adj.* unhealthy 1.4.572, 2.14.78

vnhelthe, *n.* ill health 1.4.565

vnheyle, *n. or adj.* ill health; unhealthy 1.4.340

vnmiȝty, *adj.* powerless 1.3.202, *vnmyȝty* 2.3.606, *vnmyghty* 3.18.37

vnmyȝtyhede, *n.* impotence, powerlessness 2.3.606

vn(n)eþe(s), *adv.* hardly, scarcely, with difficulty 1.3.132, 2.3.3, 2.3.815, 2.12.41, *on(n)eþes* 2.3.516, 3.6.24; *quasi-adj.* ~ *of* hardly any 3.19.159

vnpropre, *adj.* of planetary motion: against the direction of firmament 2.6.145

vnpropurly, *adv.* incidentally, accidentally 1.4.528, 2.2.70; incorrectly, not using the proper terms 2.2.358, 2.3.431, *vnpropurlik* 2.2.357, *vnproperly* 2.3.476

vnpur(e), *adj.* thick, raw, unrefined 2.7.206, 2.10.115

vnshaply, *adj.* without proper form, ill-formed 2.4.315

vnskilful, *adj.* of animals: lacking reason 2.3.727

vnstablenes, *n.* instability, variability 1.4.635

vnstalede, *v.pa.ppl.* of ale, beer: unsettled, not yet clear, new 1.4.769

vnverraie, *adj.* false 2.6.116, *vnueray* 2.6.112

vnwroght, *v.pa.ppl.* unworked, unrefined 3.16.55, *vnwrogh* 1.3.217

vpbraidinges, *ger.pl.* reproaches Prol.31, *vpbraidingz* Prol.36

vp(p)on, *prep.* on, upon, based on Prol.15, 1.1.30, 1.3.233, 1.4.610; depending on 1.4.816; ~ *þat* depending on whether 1.4.817, based on or in accord with 1.4.322; *vp þat* insofar as 2.3.133; ~ *the proporcioun (quantite) of* proportional to 1.3.26, 2.2.313

vp-so-doun(e), *adj.* upside down, topsy-turvy 2.4.254, 2.12.67, *vp-so-down* 2.7.563

vrynal, *n.* a vessel for examining urine 1.4.135, 1.4.215, *vrinal* 2.10.144

†vrythides, *n.pl.* the vessels between the kidneys and the bladder, the ureters 1.3.161, 2.3.85, †*vrithides* 2.4.137, †*vrichides* 2.7.538, 2.10.138; *n.sg. vrichide* 2.10.146; † ~ *pory* (†*vrithides pori,* †*vrichides pori)* urinary passages, the ureters 1.3.161, 2.3.86, 2.7.539

vrytif, *adj.* burning 1.1.22, 1.1.24

vsual, *adj. day (dai)* ~ the period of time when the sun is above the horizon 2.6.177, 2.6.178, †*dies vsualis* 2.6.177

vtter, *comp.adj.* outer, peripheral 2.3.336, 2.8.308, *vttre* 3.16.135, *otter* 2.6.514; *sup.adj. vttereste* most extreme 3.19.35

vue, *n.* the uvula 2.7.364, †*vua* 2.7.352; †*vua* a disease of the throat involving a rattling or reverberating sound 2.7.360, 3.4.34

vuel, *n.* the uvula 2.7.352, *vuul* 2.7.361, †*vuula* 2.7.352; a disease of the throat involving a rattling or reverberating sound 3.4.34, †*vuula* 2.7.360, 3.4.33

†vulgaris, *adj. dies* ~ the artificial day, the period of time when the sun is above the horizon 2.6.177

†vulua see **value**

waies, *n.pl.* vessels, ducts, passages in the body 1.3.44, 1.3.158, 1.3.176; ~ *of þe (here) vryn* the urinary vessels, ureters and urethra 1.4.271, 2.2.73; ~ *of blode* veins 2.3.224; ~ *of þe sparme* seminal vessels 2.13.88

walmeth, *v.pr.3sg.* of flame: surges, shoots up 2.9.121; *pr.pl. walme(n)* pour forth, gush 2.8.308, 3.16.265, *walmyn* 1.4.607; *pr.ppl. walmand* 2.2.177, 2.4.104

walmyng, *ger.* a churning or gushing of substances in the body 2.2.64, 2.10.132, 2.12.29

w(h)an, *adj.* dim, leaden, discoloured 1.4.537, 2.2.24, 2.10.208

wand(e)rand, *v.pr.ppl.* wandering, erratic 1.4.247, 2.6.120, *wandrawnt* 2.6.122

wannys(s)h(e), *adj.* somewhat wan 1.4.701, 2.3.569, 2.10.29, 3.8.39, *wannissh* 2.4.245

wanysshede, *v.pa.ppl.* wasted away, diminished 2.8.353, *wanysshid* 3.10.96

wanys(s)hyng, *ger.* wasting away, diminution 2.4.282, 2.8.9, *wanysyng* 2.4.262, *anysshing* 2.9.146, *wanesshyng* 2.4.285, *waneshing* 2.7.237, *wanisshyng* 2.4.262

wap(p)ed(e), *v.pa.sg.* wrapped 2.7.63; *pa.ppl.* 1.1.44, 2.3.191

war(e), *adj.* skilful, knowledgeable 1.4.4, 1.4.819; alert 2.13.110

wark, *n.* work, task, deed Prol.9, Prol.40

warmehede, *n.* warmth 2.3.718

warres, *n.pl.* thickened swellings 3.18.74

wars(s)hing, *ger.* recovery, healing 2.2.82, 2.2.204, *wars(s)hyng* 2.2.129, 2.2.236, *warsching* 2.2.162, *warschyng* 1.4.73, *warisshing* 2.8.177, *warisshyng* 2.2.79; *perilouse warsching* recovery that is still at risk of relapse 2.2.194

wasschyng, *ger.* washing, bathing 1.4.680

wasshen, *v.pa.ppl.* washed 1.1.40, *wesschen* 1.1.29

wasteþ, *v.pr.3sg.* destroys (sth.), causes (sth.) to waste away 2.8.225, 2.8.238

wastour, *n.* a wasteful or lavish person 1.4.373

wasty(i)ng, *ger.* wasting away, drying up 1.4.97, 2.1.26, 2.2.152; *n.pl. wastinges* particles produced by the wasting away of the lungs 2.8.290

water, *n.* the element water 1.4.292, 1.4.299; excreted fluid, urine 1.1.35, 1.2.5

wat(e)rishede, *n.* wateriness 2.4.31, 3.4.9

wat(e)ris(s)h(e), *adj.* pale, watery 1.4.789, 2.3.8, 2.4.207, 3.19.44, *waterisse* 1.4.701

water-wan, *adj.* pale or dilute as water, watery 3.3.30

wat(e)ry, *adj.* watery, diluted 1.4.43, 2.4.214, *watri(e)* 2.4.6, 2.7.168, *watre* 3.3.37

wat(t)rihed(e), *n.* wateriness 1.4.800, 2.4.30

wawh, *n.* a wall; *wombe-ȝate ~* the hymen 2.7.556; *n.pl. wawes* 2.7.53, *wawis* 2.7.51

waxen, *v.* to grow, to become, to increase 1.4.341; *pr.3sg. waxeþ* 1.4.400, 2.2.24; *pr.pl. wax(e)(n)* 1.4.552, 2.3.373, 2.3.815; *pr.subj. wax(e)* 2.2.331, 2.2.335, 2.12.50; *pa.ppl. waxen* 3.11.23, 3.11.62

waxing, *ger.* increase, growth 1.4.270, 2.3.763; of a sickness: the period in which an illness worsens (Lat. *augmentum*) 2.2.283, 2.4.262

web(be), *n.* a film or cloud over the eye, cataract or some other ailment 1.1.33; a membrane 2.2.182, 2.4.34; *webbes of þe (the) lyuer* membranes around the liver 3.7.26, 3.7.29; *arayne (areyn, areyns) ~* spider web 3.5.4, 3.8.62, 3.20.179

webby, *adj.* membranous 3.15.37

weif, *n.* an odour; *wicked ~* a bad smell 2.12.96

wel, *n.* a well, a source (*fig.*) 1.3.97, 2.4.248, 3.20.4

welde, *n.* control, move 2.12.104

wending, *ger.* moving, turning 2.6.280

wendiþ, *v.pr.3sg.* changes, alters 2.13.29

wengede, *adj.* lobed 2.7.403

wenges, *n.pl.* lobes of the lungs or liver 2.7.399, 2.7.459

werr(e), *comp.adj.* worse 2.6.271, 2.7.461

weryhede, *n.* weariness 1.4.521

wesand(e), *n.* the esophagus 2.7.353, 2.7.376, *wesonde* 2.7.367

wes(s)el(e), *n.* a weasel 2.14.46, 2.14.47

wete, *adj.* wet 1.2.36, 1.4.437

wet(e), *v.* to know, to learn, to ascertain 1.1.4, 2.3.802; *pr.3sg. wote* 1.4.122, 3.17.49; *pr.pl. witen* 1.4.125; *pr.sg.subj. wete* 2.13.210; *impv. wet(e)* 2.4.153, 2.2.236, 3.19.91, *witt* 2.14.121

whei(e), *n.* whey 1.2.17, 1.2.33, 3.20.253

whelkes, *n.pl.* pustules 3.16.215, *welkes* 3.16.213

wherof, *conj.* from where, whence Prol.97

whet, *pron.* what 2.8.181

whete, *n.* wheat 1.4.740, 2.3.689

wheþer, *pron.* ~ *it be* whichever (of two things) is 1.4.47, 2.5.43; whichever it may be 2.9.31, 3.19.47

whiei, *adj.* like whey, whey-ish 3.20.252

whil(e), *conj.* ~ *þat* whereas Prol.38; ~ *er(e)* previously 1.3.170, 2.10.99

whilk(e), *pron.* which, what kind (of thing) 1.4.6, 1.4.13

whirlebon(e), *n.* a bone joined with another bone, in general or specifically the hip bone 3.16.135, 3.16.152, 3.18.130

whitishede, *n.* whiteness 2.3.605

whitis(s)h(e), *adj.* off-white, somewhat white 1.4.278, 2.4.215, 2.5.3, 3.16.54, *whitissch* 1.4.268, *whitisse* 1.4.695

whyte, *adj.* of persons: pale, of fair complexion 1.4.380

wi(c)k(e), *adj.* wicked, harmful 2.2.179, 2.6.508, 3.11.19

wil, *adv.* well, very 3.7.56, *wol* 3.19.229, 3.20.54; ~ *onneþes* with great difficulty, very uncommonly 3.16.121

wilhede, *n.* wildness 3.20.37

wilt(e), *v.pr.2sg.* will, want to 1.1.4, 1.4.3

wirke(n), *v.* to work 1.4.178, 1.4.718, *wirk* 1.4.611, *wyrken* 1.1.11, *wirch* 1.4.610; *pr.3sg. wirkeþ* 1.3.103, *wirketh* 2.2.273; *pr.pl. wirke(n)* 1.3.185, 1.4.36; *pr.ppl. wirk(e)and* 2.6.24, 3.16.81; *pa.ppl. wroʒt* caused, effected, produced, made 1.2.30, *wroght* 1.2.25 *wrogh* 1.4.244; *wirkeþ into* introduces (sth.) into (sth.) 1.4.47; *wroʒt into* had an effect on 1.3.220

wirkyng, *ger.* working, operation 1.4.83, *wirking* 2.7.279, *wirching* 1.4.35, *wirchyng* 1.4.46, *werkyng* 1.3.83, *wyrkyng* 1.3.189; ~ effect 1.4.251; ~ processing 1.2.18, 1.2.46

wirst(e), *n.* the wrist 2.1.82, 2.3.109; *n.pl. wristes* 2.1.81, 3.16.88

wise, *n.* manner, way 1.2.43, 1.3.2, *wyse* 1.3.86; *n.pl. wise* 1.4.49

wissen, *v.pr.pl.* reveal, show 3.1.14

withinforþe, *adv.* inside, within Prol.61

wiþ, *prep.* by Prol.30

wiþhalt, *v.pr.3sg.* withholds, restrains 1.4.42

wiþinward, *adv. fro* ~ from within 1.4.560, 1.4.822

wiþout(e)ward(e), *adv. fro* ~ from outside 1.4.252, 1.4.527, 2.7.288, 2.7.302

wiþoutforth, *adv.* outside Prol.61

wiþset, *v.pa.ppl.* hindered, blocked 2.7.147

wiþstant, *v.pr.3sg.* withstands, opposes 2.4.333, 2.6.59; *pa.ppl.* opposed, resisted, withstood 2.6.343

wiþstoppeþ, *v.pr.3sg.* obstructs 2.7.106

witty, *adj.* clever, learned Prol.14

wlateþ, *v.pr.3sg.* cannot keep down (food), is nauseated by 2.13.193; *pa.pl. wlatede* nauseated 2.7.60

wlating, *ger.* nausea 2.7.593; ~ *of* nausea at (food) 3.20.167

wlgare, *adj. as n.* vernacular language Prol.8, Prol.64

wlispe, *v.* to lisp 2.3.219; *pr.3sg. wlispeþ* 2.3.215

wlisper, *n.* someone who lisps (as term for a vocal nerve) 2.3.215

wode, *adj.*[1] wooded, woody 1.4.576

wode, *adj.*[2] see **wo(o)de**

wolly, *adj.* woolly, shaggy 2.3.640, 2.7.472

wom(b)e, *n.* the stomach 1.4.667, 1.4.668, 2.10.70; *wombe sak* the caecum 1.3.66; ~ *ʒate* the vulva as the "gate" to the uterus 2.3.697, 2.3.711; *wombe-ʒate wawh* the hymen 2.7.556; *wome-ʒate tunge* the clitoris (poss. with confusion with the hymen) 2.7.557; ~ *flux* pathological flow of blood or other material from the stomach, as in dysentery, diarrhea, etc. 2.3.12, 2.3.382, 2.7.212

wombed, *adj.* having a stomach of a certain quality; *sad- (hard-) wombed(e)* constipated 2.8.338, 3.11.75

wonden, *v.pa.ppl.* wound, wrapped around 1.1.43

wone, *adj.* customary 2.14.76

woneþ, *v.pr.3sg.* dwells, stays 2.6.323; *pa.ppl. wont(e)* accustomed Prol.68, Prol.76

wo(o)de, *adj.* of an illness or symptoms: intensely painful, fierce, severe 2.2.287, 2.12.46; of a dog: mad, rabid 2.3.686; of persons: mad (with sexual desire) 3.16.249

wo(o)d(e)hed(e), *n.* ferocity, painful intensity 2.6.534; madness 2.12.67, 3.20.79

wo(o)dnes(se), *n.* madness 3.2.126, 3.20.99; intense sexual desire 3.16.67

word(e), *n.* ~ *for* ~ verbatim, literally 1.3.262, 1.4.180

wortes, *n.pl.* herbs, greens 1.4.750

worþihede, *n.* value, importance 2.2.36

wortyng, *ger.* of a pig: digging in the earth with the snout 1.3.260

woses, *n.pl.* muddy waters 1.4.579

wosie, *adj.* moist 3.16.247

wringeþ, *v.pr.3sg.* squeezes, compresses 1.3.30; *pa.ppl. wrongen* 1.2.17, 1.2.20

wroght, wroȝt see **wirke(n)**

wronge, *ppl.adj.* bent, crooked, twisted 2.2.331, 2.3.440

wroþþi, *adj.* easily angered 1.4.373

wrottes, *n.pl.* animal snouts 3.18.72

wrowe, *adj.* difficult (of resolution), doubtful, problematic 3.16.39

wryn, *n.* urine 3.20.64

wymble, *n.* a wimble, a gimlet 2.7.113

wyndowede, *ppl.adj.* of urine: having alternating dark and light regions 2.4.22

wyrken see **wirke(n)**

wytte, *n.* wit, intellect, understanding 1.4.380, *witt(e)* Prol.12, 2.7.248; *n.pl. wyttes* the (five) senses 2.4.376, *wittes* 1.4.248, *wyttz* 2.3.180

wytterly, *adv.* certainly 1.1.4, 1.4.224

Y, *pron.1sg.nom.* I Prol.6, Prol.12

ydiotes, *n.pl.* illiterate or ignorant people Prol.29

ydropisi(e), *n.* dropsy 1.1.27, 2.3.609, *ydropisy(e)* 2.3.609, 2.10.82, *ydropsi* 2.10.88, *ydropesie* 2.10.77, *ydropesy* 2.10.87, †*ydropisis* 2.4.28

yeme, †*yemps,* †*yems* see **hyeme**

yifen, *v.* to give 1.3.99, *ȝif* 2.3.155; *impv. ȝif* 1.4.164

yle, *n.*[1] essence (Gr. *hyle*) 2.13.103; ~ the kidneys and loins (as a source of life) 2.13.104, 2.13.107

yle, *n.*[2] a gouty illness of the kidneys and loins 3.16.144, 3.16.145

†yli(a)ca, *adj.* pertaining to the ileum; ~ *(iliaca) passio* intestinal pain caused by obstruction in the ileum 1.3.75, 2.7.97, 2.7.144; *adj. as n. yliaca* an aposteme of the kidneys 2.13.101, 2.13.102

†yliacus, *n.* someone suffering from pain in the kidneys 2.13.119, *ylycus* 2.13.107

†yliale, *adj.* pertaining to the ileum; *malum* ~ intestinal pain caused by obstruction in the ileum 3.16.140; *adj. as n.* 3.16.147, *iliale* 3.16.144

ylio(u)n, *n.* the ileum, the small intestines 1.3.72, 1.3.74, 2.7.98; *n.pl.* **†yliones** 1.3.72, 2.7.106

ymaginacioun, *n.* the mental faculty of forming images 2.7.257, 2.7.283; *vppon* ~ in the mind's eye, when considered mentally 2.3.3

ymaginatif, *adj. as n.* the first of three cells of the brain, where images are formed 2.7.281, 2.7.285, **†ymaginatiua** 2.7.280

ymagynede, *v.pa.ppl.* envisioned, conceived in images 2.7.311

ymped(e), *v.pa.ppl.* added, inserted 2.6.232, 2.6.337

ynogh, ynow see **anogh**

†ypigozontamen see **†epigozontaymenon**

ypocondre, *n.* one of the hypochondria, the lateral abdominal regions below the ribs 2.3.610, 2.3.613, 2.8.176, *ypocundre* 3.20.61, *ypicondre* 2.3.608, 2.8.162; *n. pl.* **†ypocondria** 2.3.610, 2.7.194, **†ypocondri** 2.9.126

yposarc, *n.* a form of dropsy 2.4.44, *yposark* 2.4.28, **†yposarca** 2.4.28

†yposarchicus, *n.* a person suffering from *yposarca* 2.4.42

ypostasy, *n.* hypostasis, precipitated or suspended matter in the lower portion of a urine sample, residing properly at the bottom of the urinal but able to move upward at times 1.3.200, 3.9.3, *ypostasi* 2.2.368, **†ypostasis** 1.3.180, 1.3.182

yren, *n.* iron 1.3.34, 3.20.189

yrke, *adj.* weakened, distressed 2.13.233

†ysmonia see **ismonie**

†ysmonicus, *adj. as n.* a person suffering from *ismonie* 2.7.395

†ysophagus, *n.* the esophagus 2.7.195, 2.7.196

ʒa, *interj.* yes Prol.30, *ʒe* Prol.45

ʒate, *n.* gate, doorway, exit 1.4.493; *mylk(e)* ~ the jejunum (*lactea porta*) 1.3.53 (see n.); the portal vein (*vena ramosa* or *lactea porta*) 2.3.57; the rectum 2.3.63; *water ʒatʒ* vessels carrying urine to the bladder, the ureters 2.10.137; *maw(e)* ~ the opening at the bottom of the stomach, the pylorus 1.3.20, 1.3.29; *wom(b)e* ~ the vulva 2.3.697, 2.3.711, 2.7.556, 2.7.557

ȝede, *v.pa.sg.* went 3.8.111

ȝelow(e)hed(e), *n.* yellowness 2.5.6, 2.5.10, 2.7.17; *ȝalowhede* 2.4.251

ȝelowishede, *n.* yellowishness 3.6.62

ȝelowisshe, *adj.* yellowish, somewhat yellow 1.4.278

ȝerde, *n.* the penis 1.1.32, 1.3.159, *ȝerdes ende* tip of the penis 3.10.8, *eye of þe ~* the opening of the urethra 3.17.21

ȝerded, *v.pa.ppl.* streaked, full of bright rays 2.4.22

ȝeueþ, *v.pr.3sg.* gives, imparts (knowledge), conveys 1.2.27, 1.4.502, *ȝiffeþ* 1.3.109, *geuyþ* 2.3.254; *pr.pl. ȝeuen* 1.2.28, 1.4.719

ȝicching, *ger.* itching 3.16.212, *ȝykyng* 1.4.107

ȝif see yifen

ȝilden, *v.pr.pl.* give back 1.4.719

ȝisty, *adj.* frothy, thick, yeasty 2.7.598

ȝit(t), *adv.* yet, still 1.4.206, 2.2.337, *ȝitte* 1.4.4, *ȝet* 3.6.42 (see n.)

ȝolk(e), *n.* yolk (of an egg) 2.8.70, 2.13.350

ȝolwe, *adj.* yellow 2.14.43

ȝond-half, *n.* yonder half, regions beyond (e.g., the Continent, regions beyond Rome) 2.6.250

ȝondrast, *sup.adj. as n.* the furthest (away) 2.6.413

ȝong(e), *adj.* young 1.4.272, 3.11.38

ȝyche see ic(c)he

ȝykyng see ȝicching

ȝyuyng, *ger.* emission (of sperm) 2.3.728

†zirbus, *n.* the uppermost of two membranes around the liver 2.4.36 (see n.), 2.4.37, 2.7.519

Guide to Proper Names

Proper nouns used in the *Liber Uricrisiarum* – aside from those that appear in forms identical or very similar to their modern forms – are listed below under their most common Middle English spelling, followed by variant Middle English spellings and Latin forms. These nouns include the names of persons, places, works, winds, and ecclesiastical feasts. References are by book, chapter, and line number and usually include all occurrences of the names and titles in the text, except for extremely common names such as Ypocras, Galienus, Isaac, Giles, the Commentor on Giles, and Gilbert. Dates given are of the Common Era (CE), unless indicated as before the Common Era (BCE).

Afforismis, Afforismys, Affurmis see **Ypocras**

Affricus the south-southwest wind 1.4.589, **Aufricus** 1.4.591

Albert Albertus Magnus, OP (c. 1200–1280), theologian and philosopher

– **þe 5 boke of Albert** *Of Preciouse Stones Mineralium libri V* 2.7.78

Alexandre Alexander of Tralles (Alexander Trallianus, c. ?500–c. ?560), Byzantine physician and medical writer 3.11.34

Almagest, Almagesti, Almagisti see **Ptholomeus**

Anathomys, Anatomyes, Liber Anathomiarum see **Galien**

Antitodarie see **Constantyn**

Aquilo the north-northeast wind 1.4.590, 1.4.593

Araby Arabia, the Islamicate world 2.14.16

Aristotel Aristotle (384–322 BCE) 2.8.188, **Aristotil** 1.4.667, 3.16.351

– *Methaphisice Metaphysics* Prol.70

– *Elenchorum Sophistical Refutations* Prol.74

– *Boke of Kynd(e) of Bestes History of Animals* 2.3.768, 2.3.846

Aueroys the al-Andalus philosopher Averroës (Abu l'Walīd Muhammad ibn Ahmad ibn Muhammad ibn Rushd, 1125–1198) Prol.15

Aufricus see **Affricus**

Auicen Avicenna (Abū 'Ali al-Husayn ibn 'Abd Allāh ibn Sīnā, 980–1037), Persian philosopher and scientist 2.3.441, 2.3.537, 2.4.201, 2.6.23, 2.6.510, 3.16.53

– *Bok of Vrynes* 1.4.510 (see n.)

Augustus Cesar Caesar Augustus, Roman emperor (Octavian; 63 BCE–14 CE) 2.6.332

Auster the south wind 1.4.583, 1.4.584

Austyn Augustine of Hippo, bishop, theologian, exegete (354–430)

– *pistel ... to Seynt Jerom* 2.3.759 (see n.)

Bartholome, Maistre Master Bartholomew, misattributed author of the *Liber Geneciarum* (see *Genecyis, Boke of*) 3.16.363 (see n.)

Bartholomeus (St) Bartholomew's (Eve, Day: 23, 24 Aug.) 1.4.423, *Bartho* (abbrev.) 1.4.428

Borea the north wind 1.4.583, 1.4.585

Breuiarie of Medycyn, Breuiarius medicine see **Johan de Sancto Paulo**

Calabre Calabria 2.13.2

Cathedra Sancti Petri the feast day of the Chair of St Peter (22 Feb.) 1.4.421, 1.4.425

Chorus the west-southwest wind 1.4.589, 1.4.592

Circius the north-northwest wind 1.4.590

Clementz (St) Clement's (Eve, Day: 22, 23 Nov.) 1.4.424, 1.4.425, *Clemens* 1.4.428

Comentour vp(p)on Giles, þe the author of the Standard Commentary on Giles of Corbeil's *Carmen de urinis* (see n. to 1.1.30; fl. first half of 13th cent.) 2.4.161, 2.4.344, þe **Comentour** 3.9.30, 3.10.34, þe **Comentoure vpon Gyles** 1.1.30

Coment vpon Giles (Gilis), þe the Standard Commentary on Giles of Corbeil's *Carmen de urinis* (see n. to 1.1.30) 3.10.2, 3.11.62, þe **Coment of Gilis** 3.8.66, **Giles in þe Coment** 3.7.5

coment, comentour see **Constantyn; Galien; Gilbert;** *Lapidarie*

Compote, Maister of John of Sacrobosco, Parisian master and author of mathematical, astronomical, and calendric texts (d. after 1236) 2.6.272

– *Boke of Compote Compotus ecclesiasticus* (*De anni ratione*) 2.6.272

Constantyn Constantinus Africanus (Constantine the African), translator of Arabic medical texts into Latin (d. before 1098 or 1099) 2.10.88, 2.11.44, 3.16.120, 3.16.162, **Constantinus** 2.8.241, 2.12.99

– *Boke of Medycyns* Constantine's translation of ibn al-Jazzār's *Viaticum* 2.14.119, 3.2.137, 3.11.81, *Antitodarie* 3.16.97, 3.16.103

– Constantyn in his coment 2.7.272

Danyel, Henry Henry Daniel, author of *Liber Uricrisiarum* (fl. c. 1379) Prol.3, **Henricus Daniel** 3.20.411

– *Liber Vricrisiarum* (**Þe Boke of Demyng of Vryn**) Prol.62–3

Elenchorum see **Aristotel**

Eluenden Walter Elveden, alumnus of Gonville Hall, Cambridge (MA by 1348, DCL by 1350), diocesan official in Norwich, donor of medical and legal MSS to Gonville Hall (d. by 1360)

– **Eluenden in his** *Kalender* Elveden's *Kalendarium* for the years 1330–86 2.6.494

Empidijs see **Ypocras**

Ethiop Ethiopia 2.1.20, 2.2.5

Eurus the east wind 1.4.583, 1.4.584

Fauonius the west-northwest wind 1.4.589, 1.4.592

Ferare, Maistre Ferrarius of Salerno, physician (fl. 12th cent.) 2.10.155

Galien Galen of Pergamum, Greek physician and prolific medical author, to whom many pseudonymous works were also attributed (c. 129–after 216?) 1.3.181, 2.2.348, **Galienus** 2.2.344

– Galien … vppon *Empidijs* Galen's *Commentary on Hippocrates'* Epidemic Diseases 2.2.341

– **þe comentour, i. expositour … vppon Ypocras** *Afforismys* Galen's *Commentary on Hippocrates'* Aphorisms 2.3.435, **þe same comentour** 2.3.451

– [ps.-]Galien, *Bok(e) of Anathomyes* the anonymous Salernitan treatise *Anatomia porci* (attributed to Copho of Salerno in the Renaissance and much modern scholarship) 2.1.77, 2.3.695, *Anatomis* 1.3.111, *Anatomyes* 2.4.32, **Galienus in his** *Bok(e) of Anathomyes* 2.1.77, 2.7.393, … in *Libro anathomiarum suarum*, in þe *Boke of his Anathomy* 1.3.23, … in *Libro anathomiarum suarum* 2.7.349

– þe auctour of *Anathomys* 1.3.43, 2.7.361, þe *Bok of Anathomis* 1.3.82, þe *Boke of Anathomyes*, i. in þe *Boke of þe Exposisioun of þe Inder Parties of Mannes Body* 2.7.259 (these anonymous citations also refer to the ps.-Galenic *Anatomia porci*)

Garlandus Gerlandus "the Computist," author of a treatise on calculating ecclesiastical dates (fl. 11th cent.) 2.6.287

Genecyis (Genecyes), Bok(e) of Trotula (attrib. author of medieval gynecological texts), *Liber de sinthomatibus mulierum* (*Book on the Conditions of Women*), misattributed by Daniel to "Maistre Bartholome" 2.3.655, 3.16.363, *Liber geneciarum* 2.3.654

Gilbert Gilbertus Anglicus (Gilbert the Englishman), author of a commentary on Giles of Corbeil's *Carmen de urinis,* as well as other medical treatises (b. after 1210–d. after c. 1260) 1.1.33 (see n.), 1.2.27, 1.4.5, **Gilbertus** 2.13.17

– **Gilbert in his coment vpon Giles (Gilis)** Gilbert's *Comment on Giles of Corbeil's* Carmen de urinis Prol.15, 2.7.270, 3.19.148, **Gilbert ... in his coment** 3.3.53, 3.11.66, **Gilbertus in his coment vpon Giles** 1.4.802

Giles, Gilis, Gyles Giles of Corbeil (Gilles de Corbeil, Aegidius Corboliensis), Salerno-trained physician, teacher of medicine at Paris, author of the *Carmen de urinis* and other versified medical treatises (c. 1140?–c. 1224?) 1.4.5, 2.4.283, 2.4.288, 2.10.157, 2.13.422, 3.9.30, **Egidius** 2.12.82

– **Giles in his texte** [the *Carmen de urinis*] 1.2.2

– *Pouses, Tretee of* Giles's versified treatise *De pulsibus* 2.13.135

– See also **(þe) Comentour vp(p)on Giles**

Gregorie Pope Gregory I (c. 540–604)

– **glose vpon þe 3 boke of Holy Write** 2.3.770

Grew(e) Greek, the Greek language 1.1.14, 2.3.77, *Gru(e)* 2.3.356, 2.4.192

Haly in his *Persectif* a confused reference to an Arabic author named 'Alī, possibly 'Alī ibn 'Abbās al-Majūsī (Haly Abbas), author of the *Pantegni* (or *Liber regalis*) or 'Alī ibn Ridwān, an important commentator on Galen's *Ars parva* or *Tegni* 2.6.520 (see n.)

Holy Writ(te) the Bible, Scripture Prol.27, 1.4.393, 2.6.167, 2.7.546, 2.7.553, **Holy Write** 2.3.771, **Holy Scripture** 3.16.240, **Scriptures** Prol.25

Isaac Isaac Israeli (Ishāq ibn-Sulaymān al-Isra'īlī), philosopher, physician, and author of medical works on urines, fevers, diet, etc. (c. 855–c. 955) Prol.148, 1.3.42, 1.3.81, **Ysaac** 1.2.28, 1.4.168, 2.4.199

– **Isaac ... in þe laste ende of his** *Bok of Vryn* 3.20.2, **Isaac ... in þe 10 bok of his** *Vryns* 3.20.9, **Ysaac ... in þe 10 partie of his** *Boke of Vryns* Prol.102, **Ysaac ... in þe laste boke of his** *Vryns* 3.20.393

– **Isaac in þe 4 boke** *De febribus* 2.2.34, **Isaac in þe same boke** 2.2.268, **Isaac in þe forsaide boke** 2.2.307, **as Isaac seiþ, þe 4 bok** *De febribus* 2.2.321, **Ysaac ... in þe 4 boke** *Of þe Febre* 2.2.191, **Ysaac in þe 4 boke** *Of Febres* 2.13.204, 2.13.393

Jerom St Jerome, biblical translator, commentator, polemicist (c. 347–419/420) 2.3.760

Johan de Sancto Paulo, Maistre John of St Paul (12th to early 13th cent.), medical writer associated with the School of Salerno 2.10.156

– John de Sancto Paulo, *Boke of Phisik Medycynal De simplicium medicinarum virtutibus* 1.4.785

– *Breuiarie of Medycyn, Breuiarius medicine* John of St Paul's *Breviarius medicine* 1.4.122, 1.4.123

Johannicius (Johannitius) Hunayn ibn 'Ishāq al-'Ibādī, Nestorian Christian physician, medical author, and translator of Greek medical texts into Arabic (808–873)

– *De ysagogis Isagoge ad Tegni Galieni* (a brief introduction to Galenic medicine) 1.4.739, *Ysigogis* 2.5.45, *Boke of Ysagogis* 2.8.60

John de Sancto Paulo see Johan de Sancto Paulo

Julius Cesar Julius Caesar, Roman emperor (100–44 BCE) 2.6.330

Ketoun Ketton, Rutland, UK Prol.5

Lapidarie, þe Coment vppon þe a commentary on a treatise on stones 2.7.79 (see n.)

Mathies (Mathiez, Mathis), Seynt St Matthias (feast day 24 Feb.), 2.6.233, 2.6.244, 2.6.262

Medycynarie, our Henry Daniel's planned work on medical remedies (poss. his herbal, the *Aaron Danielis,* written after the *Liber Uricrisiarum*) 3.16.369

Mesondeu, Maistre of þc Petrus Musandinus, Salernitan physician and master, author of works on diet and practical medicine (fl. c. 1180?) 2.10.158

Methaphisice see Aristotel

Nothus the south-southeast wind 1.4.589, 1.4.591

Peyto Poitou 1.1.45 (see n.)

Platearye, Maistre Platearius, Salernitan physician and master (fl. mid-12th cent.) 2.10.155

Poule, Seynt Paul of Tarsus, author of New Testament epistles (c. 5–c. 67) Prol.94

Pouses, Tretee of see Giles

Pronostik(e)s see Ypocras

Ptholomeus Claudius Ptolemy, Alexandrian astronomer (c. 100–c. 175) 2.6.389, 2.6.407, Ptholome 2.6.428

– Ptholomeus in his bok ... *Almagisti* 2.6.148, Ptholomeus in libro *Almagesti ...* þat he calleþ *Almagest* 2.6.381

Sarasyn(e)s Saracens, Muslims 2.6.169, 2.14.17, *Sarasenis* 2.6.495

Scripture(s) see **Holy Writ(te)**

Stawnford Stamford, Lincolnshire, UK 2.7.49

Subsolanus the east-southeast wind 1.4.589, 1.4.590

Tadeus prob. Thaddeus (Taddeo) Alderotti, Florentine-born physician and professor of medicine at the University of Bologna (c. 1210–1295) 3.5.12, 3.7.46, **Thade** 2.10.89, 2.14.94

Theophilus Theophilus Protospatharius, Byzantine author of a treatise on urine (?7th cent.) 2.7.228, 2.13.8, 2.13.425, 3.15.32, **Theophile** 1.2.28

– **Theophilus** in his *Boke of Vryns* 2.2.362, **Theophilus** in his *Bok of Vryns* 2.10.86

– **Theophile** in his *Vryns* 2.4.338

– **Þeophil** in his *Boke of Vryns* 2.4.110

Turnour, Walter Walter Turnour of Ketton (Rutland), dedicatee of the *Liber Uricrisiarum* and colleague (*socius/felowe*) of Henry Daniel (dates unknown) Prol.5

Vesper Venus as the evening star 2.6.221

Vrbanes (St) Urban's (Eve, Day: 24, 25 May) 1.4.422, *Vrbanus* 1.4.427

Wlturnus the east-northeast wind 1.4.588, 1.4.590

Ynde India 3.1.58

Ypocras Hippocrates of Kos, Greek physician (5th to 4th cent. BCE) 2.2.238, 2.3.305, 2.3.645

– **Ypocras** *Afforismys* Aphorisms 2.3.435, **Ypocras** in his *Afforismis* 2.4.74, **Ypocras** eke in his *Affurmis* 2.4.338, **Ypocras** in þe laste ende of þe 4 boke of *Afforismis* 2.7.180, **Ypocras** ... in his *Afforismis* 3.4.44, **Ypocras** in the ende of þe 4 particule of *Afforismys* 3.7.15, **Ypocras** in *Afforismis* 3.12.14, **Ypocras** in his boke of *Afforismis* 3.16.286

– **Ypocras** ... in his *Bok(e) of Pronostik(e)s* Prognostics 2.10.84, 2.11.81, **Ypocras** in his *Pronostikes* 2.13.423

– **Ypocras** in his *Empidijs* Epidemic Diseases 2.2.254

Ysaac see **Isaac**

Ysagogis, Ysigogis see **Johannicius**

Ysodre Isidore of Seville, early medieval bishop and encyclopedist (c. 560–636)

– boke of *Ethimologies* Etymologiae (*Etymologies*) 2.8.155, bok of *Ethimologyis* 2.14.107

Ȝol(e) Yule, Christmas 2.6.271, ~ *day* Christmas Day 2.6.269

Zephirus the west wind 1.4.584, 1.4.586, *Zepherus* 1.4.583

Works Cited

Albertus Magnus. 1890. *Mineralium libri V*. In *B. Alberti Magni Opera omnia*, ed. Auguste Borgnet, 5: 1–103. Paris: Vivès.

Alexander of Tralles. See Langslow, ed. and trans. 2006.

Alfraganus (Abū al-'Abbās Aḥmad ibn Muḥammad ibn Kathīr al-Farghānī; Latin: Alfraganus). See Carmody, ed. 1943.

Alonso Guardo, Alberto. 2001. "*Febris augmastica, febris homotena y febris epaugmastica*: Origen y evolución de tres términos aplicados a la fiebre durante la Edad Media." *Praktika: Proceedings of the Eleventh Congress of the International Federation of Associations of Classical Studies* (Kavala 1999). 3 vols., 1: 24–37. Athens: International Federation of Associations of Classical Studies.

Anglo-Norman Dictionary. See Rothwell et al., eds. 2006– .

Anon. Standard Commentary on Giles of Corbeil, *Carmen de urinis*. BL, Sloane MS 282, ff. 19v–46v; Bodl., MS Laud lat. 106, ff. 209vb–229rb; London, Wellcome Library, MS 547, ff. 146r–166v.

Aristotle. *History of Animals*. Trans. d'A.W. Thompson. In Barnes, ed. 1984, 1: 774–993.

– *Metaphysics*. Trans. W.D. Ross. In Barnes, ed. 1984, 2: 1552–1728.

– *Nicomachean Ethics*. Trans. W.D. Ross, rev. J.O. Urmson. In Barnes, ed. 1984, 2: 1729–1867.

– *Sophistical Refutations*. Trans. W.A. Pickard-Cambridge. In Barnes, ed. 1984, 1: 278–314.

Ars medicinae [*Articella*]. c. 1300. BL, Harley MS 3140.

Articella seu thesaurus operum medicorum antiquorum. 1483. Venice: Hermannus Liechtenstein.

Augustine of Hippo. See Mosher, trans. 1982.

Ausécache, Mireille. 1998. "Gilles de Corbeil ou le médecin pédagogue au tournant des XIIe et XIIIe siècles." *Early Science and Medicine* 3 (3): 187–215.

– ed. 2017. *Gilles de Corbeil, Liber de uirtutibus et laudibus compositorum medicaminum: Édition et commentaire*. Florence: SISMEL.

Avicenna (Abu 'Alī al-Husayn ibn 'Abd Allāh ibn Sīnā). 1522. *Liber canonis totius medicine*. Lyons: Jacobus Myt.

Bacon, Roger. *Opus maius*, part 4. See Bridges, ed. 1900; Burke, trans. 1962; Jebb, ed. 1733.

Barnes, Jonathan, ed. 1984. *The Complete Works of Aristotle*. Princeton: Princeton University Press.

Bede. *The Reckoning of Time*. See Wallis, trans. 1999.

Benskin, Michael. 1982. "The Letter <þ> and <y> in Later Middle English, and Some Related Matters." *Journal of the Society of Archivists* 7 (1): 13–30.

Benskin, Michael, and M.L. Samuels, eds. 1981. *So Meny People Longages and Tonges: Philological Essays in Scots and Mediaeval English Presented to Angus McIntosh*. Edinburgh: Middle English Dialect Project.

Bernard de Gordon. 1574. *De urinis*. In *Lilium medicinae*. Lyons: Rovillius, 728–824.

Biblia sacra iuxta vulgatam versionem. 1969. Ed. Robert Weber, Boniface Fischer, et al. 2 vols. Stuttgart: Württembergische Bibelanstalt.

Bridges, John Henry, ed. 1900. *The "Opus Majus" of Roger Bacon*. 3 vols. London and Oxford: Williams and Norgate.

Brown, George Hardin, and Linda Ehrsam Voigts, eds. 2010. *The Study of Medieval Manuscripts of England: Festschrift in Honor of Richard W. Pfaff*. Medieval and Renaissance Texts and Studies 384. Tempe: Arizona Center for Medieval and Renaissance Studies.

Burke, Robert Belle, trans. 1962. *The "Opus Majus" of Roger Bacon*. 2 vols. New York: Russell & Russell.

Burrow, J.A. 1986. *The Ages of Man: A Study in Medieval Writing and Thought*. Oxford: Clarendon Press.

Carmody, Francis J., ed. 1943. *Al Farghani Differentie scientie astrorum (= Elements of Astronomy)*. Berkeley: n.p.

Carrillo Linares, María José, ed. 2006. "De Humana Natura (*Liber cerebri*)." In Tavormina, ed. 2006, 1: 249–75.

Chaucer, Geoffrey. 1987. *The Riverside Chaucer*. Gen. ed. Larry D. Benson. Boston: Houghton Mifflin.

Choulant, Louis, ed. 1826. *Aegidii Corboliensis Carmina medica*. Leipzig: Voss. ("Liber de urinis metrice compositus": 1–18; "Liber de pulsibus metrice compositus": 19–43.)

Collins, Kenneth, Samuel Kottek, and Helena Paavilainen, eds. 2015. *Isaac Israeli: The Philosopher Physician*. Jerusalem: Muriel and Philip Berman Medical Library, Hebrew University.

Constantinus Africanus. 1515a. *Pantegni* (Theorica and Practica; trans. of ʿAlī ibn al-ʿAbbās al-Majūsī, *Kitāb Kāmil al-ṣināʿah al-ṭibbīyah*). In *Omnia opera Ysaac* 2: 1ra–144ra.

– 1515b. *Viaticum* (trans. of ibn al-Jazzār, *Zād al-musāfir*). In *Omnia opera Ysaac* 2: 144rb–171vb.

Corner, George W., ed. and trans. 1927. *Anatomical Texts of the Earlier Middle Ages: A Study in the Transmission of Culture, with a Revised Latin Text of "Anatomia Cophonis" and Translations of Four Texts.* Carnegie Institution of Washington Publication No. 364. Washington, DC: Carnegie Institution of Washington.

Corpus of Middle English Prose and Verse. 2000–6. https://quod.lib.umich.edu/c/cme.

Daniel, Henry. *Liber Uricrisiarum* (Latin). Glasgow UL, Hunterian MS 362, ff. 1r–83v.

– *Herbal* (*Aaron Danielis*). BL, Add. MS 27329, ff. 4ra–236rb.

– *Herbal.* BL, Arundel MS 42, ff. 3r–92r.

– ?1527. *The Judycyall of Vryns.* ?Southwark: P. Treveris.

– See Hanna, ed. 1994; Jasin, ed. 1983; Johannessen, ed. 2005; Mäkinen, ed. 2002.

Darby, Peter. 2012. *Bede and the End of Time.* Burlington, VT: Ashgate.

Dase, Sonya, ed. 1999. *"Liber urinarum a uoce Theophili": Edition einer Übersetzung des 12. Jahrhunderts mit ausführlichem Glossar.* Edition Wissenschaft, Reihe Sprachwissenschaft 20. Diss. Osnabrück 1997. Marburg: Tectum Verlag.

De Renzi, Salvatore, ed. 1852–9. *Collectio salernitana, ossia Documenti inediti, e trattati di medicina appartenenti alla Scuola medica salernitana.* 5 vols. Naples: Filiatre-Sebezio.

Demaitre, Luke. 2013. *Medieval Medicine: The Art of Healing, from Head to Toe.* Santa Barbara: Praeger.

Dendle, Peter, and Alain Touwaide, eds. 2008. *Health and Healing from the Medieval Garden.* Woodbridge: Boydell.

Dictionary of Medieval Latin from British Sources. 1975–2013. Ed. R.E. Latham, D.R. Howlett, and R.K. Ashdowne. Oxford: British Academy. https://logeion.uchicago.edu. (*DMLBS*)

Dictionary of the Scots Language. 2001–4. https://dsl.ac.uk.

Dove, Mary. 1986. *The Perfect Age of Man's Life.* Cambridge: Cambridge University Press.

Edwards, A.S.G., ed. 2008. *English Manuscript Studies 1100–1700.* Vol. 14: *Regional Manuscripts 1200–1700.* London: The British Library.

English Dialect Dictionary. 1898–1905. Ed. Joseph Wright. 6 vols. London: Frowde.

al-Farghānī, Abū al-ʿAbbās Aḥmad ibn Muḥammad ibn Kathīr. See Carmody, ed. 1943.

Fontana, Eugenio, ed. and trans. 1966. *Il libro delle urine di Isacco l'Ebreo tradotto dall'arabo in latino da Costantino Africano.* With Italian translation. Pisa: Giardini.

Friedman, John B. 1994. "The Friar Portrait in Bodleian Library MS. Douce 104: Contemporary Satire?" *Yearbook of Langland Studies* 8: 177–85.

Frutos González, Virginia de, ed. 2010a. "Edición crítica del *Regimen sanitatis salernitanum* transmitido por los manuscritos Add. 12190 y Sloane 351 de la British Library de Londres." *Minerva: Revista de filología clásica* (Valladolid) 23: 143–95.

– ed. 2010b. *Flos medicine: Regimen sanitatis salernitanum: Estudio, edición crítica y traducción.* Valladolid: University of Valladolid.

Galen. Comment on Hippocrates, *Aphorisms.* In *Articella* 1483, ff. 8r–45vb.

– 1490. *De iuuamentis membrorum* and *De crisibus* [*De crisi*]. In *Galienus Pergamensis medicorum omnium principis Opera.* 2 vols. Venice: Pincius, vol. 1, sigs. cc j recto (a)–gg j recto (b), mm vij recto (a)–oo viij verso (b).

– 1565. *Omnia quae extant opera in Latinum sermonem conuersa.* 11 vols. Venice: Giunta.

ps.-Galen. *Anatomia porci.* In Corner, ed. and trans. 1927, 48–53.

Gauthier, René Antoine, ed. 1972–4. *Ethica Nicomachea.* 5 vols. Aristoteles Latinus, 26.1–3. Leiden: Brill.

Gerlandus. See Lohr, ed. 2013.

Getz, Faye Marie. 1990. "Charity, Translation, and the Language of Medical Learning in Medieval England." *Bulletin of the History of Medicine* 64: 1–17.

Getz, Faye Marie, ed. 1991. *Healing and Society in Medieval England: A Middle English Translation of the Pharmaceutical Writings of Gilbertus Anglicus.* Madison: University of Wisconsin Press.

Gilbertus Anglicus. Comment on Giles of Corbeil, *Carmen de urinis.* Wellcome Library, MS 547, ff. 104r–145v; Biblioteca Apostolica Vaticana, MS Vat. lat. 2459, ff. 51r–63v.

Giles of Corbeil. *Carmen de pulsibus.* See Choulant, ed. 1826.

– *Carmen de urinis.* See Choulant, ed. 1826; Vieillard, ed. 1903.

– *Liber de uirtutibus et laudibus compositorum medicaminum.* See Ausécache, ed. 2017.

– *Viaticus de signis et symptomatibus aegritudinum.* See Rose, ed. 1907.

Gillespie, Vincent, and Anne Hudson, eds. 2013. *Probable Truth: Editing Medieval Texts from Britain in the Twenty-First Century.* Turnhout: Brepols.

Glaze, Florence Eliza, and Brian K. Nance, eds. 2011. *Between Text and Patient: The Medical Enterprise in Medieval and Early Modern Europe.* Florence: SISMEL.

Glossa Ordinaria. 1617. *Biblia Sacra cum Glossa Ordinaria ... et Postilla Nicolai Lyrani ... .* 6 vols. Douai: Baltazar Bellerus, vol. 1; Antwerp: Johannes Keerbergius, vols. 2–6.

Goldstein, Bernard R., ed. and trans. 1967. "The Arabic Version of Ptolemy's Planetary Hypotheses." *Transactions of the American Philosophical Society* n.s. 57 (4): 3–55. Philadelphia: American Philosophical Society.

Goyens, Michèle, Pieter De Leemans, and An Smets, eds. 2008. *Science Translated: Latin and Vernacular Translations of Scientific Treatises in Medieval Europe*. Leuven: Leuven University Press.

Grant, Edward. 1994. *Planets, Stars, and Orbs: The Medieval Cosmos, 1200–1687*. Cambridge: Cambridge University Press.

Green, Monica H., ed. and trans. 2001. *The Trotula: A Medieval Compendium of Women's Medicine*. Philadelphia: University of Pennsylvania Press.

Green, Richard Firth. 1997. "Friar William Appleton and the Date of Langland's B Text." *Yearbook of Langland Studies* 11: 87–96.

Hanna, Ralph. 1996. *Pursuing History: Middle English Manuscripts and Their Texts*. Stanford: Stanford University Press.

– 2013. "Editing Texts with Extensive Manuscript Traditions." In Gillespie and Hudson, eds. 2013, 111–29.

– 2015. "The Sizes of Middle English Books, ca. 1390–1430." *Journal of the Early Book Society* 18: 181–91.

Hanna, Ralph, ed. 1994. "Henry Daniel's *Liber Uricrisiarum* (Excerpt)." In Matheson, ed. 1994, 185–218.

– 2008. *Speculum Vitae: A Reading Edition*. 2 vols. EETS o.s. 331–2. Oxford: Oxford University Press.

Hanna, Ralph, and Sarah Wood, eds. 2013. *Richard Morris's "Prick of Conscience": A Corrected and Amplified Reading Text*. EETS o.s. 342. Oxford: Oxford University Press.

Harvey, E. Ruth. 1998. "The Judgement of Urines." *Canadian Medical Association Journal* 159: 1482–4.

Harvey, John H. 1972. "Mediaeval Plantsmanship in England: The Culture of Rosemary." *Garden History* 1 (1) (Autumn): 14–21.

– 1974. *Early Nurserymen: With Reprints of Documents and Lists*. London: Phillimore.

– 1987. "Henry Daniel: A Scientific Gardener of the Fourteenth Century." *Garden History* 15 (2) (Autumn): 81–93.

– 2004. "Henry Daniel Henry (fl. 1379)." *Oxford Dictionary of National Biography Online*. Oxford University Press. https://www.oxforddnb.com/view/article/7116.

Hippocrates. 1923–2012. *Works* (Greek and English). 10 vols. Loeb Classical Library. Cambridge, MA: Harvard University Press. (*Airs Waters Places*: 1: 65–137, trans. W.H.S. Jones; *Prognostic*: 2: 1–55, trans. W.H.S. Jones; *Aphorisms*: 4: 97–221, trans. W.H.S. Jones.)

– *Aphorisms*. In *Articella* 1483, ff. 8r–45vb.

– *Prognostics*. In *Articella* 1483, ff. 46r–75rb.

Hunt, Tony. 1989. *Plant Names of Medieval England*. Cambridge: Brewer.

Ideler, Julius Ludwig, ed. 1841–2. *Physici et medici Graeci minores*. 2 vols. Berlin: Reimer.

Isaac Israeli (Isaac Judaeus, Abū Yaʿqub Isḥāq ibn Sulaymān al-Isrāʾīlī). 1515. *Omnia opera Ysaac*. 2 vols. Lyons: Bartholomeus Trot.

– *Liber Febrium*. In *Omnia opera Ysaac* 1515, 1: 203va–226vb.

– *Liber Urinarum*. In *Omnia opera Ysaac* 1515, 1: 156rb–203rb.

– *Liber Urinarum*. See Peine, ed. 1919; Fontana, ed. and trans. 1966.

Isidore of Seville. See Lindsay, ed. 1911.

Jacquart, Danielle. 1986. "A l'aube de la renaissance médicale des XIᵉ–XIIᵉ siècles: *L'Isagoge Iohannitii* et son traducteur." *Bibliothèque de l'École des chartes* 144: 209–40.

Jacquart, Danielle, and Agostino Paravicini Bagliani, eds. 2007. *La Scuola Medica Salernitana: Gli autori e i testi*. Florence: SISMEL.

– eds. 2008. *La "Collectio Salernitana" di Salvatore De Renzi*. Florence: SISMEL.

Jasin, Joanne. 1993a. "The Compiler's Awareness of Audience in Medieval Medical Prose: The Example of Wellcome MS 225." *Journal of English and Germanic Philology* 92: 509–22.

– 1993b. "The Transmission of Learned Medical Literature in the Middle English *Liber Uricrisiarum*." *Medical History* 37: 313–29.

Jasin, Joanne, ed. 1983. "A Critical Edition of the Middle English *Liber Uricrisiarum* in Wellcome MS 225." Diss. Tulane University.

Jebb, S., ed. 1733. *Fratris Rogeri Bacon, Ordinis minorum, Opus majus ad Clementem Quartum*. London: William Bowyer.

Johannessen, Tom Arvid, ed. 2005. "The *Liber Uricrisiarum* in Gonville and Caius College, Cambridge, MS 336/725." Master's Thesis, University of Oslo.

Johannitius ('Abū Zayd Hunayn ibn 'Isḥāq al-ʿIbādī). *Isagoge ad Techne Galieni*. See Maurach, ed. 1978. Also in *Articella* 1483, ff. 2ra–4va.

John of St Paul. *Breviarius medicine* (= *Breviarius Ypochratis*). Montreal, McGill University Library, Osler MS 7627, ff. 1r–70r. Ebook. https://mcgill.worldcat.org/title/breuiarius-ypochratis-latin-medical-notes-beginning-theorica-est-perfecta-noticia-rerum/oclc/429188580.

– *De simplicium medicinarum virtutibus*. See Kroemer, ed. 1920.

Jones, Peter Murray. 2008. "The 'Tabula medicine': An Evolving Encyclopedia." In Edwards, ed. 2008, 60–85.

– 2011. "Mediating Collective Experience: The *Tabula Medicine* (1416–1425) as a Handbook for Medical Practice." In Glaze and Nance, eds. 2011, 279–307.

– 2016. "The Medicine of the Friars in Late Medieval England." History of Pre-Modern Medicine Seminar, Wellcome Library, 2 February.

Kaeppeli, Thomas. 1970–93. *Scriptores Ordinis Praedicatorum Medii Aevi*. 4 vols. Rome: Istituto Storico Domenicano.

Keiser, George R. 1996. "Through a Fourteenth-Century Gardener's Eyes: Henry Daniel's Herbal." *Chaucer Review* 31 (1): 58–75.

– 1998. *A Manual of the Writings in Middle English 1050–1500.* Vol. 10: *Works of Science and Information.* New Haven: Connecticut Academy of Arts and Sciences.

– 2008. "Rosemary: Not Just for Remembrance." In Dendle and Touwaide, eds. 2008, 180–204.

Ker, N.R., with Ian Campbell Cunningham and Andrew G. Watson. 1969–2002. *Medieval Manuscripts in British Libraries.* 5 vols. Oxford: Clarendon Press.

Kibre, Pearl S. 1985. *Hippocrates Latinus: Repertorium of Hippocratic Writings in the Latin Middle Ages.* Rev. ed. New York: Fordham University Press.

Kroemer, Georg Heinrich, ed. 1920. "Johanns von Sancto Paulo: *Liber de simplicium medicinarum virtutibus* und ein anderer Salernitaner Traktat: *Quae medicinae pro quibus morbis donandae sunt* nach dem Breslauer Codex herausgegeben." Diss. Leipzig. Borna-Leipzig: Noske.

Kühn, Karl Gottlob, ed. 1821–33. *Claudii Galeni opera omnia.* 20 vols. Leipzig: Cnobloch.

Langslow, D.R., ed. and trans. 2006. *The Latin Alexander Trallianus: The Text and Transmission of a Late Latin Medical Book.* Journal of Roman Studies Monographs 10. London: Society for the Promotion of Roman Studies.

Lewis, Robert E., ed. 1978. *Lotario dei Segni (Pope Innocent III): De miseria condicionis humane.* Chaucer Library. Athens: University of Georgia Press.

Liber de sinthomatibus mulierum. In M.H. Green, ed. and trans. 2001, 70–115.

Lindsay, W.M., ed. 1911. *Isidori Hispalensis episcopi Etymologiarvm sive originvm libri XX.* 2 vols. Oxford: Clarendon Press.

Lohr, Alfred, ed. 2013. *Der "Computus Gerlandi": Edition, Übersetzung und Erläuterungen.* Sudhoffs Archiv, Beihefte 61. Stuttgart: Steiner.

– ed. 2015. *Opera de computo saeculi duodecimi.* Corpus Christianorum Continuatio Mediaeualis 272. Turnhout: Brepols.

Lotario dei Segni. See Lewis, ed. 1978.

Mäkinen, Martti, ed. 2002. "Henry Daniel's Rosemary in MS X.90 of the Royal Library, Stockholm." *Neuphilologische Mitteilungen* 103: 305–27.

Matheson, Lister M., ed. 1994. *Popular and Practical Science of Medieval England.* East Lansing: Colleagues Press.

Maurach, Gregor, ed. 1978. "Johannicius: Isagoge ad Techne Galieni." *Sudhoffs Archiv* 62: 148–74. Trans. in Wallis, ed. 2010, 139–56.

Maxwell-Stuart, P.G. 1981. *Studies in Greek Colour Terminology.* 2 vols. (*Glaukos*; *Charopos*). Leiden: Brill.

McIntosh, Angus, M.L. Samuels, and Michael Benskin. 1986. *A Linguistic Atlas of Late Mediaeval English.* 4 vols. Aberdeen: Aberdeen University Press. (*LALME*) Electronic version. Rev. and suppl. by Michael Benskin and Margaret Laing. 2013. http://www.lel.ed.ac.uk/ihd/elalme/elalme.html. (*eLALME*)

McVaugh, Michael R. 1997. "Bedside Manners in the Middle Ages." *Bulletin of the History of Medicine* 71: 201–23.

– 2010. "Who Was Gilbert the Englishman?" In Brown and Voigts, eds. 2010, 295–324.

Means, Laurel. 1992. "'Ffor as moche as yche man may not haue þe astrolabe': Popular Middle English Variations on the Computus." *Speculum* 67: 595–623.

Middle English Dictionary. 1952–2001. Ann Arbor, MI. https://quod.lib.umich.edu/m/middle-english-dictionary. (*MED*)

Montford, Angela. 2003. "Dangers and Disorders: The Decline of the Dominican *Frater Medicus.*" *Social History of Medicine* 16: 169–91.

– 2004. *Health, Sickness, Medicine and the Friars in the Thirteenth and Fourteenth Centuries.* Aldershot: Ashgate.

Mosher, David L., trans. 1982. Augustine of Hippo, *Eighty-Three Different Questions.* Fathers of the Church, vol. 70. Washington, DC: Catholic University of America Press.

Moulinier-Brogi, Laurence. 2008. "L'uroscopie en vulgaire dans l'Occident médiéval: un tour d'horizon." In Goyens et al., eds. 2008, 221–41.

– 2012. *L'Uroscopie au Moyen Âge: "Lire dans un verre la nature de l'homme".* Paris: Champion.

Norri, Juhani. 1992. *Names of Sicknesses in English, 1400–1550: An Exploration of the Lexical Field.* Helsinki: Suomalainen Tiedeakatemia.

– 1998. *Names of Body Parts in English, 1400–1550.* Helsinki: Academia Scientiarum Fennica.

– 2016. *Dictionary of Medical Vocabulary in English, 1375–1550: Body Parts, Sicknesses, Instruments, and Medicinal Preparations.* 2 vols. Abingdon: Ashgate.

Ogden, Margaret S., ed. 1971. *The Cyrurgie of Guy de Chauliac.* EETS o.s. 265. London: Oxford University Press.

Omnia opera Ysaac. 1515. See Isaac Israeli 1515.

O'Neill, Ynez Violé. 1970. "Another Look at the 'Anatomia Porci.'" *Viator* 1: 115–24.

Oxford Dictionary of National Biography Online. 2017. Ed. David Cannadine. Oxford: Oxford University Press. Available by subscription. https://www.oxforddnb.com.

Oxford English Dictionary, 2nd ed. 1989. Oxford: Oxford University Press. Updated online version (2000–), chief ed. Michael Proffitt. Available by subscription. https://www.oed.com. (*OED*)

Pedersen, Olaf. 1985. "In Quest of Sacrobosco." *Journal for the History of Astronomy* 16: 175–221.

Peine, Johannes, ed. 1919. "Die Harnschrift des Isaac Judaeus." Diss. Leipzig. Borna-Leipzig: Noske. Rpt. in *Isḥāq ibn Sulaymān al-Isrā'īlī (d. c. 325/935): Texts and Studies*, ed. Fuat Sezgin. *Islamic Medicine* 35 (1996). Frankfurt am

Main: Institute for the History of Arabic-Islamic Science, Johann Wolfgang Goethe University, 41–121. [Transcribed from *Opera omnia Ysaac* 1515 edition, with minor collations from a Leipzig MS.]

Plomer, Henry R. 1907. *A Dictionary of the Booksellers and Printers Who Were at Work in England, Scotland and Ireland from 1641 to 1667*. London: Blades, East and Blades.

Ptolemy, Claudius. *Almagest*. See Toomer, ed. and trans. 1984.

– *Tetrabiblos*. See Robbins, ed. and trans. 1980.

Recio Muñoz, Victoria, ed. and trans. 2016. *La "Practica" de Plateario: Edición crítica, traducción y estudio*. Edizione nazionale dei testi mediolatini d'Italia 40 (ser. II, 18). Florence: SISMEL, Edizioni del Galluzzo.

Redeker, Franz, ed. 1917. "Die 'Anatomia Magistri Nicolai phisici' und ihr Verhältnis zur *Anatomia Chophonis* und *Richardi*." Diss. Leipzig. Borna-Leipzig: Noske.

Riddle, John M., ed. 1977. *Marbode of Rennes' "De lapidibus" Considered as a Medical Treatise, with Text, Commentary, and C.W. King's Translation*. Wiesbaden: Steiner.

Robbins, F.E., ed. and trans. 1940; rpt. 1980. *Ptolemy: Tetrabiblos*. Loeb Classical Library 435. Cambridge, MA: Harvard University Press.

Robertus Anglicus. See Thorndike 1949.

Roger de Barone. 1519. *Practica magistri Rogerii*. In *Cyrurgia Guidonis de Cauliaco: et cyrurgia Bruni. Teodorici. Rolandi. Lanfranci. Rogerii. Bertapalie*. Venice: Venetus de Vitalibus, ff. 211ra–234vb.

Rose, Valentin, ed. 1907. *Egidii Corboliensis Viaticus de signis et symptomatibus aegritudinum*. Leipzig: Teubner.

Rothwell, W., D.A. Trotter, G. De Wilde, et al., eds. 2006– . *Anglo-Norman Dictionary*, 2nd ed. Online edition. http://www.anglo-norman.net. (*A-ND*)

Sacrobosco, Johannes de. *Compotus*. In BL, Harley MS 3647, ff. 33v–54v. Also as *Computus ecclesiasticus* in Wittenberg 1543 ed.

– 1543. *Libellvs de sphaera: accessit eivsdem autoris Compvtvs ecclesiasticvs*. With prefaces by Philip Melancthon. Wittenberg: Seitz. [*Computus ecclesiasticus* in second half of book, with new signature series A.1–H.4.]

Samuels, M.L. 1981. "Spelling and Dialect in the Late and Post-Middle English Periods." In Benskin and Samuels, eds. 1981, 43–54.

Sears, Elizabeth. 1986. *The Ages of Man: Medieval Interpretations of the Life Cycle*. Princeton: Princeton University Press.

Siraisi, Nancy G. 1981. *Taddeo Alderotti and His Pupils: Two Generations of Italian Medical Learning*. Princeton: Princeton University Press.

Star, Sarah. 2016. "*Anima Carnis in Sanguine Est*: Blood, Life, and *The King of Tars*." *JEGP: The Journal of English and Germanic Philology* 115 (4): 442–62.

– 2018a. "Henry Daniel, Medieval English Medicine, and Linguistic Innovation: A Lexicographic Study of Huntington MS HM 505." *Huntington Library Quarterly* 81 (1): 63–105.

– 2018b. "The Textual Worlds of Henry Daniel." *Studies in the Age of Chaucer* 40: 191–216.

Sudhoff, Karl. 1929. "Commentatoren der Harnverse des Gilles de Corbeil." *Archeion: Archivo di storia della scienza* (Rome) 11: 129–35.

ps.-Taddeo (Alderotti). "Noua reportata super Egidium de vrinis." Paris, Bibliothèque de l'Arsenal, MS 1024, ff. 1ra–12va. https://archivesetmanuscrits.bnf.fr/ark:/12148/cc79033f.

Talbot, C.H., and E.A. Hammond. 1965. *The Medical Practitioners in Medieval England: A Biographical Register*. London: Wellcome Historical Medical Library.

Tavormina, M. Teresa. 2014. "Uroscopy in Middle English: A Guide to the Texts and Manuscripts." *Studies in Medieval and Renaissance History*, ser. 3, 11: 1–154.

Tavormina, M. Teresa, ed. 2006. *Sex, Aging, and Death in a Medieval Medical Compendium: Trinity College Cambridge MS R.14.52, Its Texts, Language, and Scribe*. 2 vols. Medieval and Renaissance Texts and Studies 292. Tempe: Arizona Center for Medieval and Renaissance Studies.

– ed. 2019. *The Dome of Uryne: A Reading Edition of Nine Middle English Uroscopies*. EETS o.s. 354. Oxford: Oxford University Press.

Theophilus Protospatharius. *Liber urinarum*. See Dase ed., 1999. Also in *Articella* 1483, ff. 5rb–7vb.

Thorndike, Lynn. 1949. *The Sphere of Sacrobosco and Its Commentators*. Chicago: University of Chicago Press.

– 1955. "Unde versus." *Traditio* 11: 163–93.

Toomer, G.J., ed. and trans. 1984. *Ptolemy's Almagest*. New York: Springer Verlag.

Töply, Robert. 1902. *Anatomia Ricardi Anglici (c. a. 1242–1252)* [= ps.-Galen, *Anatomia vivorum*]. Vienna: Joseph Šafář.

van Helden, Albert. 1985. *Measuring the Universe: Cosmic Dimensions from Aristarchus to Halley*. Chicago: University of Chicago Press.

Veit, Raphaela. 2015. "Isaac Israeli: His Treatise on Urine (*De Urinis*) and Its Reception in the Latin World." In Collins et al., eds. 2015, 77–113.

Vieillard, Camille. 1903. *L'Urologie et les médecins urologues dans la médecine ancienne: Gilles de Corbeil, sa vie, ses oeuvres, son poème des urines*. Paris: Rudeval. (Edition and French translation of *Carmen de urinis*: 267–301.)

Visi, Tamás. 2015. "Tradition and Innovation: Isaac Israeli's Classification of the Colors of Urines." In Collins et al., eds. 2015, 39–66.

Voigts, Linda Ehrsam, and Patricia Deery Kurtz. 2019. *Scientific and Medical Writings in Old and Middle English: An Electronic Reference*. Exp. and rev. ed. https://cctr1.umkc.edu/cgi-bin/search. (eVK2)

Wallis, Faith. 2015. "What a Medieval Diagram Shows: A Case Study of *Computus*." *Studies in Iconography* 36: 1–40.

Wallis, Faith, ed. 2010. *Medieval Medicine: A Reader*. Toronto: University of Toronto Press.

Wallis, Faith, trans. 1999. *Bede: The Reckoning of Time*. Liverpool: Liverpool University Press.

Walsh Morrissey, Jake. 2014a. "Anxious Love and Disordered Urine: The Englishing of *Amor Hereos* in Henry Daniel's *Liber Uricrisiarum*." *Chaucer Review* 49: 161–83.

– 2014b. "An Unnoticed Fragment of *A Tretys of Diverse Herbis* in British Library, MS Sloane 2460, and the Middle English Career of Pseudo-Albertus Magnus' *De virtutibus herbarum*." *Neuphilologische Mitteilungen* 115: 153–61.

Walther, Hans. 1963–86. *Proverbia sententiaeque latinitatis medii ac recentioris aevi*. 9 vols. Göttingen: Vandenhoeck and Ruprecht.

Warner, George F., and Julius P. Gilson. 1921. *Catalogue of Western Manuscripts in the Old Royal and King's Collections*. 4 vols. London: British Museum.

Whiting, B.J. 1968. *Proverbs, Sentences, and Proverbial Phrases from English Writings Mainly before 1500*. Cambridge, MA: Harvard University Press.

Index

The Index contains the names of persons, places, works, and selected subjects mentioned in the Introduction, Appendices (excluding texts presented therein), and Explanatory Notes. It does not index the *Liber Uricrisiarum* text proper, nor does it include the names of modern scholars cited in the book. The latter can be found in the Works Cited list.

For reasons of space, we have not attempted to index every medical term that Daniel uses in the course of his massive work. The General Glossary can serve as a proxy index to more of Daniel's medical terminology, though it does not provide exhaustive lists of illustrative citations and excludes easily recognized terms.

The symbol ° preceding an entry indicates that the person, place, or work also appears in the Guide to Proper Names, with references there to relevant lines in the Middle English text. Pseudonymous works (e.g., ps.-Galen) are alphabetized under their attributed author.

Milton Keynes UK
Ingram Content Group UK Ltd.
UKHW011253210424
441408UK00003B/32/J